■ The Ethics of Sport

The Ethics of Sport

Essential Readings

EDITED BY

Arthur L. Caplan and Brendan Parent

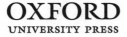

OXFORD
UNIVERSITY PRESS

OXFORD
UNIVERSITY PRESS

Oxford University Press is a department of the University of Oxford. It furthers
the University's objective of excellence in research, scholarship, and education
by publishing worldwide. Oxford is a registered trade mark of Oxford University
Press in the UK and certain other countries.

Published in the United States of America by Oxford University Press
198 Madison Avenue, New York, NY 10016, United States of America.

© Oxford University Press 2017

Library of Congress Cataloging-in-Publication Data
Names: Caplan, Arthur L., editor. | Parent, Brendan., editor.
Title: The ethics of sport : essential readings / edited by Arthur L. Caplan and
Brendan Parent.
Description: New York : Oxford University Press, [2017] Identifiers: LCCN 2016006208 |
ISBN 9780190210991 (pbk. : alk. paper) | ISBN 9780190210984 (hardcover : alk. paper)
Subjects: LCSH: Sports—Moral and ethical aspects.
Classification: LCC GV706.3 .E866 2016 | DDC 796.01—dc23
LC record available at http://lccn.loc.gov/2016006208

This reader is dedicated to Meg Caplan and Jane Pucher.

■ CONTENTS

■ ACKNOWLEDGMENTS

The editors would like to thank Jessica Wico of the NYU Langone Medical Center, Division of Medical Ethics; Emily Sacharin and Peter Ohlin of Oxford University Press; Dena Burke of the NYU School of Professional Studies; Dennis Di Lorenzo, Dean of the NYU School of Professional Studies; and Mark Gourevitch, MD, and Robert Grossman, MD, of the NYU Langone Medical Center. They would also like to thank Scott Briggs and Jason Chung for their work in compiling and editing this volume. They give special thanks to NYU Sports and Society, especially its chair, Arthur R. Miller.

PART I
What Is Sport?

What makes something a sport as opposed to an exhibition, recreation, or a hobby? To know what ought to happen and what ought to be prevented in and around sport—the ethics of sport—we should know not only the rules but also the essence of sport. We all have our intuitions, but crafting a good definition is difficult. For every quality that seems essential to the meaning of sport, there is at least one activity without that quality that is called a sport.

Do sports need teams? There are several sports that can be played between individuals—tennis, running, cycling, boxing. Do sports need winners and losers? We do not always keep score. The "sportness" of basketball, or ultimate Frisbee, or squash does not disappear if you lose track of the points. Do sports need competition between people? One can play many sports completely alone—racquetball, golf, sailing. Some might say that when playing alone, one is competing with oneself to improve time or score. If the sole player is not looking to improve, though, does the activity stop being a sport and become recreation? What about strategy? It often helps individuals and teams win, but playing without following steps in the winning plan does not mean you are no longer engaging in the sport.

Do sports need physical exertion? Many argue that competitive video-game playing is a sport. It even carries the name "E-sports." Many also believe that "speed cubing" is a sport, which involves solving versions of the Rubik's Cube in record time. Do these competitors need to get their heart rates up, or use as many muscle groups as soccer players or jai alai players, for their activities to be considered sports?

Maybe sports require entertainment value. While there are some sports that have few spectators, all sports usually entertain their participants. However, we all know of "blowouts," during which one side loses badly and feels far from entertained. Furthermore, there are countless entertaining activities that we would not call sports, so entertainment value is not sufficient by itself.

In chapter 1, a selection from Roland Barthes's "What is Sport?" several of these qualities are described in sports, which make them reflect human desire and struggle. The author's epic descriptions illustrate how sports mirror society. They give us a space to play out our passions and face our fears without the consequences imposed by "real" life, a form of escape. Yet, sports can carry serious consequences when they cause permanent injury to players and fans, start riots, damage relations between countries, or become venues for terrorism. So, sports might be too intertwined with reality to be strictly a form of escapism.

Sigmund Loland, in chapter 2, proposes several theories of sport based on different qualities. First, he offers that sports are an instrument to achieve goals, whether political, social, or cultural. This quality is clearly not sufficient because many nonsport activities are instrumental in this way, but is it even necessary? Can a sport be played simply for its intrinsic enjoyment? According to the performer theory, the answer is yes. The key quality here is that sports serve as a source of satisfaction for the athlete.

Loland provides another alternative: that sports might be the demonstration and improvement of performance. We love seeing athletes break records and create new strategies for excellence. Yet, prioritizing this quality can be dangerous: there is no logical end to making athletes and their sports bigger, faster, and stronger, while there are limits to how much physical impact the human body can take. Furthermore, the rules of a sport begin to look less important if we care too much about performance power. As rules break down the sport loses structure, and the body in which the spirit of sport lives dissolves. So perhaps rules of play are essential to sport.

After establishing some core qualities, we can begin questioning how to preserve and promote them to make sports better. What makes a good team? How can athletes be virtuous winners and losers? How should we balance risk with safety? At what point does the focus on entertainment detract from the integrity or purity of the game? What is fair competition? Who should have access to the game? Under what circumstances can the rules be broken?

Questions like these are the focus of this reader. The answers are nuanced, different for each sport, and perhaps some questions are unanswerable. Sports have great power to promote human flourishing and cause suffering. Seeking the answers to ethical questions in sport and acting on them is our duty as fans and participants, so that we might enable sports to better serve those who engage in them.

1 | Selection from *What is Sport?*

■ ROLAND BARTHES

[Translated by Richard Howard]

What need have these men to attack? Why are men disturbed by this spectacle? Why are they totally committed to it? Why this useless combat? What is sport?

Bullfighting is hardly a sport, yet it is perhaps the model and the limit of all sports: strict rules of combat, strength of the adversary, man's knowledge and courage; all our modern sports are in this spectacle from another age, heir of ancient religious sacrifices. But this theater is a false theater: real death occurs in it. The bull entering here will die; and it is because this death is inevitable that the bullfight is a tragedy. This tragedy will be performed in four acts of which the epilogue is death.

First, passes of the cape: the torero must learn to know the bull—that is, to play with him: to provoke him, to avoid him, to entangle him deftly, in short to ensure his docility in fighting according to the rules.

Then the picadors: here they come, on horseback at the far end of the ring, riding along the barrier. Their function is to exhaust the bull, to block his charges in order to diminish his excess of violence over the torero.

Act three. The banderillas.

A man alone, with no other weapon than a slender beribboned hook, will tease the bull: call out to him . . . stab him lightly . . . insouciantly slip away.

Here comes the final act. The bull is still the stronger, yet will certainly die . . . The bullfight will tell men why man is best. First of all, because the man's courage is conscious: his courage is the consciousness of fear, freely accepted, freely overcome.

Man's second superiority is his knowledge. The bull does not know man; man knows the bull, anticipates his movement, their limits, and can lead his adversary to the site he has chosen, and if this site is dangerous, he knows it and has chosen it for this reason.

There is something else in the torero's style. What is style? Style makes a difficult action into a graceful gesture, introduces a rhythm into fatality. Style is to be courageous without disorder, to give necessity the appearance of freedom. Courage, knowledge, beauty, these are what man opposes to the strength of the animal, this is the human ordeal, of which the bull's death will be the prize.

Furthermore what the crowd honors in the victor, tossing him flowers and gifts, which he graciously returns, is not man's victory over the animal, for the

3

bull is always defeated; it is man's victory over ignorance, fear, necessity. Man has made his victory a spectacle, so that it might become the victory of all those watching him and recognizing themselves in him.

And what do they recognize in the great car racer? The victor over a much subtler enemy: time. Here all of man's courage and knowledge will be focused on one thing: the machine. By the machine man will conquer, but perhaps by the machine he will die. So that here the relation between man and the machine is infinitely circumspect: what will function very fast must first be tested very slowly, for speed is never anything but the recompense of extreme deliberation; first of all, the gears must be verified, for a great deal will be asked of them: up to 2500 changes of speed an hour; the site of the competition must also be carefully checked, the track first of all, its angles, its curves, its levels . . .

Next, in order to try it out, to race alone, with no other enemy but time, and to confront in this effort both the machine and the terrain together, for it is all three at once that the racer must first of all conquer before triumphing over his human rivals.

Finally and above all it is the engine that must be prepared and where we find an embarrassment of riches, much like those found in an inspired brain: here twelve sparkplugs must be changed every five laps.

We are at Sebring in Florida; this is a twelve-hour race among different types of cars. Once the race starts, an implacable economy will govern each atom of movement, for time is henceforth everywhere.

On straight drives, it is the motor's effort that is most important, yet this effort remains human in its way: in it are deposited the labor, the inventiveness, and the care of dozens of men who have prepared, refined, and checked the most difficult of equations: an extreme power, a minimal resistance, whether of weight or of wind.

But on the turns, apart from the machine's suspension, it is the racer who does everything; for here, space is against time. Hence the racer must be able to cheat space, to decide whether he can spare it . . . or if he will brutally cut it down; and he must have the courage to drive this wager to the brink of the impossible.

It is not only the racer who struggles against time, it is his whole team. At Sebring, the track is a former airfield, on which tires are quickly worn down; some teams manage to change them in a minute and a half: to them too belongs a share of the final victory. In this combat against time, terrible as the consequences may sometimes be, there is no fury, only an immense courage focused on the inertia of things. Hence the death of a racer is infinitely sad: for it is not only a man who dies here, it is a particle of perfection which vanishes from this world. But it is precisely because such perfection is mortal that it is human. No sooner is everything lost in one place than other men will begin again in another.

Here is the start of one of the world's Grand Prix races: it is a crucial test, because the more powerful the machine, the heavier it is, and from this paradox the greatest speed must be derived: hence there is no starter on these cars: to suppress a few kilos is to gain a few seconds.

It is these preparations for starting that give the car race its meaning: that of a victory over weight and the inertia of things. At rest, these cars are heavy, passive, difficult to maneuver: as with a bird hampered by its wings it is their potential power that weighs them down. Yet once lined up, approaching their function, which is combat, they already become lighter, grow impatient.. . . Once started, these machines will gradually transform their mass into agility, their weight into power; no sooner are they in their element, which is speed, than they will wrap the entire world in it, on the most varied tracks and circuits: at Nürburgring, the most dangerous; at Monaco, the most torturous; from Monza, the most exhausting, to Spa, the fastest.

To stop is virtually to die. If the machine fails, its master must be informed of the fact with a certain discretion. For a great racer does not conquer his machine, he tames it; he is not only the winner, he is also the one who destroys nothing. A wrecked machine generates something like the sadness caused by the death of an irreplaceable being, even as life continues around him.

This is the meaning of a great automobile race: that the swiftest force is only a sum of various kinds of patience, of measurements, of subtleties, of infinitely precise and infinitely demanding actions.

What this man has done is to drive himself and his machine to the limit of what is possible. He has won his victory not over his rivals, but on the contrary *with them*, over the obstinate heaviness of things: the most murderous of sports is also the most generous.

2 Normative Theories of Sport
A Critical Review

■ SIGMUND LOLAND

My address today will be another contribution to what can be considered a classic topic in the social sciences and humanities of sport, namely the (possible) relationship between sport and value. More specifically, my paper can be seen as a prolongation of the philosophical discourse on these issues that can be found, among other places, in Bob Simon's and Nick Dixon's presidential addresses from 2000 and 2002, respectively [30, 8]. In his address, Simon drew a basic distinction between an externalist point of view in which sport is seen as mirroring or enforcing the values of wider society and variants of internalism in which sport is seen as having a significant degree of normative autonomy and as a source of value within itself. Simon argued in favor of what he called broad, interpretive internalism built on articulation of the particular normative principles that seem to underlie sport. Dixon built on Simon's distinctions and presented an interpretation of a broad, interpretive internalism on moral-realist foundations.

The distinction between internalist and externalist theories will be of relevance in what I will say here. However, I will not to the same extent as Simon and Dixon dwell on the philosophical and metaethical premises of these theoretical possibilities. Instead, I will attempt to flesh out in more substantial detail what externalist and internalist theories of sport might look like and what their consequences might be. More specifically, I will describe what I take to be three ideal-typical kinds of normative theories of competitive sport and discuss critically some of their ethical implications and their potential in the understanding of sport as a normative sphere.

▨ INSTRUMENTALISM

Views on the relationships between sport and value take many forms. One of the more rudimentary forms is instrumentalism. The terminology is self-explanatory. Instrumentalist views are externalist views in the sense that sport is considered to have no particular value by itself but is attributed value from interests on the outside. Simply put, instrumental views consider sport a means, or an instrument, toward external goals.

What, then, are these goals? Sport has been used for religious, social, and political purposes from its very beginning. For example, the ancient Greek Olympic Games were parts of a religious cult and served as a cultural and political celebration of Greek identity, or Greekness [10]. Strict instrumentalism, such as the deliberate use of sport to reach political goals, seems to arise with modern sport in the 19th and 20th centuries [16, 28]. A paradigmatic case can be the former German Democratic Republic (GDR), which together with other communist countries saw the role of sport as the demonstration of the superiority of communist over capitalist man [27]. Although the external goal is different, the instrumental view seems predominant in the commercial sport entertainment industry, as well. Sport seems to matter only insofar as it has commercial potential. In an essay on sport broadcasting, Paul Klein of ABC (American Broadcasting Company) is quoted in describing commercial sport television as "the business of selling audiences to advertisers" [6]. Sport is not even part of the formula.

It should be added, however, that instrumentalism deals not only with rewards in terms of prestige and profit but also with social and, to a certain extent, moral goals, as well. Today there are many projects by public and ideal operators in which sport is used as a means to reach social goals, for instance in the treatment of adolescents with psychosocial problems, in the integration of minority groups into larger society, or, more ambitiously, in the development of democratic virtues and civic society.[1] Moreover, to an increasing degree in the Western world, sport and physical activity are seen as key means in maintaining and improving health and fitness levels in the population.

What are the implications of instrumentalist views for sport ethics? The answer is simple. The moral relevance of sport has to be judged on the basis of the goals it is supposed to serve. If sport is intended to serve nonmoral goals such as political or commercial payoff, moral ideals in sport are usually given little weight. Examples can be the systematic drug use in the former GDR or deeply problematic personal histories from the commercial sport scene such as that of heavyweight boxer Mike Tyson. What counts here is ideological prestige, or public attention and profit, no matter what the human costs. If the external goals are moral goals, such as the all-round education of the individual, social integration of marginalized groups, or the development of democratic ideals and civic society, moral ideals are usually taken more seriously. In youth sport, for example, references to moral education and the ideal of fair play are frequent, and it seems reasonable to assume that these ideals have an impact on practice [20].

How can instrumentalist views be critically assessed? What is their potential in the understanding of sport as a normative sphere? To a certain extent, their reputation is worse than they deserve. Instrumentalism has a certain common-sense appeal. It provides ready and concrete answers to questions such as "What is sport good for?" Moreover, instrumentalist views challenge idealist conceptions of sport as a politically neutral and ideal sphere of universal value, views not uncommon in the traditional rhetoric of sport leaders and politicians.

On the other hand, when it comes to the understanding of sport as a normative sphere, instrumentalism has little or no explanatory force. I shall not spend time on reviewing the elaborate and extensive critique of externalist theories in general and of neo-Marxist theories in particular offered by, among others, Morgan [23]. Let me just mention one obvious point. The efficient use of sport to reach various goals, whether we talk of socially and morally desirable ones or not, depends on people being motivated for, engaged in, or at least interested in, sport in itself. Take as an example the sociohygienic goal of increasing the fitness level of a population. If sport is to be an efficient means in this respect, there is a need for knowledge of what kinds of sport will serve the purpose, of the optimal frequency and intensity of the activity, and, most important, of motivational aspects and perceived values of the various activities among those who take part. Instrumentalism builds on the premise that people value sport. In its ideal-typical versions, however, instrumentalism offers no conception of this valuing at all and seems ignorant of its own very raison d'être.

This is an explanatory weakness that might have serious practical consequences. If sport fails to realize the goals to which it is considered a means, instrumentalist views offer no help whatsoever. There are no resources here for critical reflection on sport itself and its failure, and hence, what can be done about it. I turn now to theories that offer more substantial theses on sport-specific norms and values and in which sport is considered a relatively autonomous normative field. That is, I turn now to internalist theories.

▪ PERFORMANCE THEORIES

Some internalist theories see the core values of sport as being the demonstration and constant improvement of performance. Hence, I will call them performance theories.

The idea of sport as a constant search for improved performance stands strong in much of current sport practice. Especially in elite sport, the performance principle seems to be the social logic around which everything else is organized [15]. For instance, in a seminar on the possibilities for new records in athletics, the coach Frank Dick stated that "limits are (the misconceived) products of the human mind" and that predictions on limits of human performance are foolish and doomed to fail [7]. I am sure he spoke for more than himself. This understanding echoes ideas in the theorizing about sport. Pierre de Coubertin talked of the sporting record as having the same function in Olympism as the law of gravity in Newtonian mechanics—it is "the eternal axiom" [21]. With its emphasis on measurable, individual performance and quantification of growth, sport can be seen as a paradigmatic expression of the core values of modernity: freedom, rationality, and progress [14, 26]. At its best, sport demonstrates human freedom and possibility and transcendence of what have previously been thought of as traditional ideas of human limitations.

Some sport philosophers have developed these ideas into more reflective and systematic philosophical theses. I will look into two examples here. Based on a classic liberal framework from John Stuart Mill, Tamburrini [32] argues against sport essentialism and in favor of a nonpaternalist approach with individual freedom to continuous improvement of performance as a key principle. In a new collection of essays, Gebauer [12] suggests that we should see sport as part of what French situationist Guy-Ernest Debord calls la société du spectacle—the society of the spectacle. In sport, the free postmodern subject appears, seeking its chance and constructing itself through the maximization of its performance potential with whatever means seem appropriate.

What are the implications of performance theories for sport ethics? Because of the focus on improvement and progress, performance theories usually imply strong requirements on precise performance measurements. In Tamburrini in particular, a primary ideal is fairness understood as equality of external conditions and development of advanced measurement techniques.

However, the fairness ideal is given limited validity. Performance theories accept few or no limitations and regulations on performance enhancement outside of the competitive setting. For instance, within his liberal framework, Tamburrini rejects the rationale for sex classifications. Let those compete who can challenge and match each other independent of sex! Both Tamburrini and Gebauer are skeptical as to general moral evaluations of cheating. On rationalistic, utilitarian grounds, Tamburrini defends Diego Maradona's handball goal in a 1986 World Cup game against England as "blameful rightdoing." Cheating in games is not defensible as a general norm because this would deprive sport of (utilitarian) value. In the longer run, however, Maradona's particular handball can be expected to add a certain "agonistic flavor" and increase the overall joy and excitement over matches between England and Argentina. From this point of view, Maradona's handball was the right thing to do. Gebauer reaches radical conclusions, too. Athletes search for their chance in sport, and competitions are radical challenges in which they try to overcome each other with whatever means possible. The athlete who can "bend" the rules when necessary is the free and creative athlete with potential for innovative performance. Moreover, both Tamburrini and Gebauer pose critical questions to restrictions on the use of performance-enhancing biochemical substances and medical technology. Although they do not endorse the use of drugs, both consider the justification of a ban problematic and, in Tamburrini's case, unjustifiable. In the discussion of the use of genetic technology, Tamburrini takes a step farther and writes of a world of genetically engineered athletes in which unfair genetic and biological inequalities are overcome and human character can flourish in its pure form.

As is evident from what is said so far, performance theories imply a significant skepticism toward traditional sport ethics. Whereas Tamburrini is critical of most regulations on performance enhancement outside of competitions, Gebauer is skeptical about the whole idea of sport ethics. According to Gebauer's strong internalist view, it is unfair and intellectually dishonest to imply or judge a practice based on some kind of theoretically deduced ethical system with origins outside of sport itself. What counts in sport is not ethical reflection but practical action. Tamburrini and Gebauer unite in the idea that there is no human essence, or telos. Or rather, what is uniquely human is the ability to perform, expand, and transcend.

To what extent do performance theories provide insights into sport as a normative sphere? Different from instrumentalism, these are substantial normative theories. Competitive sport is about the constant improvement of performance and the transcendence of limits. Moreover, performance theories reject, to a certain extent with strong arguments, traditional ideas of restrictions on performance such as on the use of certain drugs and biotechnological means.

Still, performance theories are open to several lines of critique. One possible critique concerns their simplicity. Performance theories do not really seem to take account of the many and diverse social realities of sport. For instance, there are few signs here of an understanding of the complex values and motivational structures in individual and collective interest in sport. As Morgan [24] points out in his critique of Gebauer's position, there is no emphasis here on sport as a social practice with a history and with particular traditions and ideals. People seem to value competitive sport because, among other things, it gives experiences of excitement, challenge, and mastery, of a sense of belonging, of identity, of symbolic conflict, and so forth. It seems as if very few of those engaged and interested in sport, even at the highest level, would subscribe to the idea that sport is about performance and progress only.

Another criticism is that, in their strong internalism, performance theories seem to take the form of some kind of reversed instrumentalism. The goal of performance enhancement seems to overrule all other social, cultural, and moral norms and values. Enhanced performance seems to be considered the goal that justifies all means—the surrounding world becomes a smorgasbord of options open to athletes' free choice. It is difficult to understand why performance is given clear-cut normative superiority here—there are few or no real strong normative arguments to support it. Moreover, the strong emphasis on performance might seem irrational with regard to some of its consequences. Let us look at the case of performance-enhancing drugs.

Most performance-enhancing drugs have a cost in terms of a risk for harm. Performance theorists such as Tamburrini and Gebauer would probably agree that the optimal solution is no use of potentially harmful drugs. Still, their view is, and here I am talking of Tamburrini in particular, that the ban on drugs implies unjustified restrictions on individual freedom and is an expression of strong paternalism. Therefore, the ban should be lifted. However, the use of efficient performance-enhancing drugs by one athlete or team exerts a coercive force on competing athletes and teams [3, 25]. In a no-ban situation, drug-using athletes gain a competitive advantage. To be able to compete, nonusers are more or less forced to change strategy into use. At least in this scenario, it is possible to argue that the liberal attitude to performance-enhancing means and methods leads to more severe restrictions on individual freedom and self-determination than in the current situation with a ban on drugs.

The final but perhaps most radical criticism of performance theories is their inclination toward the extreme. These theories link with a perfectionist tradition in ethics in which individuals and their actions are judged by a maximal standard of achievement. This is reminiscent of technological optimism of various kinds, such as that of midwar Italian futurists with their deep fascination with speed and the merging of humans and machines or today's optimistic beliefs in artificial intelligence (AI) and in the potential values of the cyborg. For instance, in an essay on the philosophy of technology, Cooper [4] refers to AI researcher Marvin Minsky, who argues against anthropological essentialism and talks provocatively of the human brain as a meat-machine. Minsky suggests that future generations should enhance performance by inserting microchips in the brain, cyborg style so to speak. The alternative, Minsky says, is to continue to walk around as "dressed-up chimpanzees." In this way, Minsky can be seen to provide a possible rationale for Tamburrini's ideas of the ultimately fair conditions of a future gene-manipulated performance sport.

Perfectionism, combined with sociological naiveté and technological optimism, can become deeply problematic. In his recent book with the telling title Better than Well—American Medicine Meets the American Dream, Elliot [9] describes American subcultures that take the new medical technology as their opportunity to transcend limitations of all kinds and pursue what to most of us appear to be more or less twisted ideas of self-realization. For instance, there is a group of voluntary amputees who, in their feeling of not being at home in their bodies, amputate an arm or a leg to feel "real." Elliot talks of "the tyranny of happiness." As a critical comment on performance theories, we could perhaps talk of a similar "tyranny of the record."

These criticisms can be countered, of course. A response to the point on simplification is more or less implicit in the writings of Tamburrini and Gebauer. They are both concerned with understanding sport as a sphere of value in itself and are skeptical about contextualization in which sport is linked with traditional values. We find similar responses to the question of unintended social consequences and extreme perfectionism. What seems sociologically naïve and technologically problematic today might look different tomorrow. For instance, in a few decades current expert medical knowledge might be common knowledge. Drugs designed according to individual genetic profiles might be used knowledgeably by most of us, and biochemical and gene-technological means might be part of everyday life inside and outside of sport. In such a context, currently banned biomedical technology might appear as legal means that empower the individual and make way for new understandings of what sport, athletic performances, and, in fact, human life are all about.

■ PERFORMER THEORIES

The critiques of performance theories are derived primarily from theorists who interpret the values of sport quite differently. I turn now to what I will call performer theories of sport. Again, at least to a certain extent, the reference is internalist in the sense that sport is considered to have a source of value from within. In addition, sport is considered to have the potential of generating values other than those of the society of which sport is a part. Sport has a relative autonomy and its own particular normative logic. Performer theories are built on a broader interpretation of the value of sport. More specifically, these theories link sport to moral ideals of human development. What is at stake here is not the improvement of performances but the improvement of performers.

A comment is warranted on the relationship in performer theories between sporting values and more general ideals. Moral ideals of human development, whether we talk of Aristotelian, Kantian, or other interpretations, are developed independent of and outside of sport. Does this not make performer theories into externalist, instrumental theories, really? This is not necessarily the case. As will be shown below, in performer theories, general ideals and sport-specific values are considered to be interwoven and interdependent on each other. For instance, several scholars have seen the values of sport as dependent on the realization of internal goods in MacIntyre's sense of the term [22]. These are goods that can be realized only in practicing sport according to its particular standards of excellence. Through the realization of internal goods, the path lies open to the development of more general moral virtues and moral character. There is a typical Aristotelian thought here. One becomes good by becoming a good chooser and doer. This is done not just by choosing or doing the right actions for instrumental reasons but by choosing and doing them in the right way. In the good life, each particular action reflects the whole and the whole is reflected in its parts [5]. Hence, the realization of ideals of human development in performance theories depends on the realization of values originating in sport itself, which again is a characteristic of internalist theories of sport.

There are many versions of performer theories of sport. Historically, a thick interpretation of de Coubertin's Olympism in which sport is seen as a sphere for education and moral development can be one example [21]. The amateur ideology of last century's England is another. According to amateurism, if practiced according to a certain disinterested and impartial attitude, sport is considered to cultivate dignity in defeat and modesty in victory—characteristics of the moderate, sensible person [1, 31]. Current developments of performer theories in sport philosophy can be found in, for instance, works of Fraleigh [11], Simon [29], Morgan [23], and Loland [19]. I shall outline briefly my own ideas.

One key idea in performer theories is that, if practiced in the right manner, sport has the potential to become a sphere of human flourishing in which individuals can realize their particular talents and abilities through their own efforts. A relevant presupposition in this respect, agreed on in most ethical theories, is that we should not treat people differently in significant matters based on inequalities that they cannot influence or control in any significant way and for which they therefore cannot be held responsible [2]. In other words, to secure equal opportunity to perform in sport, we should eliminate or compensate for what from a moral point of view are nonrelevant inequalities. In what follows, I will call this the fair-opportunity principle (FOP). In a sense, my theory of fair play [19] is an articulation of the particular normative interpretations and implications of FOP in sport.

First, and in agreement with performer theories, performance theories include strict demands on equality of opportunity. However, the justification of FOP is rooted in different ideals and has more far-ranging consequences. In performer theories, equality of opportunity means more than concern for exact, objective measurements under standardized conditions. There is a further interest in individual and system inequalities.

In many sports, competitors are classified according to athletes' sex and age. Based on FOP, performer theories offer a critical perspective in this respect. In some sports, this seems justifiable, in other sports not. Think of a continuum here. At the one end there are sports such as 100-meter sprint running in which basic biomotor abilities such as explosive strength and speed are crucial. Statistically, and because of biological inequalities between the sexes, young men have an advantage over women and older men. Classification seems justified. At the other end of the continuum sports such as archery, shooting, sailing of various kinds, and curling can be found. Here, technical and tactical skills seem far more important, and, depending on equal access to resources, women can compete on an equal level with men, and older people with younger people.

In other sports, there seems to be too little classification. In boxing, the martial arts, and weight lifting, body mass is crucial to performance, and there are classes accordingly. In sports such as basketball and volleyball, height has significant and systematic impact on performance. In gymnastics, being small seems equally important. In line with FOP, in these sports competitors should be classified according to body size, or, more specifically, according to body height.

Performer theories usually also imply regulations on inequalities in supporting systems: the economic, technological, scientific, and human performance-enhancing support of an athlete or a team. Inequalities in system strength cannot be controlled or influenced by the individual in any significant way, and, if exerting significant impact on performance, they ought to be eliminated or compensated for. Inequalities in equipment and technology can be eliminated or at least compensated for by strict standardization procedures. In the throwing events in athletics, for instance, or in most sailing classes, rules define strictly the standards of the equipment such as javelins, discus, hammers, and boats. In other sports such as skiing, standardization procedures are critically missing. Other things equal, skiers with the best ski sole [ski base] and the best waxing experts will win. Similar inequalities between competitors can be found in economic strength, as seen in among other places international soccer. Here, a few wealthy clubs control the market of star players. From the perspective of performer theories, these inequalities ought to be compensated for by federations distributing economic resources equally among all clubs competing in the same series. The same ideal would hold for inequalities in scientific know-how. Performer theories would support open publication of all findings linked to performance enhancement in sport.

If FOP is followed in practice, athletic performance becomes primarily the result of each individual's unique dealing with his or her talent and potential. In this way, the argument goes, sport becomes a sphere of individual development through athletes' own efforts and of individual freedom and responsibility. Hence, sport can be counted as one among many elements in human flourishing and in a good life.

How can performer theories be assessed with regard to providing an understanding of sport as a normative sphere? As in the discussion of performer theories, we can take a closer look at the ban on performance-enhancing drugs. Most performer theories would support the banning of such drugs, because they tend to move the responsibility for performance from the individual athlete toward external biomedical-expert systems. Alas, the potential of sport as a sphere for individual development through athletes' own efforts is reduced. More generally, performer theories imply skepticism toward performance-enhancing regimes in which individual athletes become strongly dependent on external expertise. The possibilities for individual development and flourishing are significantly reduced, and, as Hoberman has so vividly demonstrated [17], the possibilities for being treated as a means toward the realization of system interests increase.

Performer theories have their critics, as well. One main criticism is that these theories are based on premises that take too much for granted. To a certain extent, performer theories are marked by conservatism and moral conventionalism. For example, their restrictions on performance enhancement build on anachronistic views of human nature and performance potential [32]. The Olympic history of the amateur paragraph is the standard historical example of these shortcomings [13]. The current example is the enforcement of antidoping policies that by critics are considered unfair and repressive. For instance, in cross-country skiing, athletes from strong support systems use high-altitude chambers and high-altitude training to balance accurately the limitations on biochemical levels in the blood set by the international federation FIS. Athletes from systems with fewer resources have no chance of doing this. However, with the systematic and controlled use of erythropoietin (EPO) they can reach the same levels as their competitors. The problem is that EPO is banned, and the differences between the rich and the poor tend to increase. Critics such as Tamburrini and Gebauer talk of the need for liberation from biological, social, and cultural essentialism and for an open and nonprejudiced approach to new technological possibilities.

A further criticism points toward the complexity of what to a certain extent are contradictory norms and values that are under constant change and revision and on which there is constant disagreement in the sports community. For instance, the social logic of sport is to measure, compare, and rank competitors according to performance. Athletes undergo extreme training regimes with special diets, advanced medical testing, high-altitude training, and so forth. Certain means, however, such as use of drugs on the doping list, are banned, even if these means can be used under medical control and without serious risks for harm. The distinctions between the acceptable and the nonacceptable seem contingent and random. The understanding of sport as a normative sphere, it is argued, is unclear and confused.

As with performance theories, however, performer theorists respond to the criticism. As said above, the ban on drugs is justified because it is seen to protect individual freedom and responsibility in sport. Moreover, proponents of performer theories could argue that ambiguity and complexity should not be interpreted as weaknesses but as a sign of the strength of their position. These theories provide a dynamic ethical understanding of the rapid developments of sport in the early 21st century.

▪ CONCLUDING COMMENTS

I have outlined what I consider to be three ideal-typical kinds of normative theories of sport, and I have discussed critically some of their ethical implications and their potential for contributing to an understanding of sport as a normative sphere.

A first position, the instrumentalist one, is of little value in this regard. Instrumentalism might function to a certain extent in political rhetoric but provide little or no insight into the norms and values of sport per se. A second position, exemplified by performance theories, is built on the internalist premise that sport is a particular source of value in itself. The core value set of sport is held to be performance, progress, and transcendence, more or less by any means possible. A third kind of theory consists of what I called performer theories. Similar to performance theories, these are internalist theories and articulate what are considered to be a particular set of values of sport itself. In contradistinction to performance theories, however, the focus here is on the possible development of the performer as a moral subject.

Both performance and performer theories have significant things to say about sport and values in general and about sport ethics in particular. In summing up, the question arises as to whether it is possible to rank them according to their merits when it comes to normative understandings of sport. As should be evident from my other writings, I am skeptical about what I take to be the simplistic aspects and the lack of moderation found in performance theories, and I consider performer theories as offering a more nuanced and useful framework for normative reflection on sport. However, there is of course no Archimedean point here to settle the dispute. I accept that, if developed in reflective, consistent, and systematic ways, as is more or less the case with Tamburrini and Gebauer, performer theories constitute viable philosophical alternatives that ought to be taken seriously. The tensions between performance and performer ideals are key tensions in sport ethics, and there is no reason to believe that their actuality will decrease in the time to come.

A final question to be commented on concerns the practical relevance of my discussion. What is the status of the various alternatives? What are the predominant normative theories in today's world of competitive sport? At first sight, commercial, political, and ideological interests in sport seem stronger than ever, and various versions of instrumental theories, blended to some extent with the ideals of groundbreaking performances and the setting of records, seem predominant. In elite sport at least, performer theories as sketched above seem marginalized and on their way to becoming anachronistic expressions of a time gone by.

There are, however, alternative interpretations of the development. One such interpretation is that performer theories face revitalization and new actuality. There seems to be here a certain self-destructive logic in instrumental theories and in a one-sided emphasis on performance enhancement [18]. Sport cultures with cynical winning attitudes, or sports with highly specialized and standardized demands on performance, might lose their human touch and their attractiveness to the general public. Interestingly, new sports in which the focus is on the particular qualities of the individual performer are appearing on the scene. The so-called board sports such as surfing, skateboarding, and snowboarding are good examples. With relatively nonprecise measurements of technically (and tactically) complex performances, and with emphasis on aesthetic qualities and individual expression, these sports can be seen to represent an upbeat and new version of performer theories that might become the predominant sporting paradigm in the time to come.

■ **ABOUT THE AUTHOR**

Sigmund Loland (sigmund.loland@nih.no) is with the Norwegian University for Sport and Physical Education, Oslo. This paper was delivered as the Presidential Address at the 2003 meeting of the International Association for the Philosophy of Sport, and was reviewed by members of the JPS Editorial Review Board prior to its original publication.

▣ NOTE

1. In most sport policy documents written within the last decades, references to instrumental goals are predominant. See, for example, the official policy documents of the Norwegian sport, *Stortingsmelding nr. 14 (1999–2000): Idrettslivet i endring. Om statens forhold til idrett og fysisk aktivitet.*

▣ REFERENCES

1. Allison, L. *Amateurism in Sport: An Analysis and a Defense.* London: Frank Cass, 2001.
2. Beauchamp, T. L. *Philosophical Ethics: An Introduction to Moral Philosophy.* 2nd ed. New York: McGraw-Hill, 1991.
3. Breivik, G. "The Doping Dilemma—Game Theoretical Considerations." *Sportwissenscaft* 17(1), 1987, 83–94.
4. Cooper, D. E. "Technology: Liberation or Enslavement?" In *Philosophy and Technology*, D. Fellows (Ed.). Cambridge, MA: Cambridge University Press, 1998, 7–18.
5. Cooper, J. M. *Reason and Human Good in Aristotle.* Cambridge, MA: Harvard University Press, 1975.
6. Danner, M. "The Lost Olympics." *The New York Review of Books* 17, 2000, 66–67.
7. Dick, F. "No Limits." Paper presented at the IAF-seminar "Human Performance in Athletics: Limits and Possibilities," Budapest, Hungary, October 11–12, 1997.
8. Dixon, N. "Canadian Figure Skaters, French Judges, and Realism in Sport." *Journal of the Philosophy of Sport* XXX, 2003, 103–116.
9. Elliot, C. *Better Than Well. American Medicine Meets the American Dream.* New York: W.W. Norton, 2003.
10. Finley, M. I., and Pleket, H. W. *The Olympic Games: The First Thousand Years.* London: Chatto and Windus, 1976.
11. Fraleigh, W. P. "Right Actions in Sport. Ethics for Contestants." *Journal of the Philosophy of Sport* XI, 1985, 83–88.
12. Gebauer, G. *Sport in der Gesellschaft des Spektakels.* Sankt Augustin, Germany: Academia Verlag, 2002.
13. Glader, E. A. *Amateurism and Athletics.* West Point, NY: Leisure Press, 1978.
14. Guttmann, A. *From Ritual to Record. The Nature of Modern Sports.* New York: Columbia University Press, 1978.
15. Heikkila, J. "Discipline and Excel: Techniques of the Self and Body and the Logic of Competing." *Sport Sociology Journal* 10, 1992, 397–412.
16. Hill, C. R. *Olympic Politics.* Manchester, UK: Manchester University Press, 1992.
17. Hoberman, J. M. *Mortal Engines. The Science of Performance and the Dehumanization of Sports.* New York: Free Press, 1992.
18. Loland, S. "Record Sports: An Ecological Critique and a Reconstruction." *Journal of the Philosophy of Sport* XXVIII, 2001, 127–139.
19. Loland, S. *Fair Play in Sport: A Moral Norm System.* London: Routledge, 2002.

20. Loland, S., and Ommundsen, Y. "Values and Ideologies of Norwegian Sport as Perceived by the General Population." *European Physical Education Review* 2, 1996, 133–142.
21. MacAloon, J. J. *This Great Symbol. Pierre de Coubertin and the Origins of the Modern Olympic Games.* Chicago: Chicago University Press, 1981.
22. McNamee, M. "Sporting Practices, Institutions, and Virtues: A Critique and Restatement." *Journal of the Philosophy of Sport* XXII, 1995, 61–82.
23. Morgan, W. J. *Leftist Theories of Sport: A Critique and Reconstruction.* Urbana: University of Illinois Press, 1994.
24. Morgan, W. J. "Hvordan man ikke bør løse etiske dilemmaer i idrett." In *I bevegelse— et festskrift til Gunnar Breivik på hans 60 årsdag,* V. Fusche-Moe and S. Loland (Eds.). Oslo: Gyldendal, 2003.
25. Murray, T. H. "The Coercive Power of Drugs in Sport." *The Hastings Center Report* XIII, 1983, 24–30.
26. Østerberg, D. *Det moderne—et essay om vestens kultur.* Oslo: Gyldendal, 2000.
27. Riordan, J. "The Impact of Communism on Sport." In *The International Politics of Sport in the 20th Century,* J. Riordan and A. Krüger (Eds.). London: EF & N Spon, 1999.
28. Riordan, J., and Krüger, A. (Eds.). *The International Politics of Sport in the 20th Century.* London: EF & N Spon, 1999.
29. Simon, R. L. *Fair Play. Sports, Values, and Society.* Boulder, CO: Westview Press, 1991.
30. Simon, R. L. "Internalism and Internal Values in Sport." *Journal of the Philosophy of Sport* XXVII, 2000, 1–16.
31. Skillen, A. "Sport Is for Losers." In *Ethics in Sport,* M. J. McNamee and J. Parry (Eds.). London: E & FN Spon, 1998.
32. Tamburrini, C. M. The "Hand of God." *Essays in the Philosophy of Sport.* Gothenburg, Sweden: Acta Universitatis Gothoburgensis, 2000.

PART II

Categories and Discrimination

Categories make organized sports interesting and fair. In youth sports like Little League Baseball, an eleven-year-old is not allowed to compete on a team of six- and seven-year-olds. The older child has biologically superior coordination, discipline, and muscle formation, which grants her team an unfair advantage. Vastly uneven odds make a competition less engaging for players and fans, and they warp the framework in which sport skills like patience and perseverance can be acquired. How can we teach a child to get back on the horse and try again if the next outcome and the one after are certain failure? This is why leagues have algorithms for determining team placement according to categories like age, weight, and skill level. These are not perfect—there will always be some lopsided games—but having a process for selection decreases the capacity to predict who will win, which improves fairness.

The amateur distinction for college athletes was designed to ensure the prioritization of academics. Sports were largely instituted as a means of enhancing the social component of education at a time when no one imagined that athletes would ever get paid to play. While all colleges and universities outwardly exist to educate, several schools that compete in the NCAA's Division I have become beholden to the massive wealth that their sports programs generate and the alumni gifts they produce. Athletes at these institutions are often pressured to sacrifice both academics and social life to increase the chances of a winning team record, which brings the school more money. Many of these athletes dream of playing professionally, but only about 1 percent will actually make it.

In chapter 4, as Glenn Wong explains, this creates a quagmire of contradictions for young athletes. They are encouraged to aspire to professional sports, but are heavily penalized for getting any sports-related compensation or representation while still in college. They are expected to be students first, but are required to commit the vast majority of their hours to athletics. The category of amateurism was designed to promote the social value of education, but instead subjugates athletes to grueling college sport schedules that undermine their academic pursuits and encourage young athletes to depart early from school to pursue often unfruitful professional sport fantasies.

Even seemingly benign sport categories, like gender, must be ethically questioned. On average, being biologically male confers the advantage of higher testosterone levels, which is correlated with greater speed and strength. This advantage becomes more consistent as athletes specialize and enter prime competition years. Accordingly, there are some sports that might benefit from gender segregation for safety and fairness, such as boxing and mixed martial arts, especially at the professional level. However, there is no conclusive evidence that being male or female confers advantage in other sports-related abilities like discipline, pain tolerance, stability, or strategizing. In some sports like sailing, long-distance swimming, ultra-long-distance running, archery, and several equestrian events, men and women exhibit equal ability. It begs the question of why competitors in some of these events are still separated by gender. As Katrina Karkazis's article, chapter 6, demonstrates, the category of gender itself is not clearly defined. Deciding whether males and females should compete together, and whether someone's hormone levels are "too male" to compete against females, are not just matters of fairness in sports but also reinforce social gender expectations in other arenas like employment, politics, and education. These decisions should still consider safety and fair competition, but also should consider evolving statistics about female ability, and most important, should prioritize equal access and opportunity.

As a sport category, race is more tenuous than gender because it is even less well characterized. There are some demographics defined by a combination of geography and culture that seem to demonstrate superior skill in certain sports, like the Kalenjin of Kenya, a tribe that has produced many of the world's best long-distance runners. The Kalenjin have biological and cultural commonalities that provide many of them with an advantage. Race, however, is not biological and is too broad in terms of culture to show meaningful correlation with sport ability. If you select any two people, one who identifies as black and the other as white, it is possible that these two are more similar to each other in terms of culture *and* genetics than two people who both identify as black or two people who both identify as white. Accordingly, there are no reasons to segregate sports on the basis of race. In light of present and past social inequities, there are reasons to promote opportunities for people of color to play, organize, and lead sports that have always been dominated by whites.

As with both race and gender, social inequity impels the sports world to create opportunities for individuals with disabilities. However, defining these opportunities is complicated by the complexity of disability. For example, how do we determine fair competition categories for individuals capable of swimming, but who are unable to swim in traditional styles or at age-commensurate levels? Is it fair to pit a swimmer with developmental delays against a swimmer with one leg? How about a swimmer who is missing the lower part of her leg against another swimmer who is missing her whole leg? It is incredibly difficult to determine the appropriate expected ability range for an individual with a disability, not to mention the appropriate response when such a person defies expectations and demonstrates skill associated with traditional bodies, as D. A. Baker's article, chapter 9, discusses. Oversight committees have created careful taxonomies to group competitors in the Paralympics, and in the Special Olympics according to similar qualifying scores, but does not prevent anyone from entry. Both have thankfully evolved from assessment of handicap toward determination of ability. To make sense and be ethical, these groupings must continue to adapt to developments in assistive technology with an emphasis on promoting inclusion and ensuring fairness.

A. Professional vs. Amateur

3 Uneven Bars

Age Rules, Antitrust, and Amateurism

in Women's Gymnastics

■ RYAN M. RODENBERG AND
ANDREA N. EAGLEMAN

■ I. INTRODUCTION

> We respect the [gymnastics minimum-age] rules and some
> countries don't.
>
> —*U.S. national team coach Martha Karolyi*[1]

Ten years. That is how long it took Dominique Dawes, one of the most decorated American gymnasts ever, to receive the bronze medal she and her 2000 Olympic Games (Olympics or Games) teammates deserved.[2] In Sydney, Australia—the site of the 2000 Olympics and the first Games to be held since stricter minimum-age rules were imposed in the sport of women's gymnastics—Team USA won no medals but showed improvement over their 1999 World Championship performance by placing fourth as a team.[3] However, a decade later, the 2000 team was retroactively awarded the bronze medal because the medal-winning Chinese team was disqualified for knowingly having an underage athlete on the team.[4] Upon receiving her medal, Dawes said: "[T]he truth has been revealed."[5]

Precocity and elite-level gymnastics have a long history. In 1976, fourteen-year-old Nadia Comaneci of Romania dazzled viewers with the first set of perfect scores ever in Olympic competition.[6] Twenty years later, fellow fourteen-year-old Dominique Moceanu was a key member of the "Magnificent Seven," which became the first American squad to claim the team gold at the Olympic Games.[7] However, neither Comaneci nor Moceanu would be permitted to compete under the now-current age rules enacted in 1997.[8] Further, as evidenced by numerous cases of state-sponsored age falsification, compliance with the minimum-age rule has been mixed and enforcement of the rule has been lacking.[9] As a result, concerns about an uneven playing field between compliant and noncompliant nations have arisen.[10] Similarly, the more stringent minimum-age policy has, in an unintended way, facilitated increased age-related fraud and moved women's gymnastics further away from its amateurism ideals, damaging the sport's credibility.[11]

The history of elite-level gymnastics is replete with numerous examples of fifteen-year-old girls or younger who can achieve success on the biggest stage.[12] However, to date, no gymnast has filed a lawsuit challenging the mandates of the age eligibility rule. The primary purpose of this article is to establish the legal framework by which such a claim would be analyzed. The secondary purpose of this article is to explain how gymnastics' age rule has helped further the demise of the sport's amateurism principles. Section II of this paper provides a historical overview of elite-level gymnastics, with an emphasis on both the interrelationship between the governing bodies and the current age rule. Section III addresses the overlap between antitrust law and sports, explains how eligibility rules in sports are treated by the courts, and analyzes the antitrust legality of minimum-age rules in gymnastics. Section IV concludes with an outline of the important policy implications stemming from the mixed enforcement of gymnastics' minimum-age rule and the resulting impact on amateurism.

▪ II. OVERVIEW OF ELITE-LEVEL GYMNASTICS

A. Historical Development and Current Status

The sport of gymnastics has existed in the United States since the 1830s, when it was introduced by European immigrants.[13] Originally controlled by the Amateur Athletic Union (AAU), USA Gymnastics (formerly known as the United States Gymnastics Federation) took over as the sport's national governing body in 1970 and has presided over the sport in the U.S. ever since.[14] Based in Indianapolis, Indiana, USA Gymnastics is responsible for setting policies for gymnastics in the United States, selecting national teams, promoting the sport of gymnastics, enforcing International Olympic Committee (IOC) and Federation Internationale de Gymnastique (FIG) rules, and serving as a resource for its member clubs, professional members, athletes, and fans.[15]

The first U.S. women's team competed in the Olympic Games in 1936, thus marking the international emergence of American elite-level women's gymnastics.[16] The United States, which initially was not a strong contender for Olympic medals in women's gymnastics, won its first medal in 1948, a team bronze.[17] The women did not win another medal for thirty-six years, when the traditionally dominant Russians boycotted the 1984 Los Angeles Olympic Games, and the U.S. team finished with the silver medal behind Romania.[18] One U.S. gymnast at those Games, Mary Lou Retton, was the first-ever U.S. woman to win the all-around gold medal and became an "American folk heroine," as the New York Times referred to her following that Olympics.[19] Retton was coached by Bela Karolyi, the same man who guided Romanian Nadia Comaneci to a gold medal in 1976.[20] Karolyi, a Romanian citizen who defected to the United

States in 1981, established the United States as a powerful contender for World and Olympic medals after being named its national-team coach.[21] Women from the United States went on to win five medals at the 1992 Barcelona Olympics and four medals at the 1996 Atlanta Olympics (including the team gold medal), after which Karolyi retired from coaching.[22] Following a poor showing by the U.S. women at the 1997 World Championships,[23] Karolyi was retapped to lead the team for the 2000 Sydney Olympics.[24]

After the 2000 Olympics, Martha Karolyi replaced her husband as national-team coordinator.[25] Martha implemented a semicentralized training system for the U.S. team. Under this system, gymnasts train with their hometown coaches but convene at the Karolyis' ranch in Texas several times a year for national team training, where Martha Karolyi and the national team training staff assess the progress of the gymnasts.[26] The semicentralized system continues today, and since its implementation in 2001, the U.S. women's team has won a team medal at all subsequent World Championships and Olympic Games.[27] Individual gymnasts have also found success, with Carly Patterson and Nastia Liukin winning the all-around gold medal at the 2004 and 2008 Olympics, respectively.[28]

B. FIG and USA Gymnastics Governance

The IOC and its officials recognize the FIG as the supreme authority on international gymnastics.[29] The FIG, based in Lausanne, Switzerland, is the oldest governing body for the sport of gymnastics. It began in 1881 as the European Federation of Gymnastics and was renamed in 1921 when countries outside of Europe were first added to the federation.[30] In 2010, the FIG reported having 130 member federations, one of which is USA Gymnastics.[31] The FIG's governance structure consists of a rule-making congress, a twenty-three-person executive committee (of which two members are from the United States), a twenty-one-person council (of which one is from the U.S.), six technical committees, two auditors, and thirteen content-specific commissions.[32]

The FIG is the highest authoritative power in the sport of gymnastics, as it governs gymnastics competitions at the Olympic Games, World Games, World Championships, and all other multi-continental events.[33] All member national federations, such as USA Gymnastics, must follow FIG rules and regulations regarding athlete eligibility in order to field a team for international competition and, more generally, in order to maintain their membership status in good standing.[34] National federations who are members of the FIG are entitled to vote, submit proposals, and participate in official FIG events.[35] The FIG retains the authority, however, to suspend or expel a member federation for rule violations.[36]

USA Gymnastics is designated as the sole national governing body of gymnastics by the IOC and the FIG.[37] It became a member federation of the FIG in 1970.[38] "USA Gymnastics sets the rules and policies that govern gymnastics in the United

States . . . [and] has many responsibilities, including selecting and training the U.S. Gymnastics Teams for Olympic Games and World Championships."[39] The organization is governed by a president and chairman, a twenty-person board of directors, and an advisory council.[40]

The FIG is most involved in USA Gymnastics' governance of athletes who compete at an elite international level.[41] Athletes on the national team routinely represent the U.S. in international competitions.[42] The national team consists of approximately twenty-eight athletes, both junior (gymnasts under the age of sixteen) and senior (gymnasts who are sixteen years old and older).[43] National teams are selected at the annual national championships.[44] Gymnasts may also become members of the national team via approved petitions.[45] Any gymnastics event in which U.S. athletes compete with competitors from more than one nation must follow FIG regulations, as stated in Section II of the Sanctioning Procedures section of the USA Gymnastics 2010–2011 Women's Program Rules and Policies document.[46] Historically, the relationship between USA Gymnastics and the FIG has been harmonious, as USA Gymnastics has never publicly deviated from FIG-imposed policy.

C. Enactment and Administration of Minimum-Age Rule

Prior to 1980, female gymnasts were required to be fourteen years or older in order to compete as senior gymnasts in international competitions.[47] In 1980, the FIG enacted a new minimum-age rule, which stated that the gymnast must turn fifteen years old in the same calendar year as the competition in order to be eligible to compete as a senior gymnast.[48] The rationale behind this decision was to emphasize and promote the artistry of the sport, which was more commonly associated with older gymnasts, than the acrobatic elements performed by younger gymnasts.[49] In 1997, the FIG increased this standard to sixteen years of age, which remains the current age minimum in women's artistic gymnastics.[50] The increase from fifteen to sixteen years of age stemmed from the FIG's increased concerns about "musculoskeletal development of young competitors, lengthening gymnastics careers, preventing burnout, and in order to redirect the image of the sport positively for the public, spectators and media."[51] FIG's concerns mirrored issues raised by researchers, who keyed in on societal and health risks of elite-level youth sports such as mental burnout, overbearing parental and coach involvement, inhibited motor skill development, early-onset osteoporosis, amenorrhea, and eating disorders such as anorexia and bulimia.[52] Along with these documented health risks, commentators also have cited child-labor issues that arise when young elite athletes turn professional.[53] Another researcher brought attention to several ethical issues involved with elite-level training for young athletes and urged governing bodies to answer elucidating questions: "What are the risks—physical, psychological, social—for children in elite sports? How common are they?"[54] The aforementioned health, well-being, and ethical risks for young elite athletes provided the basis for the FIG's decision to enact minimum-age rules in the sport of gymnastics.[55]

Since the implementation of minimum-age rules, there have been several instances of nations falsifying the age of their gymnasts.[56] For example, even when the age minimum was set at fifteen years old, North Korea was found to have falsified the age of gymnast Kim Gwang Suk, who won the gold medal on the uneven parallel bars at the 1991 World Championships.[57] North Korea was banned from competing in the 1993 World Championships as a result of the fraud.[58] More recently, as alluded to above, the 2000 U.S. women's gymnastics team received a bronze medal ten years after the team finished fourth in the Sydney Olympics because officials discovered that a gymnast from the medal-winning Chinese team did not meet the minimum age of sixteen in 2000.[59] Similarly, the Chinese women's team received heavy media scrutiny in 2008 when cybersleuths uncovered online documents that showed at least two gymnasts were underage.[60] The documents later disappeared from the internet, and the FIG launched an investigation into the matter. Ultimately, the FIG decided that the age verification documents provided by China were accurate and the gymnasts had not violated the age-minimum rule.[61] Finally, in November 2010 the FIG announced a two-year suspension for the entire North Korea team after one of its gymnasts was found to have used three different birthdates in international competitions from 2003 to 2010.[62] The FIG explained that its decision "is a clear signal to those who would willfully disregard the current rules surrounding gymnast age. The health of its athletes and respect for the law are among [our] highest priorities."[63]

In an effort to better track the age of gymnasts competing internationally and reduce the prevalence of age fabrication, the FIG introduced a license (also called a "gymnastics passport") at the start of 2009.[64] All gymnasts must present this license in order to be eligible for international competitions.[65] The license must be renewed every two years, and it requires gymnasts to provide detailed personal information such as their full name, home address, email address, passport number, gender, date of birth, and the signature of both the gymnast and a representative from her national federation.[66]

■ III. LEGALITY OF GYMNASTICS' MINIMUM-AGE RULE

A. The Overlap of Antitrust Law with Sports

Legal challenges to age-eligibility rules in sports usually take the form of antitrust lawsuits. The Sherman Antitrust Act of 1890 (Sherman Act) is the primary federal antitrust statute in the United States.[67] Section I of the Sherman Act prohibits "[e]very contract, combination[,] . . . or conspiracy, in restraint of trade or commerce among the several states."[68] Recognizing that a plain-language reading of the Sherman Act could render almost all business agreements that crossed state lines illegal, the Supreme Court of the United States adopted a "rule of reason" test in its seminal Sherman Act opinion *Standard Oil Co. v. United States* over 100 years ago.[69] In *Standard Oil*, the Justices deemed that interstate commercial agreements would only be labeled illegal if they "unreasonably" restrained trade.[70] Later clarifications by the Supreme Court introduced an antitrust balancing test whereby the procompetitive effects of the regulation are considered vis-à-vis the restraint's detrimental impact on competition.[71] The rule of reason balancing test is not always employed. The Supreme Court has determined that certain types of egregious anticompetitive activity to be per se illegal. Examples include horizontal price fixing,[72] tying arrangements,[73] and market division between direct competitors.[74] Nevertheless, with a few notable exceptions discussed *infra*, a perusal of the relevant case law reveals that most sports-related antitrust issues are evaluated under the rule of reason standard.[75]

The interaction between sports and antitrust began inauspiciously. In 1922, the Supreme Court granted Major League Baseball an antitrust exemption based on a finding that the interstate commerce aspects of the sport were merely incidental to the staging of professional ballgames.[76] Although subsequently described as an "anomaly,"[77] an "aberration confined to baseball,"[78] and a "derelict in the stream of law,"[79] the 1922 *Federal Baseball Club of Baltimore v. National League of Professional Baseball Clubs* case has yet to be explicitly overruled by Congress or the Supreme Court.[80] Baseball's peculiar antitrust exemption did not extend to other sports, however. In *International Boxing Club v. United States,* the Supreme Court concluded that there was no unique aspect in sports meriting an across-the-board exemption from federal antitrust laws.[81] After boxing was found nonexempt, other sports were similarly deemed subject to antitrust scrutiny, including basketball,[82] football,[83] hockey,[84] golf,[85] and tennis.[86]

B. Antitrust Principles Applied to Sports Eligibility Rules

Eligibility issues in the sports industry have been a frequent subject of litigation.[87] The vast majority of plaintiffs have looked to the Sherman Act when filing lawsuits challenging sports eligibility rules.[88] Such rules are challenged on the basis that they constitute an impermissible concerted refusal to deal or group boycott.[89] Early Supreme Court cases found concerted refusals to deal and group boycotts to be per se illegal.[90] However, the Supreme Court has looked to the rule of reason standard in more recent decisions.[91]

The mode of analysis adopted in sports-eligibility rule cases has been somewhat of a mixed bag, with both the per se and rule of reason standards being adopted.[92] Cases that found eligibility rules to be illegal per se include *Boris v. United States Football League* (age and education rule),[93] *Blalock v. Ladies Professional Golf Ass'n* (twelve-month suspension of player–member for on-course rule violation),[94] *Haywood v. National Basketball Ass'n* (four-year college eligibility rule),[95] and *Linseman v. World Hockey Ass'n* (minimumage rule of twenty).[96] In contrast, a number of other cases looked to the rule of reason standard when evaluating the antitrust legality of specific sport eligibility rules. In *Deesen v. Professional Golfers Ass'n*, the court upheld league rules requiring players to meet certain performance thresholds for future eligibility.[97] Similarly in *Neeld v. National Hockey League*, the court deemed a league rule requiring all players to have sight in both eyes to be a reasonable restraint given the accompanying safety issues.[98] Finally, the court in *Molinas v. National Basketball Ass'n* found that the association's antigambling rules were reasonable and justified the suspension of a player who gambled.[99]

The Supreme Court has yet to decide a player eligibility case within the context of an individual (that is, non-team) sport. As such, there is no direct precedent how such a case would be decided.[100] The Supreme Court lends some guidance, however, in two sports-industry cases: *National Collegiate Athletic Ass'n v. Board of Regents*[101] (*NCAA*) and *American Needle, Inc. v. National Football League*.[102] Both decisions support the proposition that a court would likely evaluate an antitrust challenge to a minimum-age rule in individual sports under the rule of reason standard.[103] In *NCAA*, the Justices recognized the unique nature of sports in the context of an antitrust challenge to the NCAA's limits on television exposure for certain member schools, finding that the "case involve[d] an industry in which horizontal restraints on competition are essential if the product is to be available at all."[104] In its reasoning, *NCAA* distinguished between eligibility rules, which are restrictive but potentially procompetitive, and anticompetitive television broadcast limitations.[105] The Court in *American Needle* similarly deemed the rule of reason to be the correct analytical standard when considering the NFL's licensing activities.[106] Justice Stevens, the author of the unanimous *American Needle* decision in 2010, rationalized that there are a number of reasons in the sports industry that "provide[] a perfectly sensible justification for making a host of collective decisions."[107] Further, *American Needle* cited *NCAA* for the proposition that "[w]hen 'restraints on competition are essential if the product is to be available at all,' *per se* rules of illegality are inapplicable, and instead the restraint must be judged according to the flexible Rule of Reason."[108]

C. Proposed Antitrust Analysis Extended to Gymnastics' Minimum-Age Rule

If an underage gymnast seeking a place on the U.S. Olympic team or other elite-level national team is inclined to file a lawsuit challenging gymnastics' age rule, she would likely file her claim under section I of the Sherman Act.[109] USA Gymnastics, as the national governing body exclusively charged with administration of the sport and enforcement of its rules, would be the defendant.[110] It is conceivable that the FIG, the governing body that formally enacted the age rule in 1997, could also be a possible target defendant. Although a trilogy of cases addressed the issue of extraterritorial jurisdiction in antitrust litigation,[111] the ability of an American plaintiff to have jurisdiction over the FIG, a Swiss entity with few contacts in the United States, is uncertain.[112] Accordingly, the focus here will be on USA Gymnastics, which has dutifully enforced gymnastics' age rule since the current policy was enacted in 1997.[113]

Jurisdiction-related reasons notwithstanding, an underage gymnast plaintiff would be presented with a difficult antitrust case. As described *supra,* the rule of reason standard would probably govern, with the court balancing the procompetitive effects of the age rule with the rule's anticompetitive impact.[114] Under this analytical standard, the court would be receptive to expert testimony and inquire "whether the restraint imposed is such as merely regulates and perhaps thereby promotes competition or whether it is such as may suppress or even destroy competition."[115] The Supreme Court has made clear that "the antitrust laws were passed for the 'protection of competition, not [individual] competitors.' "[116] Like other sports, organized women's gymnastics requires some degree of central rulemaking to establish uniformity regarding scheduling, scorekeeping, competition rules, and athlete eligibility. In addition to that uniformity, health and safety rationales, which were cited as impetuses for the current age rule's enactment in 1997,[117] also justify some degree of central rulemaking. Empirical evidence analyzing the careers of gymnasts that emerged after the enactment of the current rule may yield additional evidence of the rule's efficacy.[118]

A plaintiff challenging the minimum-age rule would likely advance two arguments. First, she would claim that the age restrictions are per se illegal as a group boycott or concerted refusal to deal.[119] For the reasons detailed at length above, the possibility of such a per se argument being successful is slim.[120] Second, she would posit that there are less restrictive alternatives to the bright-line rule age policy currently in place.[121] In this second prong of her argument, the underage gymnast would look to other women's sports leagues that impose minimum-age rules but administer such rules much more liberally. In women's tennis, the governing body (WTA Tour) has an age rule that prohibits those fourteen and under from competing.[122] From the ages of fourteen to seventeen, players may compete in a limited number of events per a sliding scale that is more permissive each year.[123] At age eighteen, players may play as much or as little as desired.[124] In women's golf, the LPGA Tour's age rule mandates that players be at least eighteen.[125] However, the LPGA Tour rule includes a mechanism where exceptions to the policy are granted on a case-by-case basis after a careful evaluation of the applicant's intelligence, financial stability, maturity, and playing ability.[126] The LPGA Tour's approach is analogous to the one seemingly proposed by U.S. national-team coordinator, Martha Karolyi, who opined, "I'd like the FIG to look at the preparation of the child and let the country decide who is best to compete."[127]

While plausible, these twin claims would be difficult to argue persuasively for at least three reasons. First, gymnastics, like all sports, can only function if uniform rules are applied. Eligibility rules would almost certainly be categorized as a core function of a governing body, as alluded to, and seemingly exempted in, *American Needle, Inc. v. National Football League*.[128] Second, given the dearth of empirical evidence analyzing the efficacy and effect of the 1997 rule change, an antitrust plaintiff with the burden of proof would have a difficult time positing that the anticompetitive effects of the rule outweigh the possible procompetitive and beneficial aspects of the rule.[129] Indeed, gymnastics' age rules were primarily enacted to protect young athletes from a host of health-related maladies.[130] Third, defendant USA Gymnastics may be able to avoid litigation altogether on jurisdictional grounds, arguing that the FIG is the appropriate (and sole) target of any antitrust claim given that the Swiss-based body is the entity that enacted the policy, is charged with the duty to investigate rule-breakers, and levies punishment against athletes and national federations in violation of the minimum-age rule.[131]

IV. CONCLUSION

While gymnastics' current minimum-age rule would likely survive an antitrust challenge, the rule's policy impact has been profoundly negative in two distinct ways. First, as predicted by Martha Karolyi,[132] the enactment of the current age rule has helped usher in an era of increased corruption related to age fabrication. As the recent cases in China and North Korea evidence, the nefarious conduct reached governmental levels, where officials knowingly altered documents to further the fraud.[133] Second, the countries that falsify such documents as a way to circumvent the age rule have created an unlevel playing field vis-à-vis those countries that follow the rule.

Jennifer Sey, the 1986 U.S. national champion and seven-time national team member, cited the lightness and lack of fear of younger gymnasts as two key reasons why countries enlist underage gymnasts in international competitions; both factors allow gymnasts to perform difficult skills with greater ease.[134] Similarly, in the book *Little Girls in Pretty Boxes*, a 1995 exposé on gymnastics and figure skating, author Joan Ryan claimed that female gymnasts are "racing against puberty" to reap the benefits of having a smaller, lighter body in gymnastics.[135] Additionally, offering credence to the idea that smaller, lighter, and younger gymnasts are viewed as the ideal, Ryan posited, "The window of opportunity is so narrow: from about thirteen to the onset of puberty."[136]

By developing sophisticated methods to bypass the FIG's minimum-age rule, certain countries have contributed to the decay of amateurism ideals in both gymnastics and the Olympics. This increase in age-related corruption has resulted in the counterfeiting of government documents such as birth certificates and passports,[137] which has forced preteen amateur athletes to lie about their ages because of directives from their coaches and government-run national federations.[138] It is irresponsible of these adults in powerful positions to compel young amateur athletes to knowingly misstate their ages. In addition, it is unjust in the sense that a deserving and genuinely eligible athlete who meets the age requirement is shut out of competition and replaced by an underage teammate who is considered more valuable by her nation's coaches and sport administrators.

Although the FIG recently implemented a new gymnastics "passport" licensing system, gymnastics experts pointedly question its efficacy.[139] For example, Bela Karolyi, who is now an NBC gymnastics commentator and no longer holds any official affiliation with USA Gymnastics,[140] offered the following solution: "The only way to stop this is to take off the age limit. To force honest countries to hold back [talented, but underage, gymnasts] and allow other countries, [who are] not so honest, to push them forward, it's not fair."[141] Karolyi's point is timely and relevant: if the FIG is unable or unwilling to effectively implement and enforce the rule, the sport of gymnastics might benefit from having no minimum-age requirement at all. This would level the playing field between countries in international competition and provide more opportunities for gymnasts who might otherwise miss their window of opportunity to compete internationally. Under the current rule, an athlete's birthday can drastically affect her ability to compete in World Championships and the Olympics. Karolyi opined on this point: "Think how many kids are ineligible because of a month or two? Where will they be in four years? Not in the same place. The window is small for gymnastics. Is it fair that they missed their chance at the Olympics by months or weeks?"[142]

In any discussion of minimum-age rules, the health effects of elite gymnastics is a germane corollary conversation.[143] Despite the actions of certain noncompliant countries, the average age of gymnasts competing in the World Championships and Olympic Games is higher now than it was pre-1997.[144] However, this fact does not necessarily mean that younger gymnasts are no longer competing at a high level. The difference now is that gymnasts under the age of sixteen are considered "junior elite" gymnasts rather than "senior elite."[145] The distinction is illusory, however, as the younger gymnasts follow training and competition schedules analogous to their elders.[146] Revealingly, Kelli Hill, a prominent American gymnastics coach, stated, "Sometimes our top juniors are better than some of our seniors."[147] As such, retracting the minimum-age rule would not force gymnasts to reach the elite level any earlier than they already are. Rather, it would provide greater international competition opportunities for all elite gymnasts regardless of their chronological age. Scholar Maureen Weiss emphasized this point:

[C]hronological age is not equivalent to social, emotional, cognitive, and anatomical age. . . . Two adolescents of the same age can be widely different in terms of social and emotional types of maturity. . . . So the implication of this idea is that age eligibility rules and policies need to consider the wide variety of individual differences in these various age indices and strategize ways of ensuring that the adolescent phenom is ready for the transition to professional.[148]

The trend in which some countries follow the minimum-age rule while others repeatedly break it has resulted in the rule operating as an uneven bar on the issue of eligibility. National teams now compete in a competitive realm that is unequal. The uptick in age-related fraud has caused disintegration of the amateur ideals of the sport, which conflicts with the integrity-preserving impetus for the rule. However, it is unlikely that antitrust litigation would be successful in over-turning the minimum-age rule. Instead, the FIG should revisit the minimum-age rule from a policy perspective that is centered on restoring amateurism ideals and improving athlete health as a way to ensure that it can be enforced prop-erly (to the extent it is retained at all) and all countries are in compliance. But, if the FIG, in collaboration with national-level governing bodies such as USA Gymnastics, determine such a policy goal to be unreachable, the rule should be eliminated to allow all gymnasts and countries the opportunity for greater parity and fairness in elite-level international competition.

■ NOTES

1. Eddie Pells, *US Gymnastics Still Unhappy About Age Rules*, USA TODAY (Aug. 16, 2010, 5:20 PM), http://www.usatoday.com/sports/olympics/2010-08-16-4215111810_x.htm.

2. *2000 Olympic Team Receives Bronze Medal at Visa Championships*, USA GYMNASTICS (Aug. 11, 2010), http://www.usa-gymnastics.org/pages/post.html? PostID=6001.

3. Pells, *supra* note 1; Diane Pucin, *U.S. Olympics Gymnastic Team Gets Bronze, 10 Years Later*, L.A. TIMES (Apr. 28, 2010), http://articles.latimes.com/print/2010/apr/28/sports/la-sp-gymnasts-bronze-20100429.

4. Pucin, *supra* note 3.

5. *USA Gymnastics Statement Regarding the IOC's Decision to Award 2000 Olympic Bronze Medal to USA*, USA GYMNASTICS (Apr. 28, 2010), http://www.usagymnastics.org/pages/post.html?PostID=5280&prog=h.

6. Dan Wetzel, *The Olympics' Age-Old Problem*, YAHOO! SPORTS (Aug. 14, 2008, 8:51 PM), http://sports.yahoo.com/olympics/beijing/gymnastics/news?slug=dw-gymnasts age081408.

7. *USA Gymnastics Names 2010 Hall of Fame Inductees*, USA GYMNASTICS (Mar. 23, 2010), http://www.usa-gymnastics.org/pages/post.html?PostID=5069.

8. Pells, *supra* note 1; Tom Weir, *Tinkering with Rules has Tinkerbells Left Out*, USA TODAY, July 23, 1996, at 8E.

9. *See* Pells, *supra* note 1.

10. *Id.* ("[Martha] Karolyi and her husband, Bela, have long believed in scrapping age limits for senior events, saying that, among other things, they create an uneven playing field between countries that adhere to the rules and those that try to skirt them.").

11. Wetzel, *supra* note 6.

12. *See* Christopher Clarey, *Miller Adds Maturity and Difficulty to Her Repertory*, N.Y. TIMES, July 18, 1996, at B9.

13. *History of Artistic Gymnastics*, USA GYMNASTICS, http://www.usagymnastics.org/pages/home/gymnastics101/history_artistic.html?prog=pb (last visited May 14, 2011).

14. *About USA Gymnastics*, USA GYMNASTICS, http://www.usa-gymnastics.org/pages/aboutus/pages/about_usag.html (last visited May 14, 2011); *Former Women's National*

Champions, USA GYMNASTICS, http://www.usa-gymnastics.org/pages/pressbox/history/nationalchamps_women.html (last visited May 14, 2011).

15. *About USA Gymnastics, supra* note 14.

16. *History of Artistic Gymnastics, supra* note 13.

17. *U.S. Medalists at Olympic Games—Men & Women Artistic Gymnastics*, USA GYMNASTICS, http://www.usa-gymnastics.org/pages/pressbox/history/olympics_medalists_artistic.html (last visited May 14, 2011).

18. *Id.*; *United States Olympic Committee Names Judge Charles Carter Lee as Chef de Mission for 2008 Olympic Games*, USA GYMNASTICS (Apr. 30, 2008), http://www.usa-gymnastics.org/pages/post.html?PostID=2149&prog=h.

19. Dave Anderson, *'I Was Thinking, Stick, Stick'*, N.Y. TIMES, Aug. 5, 1984, § 5, at 3.

20. *Id.*

21. *Karolyi Named National Team Coordinator for USA Women*, USA GYMNASTICS (Nov. 16, 1999), http://www.usa-gymnastics.org/pages/post.html?PostID=1354&prog=h.

22. *Id.*; *U.S. Medalists at Olympic Games—Men & Women Artistic Gymnastics, supra* note 17.

23. *See 33rd World Championships Artistic Gymnastics*, GYMNASTICRESULTS.COM, http://www.gymnasticsresults.com/w1997w.html (last visited May 14, 2011).

24. *Karolyi Named National Team Coordinator for USA Women, supra* note 21.

25. *Martha Karolyi Named National Team Coordinator Through 2004 Olympic Games*, USA GYMNASTICS (Feb. 20, 2001), http://www.usa-gymnastics.org/pages/post.html?PostID=1301&prog=h.

26. Alice Park & Kristin Kloberdanz, *Inside Camp Karolyi*, TIME, Aug. 16, 2004, at 64, *available at* http://www.time.com/time/magazine/article/0,9171,994881-2,00.html.

27. *U.S. Women Win Team Silver Medal at 2010 World Championships*, USA GYMNASTICS (Oct. 20, 2010), http://www.usa-gymnastics.org/pages/post.html? PostID=6558; *USOC Designates USA Gymnastics National Team Training Center at Karolyi Ranch as Newest U.S. Olympic Training Site*, USA GYMNASTICS (Jan. 26, 2001), http://www.usa-gymnastics.org/pages/post.html?PostID=6979&prog=h.

28. *Patterson Wins GOLD in All-Around*, USA GYMNASTICS (Aug. 27, 2004), http://www.usa-gymnastics.org/pages/post.html?PostID=1194&prog=h; Michael David Smith, *Olympic Gymnastics: USA's Nastia Liukin Wins Gold, Shawn Johnson Silver*, FANHOUSE (Aug. 15, 2008), http://olympics.fanhouse.com/2008/08/15/olympic-gymnastics-usas-nastia-liukin-wins-individual-all-arou/.

29. *See International Gymnastics Federation*, OLYMPIC.org, http://www.olympic.org/fig-artistic-gymnastics (last visited May 14, 2011); USA Gymnastics: Our Role in the Olympic Family, *About USA Gymnastics*, USA GYMNASTICS, http://www.usagymnastics.org/pages/aboutus/pages/about_usag.html (last visited May 14, 2011); *see also* STATUTES OF FÉDÉRATION INTERNATIONALE DE GYMNASTIQUE (2011), *available at* http://figdocs.lx2.sportcentric .com/external/serve.php?document=2549 [hereinafter FIG Statutes].

30. *Milestones in FIG History*, FÉDÉRATION INTERNATIONALE DE GYMNASTIQUE, http://www.fig-gymnastics.com/vsite/vcontent/page/custom/0,8510,5187-204412-221635-49054-313081-custom-item,00.html (last visited May 14, 2011).

31. *See id.*; *About USA Gymnastics, supra* note 14 (noting that USA Gymnastics became a member of the FIG in 1970).

32. *FIG Directory*, FÉDÉRATION INTERNATIONALE DE GYMNASTIQUE, http://www.fig-gymnastics.com/vsite/vnavsite/page/directory/0,10853,5187-188051-205273-navlist,00.html (last visited May 14, 2011).

33. *See supra* note 29 and accompanying text.

34. *See About USA Gymnastics, supra* note 14.

35. FIG STATUTES ch. 3, art. 3.1.

36. *Id.* arts. 7, 8.

37. *About USA Gymnastics, supra* note 14.

38. *Id.*

39. *Id.*

40. USA GYMNASTICS BYLAWS §§ 4.01, 4.02, 6.02(a), 7.01, 7.02 (2009), *available at* http://www.usa-gymnastics.org/PDFs/About%20USA%20Gymnastics/Govemance/usag-bylaws.pdf.

41. *About USA Gymnastics, supra* note 14.

42. *Women's Elite/Pre-Elite/TOPs Program Overview*, USA GYMNASTICS, http://www.usa-gymnastics.org/pages/women/pages/overview_elite.html (last visited May 14, 2011).

43. *About USA Gymnastics, supra* note 14.

44. *Id.*

45. *Id.*

46. USA GYMNASTICS 2010–2011 WOMEN'S PROGRAM RULES AND POLICIES pt. 4, § 2 (2010), *available at* http://usagymnastics.org/PDFs/Women/Rules/Rules%20and%20Policies/2010_2011_w_rulespolicies.pdf.

47. International Amateur Athletic Federation, *Within the International Federations*, 1980 OLYMPIC REV. 513, 520, *available at* http://www.la84foundation.org/OlympicInformationCenter/OlympicReview/1980/ore155/ORE155p.pdf.

48. *Id.*

49. Neil Amdur, *Rift over Underage Gymnasts*, N.Y. TIMES, Dec. 7, 1981, at C4.

50. *See* Weir, *supra* note 8, at 8E ("Rulesmakers hope the age limit somehow will cure the ills that cloud the seeming innocence of their sport . . . .").

51. Van Anderson, *Female Gymnasts: Older and Healthier?*, TECHNIQUE, Aug. 1997, at 14, 15, *available at* http://www.usa-gymnastics.org/pages/home/publications/technique/1997/8/female.pdf.

52. Eryn M. Doherty, Comment, *Winning Isn't Everything . . . It's the Only Thing: A Critique of Teenaged Girls' Participation in Sports*, 10 MARQ. SPORTS L. REV. 127, 128, 137–138 (1999); Lenny D. Wiersma, *Risks and Benefits of Youth Sport Specialization: Perspectives and Recommendations*, 12 PEDIATRIC EXERCISE SCI. 13, 15–18 (2000).

53. *See, e.g.*, Jenna Merten, Comment, *Raising a Red Card: Why Freddy Adu Should not be Allowed to Play Professional Soccer*, 15 MARQ. SPORTS L.J. 205 (2004).

54. Thomas W. Rowland, *On the Ethics of Elite-Level Sports Participation by Children*, 12 PEDIATRIC EXERCISE SCI. 1, 4 (2000).

55. MEN'S GYMNASTICS RULES AND POLICIES sec. VII (2011), *available at* http://www.usa-gymnastics.org/pages/men/pages/rules_policies.html. Although the focus of this article is on age rules in women's gymnastics, please note that male gymnasts must also be at least sixteen years of age in order to compete at the senior elite level. *Id.*

56. Gymnastics experts predicted that age fabrication would occur in the wake of minimum-age rules being enacted. Weir, *supra* note 8, at 8E ("Bela Karolyi[] is adamantly opposed to the age rule and believes it could inspire an onslaught of forged birth certificates.").

57. Kevin Sullivan, *In Olympic Community, N. Korea Is the Odd Neighbor*, WASH. POST, July 8, 1996, at Cl.

58. *Id.*

59. Kevin Helliker & Geoffrey A. Fowler, *China Stripped of Medal from 2000*, WALL ST. J., Apr. 29, 2010 at All, *available at* http://online.wsj.com/article/SB10001 4240527487044 23504575212053805495856.html.

60. Miguel Helft, *Internet-Age Detectives on the Trail of Gymnasts*, N.Y. TIMES, Aug. 29, 2008, at D2, *available at* http://www.nytimes.com/2008/08/29/sports/olympics/29gym-nastics.html?ref=gymnastics.

61. Juliet Macur, *Inquiry on Age Clears Some Gymnasts, Not All*, N.Y. TIMES, Oct. 2, 2008, at D1.

62. *Two Years Suspension!*, FÉDÉRATION INTERNATIONALE DE GYMNASTIQUE (Nov. 5, 2010), http://www.fig-gymnastics.com/vsite/vcontent/content/news/0,10869,5187-188805-206027-44766-311274-news-item,00.html.

63. *Id.*

64. *FIG License Check*, FÉDÉRATION INTERNATIONALE DE GYMNASTIQUE, http://www.fig-gymnastics.com/vsite/vcontent/page/custom/0,8510,5187-196741-213964-46937-297133-custom-item,00.html (last visited May 14, 2011); Marlen Garcia, *More Age Monitoring, Smaller Squad Sizes Ahead for Gymnastics*, USA TODAY (Aug. 9, 2008, 11:18 AM), http://www.usatoday.com/sports/olympics/beijing/gymnastics/2008-08-09-FIG-age_N.htm.

65. FÉDÉRATION INTERNATIONALE DE GYMNASTIQUE, FIG LICENSE RULES 1 (2010), *available at* http://figdocs.lx2.sportcentric.com/extemal/serve.php?document=2114.

66. *Id.* at 4.

67. *See* 15 U.S.C. § 1 (2006).

68. *Id.*

69. 221 U.S. 1, 63, 66 (1910).

70. *Id.* at 58.

71. *See* Nat'l Soc'y of Prof'l Eng'rs v. United States, 435 U.S. 679, 692 (1978).

72. Copperweld Corp. v. Independence Tube Corp., 467 U.S. 752, 768 (1984).

73. Int'l Salt Co. v. United States, 332 U.S. 392, 396 (1947), *abrogated by* Ill. Tool Works Inc. v. Indep. Ink, Inc., 547 U.S. 28 (2006).

74. *Copperweld Corp.*, 467 U.S. at 768.

75. *See, e.g., Nat'l Soc'y of Prof'l Eng'rs*, 435 U.S. at 691–692 (stating that unless the agreement is "so plainly anticompetitive that no elaborate study of the industry is needed to establish their illegality," it will be analyzed under the rule of reason).

76. Fed. Baseball Club of Balt. v. Nat'l League of Prof'l Baseball Clubs, 259 U.S. 200, 208–209 (1922).

77. Flood v. Kuhn, 407 U.S. 258, 282 (1972).

78. *Id.*

79. *Id.* at 286 (Douglas, J., dissenting).

80. *See generally* Toolson v. N.Y. Yankees, 346 U.S. 356, 356–357 (1952) (affirming *Federal Baseball Club of Baltimore* and noting that any change should originate in congressional legislation); Major League Baseball v. Crist, 331 F.3d 1177, 1177 n.1 (11th Cir. 2003) (following *Federal Baseball Club of Baltimore* with reservations).

81. 358 U.S. 242, 244–245 (1955).

82. Haywood v. Nat'l Basketball Ass'n, 401 U.S. 1204 (1971).

83. Radovich v. Nat'l Football League, 352 U.S. 445 (1957).

84. Phila. World Hockey Club, Inc. v. Phila. Hockey Club, Inc., 351 F. Supp. 462 (E.D. Pa. 1972).

85. Deesen v. Prof'l Golfers Ass'n, 358 F.2d 165 (9th Cir. 1966).

86. Volvo N. Am. Corp. v. Men's Int'l Prof'l Tennis Council, 857 F.2d 55 (2d Cir. 1988).

87. *See generally* Matthew J. Mitten & Timothy Davis, *Athlete Eligibility Requirements and Legal Protection of Sports Participation Opportunities*, 8 VA. SPORTS & ENT. L.J. 71 (2009) (discussing the legal frameworks behind eligibility issues at the Olympic, professional, and interscholastic levels).

88. Ryan M. Rodenberg, *Gender Policies in Golf and the Impact of Litigation*: Lawless v. LPGA, WORLD SPORTS L. REP., Dec. 2010, at 6.

89. David G. Kabbes, Note, *Professional Sports' Eligibility Rules: Too Many Players on the Field*, 1986 U. ILL. L. REV. 1233, 1234–1235; Robert B. Terry, Comment, *Application of Antitrust Laws to Professional Sports' Eligibility and Draft Rules*, 46 MO. L. REV. 797, 816 (1981).

90. Klor's, Inc. v. Broadway-Hale Stores, Inc., 359 U.S. 207, 212 (1959); Fashion Originator's Guild, Inc. v. Fed. Trade Comm'n, 312 U.S. 457, 463–464 (1941).

91. Nw. Wholesale Stationers, Inc. v. Pac. Stationary & Printing Co., 472 U.S. 284, 289 (1985); Cont'l T.V., Inc. v. GTE Sylvania, Inc., 433 U.S. 36, 59 (1977).

92. There has been a plethora of academic articles analyzing eligibility rules in sports. For general treatment, see Kabbes, *supra* note 89; Terry, *supra* note 89, at 819–825. For examples specific to certain sports, see Marc Edelman & C. Keith Harrison, *Analyzing the WNBA's Mandatory Age/Education Policy from a Legal, Cultural, and Ethical Perspective*, 3 Nw. J. L. & SOC. POL'Y 1, 21 (2008); Michael A. McCann & Joseph S. Rosen, *Legality of Age Restrictions in the NBA and the NFL*, 56 CASE W. RES. L. REV. 731, 731–744 (2006); Carter A. McGowan, *Rough Around the Edges: Professionalism, Eligibility, and the Future of Figure Skating*, 6 SETON HALL J. SPORTS & ENT. L. 501, 523–524 (1996); Bartlett H. McGuire, *Age Restrictions in Women's Professional Tennis: A Case Study of Procompetitive Restraints of Trade*, 1 J. INT'L MEDIA & ENT. L. 199, 220–251 (2007); Ryan M. Rodenberg, Comment, *Age Eligibility Rules in Women's Professional Tennis: Necessary for the Integrity, Viability, and Administration of the Game or an Unreasonable Restraint of Trade in Violation of Antitrust Law?*, 7 SPORTS LAW. J. 183, 197–212 (2000); Ryan M. Rodenberg, Elizabeth A. Gregg & Lawrence W. Fielding, *Age Eligibility Rules in Women's Professional Golf: A Legal Eagle or an Antitrust Bogey?*, 19 J. LEGAL ASPECTS SPORT 103, 110–116 (2009) [hereinafter *Age Eligibility Rules in Women's Professional Golf: A Legal Eagle or an Antitrust Bogey?*].

93. No. Cv. 83-49830 LEW, 1984 WL 894, at *1–2 (C.D. Cal. Feb. 28, 1984).

94. 359 F. Supp. 1260, 1265 (N.D. Ga. 1973).

95. 401 U.S. 1204, 1205 (1971).

96. 439 F. Supp. 1315, 1320 (D. Conn. 1977).

97. 358 F.2d 165, 170 (9th Cir. 1966).

98. 594 F.2d 1297, 1300 (D.C. Cir. 1978).

99. 190 F. Supp. 241, 244–245 (S.D.N.Y. 1961).

100. Antitrust cases pertaining to player eligibility issues that involve the major team sport leagues and accompanying labor unions are of limited precedential value in the context of gymnastics and other individual sports (e.g., tennis, golf, swimming, and track and field) since most such cases are decided on the basis of the nonstatutory labor exemption. *See, e.g.,* Clarett v. Nat'l Football League, 369 F.3d 124, 125 n.1 (2d Cir. 2004). The athletes involved in individual sports are independent contractors and not members of any labor union, rendering the nonstatutory labor exemption inapplicable. *Id.* at 130; *see*

also Age Eligibility Rules in Women's Professional Golf: A Legal Eagle or an Antitrust Bogey?, *supra* note 92, at 114.

101. 468 U.S. 85 (1984).

102. 130 S. Ct. 2201 (2010).

103. *See id.* at 2216–2217; *Nat'l Collegiate Athletic Ass'n,* 468 U.S. at 117–120. Other Supreme Court decisions also lend support to the likelihood that the rule of reason would be the prevailing standard when evaluating gymnastics' minimum-age rule. In 1977, the Court concluded that "[p]er se rules of illegality are appropriate only when they relate to conduct that is manifestly anticompetitive." Cont'l T.V., Inc. v. GTE Sylvania Inc., 433 U.S. 36, 49–50 (1977).

104. 468 U.S. at 101.

105. *Id.* at 108, 117.

106. 130 S. Ct. at 2206–2207. Dicta in *American Needle* could be persuasive in the individual, nonteam sport context. *See, e.g.,* Ryan M. Rodenberg & L. Jon Wertheim, Legal Case Brief, American Needle v. National Football League et al., *560 U.S.___(2010), 2010 WL 2025207,* 3 Int'l J. Sport Commc'n. 371 (2010).

107. 130 S. Ct. at 2216.

108. *Id.*

109. *See* 15 U.S.C. § 1 (2006).

110. There is evidence that high-ranking individual members of USA Gymnastics do not support the way that the current age rule has been enforced since its adoption in 1997. *See, e.g.,* Pells, *supra* note 1. With that said, there is no evidence in the public domain (e.g., press releases or official statements) setting forth USA Gymnastics' position on the wisdom of whether having an age rule is prudent.

111. United States v. Sisal Sales Corp., 274 U.S. 268 (1927); Am. Banana Co. v. United Fruit Co., 213 U.S. 347 (1909), *overruled by* Kirkpatrick & Co. v. Envtl. Tectonics Corp., 493 U.S. 400 (1990); United States v. Aluminum Co. of Am., 148 F.2d 416 (2d Cir. 1945).

112. Generally, a defendant must have "certain minimum contacts within the territory of the forum such that maintenance of the suit does not offend 'traditional notions of fair play and substantial justice.'" Int'l Shoe Co. v. Washington, 326 U.S. 310, 316 (1945) (quoting Milliken v. Meyer, 311 U.S. 457, 463 (1940)). For a general discussion of international antitrust litigation, see J.S. Stanford, *The Application of the Sherman Act to Conduct Outside the United States: A View from Abroad,* 11 Cornell Int'l L.J. 195 (1978).

113. Indeed, USA Gymnastics must comply with and enforce all of the FIG's applicable rules in order to ensure the continued eligibility of American gymnasts in FIG-sanctioned international competitions, including the Olympic Games. *See supra* text accompanying note 34.

114. *See supra* notes 90–92, 96–99 and accompanying text.

115. Bd. of Trade v. United States, 246 U.S. 231, 238 (1918).

116. Brooke Group Ltd. v. Brown & Williamson Tobacco Corp., 509 U.S. 209, 224 (1993) (quoting Brown Shoe Co. v. United States, 370 U.S. 294, 320 (1962)) (emphasis omitted).

117. *See supra* note 50 and accompanying text. One commentator, citing examples from figure skating and gymnastics, proposed legislation to rein in perceived exploitation of elite teen and pre-teen athletes. Rachelle Propson, Note, *A Call for Statutory Regulation of Elite Child Athletes,* 41 Wayne L. Rev. 1773 (1995).

118. *Gymnastics Too Young? FIG Says the Rumor is False*, INT'L SPORTS PRESS ASS'N (Feb. 13, 2007), http://www.aipsmedia.com/index.php?page=news&cod=830&tp=n.

119. *See* Nw. Wholesale Stationers, Inc. v. Pac. Stationary & Printing Co., 472 U.S. 284, 290 (1985).

120. *See supra* note 100 and accompanying text.

121. *See* Gabriel A. Feldman, *The Misuse of the Less Restrictive Alternative Inquiry in Rule of Reason Analysis*, 58 AM. U. L. REV. 561, 595 (2009).

122. Rodenberg, *supra* note 88, at 190.

123. *Id.* at 191.

124. *Id.*

125. *Age Eligibility Rules in Women's Professional Golf: A Legal Eagle or an Antitrust Bogey?*, *supra* note 92, at 109.

126. *Id.*

127. Pells, *supra* note 1.

128. 130 S. Ct. 2201, 2216 (2010).

129. Rodenberg, *supra* note 88, at 204–205 (quoting Smith v. Pro Football, Inc., 593 F.2d 1173, 1183 (D.C. Cir. 1978)); Jennifer Paul, Comment, *Age Minimums in the Sport of Women's Artistic Gymnastics*, 7 WILLAMETTE SPORTS L.J. 73, 77–78 (2010) (showing evidence of the effects of the 1997 rule change).

130. Paul, *supra* note 129 (citing Van Anderson, *supra* note 51, at 25–27).

131. *See* Note, *The Government of Amateur Athletics: The NCAA–AAU Dispute*, 41 S. CAL. L. REV. 464, 465 (1968).

132. Pells, *supra* note 1.

133. Helliker & Fowler, *supra* note 59, at A11; *Two Years Suspension!*, *supra* note 62.

134. Jennifer Sey, *Why are Gymnasts So Young?*, SALON.COM (Aug. 8, 2008, 12:00 PM), http://www.salon.com/sports/olympics/2008/08/08/chinese_gymnasts.

135. JOAN RYAN, LITTLE GIRLS IN PRETTY BOXES: THE MAKING AND BREAKING OF ELITE GYMNASTS AND FIGURE SKATERS 8 (1995).

136. *Id.* at 66.

137. Jeré Longman & Juliet Macur, *Records Indicate Chinese Gymnasts May Be Under Age*, N.Y. TIMES, July 27, 2006, at SP 1.

138. Wetzel, *supra* note 6.

139. Indeed, while the intent of the passport is admirable and bent on increasing integrity, the passport system's protocol presents an obvious loophole that those with the propensity for age fraud will easily exploit. Past cases of age falsification in gymnastics have commonly involved retroactive document manipulation *after* an athlete reaches an elite level. *See* Helliker & Fowler, *supra* note 59, at A11; Longman & Macur, *supra* note 137, at SP 1. Under the new passport guidelines, however, such *ex post* conduct will be replaced with a prospective *ex ante* scheme where the documentation of the youngest gymnasts (e.g., seven-year-olds) with even a glimmer of talent will be altered *before* the athlete's first FIG-mandated passport is issued.

140. Neil Campbell, *Former Gymnastics Coach Furious over Potential Underage Competitors*, EPOCH TIMES (Aug. 10, 2008), http://www.theepochtimes.com/n2/content/view/2487/.

141. Kevin Manahan, *Bela Karolyi's Solution Would End Gymnastics Age Limit*, THE STAR-LEDGER (Aug. 7, 2008, 9:59 PM), http://www.nj.com/olympics/index.ssf/2008/08/bela_karolyis_solution_would_e.html.

142. *Id.*

143. *See supra* notes 49–51.

144. Marlen Garcia, *American Gymnast Memmel Still Roaring in Her 20s*, USA TODAY (July 16, 2008, 6:13 PM), http://www.usatoday.com/sports/olympics/beijing/gymnastics/2008-07-16-chellsiememmel_N.htm.

145. *USA Gymnastics Women's Program 2011 Elite/Pre-Elite Qualification Chart*, USA GYMNASTICS, http://usa-gymnastics.org/PDFs/Women/ElitePre-Elite/10elitechart.pdf (last updated April 22, 2011).

146. *See 2011 USA Gymnastics Women's Program—Elite Calendar*, USA GYMNASTICS, http://www.usa-gymnastics.org/PDFs/Women/calendar.pdf (last visited May 14, 2011) (showing that 2011 events are split between junior and senior events).

147. Helliker & Fowler, *supra* note 59, at A11.

148. Dr. Maureen Weiss, Professor of Sport Psychology, Curry Sch. of Educ., Univ. of Va., Remarks at the Ladies Professional Golf Association Professional Athlete Forum: Phenoms to Professionals: Successful Transitions (Dec. 7, 2005) (transcript available at http://www.lpga.com/content/NYForumSuccessfulTransitionsl20705.pdf).

4 Going Pro in Sports

Providing Guidance to Student-Athletes in a

Complicated Legal and Regulatory Environment

■ GLENN M. WONG, WARREN ZOLA, AND CHRIS DEUBERT

■ INTRODUCTION

In 2008 the National Collegiate Athletic Association (NCAA) launched a national advertising campaign entitled *"Going Pro in Something Other than Sports."* As a major strategic and branding initiative by the NCAA that was years in development, this effort seeks to emphasize the academic rather than athletic abilities of collegiate student-athletes.[1] Humor captivates the audience, yet it is the campaign's tagline that the NCAA has "more than 380,000 student-athletes and most of them will go pro in something other than sports" that resonates with the viewer.[2] This declaration is true, and the promotion's purpose is clearly aimed at calling attention to the core purpose of the NCAA, which is to "govern competition in a fair, safe, equitable and sportsmanlike manner, and to integrate intercollegiate athletics into higher education so that the educational experience of the student-athlete is paramount."[3]

The reason that the NCAA feels compelled to run this campaign is to combat the high profile, occasionally controversial, and sometimes even illegal nature of the entry of many college student-athletes into professional sports. When one considers the complexities of this process, coupled with the fact that student-athletes and their families are woefully unsophisticated and unprepared to navigate the process, the lack of assistance provided by colleges and universities to their student-athletes who are preparing to join the professional ranks is shocking.

This article will discuss the existing process for this transition, the problems therein, and the urgency with which these problems need to be addressed. We then explain why it is in the best interests of all parties concerned to improve the system and make recommendations for doing so.

■ I. NAVIGATING THE PROCESS 101

Despite the NCAA's campaign, the sheer volume of former college student-athletes playing professional athletics is still enormous. About two-thirds of the 2,050 individuals drafted by the four major domestic leagues in 2010 came directly from college.[4] This does not include the 515 high school seniors drafted by Major League Baseball (MLB) and the National Hockey League (NHL) who may decide to delay their entry into these leagues by attending college.[5] The number of high school students who are now faced with major decisions related to their potential entry into the professional ranks highlights the need for earlier engagement in providing counsel. Final career decisions are often made long before a student-athlete enrolls in college, demonstrating that the traditional model of working with seniors only after their eligibility has expired is dwindling. Receiving far less attention are the large number of former college student-athletes, in a multitude of sports, who progress toward less visible leagues and the individual opportunities in professional athletics around the globe.

Many of these student-athletes do not make optimal decisions about their future during this process for a variety of reasons, including poor and conflicting sources of information, the lure of professional money, and an inability to understand the many complex issues surrounding the amateur-to-professional transition. The results of these poor decisions can be dramatic and affect a long list of stakeholders. While this article will highlight the role many organizations and people play in this process, student-athletes are, and should still be, responsible for their actions.

Although fans are most familiar with the riches and fame of professional athletes, the reality is that achieving such a lofty status is the exception and not the rule. Far more student-athletes end up as hidden victims of this flawed transition process. The athlete may suffer permanent career and financial harm while his former school may incur penalties and suffer embarrassment for any misconduct that occurred while the athlete attended the school. Furthermore, the NCAA and/or the professional league with which the athlete is now involved may have to deal with a paying public critical of their operations and constituents.

The stakes involved in professional athletics are unmistakably high and most athletes will get limited chances to make good on that potential. A failure to properly capitalize on those opportunities works to the detriment of all interested parties. To properly understand the problem, it is important to understand the current process student-athletes go through to turn professional.

A. The Current Process

For most student-athletes the process by which they contemplated pursuing a professional career in sports began long before they actually could pursue such a career. Such aspirations most likely influenced the student-athlete's choice of which high school and college to attend, the student-athlete's leisure activities, and almost certainly the student-athlete's level of interest in academia. In Division I football, 59% of student-athletes reported that athletics were the primary reason for attending their college as opposed to 24% who said academics; in men's basketball and baseball the numbers rose to 68% and 79%, respectively.[6] Additionally, 72% of Division I male student-athletes not in football, baseball, or basketball reported viewing themselves as more of an athlete than a student.[7] Even 55% of Division III male student-athletes felt the same way, as did 64% of Division I female student-athletes.[8] However, at some point whether or not the student-athlete has professional potential will no longer be evidenced by the decisions the student-athlete and his family make, but instead by the attention the student-athlete receives.

The process reaches a new level of intensity when agents, scouts, coaches, or media members begin to inquire into the student-athlete's professional goals and plans. These questions are no longer presented to just young men and women but increasingly to teenagers and adolescents. It is common today for many elite student-athletes to have been followed, graded, and interviewed since they were adolescents.[9] Amateur Athletic Union (AAU) basketball camps and teams have become particularly swarmed with coaches, recruiters, agents, and others looking for the next great college or professional star that can help their own careers.

As the process of transitioning from student-athlete to professional begins, the student-athlete may be flooded with wanted and unwanted suggestions and guidance. This transition process involves a number of important decisions, actions, and/or omissions in the latter stages of the student-athlete's college career. As will be discussed in greater detail, an athlete's agent or advisor can and should help with many of these decisions. However, the focus in this article is on the earlier decisions where a university or other entities may be positioned to provide guidance.

Other than a school's Professional Sports Counseling Panel (PSCP), which will be discussed in greater detail in Part II, a wide variety of people can and do provide a student-athlete with guidance and advice on the transition from an amateur to a professional athletic career. Certainly family members serve as an important component of a student-athlete's decision making process, yet some less actively involved relatives may see the student-athlete's budding professionalism as a cash-grab opportunity for themselves. College coaches and athletic department officials can provide an important connection to the professional world; however, they too might have the school's interests ahead of those of the student-athlete.

The sources of information and influence are never ending. Ultimately, student-athletes with professional prospects must conduct themselves in an appropriate fashion and make informed and prudent decisions throughout the process. For the vast majority of student-athletes the transition process consists of properly maneuvering through NCAA legislation so as to retain eligibility, followed by choosing an agent. Unfortunately, understanding the professional landscape they are entering is often an afterthought to be hopefully handled by their agent.

1. Maneuvering through NCAA Legislation

In the summer of 2010, a bevy of potential scandals were uncovered that jeopardized the eligibility of college football players.[10] Before a student-athlete can become a professional, he or she must properly follow NCAA rules concerning his or her amateurism.[11] Failure to do so can result in the loss of the student-athlete's ability to display his or her skills and ultimately the cessation of a career before it begins.[12] The NCAA has long been hailed as the protector of amateurism.[13] Consequently, the NCAA Bylaws have very strict and specific rules to uphold that image. In fact, Article 12 of the NCAA Division I Manual is entitled "Amateurism."[14]

While the NCAA Bylaws do not define "amateur," they state there must be a "clear line of demarcation between college athletics and professional sports."[15] "A professional athlete is one who receives any kind of payment, directly or indirectly, for athletics participation except as permitted by the [NCAA]."[16] Even if a student-athlete was never paid for his or her athletic participation, they may still be penalized if they played on a "professional" team.[17] The NCAA has a broad definition of a professional team,[18] essentially including any situation where any other player on that team received money, food, housing, apparel, transportation, or any other benefit for their athletic participation.[19] This can often be an issue for foreign student-athletes.[20]

Once a student-athlete's amateurism is established, the more difficult part is retaining it. Aiding a player in this retention is among the chief duties of any athletic department's compliance office. Compliance offices vary widely in size based on the size of the institution and also the school's history of violations and current probation status. For example, Southern Eastern Conference (SEC) schools have an average of 5 employees in their compliance departments.[21] In contrast, the Southern Conference (SoCon) members who play both Division I football and basketball have an average of 1.4 employees.[22] In addition, most of these compliance officers spend their time checking the eligibility of athletes and monitoring practice limits, rather than dealing with agents or educating student-athletes on the transition process. For perspective, Alabama's Athletic Department lists over 150 employees, including nine in the Business Office, ten in Media Relations, fourteen in the Marketing department, and nine more in something called "TIDE PRIDE."[23] While schools might avoid providing relatively substantial funding for compliance departments because they are not revenue producers, a school's failure to properly do so can easily become a massive expense.

Clearly, compliance offices almost always lack the staff, resources, and preparedness to deal with those determined to bend the rules. As a result, more and more schools are turning to outside professionals to help with the process.[24] In general, compliance offices are not staffed by attorneys, but by young professionals interested in working in college athletics.[25]

NCAA Bylaws list several activities that would cause the loss of a student-athlete's amateurism, including using his or her skills for pay, accepting a promise of pay to be received after completion of intercollegiate athletics, signing a contract to play professional athletics, receiving any kind of financial assistance from a professional sports organization without NCAA permission, competing on any professional athletics team, entering into a professional draft, and entering into an agreement with an agent.[26] The definition of "pay" per NCAA Bylaws is also quite broad, encompassing all the extraneous benefits one might foresee a student-athlete receiving because of his or her athletic skill.[27]

These Bylaws may seem plain enough, but every year hundreds and possibly thousands of student-athletes violate them, with the vast majority going undetected. In the sports most likely to attract professional attention (football, basketball, and, to a lesser extent, hockey and baseball), many talented student-athletes are not in financially stable situations.[28] Despite the scholarships and other benefits offered by the member institution,[29] student-athletes in these sports regularly accept cash, gifts, and other benefits from supporters of the school's team ("boosters"), agents, financial advisors, marketing representatives, or other people trying to win their favor.

Most student-athletes dream of being drafted into the professional ranks. Each of the major American professional team sports leagues (National Football League [NFL], Major League Baseball [MLB], National Basketball Association [NBA], and National Hockey League [NHL]), collectively known as the "Big Four," have drafts through which student-athletes enter the professional ranks. As a result of legal challenges and collective bargaining agreements, the rules of each draft have evolved over time and vary considerably in the number of players drafted, age restrictions, number of times a player can be drafted, and other issues.[30] Consequently, the NCAA Bylaws attempt to accommodate these different structures. Many of these rules have caused problems for athletes, universities, and the leagues, as will be discussed in greater detail in Part III, "Problems with the Current Process." Exhibit 1 summarizes these different rules and the interplay of the NCAA Bylaws.

2. Choosing the Right Time to Turn Professional

For the best student-athletes, one of the most important decisions will be whether or not to leave school early and begin their professional career. For the lower-tier student-athletes, an important decision is often whether or not the athlete is

Exhibit 1. Professional Drafts and Applicable NCAA Rules

	NFL	MLB	NBA	NHL
Date	April	June	June	June
Length	7 Rounds[31]	50 Rounds[32]	2 Rounds[33]	7 Rounds[34]
Number of Players[35]	255	1,520	60	210
Minimum Age	3 years since High School[36]	17 years old[37]	19 years old[38]	18 years old[39]
Pre-Draft Workouts[40]	Permissible	Permissible	Permissible	Permissible
Status if Undrafted[41]	Can Return[42]	Can Return	Can Return[43]	Can Return
Number of Times a Player Can be Drafted	Twice[44]	Four[45]	Twice[46]	Twice[47]
Team Retention Rights if Player Returns to College	One year after the date of the draft in which a player would have been in the last season of eligibility[48]	August 16 of the year of the draft[49]	One year after the date of the draft in which a player absent his becoming an Early Entry Player, first would have been eligible to be selected[50]	Expire on August 15 following the athlete's college graduation[51]

willing to try to continue his or her career overseas. As we will discuss more in Part III, the answer to that question is more frequently "Yes."

Clearly the decision to leave school early for the professional ranks can be a risky one. Leaving college early certainly can be a wise choice, and on occasion, staying in school can be a mistake from the perspective of a professional sports career. For example, wide receiver Larry Fitzgerald left the University of Pittsburgh after his sophomore year,[52] was chosen as the third overall pick in the 2004 NFL Draft, and has gone on to a sensational career. On the other hand, University of Southern California quarterback Matt Leinart chose to stay for his senior year after winning the 2004 Heisman Trophy as a junior despite being the consensus #1 overall pick in the 2005 NFL Draft. After his senior season, Leinart was selected as the tenth overall pick in the 2006 NFL Draft, a decision that arguably cost Leinart $10 million or more.[53] Yet, there are often situations where players enter the draft early only to fall into the later rounds, whereas if they had remained in school, their draft stock may have substantially improved the following year.[54] Either way, student-athletes must carefully understand this choice, its ramifications, and ways to reduce their personal risks moving forward.

As part of the decision-making process student-athletes must seek out information on their professional prospects. In recent years, approximately fifty student-athletes per year have left school and declared for the NFL draft before the expiration of their college football eligibility.[55] However, NFL players who graduate from college have, on average, longer careers than those who chose to leave early.[56] Nevertheless, it is important to point out that many of the student-athletes who leave school early do not necessarily do so because they think they are ready for the NFL, but instead are forced to leave for academic reasons.[57]

Each professional league has unique features that they have developed to assist student-athletes in making the transition from college. However, the ability to navigate through the variances can be confusing, and a college or university needs someone well versed in the nuanced differences for each sport. Football student-athletes who will be eligible for the NFL Draft following the season have the advantage of the NFL Advisory Committee, created in 1994, to assist student-athletes evaluate their potential in an upcoming NFL Draft.[58]

The student-athlete or his athletic department on his behalf may request a formal evaluation from the NFL about his potential draft prospects without jeopardizing his eligibility.[59] The Committee is comprised of general managers, personnel directors, and scouts of NFL clubs.[60] The Committee provides underclassmen who request it a draft round range in which the player could be expected to be selected. The Committee's evaluation is non-binding and certainly cannot guarantee a specific round,[61] but it can provide underclassmen with a valuable estimate of where they stand in the draft. Although the NFL and the player are to keep the evaluation confidential, a player's projection from the Committee is often revealed by the media.[62]

Obviously, the Committee does not provide a projected draft status to seniors with expiring eligibility because they have no decision to make. In reality, a student-athlete receives his professional prospect status from a variety of sources: his own coaches who may know NFL personnel, NFL scouts that are contacting the player as part of their scouting evaluations, agents who are gathering that information from friendly NFL personnel, and media who may be relying on their own projections or information they have received from NFL personnel.[63] Ultimately, each source may have its own agenda, which may strain existing relationships such as those between a student-athlete and his college or coach. Although difficult to find, it is imperative that a student-athlete and his family obtain the maximum impartial guidance available.

The deadline for early entrants to declare for the NFL draft is January 15.[64] However, within seventy-two hours of this date, student-athletes may formally remove themselves from the draft and declare their intention to resume their college career, so long as they have broken no other regulations relative to retaining their amateur status.[65] Like the NFL, the NBA has an Undergraduate Advisory Committee of general managers, player personnel directors, and scouts who will provide a confidential projection of a potential draftee's projected draft position.[66]

Again, should a player choose not to enter the draft, in order to retain the right to restore their amateur status, the student-athlete must not have signed with an agent.[67] Signing with an agent, in any sport, is a binding step, permanently shifting an individual from amateur status into the ranks of professional sports.

Nevertheless, as will be discussed, agents can provide very valuable services to an athlete during his draft preparations.

A successful entrance into and through a professional sport's leagues draft is a complicated set of regulations from the league and the NCAA. It is here, at the nexus of the two regulatory organizations, that an institution should provide a level of expertise and guidance to help navigate through the confusion.

a. The NCAA Exceptional Student-Athlete Disability Insurance (ESDI) Program

To ease the concerns that student-athletes might have in returning to college when the professional ranks become available to them, the NCAA created the Exceptional Student-Athlete Disability Insurance (ESDI) program.[68] This program was created by the NCAA to allow student-athletes with a future in professional athletics to insure against debilitating injury during their college careers.[69] The program, offered for the first time by the NCAA in 1990 for football and men's basketball, has subsequently been expanded to include men's ice hockey, baseball, and women's basketball.[70]

Student-athletes who have demonstrated that they have the potential to be selected in the first three rounds of the NFL or NHL draft, or the first round of the NBA, MLB, or Women's National Basketball Association (WNBA) draft, are eligible for the program.[71] The policy provides the student-athlete with a lump-sum payment twelve months after it has been determined that he or she has suffered permanent total disability.[72] Student-athletes are eligible for loans to pay the premiums without jeopardizing their amateur status.[73]

The NCAA's ESDI program, administered through HCC Specialty Underwriters Company, caps coverage at $5 million for projected first-round NFL draft picks and men's basketball student-athletes.[74] Coverage for baseball, men's ice hockey, and women's basketball is capped at $1.5 million, $1.2 million, and $250,000, respectively.[75] The premiums cost between $10,000 and $12,000 for each $1 million of coverage, which is a few thousand dollars cheaper than a private policy.[76] It is reported that some 80 to 100 athletes participate in the ESDI program each year, and that approximately 75% to 80% of those athletes are college football players.[77]

In addition to the ESDI program, other creative options exist through private insurers, such as "Loss of Draft Position" policies.[78] These policies provide coverage to professional prospects that are not drafted as highly as expected, making up the loss of income associated with the drop in draft status.[79] The drop in status must be associated with a serious injury causing substantial and material deterioration in his or her ability to perform.[80]

3. Choosing Competent Representation

To many people inside and outside the world of sports, agents are a leading cause of problems relating to the transition for student-athletes into professional athletes.[81] While the misconduct of agents, and/or their "runners"[82] is far-reaching, frequent, well-documented, and often litigated,[83] agents are still a necessary component of this process, and attempts to minimize their involvement or ignore their existence only exacerbates the issues. Furthermore, the vast majority of agents do follow the rules and do have the best interests of their clients at heart. Rules and processes should be tailored to reward law-abiders and enforced effectively to deter law-breakers.

It should be noted from the outset that the NCAA and member institutions have no direct regulatory power over agents. Instead agents are regulated by the players association of the particular sport in which they represent athletes.[84] In addition, there are both state and federal laws that regulate the conduct of agents,[85] though the laws are rarely enforced.[86] Furthermore, it is no longer just traditional agents that are actively recruiting players—financial advisors and marketing representatives also swarm student-athletes in hopes of providing them their services.[87]

While some may argue that there is no need for an agent until after an athlete has been drafted and negotiations with a particular team begin,[88] this position is uncommon and erroneous. Having an advisor experienced in easing the transition from the final college game to the first professional game is vital to the long-term success of any would-be professional athlete. Once a relationship is formed, a quality agent can provide valuable advice, guidance, and oversight to a professional athlete, significantly enhancing the athlete's chances of finding success in his or her career, finances, health, family, and education.

It is routine for players preparing for the NFL Draft to refer to the NFL's annual scouting combine process as "the biggest job interview of their lives."[89] In preparation for the combine and the subsequent workouts, industry competition has dictated agents must pay $10,000–$20,000 in training expenses for each player, including many who go undrafted.[90] In addition, agents are able to provide valuable information to players on what NFL teams are looking for and how the player needs to improve through their own league contacts.

When a student-athlete has eligibility remaining and is considering turning professional, they need to be exceptionally careful about their involvement with an agent.[91] As explained earlier, the NCAA has strict rules concerning the use of agents. The situation is particularly complicated in baseball and hockey, where players are often drafted out of high school but choose to attend college instead.[92] Some of these issues are discussed in greater detail in Part II.

There is both an art and a science in selecting an appropriate agent, and this is undoubtedly an area in which a modicum of education and understanding can greatly aid an individual in making a sound decision. An advisor's role is to provide guidance and resources so that student-athletes and their families interested in becoming educated about agents may do so.

There are all types of agents and it can often be a daunting task for a student-athlete and their family to sort through the pile of individuals seeking to serve as their official representative. Typically, the first step in the decision process is to understand the services that agents provide and how they are compensated.[93] Each student-athlete has unique and specific needs as they enter the professional ranks and it is important to understand how an agent's particular attributes or skills can aid those specific needs.

Beyond the compensation and negotiation of an employment contract, many agents also offer services in a spectrum of areas: marketing and endorsement deals, financial planning, community service or charitable endeavors, tax advice, media relations, legal matters, and estate planning. Finding the right level of service and support is an important determining factor in selecting the appropriate agent for an individual. Ultimately, most of the agents a student will consider are competent and trustworthy. What the student-athlete's decision most often comes down to is personality and comfort with the agent.

The rise in both salaries[94] and the visibility of professional athletes[95] has created an environment in which sound counsel is necessary to navigate a player through the opportunities available. Given the fact that a player's agent typically receives a percentage of their client's compensation,[96] competition is fierce among agents for player representation.[97] What results is an environment of competition by agents for uneducated (for these purposes) and typically naive consumers. Ultimately, as a result of this mayhem, schools are often left with NCAA violations as a result of improprieties while student-athletes, or their representatives, often find themselves making poor decisions in difficult situations.

An individual's perceived value in the upcoming draft obviously dictates the sheer volume of interest they will receive from agents. A potential first-round pick may have several dozen agents and/or firms trying to get an interview. Individuals who will potentially be drafted in the middle rounds of the NFL draft will also receive dozens of inquiries. Someone who may be on the bubble of being drafted or who falls under the "priority free agent" category may have only a few people contacting them. Finally, some student-athletes may actually need to convince an agent to represent them.

The actual process of whittling down a few agents to interview can be a daunting task but one that is necessary. When faced with dozens of agent requests and brochures that have been sent to a family or a student-athlete, typically a family will ultimately choose a few finalists (half a dozen or so) and then, when the time is right, conduct formal interviews so that the student-athlete is able to find an agent or firm to his liking. Student-athletes have the ability to, and should, negotiate with agents about their services and costs.[98]

The timing of this formal process is unique to each institution. Typically each college football program will determine a period, before, during, or after the season, in which it allows its student-athletes the ability to conduct interviews. Some schools will formally host "agent days" while others see no merit in this initiative. In addition, there is an increasing trend of schools hiring outside consultants to help them and their student-athletes with the process.[99] Nevertheless, it is not uncommon for student-athletes to ignore the rules of their school[100] and talk and meet with agents throughout the season as permitted by NCAA Bylaws.

The NCAA may be (or should be) a good resource in dealing with this selection process. In addition to NCAA rules and regulations, again primarily on the topic of eligibility, there are several helpful documents that the NCAA has developed.[101] The NCAA allows for contact between student-athletes and agents at all times,[102] and there is nothing in the rules that prohibit direct discussions at any point during a student-athlete's career. However, there is one strong restriction: no agreement, or even a promise to agree in the future, may be reached with an agent while a student-athlete is still in college.[103]

Ultimately, as Bob Ruxin correctly points out at the end of his book, *An Athlete's Guide to Agents,*[104] the onus falls upon the client for selecting the appropriate representation. This decision, while difficult and filled with potential pitfalls, is the responsibility of the student-athlete. It is their duty to use the resources available to them in order to determine their unique needs and which potential agent is the best match for them.

■ II. PROBLEMS WITH THE CURRENT PROCESS

There is an overall lack of guidance, counsel, and expertise in the transition process. With few people willing to help in the absence of a personal agenda, each year the process victimizes new crops of potential professional athletes. Over the years the amateur-to-professional transition process has only become more complex as the financial stakes have risen. To combat this problem, in 1984 the NCAA adopted legislation permitting member institutions to establish Professional Sports Counseling Panels (PSCPs).[105] This legislation "was intended to encourage member institutions to provide guidance to their student-athletes regarding future professional athletics careers."[106]

In sum, a PSCP consists of at least three panel members, the majority of which are full-time employees outside of the institution's athletic department.[107] No more than one panel member may be an athletics department staff member and no sports agent or person employed by a sports agent or agency may be a member of the panel.[108] The PSCP is permitted to:

Advise a student-athlete about a future professional career;
Provide direction on securing a loan for the purpose of purchasing insurance against a disabling injury;
Review a professional sports contract;
Meet with the student-athlete and representatives of professional teams;

Communicate directly (e.g., in-person, by mail or telephone) with representatives of a professional athletics team to assist in securing a tryout with that team for a student-athlete;

Assist the student-athlete in the selection of an agent by participating with the student-athlete in interviews of agents, by reviewing written information player agents send to the student-athlete and by having direct communication with those individuals who can comment about the abilities of an agent (e.g., other agents, a professional league's players' association); and

Visit with player agents or representatives of professional athletics teams to assist the student-athlete in determining his or her market value (e.g., potential salary, draft status).[109]

However, many universities fail to use or properly use PSCPs, thus failing to provide the appropriate level of support in this venue.[110] As a result, student-athletes often make unwise decisions at very important junctures in their lives that can have lasting and irreversible impacts, ranging from pecuniary harm to losing their professional athletic dreams altogether. The major professional sports leagues invest a significant amount of time, money, and effort into its new players.[111] However, these leagues may find their investments to be significantly frustrated by the multitude of issues confronting athletes before they even have the chance to become professional. Finally, NCAA member-institutions can suffer the "black eye" of bad publicity or the NCAA's enforcement procedures and sanctions for its or a student-athlete's faults during this transitional process.[112]

In recent years there have been several high-profile cases that highlight the problems in the transition process. Maurice Clarett, the star freshman running back on the 2002 Ohio State University National Championship football team, violated NCAA rules, was suspended for a year as a result, and decided to challenge the NFL's draft eligibility rules in court as a violation of antitrust laws. Clarett eventually lost his case, his football career, and his freedom.[113] Mike Williams, a standout sophomore receiver at University of Southern California, decided to follow Clarett's lead after Clarett was initially granted eligibility, only to see that decision reversed, forcing Williams (who had signed with an agent) to sit out a year before beginning a disappointing NFL career.[114] Similarly, Randolph Morris, a promising basketball talent at University of Kentucky, chose to leave school after his freshman year and enter the NBA draft, only to go undrafted. Unfortunately. Morris had signed with an agent and only after the NCAA found that Morris had a "clear intent to retain his college eligibility while declaring for the NBA draft," did a full-season suspension get reduced to the first fourteen games of the 2005–06 basketball season.[115] Lastly, in one recent case that has drawn a lot of attention, Andrew Oliver, a promising baseball student-athlete at Oklahoma State University had his eligibility suspended in May 2008, only to have it eventually restored by court order.[116] Oliver was suspended after it was revealed he had agents talk with the Minnesota Twins when he was drafted out of high school in 2006.[117] This case will be discussed in more detail later in the article.

The Morris situation highlights some of the difficulties in the professional basketball transition process. Beginning with the 2006 NBA draft, to be eligible, a player must be at least nineteen years old.[118] As a result, many high school players who would have gone straight to the NBA (as thirty-five did between 1995 and 2005)[119] now must attend at least one year of college or otherwise attempt to avoid the rule.[120] In reality, basketball student-athletes who know they are going to leave after just one season of college basketball ("one-and-done") can take the minimum number of classes in their first semester, barely go to class as the college basketball season winds down in their second semester, declare for the draft, and drop out of school having completed only four or five general education classes. In the five years since the implementation of the minimum age rule, there have been thirty-six "one-and-done" players, including three #1 overall picks.[121]

For the purposes of this article, at issue are not the legal ramifications, or even who is at fault in these cases, but rather an example of the level of support many student-athletes require, even before they may reach campus, in navigating their way from amateur to professional athletics. Much has been written regarding the distinction between an advisor and an agent—the former permissible, and the latter not, under the NCAA's rules.[122] As is its prerogative as a private and voluntary sports association,[123] the NCAA has defined the parameters of what it means to be an amateur in intercollegiate athletics, even though many regard the distinctions within those parameters to be farcical.[124] The challenge, as born out for Oliver and countless others on an annual basis, is that often they and/or their families are unprepared for making a seamless transition from amateur to professional. Regardless of the outcome of this particular situation, a high school senior who should be concentrating on getting ready for their prom is all too often engaged in decisions that could be made far easier with proper guidance and support.

A. Hidden Victims

When one asks "why have these problems persisted?" the answer becomes clear: there is no advocacy group for reform. The student-athletes and professional athletes are the ones that ultimately suffer the most personal and permanent harm, yet they are the least educated about the process and are in a poor position to understand the need for change when it matters most. To some extent, there is a sense that there is no true need for better guidance such as PSCPs. Either someone is talented enough to "make it" or they are not. If they are good enough, then his or her representative can help them transition to the professional league; if they do not have the talent, there is no need.

In addition, many colleges and universities stay willfully ignorant of the problems. Among the NCAA violations possible in these situations are a failure to monitor and a lack of institutional control. By not confronting and seeking out these problems, a member institution can attempt to avoid sanctions that might come had its personnel had actual knowledge and were complicit in the violations.

Often alumni who have been fortunate enough to succeed in professional athletics for a significant amount of time state how poorly they feel they were prepared for, or understood the complexities of, the business aspect of the professional sports industry. While no one could be expected to fully understand the business of the league in which they are entering, higher education, sports leagues, and unions have an obligation to provide more education and resources than they presently do.

If a school does have a PSCP, some may question the school's incentive in helping the player, having already received the bulk of their benefit from the relationship. There is also the perception that perhaps some student athletes, if encouraged, may leave school earlier than they would otherwise, thus losing years of eligibility at their institution. As a result, coaches and athletic administrators often view PSCPs as a threat rather than an opportunity to provide the student-athlete with valuable information and guidance. Why give access to their student-athletes to individuals who may help them decide to leave college early? There must be a balanced approach that recognizes in fact sometimes it *is* in the student-athlete's interests to leave school early.

The group who might benefit the most from PSCPs, student-athletes and their families, are by and large naive about this allowance by the NCAA. Certainly they have neither the ability nor the leverage to generate any pressure for a school to develop a PSCP. High school players would certainly benefit from advice (as will be shown in the *Oliver* case), but have no voice in this process. Athletic departments and coaching staffs often do not worry about a student-athlete's future in professional sports other than making the individual more proficient at their sport while in college.[125] Schools certainly are pleased when their student-athletes succeed in professional athletics yet they do very little to educate them about either entering the industry or understanding its business operations.

College student-athletes have the potential benefit of coaches, a PSCP, athletic administrative staff, and others. High school student-athletes are also an important and substantial population of potential professional athletes. Yet, colleges, professional leagues, and others do nearly nothing to provide them with the advice they need, and in fact, at times, work against allowing the student-athlete the assistance he or she may need, as is evidenced in the *Oliver* case.

B. Results of the Problems

Thus far this article has alluded to many of the problems resulting from a poor amateur-to-professional transition process. However, to properly understand the scope of the problem it is important to examine the negative effects on the diverse group of stakeholders in the situation, including the student-athlete and his or her family, the colleges and universities, the NCAA, the professional leagues and players associations, and even agents and financial advisors.

1. Student-Athletes and Their Families

As previously highlighted throughout the article, student-athletes and their families are often the interested parties that are the least sophisticated and the least understanding of the process and its potential ramifications. Yet the results of a failing transition process most directly, harshly, and permanently affects them. Ultimately if the transition process is deficient and it has a negative effect on the athlete's career it will impact the rest of his or her life.

Apart from the potential fame, glory and, hopefully, fun associated with being a professional athlete, there are obvious real world financial implications. There are dramatic salary ranges in professional sports and even though most are guaranteed at least a six-figure salary by playing professionally in America, that salary might last but a few years.[126] Studies have shown that between 60% to 78% of NBA and NFL players are in severe financial distress when surveyed within two to five years of retirement.[127] Proper handling of that income could help sustain the player and his family for the rest of their lives, but that is not often the case.

Failure to take the process seriously has resulted in many athletes being taken advantage of by unscrupulous agents and/or financial advisors.[128] Countless athletes have managed to burn through millions of dollars in poor investments, entourages, gambling, and other unnecessary expenditures.[129]

Financial mismanagement is compounded dramatically when the athlete has failed to earn his or her college degree. The National Football League Players Association (NFLPA) has repeatedly reported that players who have college degrees often have longer and hence more financially productive careers.[130] However, only about half of NFL players have their degree.[131] To encourage college programs to take their student-athletes' educations more seriously, beginning in 2005 the NCAA began tracking the academic progress and graduation success of student-athletes at member institutions.[132] Schools that fail to make sufficient progress are subject to sanctions ranging from a public warning for the first year of poor performance to restricted membership status for four consecutive years of poor performance.[133]

According to the NCAA's 2010 Report, of all student-athletes that entered college as freshmen in 2002, 79% earned a four-year degree.[134] While this number is higher than the 64% of the general student body that earns their degree in the same amount of time,[135] many people continue to point out that the graduation rates of Division I football (55%) and men's basketball (48%) student-athletes are much lower.[136]

Not surprisingly, lower rates of graduation combined with the possible lifestyle of the rich and famous has led to increased crime rates among professional athletes.[137] All of this data indicates the importance of taking the transition process seriously and understanding how the decisions therein can have a significant effect on an athlete's life.

a. *Oliver v. NCAA*

In June 2006 Andrew Oliver, a high school pitcher, was drafted by the Minnesota Twins in the seventeenth round of the MLB draft.[138] The summer following his senior year of high school, Oliver had to decide whether to enroll at Oklahoma State University (OSU) or turn professional and sign with the Twins. In compliance with NCAA Bylaw 12.3.2,[139] Oliver's family hired Robert and Tim Baratta, Major League Baseball Players Association (MLBPA) certified player agents and attorneys, as his advisors and legal counsel in February 2006.[140] Such a hiring is an extremely common practice for elite high school baseball players.

Oliver ultimately chose OSU over the Twins and after two outstanding years at OSU, Oliver notified the Baratta brothers of his intention to part ways with them and instead retained Scott Boras as his advisor.[141] The Barattas then sent Oliver a non-itemized bill for $113,750 for their services and reported possible NCAA violations to the NCAA.[142] After an investigation, the NCAA determined that the Barattas were actively involved in negotiations with the Twins on Oliver's behalf, in violation of NCAA Bylaw 12.3.2.1.[143] In fact, the Barattas talked on the phone with the Twins and were present in the Oliver home when a representative from the Minnesota Twins tendered an offer to Oliver.[144]

In May 2008 the NCAA indefinitely suspended Oliver.[145] Oliver and his family filed suit against both the Barattas and the NCAA, seeking an injunction against his suspension and permanent loss of eligibility.[146] The suit was filed in Ohio state court, where Oliver attended high school and the alleged wrongdoing by Oliver and the agents occurred. Oliver made two main claims in his lawsuit: (1) that the NCAA has no authority to promulgate a rule that would prevent a lawyer from competently representing his client and therefore violate Ohio public policy;[147] and (2) that NCAA Bylaw 12.3.2.1 is arbitrary and capricious because it does not impact a player's amateur status; rather, it limits the player's ability to effectively negotiate a contract that the player or a player's parent could negotiate.[148]

The NCAA countered: (1) that it has the right to manage its affairs and apply its bylaws, within legal limits, without interference from the judiciary, and since Oliver failed to prove that its bylaws are illegal, arbitrary, or fraudulent, the NCAA's internal affairs are presumptively correct;[149] (2) that Oliver failed to prove by clear and convincing evidence that the made by the NCAA Bylaw 12.3.2.1 was arbitrary or capricious; and (3) there was no contractual relationship between it and Oliver upon which declaratory relief could be granted.[150]

The Ohio state court granted Oliver a temporary restraining order in August 2008.[151] Unfortunately, Oliver was forced to miss OSU's chance at a Big XII Championship and participation in the NCAA College World Series.[152] In February 2009, the court granted Oliver a permanent injunction.[153] In finding that the NCAA Bylaws violated the NCAA's contractual obligation of good faith, the court emphasized that Bylaw 12.3.2.1 restricted an attorney's ability to represent a client—an action beyond the scope of NCAA power.[154] Additionally, the court found that NCAA Bylaw 19.7 "fosters a direct attack on the constitutional right of access to courts" and was consequently arbitrary and capricious.[155] This rule permits the NCAA to take punitive actions against a member institution and/or student-athlete where a student-athlete participates in an intercollegiate competition by court order and against NCAA legislation or decision.[156]

The NCAA appealed the decision and in October 2009 the parties settled, with Oliver receiving $750,000 and retaining his eligibility, while the court decision was vacated, leaving the NCAA Bylaw in question in effect.[157] The injunction permitted Oliver to play the 2009 season, which though not outstanding (5–6 record with a 5.30 ERA) helped him be drafted in the second round of the 2009 MLB Draft by the Detroit Tigers. Perhaps for obvious reasons, this time Oliver chose to sign.[158]

2. Colleges and Universities

As mentioned above, schools that do not properly advise student-athletes on the importance of an education are at risk of NCAA penalties.[159] Schools that allow or fail to prevent their athletes from dabbling impermissibly in the professional process face NCAA sanctions, ranging from the loss of a few scholarships to postseason bans, or even the dreaded "death penalty," which prohibits a team from playing at all for a year or more.[160] It is also important to point out that Conferences are an equally involved bridge between schools and the NCAA. This article discusses the problems at the institutional and NCAA level and suggests better practices—Conferences are likewise prominent in these discussions.

One of the more recent scandals involved former USC running back Reggie Bush. While at USC, "Bush, his mother and his stepfather agreed to form a sports agency with two additional partners. After the agency was formed, Bush and members of his family asked for financial and other assistance from the partners, including living rent-free in a San Diego home."[161] As a result of the violations, the USC football team was forced to vacate all wins from December 2004 through December 2005 (including the 2005 BCS National Championship), lose thirty scholarships over three years and are banned from postseason competition for two years.[162] It is debatable whether these sanctions have served as a sufficient deterrent since the number of institutions facing discipline has not changed substantially over time.[163]

In addition to providing for recovery from unscrupulous agents, thirty-four states have laws that provide a cause of action for schools against the student-athlete involved.[164] However, schools are unlikely to take advantage of this statutory option due to the fear that it would significantly hamper recruiting efforts (no student-athlete wants to go to a school that might end up suing him or her), and it could bring to light the school's own failures and improprieties.[165]

Colleges and universities undoubtedly experience surges in goodwill, applications, and donations when their athletic teams are achieving success. Yet all of those tangible and intangible assets can quickly be diminished by scandals involving the school's student-athletes. The incentives for a school to actively aid its student-athletes through the amateur-to-professional transition will be discussed in more detail in Part V.

3. The NCAA

As a result of the repeated scandals involving NCAA student-athletes, the NCAA is consistently bombarded with criticism over its established role as the guardian of amateurism.[166] NCAA revenues continue to increase, reaching $710 million in the 2009–2010 academic year, with 90% of that revenue derived from television rights fees.[167] College athletics is undeniably big business, leaving many to speculate over whether the NCAA continues to deserve its tax-exempt status,[168] whether its actions constitute violations of antitrust law,[169] and whether it treats student-athletes fairly in light of the revenues being brought in.[170]

To combat these allegations the NCAA has implemented the academic reform studies discussed earlier, and is attempting to be very transparent in explaining how NCAA revenues are being spent on educational endeavors.[171] The NCAA emphasizes a "clear line of demarcation"[172] between amateur athletics and professional sports, however a sloppy transition process only blurs the demarcation and makes the NCAA's job that much more difficult.

4. Professional Sports Leagues and Players' Associations

As a result of the poor transition process, many young athletes enter professional leagues improperly prepared for their new career. The jobs of many team, league, and union employees would be made far easier if the players entering the league were more mature, informed, and prepared for their new career. Team personnel are routinely hired and fired based on their ability to determine an athlete's potential and an increasingly important part of that evaluation is the athlete's character, mental makeup, and ability to handle the stress of professional athletics.[173]

Just as the images of the NCAA and member institutions can be tarnished by scandal, so too can those of the professional leagues and unions. Ultimately, a negative image of a league and its players leads to a less marketable product and less revenue. As a result of player conduct problems in recent years, the "Big Four" leagues have increased penalties and oversight of player conduct, most notably the NFL.[174]

Pursuant to federal labor law, these types of discipline policies must be collectively bargained with the unions.[175] Since unions have had to fight with leagues over player-conduct policies, the unions have effectively wasted one of the bullets they could have used on another issue during the collective bargaining negotiations. Furthermore, in times of labor strife, there is an important public perception battle between a league and its union.[176] The more unsavory the union's members appear or have acted, the more difficult it has been to gain public support for their side.

Although these personal-conduct policies typically only concern conduct that occurs after a player has entered the league, many professional stars have scandalous stories break from their college days long after they have left campus, such as New Orleans Saints running back Reggie Bush[177] and Chicago Bulls guard Derrick Rose.[178] If a league grows sufficiently tired of its potential players entering their league in an improper and scandalous fashion, it could collectively bargain for the right to punish those players as well. Courts have held that a union can agree to provisions that affect persons who are not yet members of the union.[179]

The unions expend tremendous resources regulating the conduct of agents, including arbitrating any disputes among agents, as well as between agents and players.[180] If athletes had better guidance, it is more likely they would be able to find and form healthy agent relationships. Also, if the process were better handled, less desirable agents would be obtaining fewer clients, resulting in less regulation violations and disputes.

Ultimately, the policies and actions of the players unions are dictated by the union members—namely, the athletes. Unfortunately, many professional athletes do not care about strictly enforcing agent misconduct or helping prevent NCAA violations. For starters, many of the players themselves might have taken cash or other benefits from agents or boosters at one time or another during their career, and they might not want to expose activities that could implicate themselves. Secondly, many professional athletes are disgruntled about the lack of guidance they received during their college career and/or the way they may have been treated by the NCAA. Consequently, convincing unions to be proactive in helping to solve these issues is very important.

5. Professional Advisors

Agents, financial advisors, marketing and insurance representatives, and other advisors who earn a living off of professional athletes are the easiest targets for those who recognize a problem with the amateur-to-professional transition. We emphasize that this category is no longer limited to the traditional definition of an agent, but instead student-athletes and athletes receive advice, guidance, and support from professionals in a wide range of industries. As a result of this proliferation, forty states have passed a form of the Uniform Athlete Agent Act (UAAA),[181] and the federal government passed the Sports Agent Responsibility and Trust Act (SPARTA) in 2004.[182] Both laws are meant to regulate the conduct of agents by broadly defining "agent,"[183] listing prohibited conduct[184] and providing for civil remedies and penalties.[185]

Diligent enforcement of these laws could potentially alleviate many of the concerns addressed in this article. However, the general perception is that there has been little to no enforcement of the state laws, and the Federal Trade Commission (FTC), the governing body in charge of enforcing SPARTA, has never brought an action based on the law.[186]

As a result, the athlete representation industry has more undesirable members than it should. In turn, the industry is more competitive and the cycle repeats. Consequently, agent frustration, litigation, and insurance premiums are all higher than necessary.

■ III. THE URGENCY OF THE PROBLEM

With 119 teams competing in the Football Bowl Subdivision and each allowed to offer 85 scholarships, each year there are as many as 10,115 student-athletes hoping to earn a living playing professional football. While the percentages are remarkably low, when you speak to a room full of freshmen on any Bowl Championship Series (BCS) conference football team,[187] and ask how many of them have aspirations of playing in the NFL, it is apparent that most believe they have a realistic chance to play on Sundays. In fact, studies have determined that 44% of African-American college student-athletes expect to play professionally, yet only 2% actually do.[188]

Not surprisingly, many student-athletes have an inflated sense of their own abilities and often fail to grasp just how difficult it is to make a living as a professional athlete.[189] Each year the "Big Four" leagues turn over only a small percentage of their rosters to rookies. Additionally, making the roster once is far from the establishment of a career, which in the "Big Four" leagues only runs an average of 3.3 to 5.6 years.[190] Nevertheless, outside of the "Big Four," professional opportunities continue to grow and as a result more and more student-athletes are becoming professional athletes.

The financial mismanagement by young professional athletes is well documented.[191] While this issue is generally left to the responsibility of the athlete's agent and financial advisor, colleges have the opportunity to provide student-athletes with a more realistic sense of their future earnings. Although dozens of student-athletes might be drafted high enough each year such that their first contract is able to provide them with a lifetime of income, the majority will not be.

Many professional athletes toil through the minor leagues, practice squads, or developmental leagues making $10,000 to $85,000 a year.[192] Even the average rookie with an average career would be lucky to clear a few hundred thousand dollars after taxes and expenses throughout his career. This is certainly not a sum enabling the athlete never to have to work again—all the more reason why the student-athlete should take his education seriously.

While many student-athletes were sought-after recruits with the ability to go to the school of their choice, they will have very little control over the location of their professional team. Furthermore, student-athletes need to be cognizant of the very real possibility of having to leave the country if they wish to make a living playing sports.

Not surprisingly, increased exposure and revenue has generated a global market for professional sports. It is becoming more common for American athletes to head overseas to compete in professional leagues, many of whom are able to offer competitive salaries compared to American leagues, particularly in hockey and basketball.[193] Just in the major four sports, new leagues are sprouting up virtually every year. At last count there are about thirteen different countries offering professional opportunities in baseball,[194] over thirty countries with professional basketball leagues,[195] and at least sixteen countries with professional ice hockey.[196] With the folding of NFL Europe in 2007, an American football player's only viable international option is the Canadian Football League (CFL).

For players who aspire to play in the NBA, they often have to choose between making between $12,000 and $24,000 per year in the NBA Developmental League (NBDL)[197] or $500,000 per year playing in Europe.[198] In addition, the Russian Continental Hockey League (KHL) has successfully persuaded several former NHL players, including Jaromir Jagr, to join their league.[199]

In basketball, if one is unable to secure a spot in the NBA, dozens of leagues around the globe exist offering professional opportunities. While the student-athletes' pursuit of international opportunities in men's basketball often occurs outside of the public eye, it should be noted that the volume of this transition dwarfs the number of former college players heading to the NBA. Amazingly, in the past five years, it is reported that 6,717 U.S. college alumni have played in professional men's basketball overseas.[200] As an example of this international growth, since 2000 former University of Massachusetts men's basketball team members have elected to play professionally in twenty-three different countries—a fact offered less for the prestige of this particular program, but more so to illustrate the broad spectrum of opportunities.[201]

Former college student-athletes are finding professional employment in athletics in a myriad of sports beyond baseball, men's basketball, football, and ice hockey. Around the globe there are professional athletes competing in just about every sport imaginable, including men's and women's soccer, track and field, women's basketball, field hockey, volleyball, softball, and lacrosse. And, as a statement of the times, no longer does the United States offer the highest level of competition or compensation in a variety of sports, including hockey, men's and women's soccer, track and field, and men's and women's basketball.

Perhaps the fastest growing class of professional athletes is women. As more and more countries outside of the United States embrace equality and female participation in athletics, so too do they embrace women's professional sports. Although women's sports leagues in the United States have had mixed success,[202] there are likely to be continued opportunities for women to play professionally here and abroad. In recent years, some of the biggest stars of the WNBA, including Diana Taurasi, Sue Bird, and Lauren Jackson, have spent their offseasons playing professionally in Russia, where they earn as much as $500,000, almost ten times their WNBA salaries.[203]

As part of its "stay in school" campaign, the NCAA has attempted to quantify the long odds against college student-athletes making it to the professional level in the sports of men's and women's basketball, football, baseball, men's ice hockey, and men's soccer.[204] The results clearly bolster the argument that the chances of success are small. According to the NCAA, in men's and women's basketball, football, and men's soccer, 2% or less of all college student-athletes will move on to play professionally.[205] The odds increase slightly for men's ice hockey to 4.1%, but this is due, in part, to the fact that there are less than 4,000 student-athletes competing in this sport.[206] Finally, while the odds of college baseball players signing a professional contract appear quite high at 10.5%, the percentage of those individuals that advance all the way through the minor leagues to the major leagues is again small.[207] It is important to point out that these NCAA estimates are grossly underestimated and probably only reflect the number of student-athletes playing professionally in the United States.[208]

However, as educators and realists we must not ignore the significant number of college student-athletes who chase their dreams of making the transition from college to the professional ranks of athletics. And, while the percentage of the participants succeeding may be low, the bottom line is that thousands of college student-athletes transition to professional sports annually.[209] In noting this fact, we must ask ourselves whether colleges and universities are preparing these student-athletes for this transition in an appropriate manner. It is our contention that colleges, universities, and the NCAA can and should do a better job of preparing student-athletes for this transition.

■ IV. REASONS FOR CHANGE

As we have detailed, there are many problems with the current process of transitioning from amateur athletics to professional sports. Perhaps more than ever before these problems are known to the public, and it has become clear that these scandals are not an occasional blip in the process, but are instead part of a systemic failure to provide meaningful guidance and support to student-athletes interested in turning professional. Furthermore, the problems persist because student-athletes are the group of people most affected by these problems, as well as the group most unaware of them and with the least amount of say in changing the process. Although solving the problem involves multiple steps and parties, there are reasons for each of the important parties involved to want to change the system.

A. Student-Athletes and Their Families

The benefits to the student-athletes and their families are the most obvious; an improved process should increase a student-athlete's chances of having a successful professional career. Many areas of information could be made more easily available and more readily explained to student-athletes and their families, including whether to remain in school, leave school, agent selection, insurance options, financial education, or dealing with the professional leagues.

B. Colleges and Universities

Among any university's basic tenets is to provide life skills for its students. Just as career services provide guidance to undergraduate students, so too should universities provide guidance to a small but incredibly visible group of students. Without a PSCP there is a void at the institutional level of an unbiased sounding board to serve as a resource for student-athletes in this process. Whether or not there is a PSCP, student-athletes will seek advice from a variety of different sources including their coaches, other athletic department staff, or personal contacts, as they ponder the decision to turn professional. While many coaches or staff administrators may be able to stay impartial while advising a student-athlete about returning to school to compete for another season, others undoubtedly suggest what is best for themselves or the institution rather than the student-athlete.

The NCAA has made it quite clear that it is "the responsibility of each member institution to control its intercollegiate athletics program in compliance with the rules and regulations of the [NCAA]."[210] Does it make sense to allow individuals who at least *may* have conflicting goals with that of the student-athlete to serve as the institution's advisor on this decision? Again, the goal of a PSCP is not to preserve eligibility and keep student-athletes in school to earn their degree—although that is often the default position—but rather to provide unbiased feedback from experts with whom they have consulted to arm a student-athlete with objective advice.

From an institutional perspective, another reason to create and use a PSCP is that alumni who succeed in professional athletics are virtually always major assets to the school's community. The earning potential and visibility of a professional athlete is enormous. From the vantage point of both advancement and public relations, schools can benefit significantly when one of their former student-athletes gains success as a professional athlete. One of the best ways in which a university may provide value to a future professional athlete is helping them enter their profession at the appropriate time to maximize their potential, both on and off the field.

Alumni relations are the lifeblood of colleges and universities across the country. When one considers the investment each institution makes in alumni and advancement efforts, it appears foolhardy to neglect such a visible and important constituency—potential professional athletes—at so many schools. Certainly, professional athletes are often listed among a college's most prominent and successful alumni. What other cohort can so easily be identified with one's alma mater and provide a tremendous benefit at such a low cost? Also, if a professional athlete does not have fond memories of his university and how it may or may not have helped him or her turn professional, that athlete is certainly less likely to recommend the school to a high school star amidst the increasingly competitive recruiting process.

A final area in which PSCPs can help a university may be crude, but remains a fact nonetheless; there is no doubt an argument could be made to create a PSCP merely because of the good will it creates for future advancement and fund-raising efforts. Again, what constituency leaving any university has greater potential for earning large income over time? As such, the potential beneficial impact that these individuals as alumni can have on an institution cannot go unnoticed. With minimal effort there is the opportunity to enhance the chances that these individuals feel that their alma mater served their interests well during their tenure in general, and in the most confusing of times in particular.

Deciding whether or not to leave school early is an incredibly important decision for a student-athlete. One of the critical services that a PSCP can provide is to gather the relevant data and resources so that student-athletes and their families can make educated decisions—decisions that are right for their unique situation and not necessarily for the university for which they compete. As important as knowing the appropriate information to consider is recognizing what information to ignore. The first question to ask when assessing the value of an opinion is whether the person offering advice has a vested interest in the decision.

Anyone working for an athletic department, such as staff and coaches, may very well be offering their honest evaluation, but they also have something to gain if an individual returns to compete for their school. At the same time, agents may try to unscrupulously convince student-athletes that "now" is the right time to turn professional.

Herein lies one of the most difficult, yet helpful, areas in which a PSCP can assist a student-athlete and their family—a realistic talent evaluation. Each professional league has different ways in which they support this decision, and knowing when and how to engage the experts is quite important.

C. The NCAA

Each year the NCAA faces costly and potentially embarrassing lawsuits over an athlete's eligibility or compliance with NCAA Bylaws. Furthermore, it must invest considerable funds into compliance, investigative and enforcement staff, in an attempt to discover violations, prosecute them, and defend them on appeal.[211] Add in the headaches resulting from annual scandals and criticism lobbed from media and other commentators, and it becomes clear that the NCAA carries a heavy burden as the guardian of amateurism. A more coherent and informed transition process could help alleviate many of these problems while also providing clarity to the "line of demarcation between college athletics and professional sports"[212] that the NCAA has stated is so important.

D. Professional Sports Leagues and Players Associations

As discussed earlier, the professional leagues and unions have also had to waste a lot of time and money on dealing with young men and women not properly prepared for the professional environment. Some of the leagues have attempted to alleviate these issues by establishing draft advisory committees and holding mandatory rookie orientations.[213] When that fails, leagues have resorted to harsh punishments as a deterrent to illegal and embarrassing behavior.[214] These professional leagues essentially treat college athletics as a form of minor leagues, from which they cultivate a product that produces nearly $20 billion annually.[215] Consequently, it only makes sense that they would invest in the simplification and legitimization of that process.

Certainly any talent evaluator in a professional sport wishes they could simply watch game-tapes to determine an athlete's potential. With an improved transition process that better educates the student-athletes on what they are facing, team personnel could potentially have to spend less time digging into a player's personal life and family history. The bottom line is that leagues invest a tremendous amount of time and money in new players. They could assure themselves a much better return on their investment if they helped facilitate a process whereby the student-athletes understood their professional prospects, opportunities, and prerequisites. In the same vein, the time and money of the unions could be better spent if their members were more self-sufficient and responsible.

Presently, none of the union's agent regulations necessarily prohibit conduct by agents that results in a student-athlete losing eligibility or being otherwise punished by the NCAA. Certainly many activities by agents that would jeopardize a player's eligibility, such as providing cash or gifts, are prohibited by the agent regulations. However, some agents will continue to talk to players in spite of school rules prohibiting such contact, which can result in the player's suspension.[216] Although the value of the relevant NCAA Bylaw's is highly questionable, the Baratta brothers did not violate MLBPA agent regulations when they helped Andrew Oliver negotiate a potential contract with the Minnesota Twins, yet their actions ultimately resulted in Oliver temporarily losing his eligibility.[217] Direct reference to NCAA Bylaws in a union's agent regulations could make the basis for an antitrust claim by any agent punishable thereunder.[218]

E. Professional Advisors

Again, agents and advisors might not be the most popular group in addressing this issue, but they are an essential part of it and any attempt to minimize their existence and role will only make them less likely to cooperate in the process. One might speculate that agents enjoy the fact that the transition process is a mess because it gives them the opportunity to prey on uneducated student-athletes. This is certainly not the approach of the leading agents in the business nor any agent who wishes to make athlete representation a long-term career.

The truth is that the best agents prefer smarter, more mature clients who understand the process. It is easier to provide services to a client who understands the process and how to conduct himself accordingly. Also, a client that takes the agent selection process seriously the first time is much less likely to fire that agent—preventing agents from expending large amounts of time and money on players from whom they may never reap any benefit, let alone have to pursue in a grievance.[219]

Whether most people believe it, most agents and financial advisors fully recognize the fiduciary relationship and responsibilities of their professions and work very hard to ensure their clients' well-being. Nevertheless, many athletes do not want to heed advice that interrupts their lavish plans and will often fire advisors until they can find one who will let them do what they want. If an athlete has some legitimate cognizance of his career and financial prospects it greatly reduces the baby-sitting an agent or financial advisor has to do.

▪ V. RECOMMENDATIONS

What this article has tried to illustrate is that there are numerous and complicated decisions which begin, for many, even before the athletes are in college. The issues for each student-athlete are different, and are far more varied than some of the cases described herein. In proposing solutions we do not suggest that one or more of them is the absolute answer—but instead we seek to start a conversation and creative thinking to solve a large-scale and multi-faceted problem in need of desperate attention.

Each sport has its own unique way of operating and the problems that come with that operation. Consequently, the recommendations we have made are meant to apply across a broad spectrum of sports and issues. As a result, we cannot expect to solve the problems of every sport. Furthermore, there might exist a variety of real-world obstacles to many of our suggestions, most notably funding. Nevertheless, this is an issue that must become more of a priority for many of the organizations mentioned throughout this article.

It is our belief that there is a clear need for more education and knowledge for these student-athletes, as well as real and tangible benefits for colleges and universities. Better educated student-athletes are more likely (although not always) to make better decisions on when to go pro, how to make legal and business decisions, and how to avoid breaking rules (NCAA and state agent legislation). If colleges and universities fail to provide proper guidance, it is likely we will see the emergence of a cottage industry of private firms offering this advice to colleges and student-athletes.[220] Seeing as how we have detailed the relatively powerless role of the student-athlete, and his or her family, in this process, the bulk of the improvements in the process must come from the other major stakeholders: colleges and universities, the NCAA, professional leagues and unions, and the agents and financial advisors.

A. Colleges and Universities

First, while a system of PSCPs is in place, not enough college and universities have PSCPs and those that do vary in terms of their use. NCAA institutions need to strongly consider using a PSCP and sufficiently funding it.

Second, colleges must increase funding for their compliance departments. A school's compliance department is its first line of defense to prevent and discover improprieties while aiding student-athletes through the complicated process. Compliance departments should be larger and universities should seriously consider hiring more attorneys to work in compliance departments as opposed to poorly paid and inexperienced graduate assistants.

Third, colleges and universities must aid in the enforcement of the Uniform Athlete Agents Act. As detailed earlier, most states have a form of the UAAA,[221] in which certain sections require that any contract between an agent and an athlete contain a warning that the player may lose his eligibility,[222] and that the agent give the school notice of the existence of a contract where the student-athlete might have eligibility remaining.[223] It is extremely unlikely that agents are complying with either of these requirements.

It is not difficult to find out which agent is representing a former student-athlete from a college or university. As soon as the agency contract is formed, that college should immediately crosscheck the agent's conduct against all applicable state laws, in particular whether that agent is registered in the state, as required by the UAAA.[224] Schools must work closely with the applicable state body to ensure consistent and diligent enforcement of state laws.

Fourth, schools should reward agents who act in an ethical manner. In addition to the UAAA, many schools ask that agents register with them as well—if an agent fails to comply with the school's demands and rules, such as when to hold a meeting and when to contact the student-athletes, schools should not help that agent in any way during the recruiting process. On the other hand, an agent who is open with the compliance department and follows the school's rules should be given access to the student-athletes when appropriate to do so and possibly even a recommendation from the athletic department.

Fifth, smaller schools without the means to improve this process must then consider doing it on a Conference level. Most NCAA member institutions only send a student-athlete into the professional ranks every few years. Consequently, they do not have the experience or incentive to properly educate themselves and their student-athletes on this process. However, these smaller schools can pool their resources and provide these services within their Conference.

B. The NCAA

Just as funding for PSCPs needs to be increased for member institutions, the NCAA also needs increased funding to combat these problems. A clear source of funding is the television deals the NCAA and the Conferences have negotiated.[225] The funding at the NCAA level could be used in a variety of ways.

First, the NCAA could create a guide of information and recommended solutions. This was done in the 1990s with a three-ring binder and can be done today with a website.

Second, the NCAA could run seminars, conferences, and webcasts to educate PSCP employees.

Third, the NCAA could hold seminars, conferences, and webcasts for the student-athletes who have a potential professional career. These could also be run on a regional and/or conference level.

Fourth, the NCAA could establish a formal grant program for institutions to establish and run PSCPs. Some of the money could go towards travel to attend a newly created PSCP conference and/or to be used in place of other university responsibilities for the chair of the PSCP.

Fifth, a course taken for college credit could be offered through the NCAA and/or member institutions that would educate student-athletes on some of the important issues involved in a professional sports career. Given the use of technology, this course could be delivered in a variety of ways, including video, delayed video, or online. Case studies using current and recent student athletes would be developed. The course could cover a variety of important issues discussed in this article and relevant to a student-athlete's professional ambitions, including: (1) NCAA rules and regulations; (2) agents; (3) contracts; (4) player unions; (5) collective bargaining agreements; (6) drafts; (7) drug testing; (8) intellectual property rights; (9) financial management; (10) the media; and (11) insurance. While there is a risk that the class could become an easy grade for student-athletes, if taken and administrated properly, it has the potential to provide a tremendous amount of important information to student-athletes in an environment where they would have to pay, at least, some attention.

Sixth, the NCAA should scrutinize and consider amending some of its Bylaws as they relate to this topic, most notably Bylaw 12.3.2, which was discussed at length in the *Oliver* case. The way in which this Bylaw relates to the use of an attorney-advisor, but not an agent, is unfair and confusing. A student-athlete needs the full scope of advice and services when considering whether to turn professional. Fortunately, it has been reported that the NCAA is considering ways in which student-athletes can utilize the services of advisors.[226]

Seventh, the NCAA needs to seriously consider the equity and long-term viability of a system where administrators, coaches, schools, and others become very wealthy in exchange for the student-athlete's complimentary education. While a discussion of the proper pay or benefits received by student-athletes is beyond the scope of this article,[227] the NCAA is currently facing serious litigation in which former student-athletes are contending that the NCAA and its member institutions have unjustly and illegally enriched themselves by misappropriating the student-athletes' rights of publicity.[228] At stake are hundreds of millions of dollars in revenue for the NCAA and its member institutions, as well as the entire business model for the NCAA and athletic departments.

If the courts determine that student-athletes are entitled to some compensation for the use of their images or likenesses in licensing arrangements, the NCAA must be ready to propose some creative options if it wishes to maintain the "clear line of demarcation between college athletics and professional sports."[229] One possibility is to use some of the money to purchase a bond, whereby if the student-athlete's wrongdoing causes the member institution or any other party any loss, the damaged party could collect on the bond.

Eighth, the NCAA must consider expanding their insurance options for student-athletes. Currently the NCAA does have a Catastrophic Injury insurance program that provides coverage to student-athletes and others injured during a covered sporting event.[230] The NCAA should consider covering student-athletes with professional potential as well. With help from the professional leagues, the NCAA could determine a certain number of athletes to cover and could even base the coverage on a graduated scale based on their potential. The premiums for the coverage could be considered loans to be forgiven if the student-athlete is not involved in any NCAA violations during his or her career. Additionally, the NCAA should consider allowing Loss of Value insurance policies for student-athletes.

Ninth, the NCAA should consider providing loans to student-athletes. To prevent student-athletes from seeking and accepting inappropriate sources of cash above and beyond their scholarship, the NCAA could provide loans to student-athletes, possibly increasing in amount as the student-athlete approaches graduation or the professional level. The loans could then be forgiven if the student-athlete is not involved in any NCAA violation during his career.

Tenth, the NCAA could consider changing the requisite burden of proof to punish a member institution for lack of institutional control. Presently, to find a school lacked institutional control, the NCAA Committee on Infractions asks whether the school "knew, or should have known" about the violations.[231] The NCAA could apply a stricter liability standard, whereby schools are punished at the same level of harshness for violations occurring under their purview, regardless of their knowledge. Ideally, this would provide an additional incentive for schools to seek out and resolve issues in this process.

Eleventh, the NCAA should consider revising some of its Bylaws and practices as they relate to recruiting at amateur competitions. In basketball in particular, assistant coaches and recruiting coordinators must regularly attend summer AAU games and camps to recruit the best players. Placing further restrictions on when or where recruiting contact may take place would help remove some of the "professional feel" that these amateur camps have taken on.

Twelfth, the NCAA should work more closely with the national federations, where they exist, such as USA Basketball and USA Hockey. These organizations are also non-profit entities that seek to develop the country's best athletes in an ethical manner. The national federations and the NCAA have many of the same goals and principles and their collaboration would be mutually beneficial.

C. Professional Sports Leagues and Players Associations

First, professional leagues and unions must be more proactive in their approach to helping their athletes. As mentioned earlier, both the NFL and NBA host rookie symposia meant to enlighten their new players on the realities of the professional sports industry. However, as discussed throughout this article there are a multitude of problems that occur well before the player even reaches the professional level. Leagues and unions should be more involved in educating prospects in high school and college, prior to any issues arising that may derail their professional dreams. "iHoops," a joint venture between the NCAA and the NBA, may serve as a valuable start or model.[232]

Additionally, each league and union must be cognizant of where their athletes come from. For instance, both the NHL and MLB need to do more to educate high school students on the amateur-to-professional transition process.

Considering the proliferation of elite leagues, tournaments, and events for high school players, it is not overly difficult to track down and begin educating these prospective student-athletes.

Second, the leagues and unions should consider collective bargaining punishment for players involved in behavior that was either illegal or against NCAA rules during their transition to the professional league. In recent years, the leagues have strengthened their enforcement and discipline of their personal conduct policies as they apply to current players. However, unethical principles can imbue in athletes far before they reach the professional ranks, drawing unwanted attention to their professional leagues when they finally do arrive. Consequently, the leagues should expand the use of their disciplinary process as a deterrent to the greatest extent possible.

D. Professional Advisors

First, agents and advisors must police themselves. No one is more aware of the new ways in which rules are being bent and broken than other agents, and arguably no one is more hurt by it than the ethical agents unable to obtain clients as a result of rule bending. Although they often lack any real proof and it might sound like sour grapes, agents should report any possible violation of law or regulation of reasonable veracity to the state, NCAA, and players' union.

Second, agents should be more forceful in defending their own rights and livelihoods through lobbying or litigation when necessary. In a highly questionable decision, the venerable Judge Posner determined that, in general, there is "nothing wrong with one sports agent trying to take a client from another."[233] Judge Posner's analysis reflects a poor understanding of the realities of the agent industry. Agents must be more vocal in explaining themselves, strive to operate in an ethical manner, and actively make suggestions to improve the current system.

■ CONCLUSION

There are a large number of student-athletes who would benefit from being educated about potential professional sports careers. While there are far more who "dream" about a professional career than actually realize one, there is still an important population of student-athletes who will pursue professional careers, and to whom colleges, universities, and the NCAA can provide valuable lessons and resources.

Student-athletes remain ultimately responsible for the decisions they make. Yet, the problems in the amateur-to-professional transition process are complex and cannot be solved by one person, one action, or one organization. While we proposed solutions relevant to each of the individual stakeholders, there must be a concerted and coordinated effort on the part of many parties to provide funding, education, enforcement, and intervention. All stakeholders should be interested in forming a Blue Panel Commission of sorts to study these issues—each stakeholder must take accountability for his or her role in this problem and be active in its solution.

■ ABOUT THE AUTHORS

Glenn M. Wong is Professor, Department of Sport Management, Isenberg School of Management, University of Massachusetts, Amherst, MA; J.D., Boston College Law School; B.A. Brandeis University. Professor Wong is the author of *Essentials of Sports Law* (4th ed., 2010) and *The Comprehensive Guide to Careers in Sports* (Jones & Bartlett Publishers, 2008).

Warren Zola is Assistant Dean, Graduate Programs, Carroll School of Management, Boston College, Chestnut Hill, MA; M.B.A., Boston College Carroll School of Management; J.D., Tulane University; B.A. Hobart & William Smith Colleges, Geneva, NY. Adjunct Professor and Chair of the Professional Sports Counseling Panel at Boston College.

Chris Deubert is Associate, Ginsberg & Burgos, PLLC, New York, NY; J.D./M.B.A., Fordham University School of Law and Graduate School of Business, New York, NY; B.S., Sport Management, University of Massachusetts, Amherst, MA.

■ NOTES

1. Marta Lawrence, *Behind the Scenes*, NCAA CHAMPION, Spring 2008, at 56, *available at* www.ncaachampionmagazine.org (follow link at bottom of page for Spring 2008 issue).

2. *Id.* NCAA Public Service Announcement developed by Young & Rubicam for the NCAA's JoJo Rinebold, NCAA's managing director of brand strategies and events.

3. NCAA.org, About the NCAA, http://www.ncaa.org/wps/wcm/connect/public/ncaa/about+the+ncaa (last visited Oct. 10, 2010).

4. The four major domestic leagues being Major League Baseball (MLB), the National Football League (NFL), the National Basketball Association (NBA), and the National Hockey League (NHL). Based on the 2010 entry drafts of the four major sports leagues there were 2,050 individuals drafted and 1,355 of them were college athletes. *See* MLB.com, 2010 MLB First-Year Player Draft, http://mlb.mlb.com/mlb/events/draft/y2010/ (last visited Oct. 8, 2010); NFL.com, 2010 NFL Draft, http://www.nfl.com/draft/2010 (last visited Oct. 8, 2010); NBADraft.net, 2010 NBA Draft, http://www.nbadraft.net/nba_final_draft/2010 (last visited Oct. 8, 2010); NHL.com, 2010 NHL Entry Draft, http://www.nhl.com/ice/eventhome.htm?location=/draft/2010 (last visited Oct.8, 2010).

5. 2010 MLB First-Year Player Draft, *supra* note 4; 2010 NHL Entry Draft, *supra* note 4.

6. 2008 NCAA Convention, THE STUDENT-ATHLETE PERSPECTIVE OF THE COLLEGE EXPERIENCE: FINDINGS FROM THE NCAA GOALS AND SCORE STUDIES, 18 (2008), http://www.ncaa.org/about/resources/research/2006-goals-study-archive (follow "The Student-Athlete Perspective of the College Experience: Findings from the NCAA GOALS and SCORE Studies" hyperlink).

7. *Id.* at 14.

8. *Id.*

9. *See* Daniel Libit, *A Basketball Program Rises by Dipping Lower*, N.Y. Times, May 7, 2010, at B19; Anne Stein, *The Best 10-Year-Old Basketball Player in America*, Chi. Trib., Mar. 31, 2010, at 1 (discussing the scouting and ranking of basketball players as early as the fifth grade).

10. The NCAA instituted several investigations. First, they examined allegations that former University of Florida lineman Maurkice Pouncey received $100,000 from an agent while still playing at Florida. The NCAA was concerned whether Maurkice's twin brother, Mike, still a lineman at Florida may have also received improper benefits. *See* ESPN.com, *Pouncey Denies Accepting Money,* July 22, 2010, http://sports. espn.go.com/ncf/news/story?id=5398414. Pouncey's agent is Joel Segal. *See* Pat Forde, *Source: NCAA Probe Allegation,* ESPN.com, July 21, 2010, http://sports.espn.go.com/ncf/ news/story?id=5392159. Second, the NCAA investigated whether several players from the Universities of North Carolina, South Carolina, and Alabama may have improperly attended a party hosted by a Miami agent. *See* Stewart Mandel, *NCAA Turning Up Heat On Agent-Player Relations with More Probes,* SportsIllustrated.com, July 19, 2010, http:// sportsillustrated.cnn.com/2010/writers/stewart_mandel/07/19/ncaa.agents/index.html; Ivan Maisel & Mark Schlabach, *Dareus May Have Attended Agent's Party,* ESPN.com, July 22, 2010, http://sports.espn.go.com/ncf/news/story?id=5396236.

11. NCAA Bylaws have been challenged many times. *See* Bloom v. NCAA, 93 P.3d 621 (Colo. App. 2004). Bloom was a college football player at the University of Colorado and also an Olympic skier. *Id.* at 622. He was paid to participate in endorsements in connection with his professional skiing career and the NCAA subsequently held Bloom to be ineligible for the final two years of his college football career. *Id.* at 622. The courts upheld the determination, finding it impossible to determine which endorsement and media activities were, in fact, unrelated to his athletic ability or prestige as Bloom contended. *Id.* at 627. Bloom was eventually drafted in the 5th round of the 2006 NFL Draft but never actually played in an NFL game during his short career. For additional cases involving eligibility, see Pryor v. NCAA, 288 F.3d 548 (3d Cir. 2002); Cureton v. NCAA, 198 F.3d 107 (3d Cir. 1999); Butts v. NCAA, 751 F.2d 609 (3d Cir. 1984); Spath v. NCAA, 728 F.2d 25 (1st Cir. 1984); Lasege v. NCAA, 53 S.W.3d 77 (Ky. 2001). For cases challenging academic standards, see Bowers v. NCAA, 475 F.3d 524 (3d Cir. 2007); Cole v. NCAA, 120 F. Supp. 2d 1060 (N.D. Ga. 2000); Tatum v. NCAA, 992 F. Supp. 1114 (E.D. Mont. 1998); Hall v. NCAA, 985 F. Supp. 782 (N.D. Ill. 1997). For a case concerning transfers, see NCAA v. Yeo, 171 S.W.3d 863 (Tex. 2005). For cases concerning financial aid, see Wiley v. NCAA, 612 F.2d 473 (10th Cir. 1979); Jones v. NCAA, 392 F. Supp. 295 (D. Mass. 1975). For cases concerning sanctions, see Regents of Univ. of Minnesota v. NCAA, 422 F. Supp. 1158 (D. Minn. 1976); NCAA v. Gillard, 352 So.2d 1072 (Miss. Sup. Ct. 1977).

12. See the discussion on Maurice Clarett *infra* Part II. *See also* cases cited *supra* note 11 (referring specifically to *Bowers, Bloom, Lasege, Hall, Wiley,* and *Hall*).

13. *See* Nat'l Collegiate Athletics Ass'n v. Bd. of Regents, 468 U.S. 85, 120 (1984). *See also* Marc Bianchi, *Guardian of Amateurism or Legal Defiant? The Dichotomous Nature of NCAA Men's Ice Hockey Regulation*, 20 Seton Hall J. Sports & Ent. L. 165 (2010); Virginia A. Fitt, *The NCAA's Lost Cause and the Legal Ease of Redefining Amateurism*, 59 Duke L. J. 555 (2009); Daniel E. Lazaroff, *The NCAA In Its Second Century: Defender of Amateurism*

or Antitrust Recidivist?, 86 OR. L. REV. 329 (2007); Christian McCormick, *The Emperor's New Clothes: Lifting the NCAA's Veil of Amateurism*, 45 SAN DIEGO L. REV. 495 (2008).

14. 2009–2010 NCAA DIVISION I MANUAL 61 (2010), *available at* http://www.ncaapublications.com/productdownloads/Dl10.pdf [hereinafter DI Manual].

15. *Id.* at § 12.01.2.

16. *Id.* at § 12.02.3.

17. The situation often occurs when European players come to play college basketball in the United States, *See* Bill Koch, *Hrycaniuk's Come Long Way for UC*, CINCINNATI ENQUIRER, Jan. 11, 2008, at Cl; Mark Lazerus, *Fumey Loses Redshirt, Year of Eligibility*, MERRILLVILLE POST-TRIBUNE, Nov. 7, 2008, at B3.

18. In hockey, Major Junior A Ice Hockey, a level of hockey played in both the United States and Canada, is considered professional, but athletes can petition for a restoration of eligibility provided they sit out at least one year of intercollegiate athletic competition. *See* DI MANUAL, *supra* note 14, § 12.2.3.2.4.

19. *See* DI MANUAL, *supra* note 14, § 12.1.2.

20. Enes Kanter is a star basketball player from Turkey. Kanter played with a professional team in Turkey but claims he refused to accept compensation specifically so he could retain his NCAA eligibility. *See* Mike DeCourcy, *Enes Kanter a Revolutionary Case for Kentucky*, NCAA, SPORTING NEWS, Apr. 14, 2010, http://www.sportingnews.com/ncaabasketball/story/2010-04-14/enes-kanter-revolutionary-case-for-kentucky-ncaa. However, NCAA Bylaw § 12.2.3.2 states that "[a]n individual shall not be eligible for intercollegiate athletics in a sport if the individual ever competed on a professional team in that sport." DI MANUAL, *supra* note 14, § 12.2.3.2. In September 2010, the General Manager of Kanter's Turkish team alleged Kanter received over $100,000 in salary and housing over a three-year period. *See* Chris Littman, *UK's Kanter Paid More Than $100K by Turkish Team*, SPORTING NEWS, Sept. 8, 2010, http://www.sportingnews.com/ncaabasketball/feed/2010-09/enes-kanter/story/report-uks-kanter-paid-more-than-100k-by-turkish-team#subnav.

21. *See* Florida Athletics Department Directory, http://www.gatorzone.com/directory/ (last visited Oct. 10, 2010) (Florida has 3 compliance employees); Georgia Bulldogs Compliance, http://www.georgiadogs.com/school-bio/compliance.html (last visited Oct. 10, 2010) (2 compliance employees); Kentucky Athletic Department Staff Directory & Contact Information, http://www.ukathletics.com/athletic-dept/directory.html (last visited Oct. 10, 2010) (4 compliance employees); South Carolina Gamecocks Administrative Directory, http://gamecocksonline.cstv.com/school-bio/scar-staff-directory.html (last visited Oct. 10, 2010) (6 compliance employees); Tennessee Compliance, http://www.utsports.com/compliance/html (last visited Oct. 10, 2010) (4 compliance employees); Vanderbilt Athletics Staff Directory, http://vucommodores.cstv.com/school-bio/vand-staff-dir.html (last visited Oct. 10, 2010) (4 compliance employees); Alabama Crimson Tide Compliance, http://www.rolltide.com/sports/compliance/main.html (last visited Oct. 10, 2010) (8 compliance employees); Arkansas Athletics—Dept. of Compliance, www.arkansasrazorbacks.com (follow "For Recruits" hyperlink; then follow "Compliance Office" hyperlink; then follow "Compliance Office Contact Information" hyperlink) (last visited Oct. 10, 2010) (5 compliance employees); Auburn Athletics Staff Directory—Compliance, http://auburntigers.cstv.com/ot/staff-directory.html#comp (last visited Oct. 10, 2010) (5 compliance employees); LSU Athletics Staff Directory, www.lsusports.net (follow "Departments" hyperlink; then follow "Compliance & Autographs" hyperlink; then follow "Staff" hyperlink) (last visited Oct.

10, 2010) (4 compliance employees); MSU Athletics Staff Directory, www.mstateath-letics.com (follow "Athletics" hyperlink; then follow "Staff Directory: hyperlink; (last visited Oct. 10, 2010) (4 compliance employees); Mississippi Athletics—Compliance, http://www.olemisssports.com/compliance/ole-compliance-staff.html (last visited Oct. 10, 2010) (5 compliance employees). Alabama has the largest compliance department, having been subjected to NCAA sanctions for major rules violations on several occasions: in 2009, the school was put on three years of probation and forced to vacate wins in which certain football student-athletes competed for receiving improper benefits; in 2002, the school was given five years of probation, banned from the postseason for 2002 and 2003 and had scholarships reduced after football student-athletes received improper gifts from boosters and for recruiting violations; and in 1995, the football team lost scholarships and was forced to forfeit wins because football student-athletes received improper benefits. *See* NCAA's Legislative Services Database, https://webl.ncaa.org/LSDBi/exec/homepage (last visited Oct. 10, 2010) (provides information about major infractions by NCAA member institutions). For more information on the history of the NCAA's infractions process and an analysis of major recent cases, see Glenn M. Wong, Kyle Skillman & Chris Deubert, *The NCAA's Infractions Appeals Committee: Recent Case History, Analysis and the Beginning of a New Chapter*, 9 VA. SPORTS & ENT. L. J. 47 (2009).

22. *See* Appalachian State Athletics Staff Directory, http://www.goasu.com/ViewArticle. dbml?DB_OEM_ID=21500&ATCLID=1546163 (last visited Oct. 10, 2010) (1 compliance employee); Chattanooga Athletics Staff Directory, http://www.gomocs.com/StaffDirectory. dbml?DB_OEM_ID=17700 (last visited Oct. 10, 2010) (2 compliance employees); Citadel Athletics Staff Directory, http://www.citadelsports.com/ViewArticle.dbml?DB_OEM_ ID=9700&ATCLID=20483698 0 (last visited Oct. 10, 2010) (2 compliance employees); Elon Athletics Staff Directory, http://www.elonphoenix.com/staff.aspx?staff & (last visited Oct. 10, 2010) (2 compliance employees); Furman Athletics Staff Directory, http://www.fur-manpaladins.com/information/directory/index (last visited Oct. 10, 2010) (1 compliance employee); Georgia Southern Athletics Staff Directory, http://www.georgiasouthernea-gles.com/SportSelect.dbml?DB_OEM_ID=18700&KEY=&SPID=10884&SPSID=95346 (last visited Oct. 10, 2010) (2 compliance employees); Samford Athletics Staff Directory, http://samfordsports.cstv.com/athletic-dept/samf-athletic-dept.html (last visited Oct. 10, 2010) (1 compliance employee); Western Carolina Athletics Staff Directory, http://www. catamountsports.com/athletic-dept/wcar-directory.html (last visited Oct. 10, 2010) (1 compliance employee); Wofford Athletics Staff Directory, http://athletics.wofford.edu/staff. aspx?tab=staffdirectory (last visited Oct. 10, 2010) (1 compliance employee).

23. Alabama Athletics Staff Directory, http://www.rolltide.com/staffdir/alab-staffdir. html (last visited Oct. 10, 2010).

24. Cornerstone Sports Consulting is run by Joe Mendes, a former NFL team and league executive and talent evaluator. Among the schools that Cornerstone is providing amateur-to-professional transition guidance are the Universities of Alabama, Southern California, and Georgia. *See* Cornerstone Sports Consulting, http://www.cornerstone-sports.com/team.html (last visited June 15, 2010); Liz Mullen, *Some Agents Question Former NFL Exec's Role with Schools*, SPORTS BUSINESS JOURNAL, Aug. 24, 2009, www. sportsbusinessjournal.com/article/63356.

25. For more on issues related to this, see Megan Fuller, *Where's the Penalty Flag? The Unauthorized Practice of Law, the NCAA, and Athletic Compliance Directors*, 54 N.Y.L. SCH. L. REV. 495 (2009/2010).

26. *See* DI Manual, *supra* note 14, § 12.1.2.

27. *Id.* § 12.1.2.1.

28. *See* Phillip C. Blackman, *NCAA's Academic Performance Program: Academic Reform or A Academic Racism?*, 15 UCLA Ent. L. Rev. 225, 242–243 (2008).

29. Throughout this article when we refer to NCAA member institutions or universities, we also mean their athletic departments and compliance staffs.

30. The drafts' rules have evolved as the result of many legal challenges over the years. For cases in the NFL, see Clarett v. Nat'l Football League, 306 F. Supp. 2d 379 (S.D.N.Y. 2004), *rev'd*, 369 F.3d 124 (2d Cir. 2004) (discussed in greater detail in Part II); Smith v. Pro Football, Inc., 593 F.2d 1173, 1183–1189 (D.C. Cir. 1978); Zimmerman v. Nat'l Football League, 632 F. Supp. 398 (D.D.C. 1986); Kapp v. Nat'l Football League, 390 F. Supp. 73 (N.D. Cal. 1974). For cases in the NBA, see Bridgeman v. Nat'l Basketball Ass'n, 675 F. Supp. 960 (D.N.J. 1987); Denver Rockets v. All-Pro Mgmt., 325 F. Supp. 1049 (C.D. Cal. 1971). For a case in the NHL, see Nat'l Hockey League Players Ass'n v. Plymouth Whalers Hockey Club, 325 F.3d 712 (6th Cir. 2003).

31. National Football League Collective Bargaining Agreement Art. XVI, §2 (a) (2006), *available at* http://images.nflplayers.com/mediaResources/files/PDFs/General/NFL%20COLLECTIVE%20BARGAINING%20AGREEMENT%202006%20-%202012.pdf [hereinafter NFL CBA].

32. Major League Baseball Rules MLR 4(b) (2008), *available at* http://www.bizofbaseball.com/docs/MajorLeagueRules-2008.pdf [hereinafter MLB Rules].

33. National Basketball Association Collective Bargaining Agreement Art. X, § 3 (2005), *available at* http://www.nbpa.org/sites/default/files/ARTICLE%20X.pdf [hereinafter NBA CBA].

34. National Hockey League Collective Bargaining Agreement Art. 8, § 8.2 (2005), *available at* http://www.nhl.com/cba/2005-CBA.pdf [hereinafter NHL CBA].

35. All numbers are approximate as the NFL, MLB and NHL drafts have systems to allow for compensatory selections on the loss of free agents and occasionally teams lose draft picks for violating league rules.

36. The NFL requires that at least "three regular seasons have begun and ended following either his graduation from high school or graduation of the class with which he entered high school, whichever is earlier." NFL CBA, *supra* note 31, Art. XVI, § 2(b). Prior to the 2006 extension of the CBA, this rule was not specifically in the CBA but instead only in the NFL Bylaws and Constitution. After the Maurice Clarett lawsuit, Clarett v. Nat'l Football League, 306 F. Supp. 2d 379 (S.D.N.Y. 2004), *rev'd*, 369 F.3d 124 (2d Cir. 2004), the NFL and NFLPA (National Football League Players Association) negotiated the inclusion of the rule into the CBA.

37. MLB does not have a specific age but instead requires that a player's high school eligibility be expired before he can sign a contract with a major or minor league club. MLB Rules, *supra* note 32, MLR 3(a) (2). However, it is important to note that players from outside of North America are not subject to the draft and are able to sign free agent contracts when they are sixteen, so long as they turn 17 prior to the end of that season or September 1, whichever is later. MLB Rules, *supra* note 32, MLR 3(a) (1) (B).

38. The NBA requires all players to be at least 19 years old; if American, at least one NBA season must have elapsed since he graduated (or should have graduated) high school. NBA CBA, *supra* note 33, Art. X, § 1(b).

39. The NHL requires all players to be at least 18 years old. NHL CBA, *supra* note 34, § 8.4.

40. An enrolled student-athlete may participate in a pre-draft workout or combine at any time, provided the individual does not miss class. The student-athlete may receive actual and necessary expenses in conjunction with one 48-hour tryout per professional team or combine. A tryout may extend beyond 48 hours if the individual self-finances additional expenses, including return transportation. A self-financed tryout may be for any length of time, provided the individual does not miss class. DI MANUAL, *supra* note 14, § 12.2.1.3. Different rules apply prior to a student-athlete enrolling. *Id.* § 12.2.1.1.

41. In any college sport other than basketball or football, a student-athlete can enter a professional league's draft once without signing with an agent and then return to college if they go undrafted and announce their intention to return within 72 hours. DI MANUAL, *supra* note 14, § 12.2.4.2.4.

42. A football student-athlete can return if he goes undrafted provided that he has not signed with an agent and declares his intention to return to intercollegiate athletics in writing within 72 hours of the draft. DI MANUAL, *supra* note 14, § 12.2.4.2.3.

43. A basketball student-athlete can enter the NBA Draft once during their career, without signing with an agent and can return to intercollegiate athletics only if they request that their name be removed from the draft list by May 8 of the year before the draft and they ultimately go undrafted. DI MANUAL, *supra* note 14, § 12.2.4.2.1.1.

44. If a player is drafted in an initial draft and does not sign with the drafting team prior to the subsequent draft, the player is eligible to be drafted by any team except the team that drafted him in the initial draft. NFL CBA, *supra* note 31, Art. XVI, §4(b) (ii).

45. A player can be drafted after high school and choose not to sign. MLB RULES, *supra* note 32, MLR 3(a) (2). If the player enters a four-year college, he cannot be drafted again until he is 21 or after his junior year. *Id.* MLR 3(a) (3)(E). Therefore, a player could be drafted after high school, his junior year of college, and then his senior year of college. In addition, some players go from high school to junior college, where you can be drafted after your second year. *Id.* MLR 3(a) (4). Hypothetically, a player could be drafted after high school, enter a junior college and be drafted after junior college, then enroll in a four-year college, be drafted after his junior year, and be drafted a fourth time after graduating from, or completing his eligibility at, the four-year college. A player does not need to enter his name into the draft, consequently avoiding some possible issues with the NCAA. A recent example of a player being drafted several times is Cincinnati Reds pitcher Micah Owings. Owings was drafted in the second round by the Colorado Rockies out of high school in 2002 but did not sign. *See* Baseball-Reference.com, Micah Owings, http://www.baseball-reference.com/players/o/owingmi01.shtml (last visited May 30, 2010). Then, he was drafted in the nineteenth round by the Chicago Cubs in 2003 after his freshman year at Georgia Tech because he was 21, but again he did not sign. *Id.* Finally, Owings was drafted the third time in 2005 after his junior year, this time at Tulane, in the third round by the Arizona Diamondbacks with whom he did sign. *Id.*

46. If a player does not sign with the team that drafts him originally, he may be drafted again in the subsequent draft. If he does not sign with the team that drafts him in the subsequent draft, he will become a free agent after the next (third) draft. NBA CBA, *supra* note 33, Art. X, § 4(b).

47. NHL CBA, *supra* note 34, Art. 8, § 8.4(ii).

48. NFL CBA, *supra* note 31, Art. XVI, § 6.

49. MLB RULES, *supra* note 32, MLR 4(d)(3). This rule only applies in cases where the drafted player has college eligibility left. As compared to the NHL, baseball players have a level of leverage unavailable to their hockey counterparts—the ability to tell a team to meet their demands or risk losing their rights. Accordingly, although not entirely the reason, there are huge differences in signing bonuses between MLB and the NHL.

50. NBA CBA, *supra* note 33, Art. X, § 6(b). If the player does not return to college, the original drafting team holds the players rights until the next draft. *Id.*, Art. X, § 4(a).

51. NHL CBA, *supra* note 34, Art. 8, § 8.6(c). If the player does not stay in college, the NHL team holds his rights until the fourth June 1 following his initial selection in the draft.

52. Fitzgerald was able to leave after just two years of college because he completed a year at a prepatory academy prior to entering University of Pittsburgh. *See* Paul Zeise, *Fitzgerald, Green Join Forces Again, Pitt's Star Receiver Third Pick of Draft*, PITT. POST-GAZETTE, Apr. 25, 2004, at D1.

53. Alex Smith, the #1 overall pick in the 2005 NFL Draft received $24 million guaranteed in his rookie contract. *See* Dennis Georgatos, *Smith Living a Dream, Rookie QB Eager to Prove He's Worth Investment*, SAN JOSE MERCURY NEWS, July 27, 2005, at 3. In contrast, Leinart received $14 million guaranteed. *See Better Late... Rookie QB Matt Leinart is Finally in Camp, and He's Raring To Go*, ARIZ. REPUBLIC, Aug. 16, 2006, at C1.

54. A notable recent example is former Ole Miss quarterback Jevan Snead. *See* Andrea Adelson, *Yo, Jevan, What Were You Thinking?*, ORLANDO SENTINEL, May 3, 2010, at C1. Snead entered the 2009 season as a junior and one of the top-rated quarterbacks in the country. However, Snead struggled through a difficult season and the consensus was that he needed to return to college to reestablish his status. Even after being given a fifth-round projection, Snead chose to enter the NFL Draft. When he was not drafted, Snead signed as a free agent with the Tampa Bay Buccaneers, was released during training camp, and faces an uphill career challenge. *Id.*

55. Fifty-three underclassmen declared for the 2010 NFL Draft. *See* Rick Gosselin, *Sizing Up the Cornerbacks for the NFL Draft*, DALLAS MORNING NEWS ONLINE, Apr. 14, 2010. Forty-six underclassmen declared for the 2009 NFL Draft. *See NFL Draft*, CHI. TRIB., Jan. 21, 2009, at 87. Fifty-three underclassmen declared for the 2008 NFL Draft. *See* Sammy Batten, *Bowl Game Could Be Last Game for Nicks as a Tar Heel*, FAYETTEVILLE OBSERVER (N.C.) ONLINE, Dec. 27, 2008.

56. *See* Brian Jaramillo, *Testing the Waters, Ways Are Sought To Give Undergraduates a Chance To Determine Their Value As Professionals Before They Give Up Their College Eligibility*, L.A. TIMES, July 25, 1993, at 3 (where NFLPA Executive Director Eugene Upshaw stated college athletes who graduated have longer professional careers); *see also* Roger Mills, *Brooks Not Super, But He is a Starr*, ST. PETERSBURG TIMES (FL), Feb. 1, 2004, at 13C (where NFLPA General Counsel Richard Berthelsen stated graduating college athletes have longer professional careers).

57. *See Indiana Opts for DiNardo as Coach*, ST. PETERSBURG TIMES (FL), Jan. 9, 2002, at 5C (mentioning ineligibility of former Georgia Tech running back Joe Burns); Matt Winklejohn, *The Draft ESPN Won't Show*, ATLANTA J.–CONST., July 12, 2007, at D2 (mentioning the ineligibility of former Georgia cornerback Paul Oliver); Evan Woodberry, *AU's McClover to Enter Draft*, MOBILE REG. (AL), Jan. 6, 2006, at C3 (discussing ineligibility of former Auburn defensive end Stanley McClover).

58. *See* Mike Chappell, *Chancy Proposition: Underclassmen who Enter Draft Weigh the Risks; Colts' Bashir Doesn't Regret Leaving School*, INDIANAPOLIS STAR, Apr. 14, 2002, at Cl; John McClain, *'Bama's Palmer to Enter Draft Now/All-America Receiver Alters Decision*, HOUS. CHRON., Jan. 11, 1994, at 3.

59. *See* Brent Schrotenboer, *Dad: Brown Will Be Back in Scarlet and Black in 2010*, SAN DIEGO UNION-TRIB., Jan. 16, 2010, at D3 (discussing decision of San Diego State wide receiver Vincent Brown to return for his senior season after receiving a projection that he would not be taken in the first three rounds); *see also* Wes Rucker, *Foster Back to Make Mark at University of Tennessee*, CHATTANOOGA TIMES (TN) ONLINE, July 19, 2008, http:// timesfreepress.com/news/2008/jul/19/foster-back-make-mark-university-tennessee/ ?print (discussing decision of Tennessee running back Arian Foster's decision to return for his senior season despite having received a second-round projection from the NFL Draft Advisory Committee).

60. *See* Randy Peterson, *Submitting Draft Paperwork Not 'Too Big a Deal' For Greene*, DES MOINES REG., Dec. 27, 2008, at C2; Nathan Warters, *Tech's Flowers, Harris Exploring NFL Draft Possibilities*, THE NEWS & ADVANCE ONLINE (LYNCHBURG, VA), Dec. 12, 2007, http://www2.newsadvance.com/sports/2007/dec/12/techs_flowers_harris_exploring_ nfl_draft_possi bili-ar-228571/.

61. There have been numerous incidents in which a player entered the NFL Draft based on the opinions of the Advisory Committee only to go undrafted. *See* Scott Hotard, *LSU's Black a Forgotten Man by NFL*, BATON ROUGE ADVOC., May 3, 2010, at Cl; Manish Mehta, *Warren Steps Up for Jets*, STAR-LEDGER (NEWARK, N.J.), May 1, 2010, at 35.

62. *See* Bob LeGere, *Injury Slowed Wootton, But NFL Will Come Calling NFL Draft Top 10 Dlinemen*, CHI. DAILY HERALD, Apr. 17, 2010, at 6 (discussing projection of Northwestern defensive end Corey Wootton as a late first or early second round pick); Susan Miller Degnan, *UM: Miami Hurricanes' Allen Bailey Back, Ready to Attack, Hurricanes Defensive Lineman Allen Bailey Passed Up the NFL Draft To Help His Teammates Improve on Last Season*, MIAMI HERALD ONLINE, July 26, 2010 (discussing projection of Miami defensive end Allen Bailey as a late first or early second round pick).

63. The best known draft projectors perhaps are ESPN's Mel Kiper and Todd McShay. However, their projections are prone to error as much as anyone else's. Famously, during the 2007 college football season McShay touted Kentucky quarterback, junior Andre Woodson, as one of the top players in the draft. It is believed that Woodson in part relied on McShay's projection in deciding to leave college early, only to be drafted in the sixth round and never to make an official NFL roster. *See* Mike Florio, *Locker Didn't Get a First-Round Grade From Advisory Committee*, NBC SPORTS PRO FOOTBALL TALK, Dec. 18, 2009, http://profootballtalk.nbcsports.com/2009/12/18/locker-didnt-get-a-first-round-grade-from-advisory-committee/.

64. *See* Chuck McGill, *Herd's Smith Wants To Play Holliday's Way*, CHARLESTON GAZETTE & DAILY MAIL (WV), Jan. 22, 2010, at 5B; Blair Kerkhoff, *OU's Peterson Dashes To NFL, Junior Forgoes Final Year After Rushing for Third-Most Yards in Sooners History*, KANSAS CITY STAR (MO), Jan. 16, 2007, at Cl.

65. DI MANUAL, *supra* note 14, § 12.2.4.2.3.

66. *See* Eric Bailey, *Jordan's TU Future Remains Unclear*, TULSA WORLD, Apr. 10, 2009, at Bl; Mike Griffith, *Hopson Makes It Clear: I'm Coming Back To Tennessee*, KNOXVILLE NEWS-SENTINEL, Apr. 16, 2010, at 503; Parrish Alford, *Ole Miss' White Will Test NBA Waters*, NORTHEAST MISSISSIPPI DAILY J. ONLINE, Apr. 10, 2010, http://www.nems360.

com/printer_friendly/7025796; Jerry Tipton, *Patterson Staying Put*, Lexington Herald-Leader Online (KY), May 9, 2009.

67. DI Manual, *supra* note 14, § 12.1.2.

68. For more information on the ESDI program, see NCAA.org, NCAA Exceptional Student-Athlete Disability Insurance Program, http://www.ncaa.org/wps/wcm/connect/ncaa/NCAA/About+The+NCAA/Budget+and+ Finances/Insurance/exceptional.html?p ageDesign=Printer+Friendly+General+Content+L ayout (last visited May 5, 2010) [hereinafter NCAA ESDI Program]. *See also* DI Manual, *supra* note 14, § 16.11.1.4; Glenn M. Wong & Chris Deubert, *The Legal and Business Aspects of Disability Insurance Policies in Professional and College Sports*, 17 Vill. Sports & Ent. L.J. 473 (2010).

69. *See generally* Wong & Deubert, *supra* note 68.

70. *See id.*

71. *Id.*

72. *Id.* at 488. Permanent total disability typically requires that the athlete be completely unable to perform their profession or sport for an entire twelve-month period after the initial injury.

73. *Id.* (citing NCAA ESDI Program).

74. *Id.* at 507.

75. *Id.*

76. *Id.*

77. *Id.*

78. *See id.* at 496–497.

79. *Id.*

80. *Id.*

81. As a demonstration of the ongoing problem in this area, noted sports attorney Bob Ruxin detailed many of the same concerns nearly thirty years ago. *See* Robert Ruxin, *Unsportsmanlike Conduct: The Student-Athlete, the NCAA, and Agents*, 8 J.C. & U.L. 347 (1982).

82. Runners can be defined as someone employed by an agent, typically a young person, whose job it is to become friendly with the student-athlete, potentially provide the student-athlete with cash, meals, clothes, or other gifts and ultimately steer the student-athlete towards the employing agent. *See* Chris Deubert, *What's a "Clean" Agent to Do? The Case for a Cause of Action Against a Players Association*, Vill. Sports & Ent. L. J. (*forthcoming*).

83. For breaches of fiduciary duties, see, e.g., Jones v. Childers, 18 F.3d 1899 (11th Cir. 1994); Lankford v. Irby, No. 04-2636, 2006 WL 2828548 (D.N.J. Sept. 29, 2006); Hillard v. Black, 125 F. Supp. 2d 1071 (N.D. Fla. 2000); Brown v. Woolf, 554 F. Supp. 1206 (S.D. Ind. 1983); In re Ekuban, No. 03-35869SAF-7, 2004 WL 1088340 (Bankr. N.D. Tex., Apr. 16, 2004). For fraud, see, e.g., Cuyahoga County Bar Ass'n v. Glenn, 649 N.E. 2d 1213 (Ohio 1995). For conflicts of interest, see, e.g., Detroit Lions, Inc. v. Argovitz, 580 F. Supp. 542 (E.D. Mich. 1984); *see also* Richard T. Karcher, *Solving Problems in the Player Representation Business: Unions Should Be The "Exclusive" Representatives of the Players*, 42 Willamette L. Rev. 737 (2006); Scott R. Rosner, *Conflicts of Interest and the Shifting Paradigm of Athlete Representation*, 11 UCLA Ent. L. Rev. 193 (2004). For unethical behavior, see Poston v. NFLPA, No. 02CV871, 2002 WL 31190142 (E.D. Va. Aug. 26, 2002); *see also* David S. Caudill, *Revisiting the Ethics of Representing Professional Athletes: Agents, "Attorney-Agents," Full-Service Agencies, and the Dream Team Model*, 3 Va. Sports & Ent.

L. J. 31 (2003); Stacey B. Evans, *Sports Agents: Ethical Representatives or Overly Aggressive Adversaries?*, 17 VILL. SPORTS & ENT. L. J. 91 (2010); Melissa Neiman, *Fair Game: Ethical Considerations in Negotiations by Sports Agents*, 9 TEX. REV. ENT. & SPORTS L. 123 (2007). For tortious interference with contractual relations, see Steinberg, Moorad & Dunn, Inc. v. Dunn, 136 Fed. Appx. 6 (9th Cir. 2005); Smith v. IMG Worldwide, Inc. 360 F. Supp. 2d 681 (E.D. Pa. 2005); Walters v. Fullwood, 675 F. Supp. 155 (S.D.N.Y. 1987); *see also* Timothy Davis, *Regulating the Athlete-Agent Industry: Intended and Unintended Consequences*, 42 WILLAMETTE L. REV. 781 (2006).

84. Only the NFLPA makes their Agent Regulations publicly available on their website. *See* NFL Players' Association Regulations Governing Contract Advisors, http://images. nflplayers.com/mediaResources/files/PDFs/SCAA/NFLPA_Regulations_Contract_ Advisors.pdf [hereinafter NFLPA Agent Regulations]. Other regulations can be viewed as a member of the Sports Lawyers Association at www.sportslaw.org, by contacting the respective players association or contacting the authors of this article.

85. For federal law, see Sports Agent Responsibility and Trust Act (SPARTA), 15 U.S.C.A. §§ 7801–7807 (2004). Some states have their own legislation, while 39 states have passed some form of the Uniform Athlete Agents Act. *See* NCAA.org,.FAQ on Uniform Athlete Agencts Act, http://www.ncaa.org/wps/wcm/connect/public/ncaa/resources/ latest+news/2010+new s+stories/july+latest+news/faq+on+uniform+athlete+agents+act (last visited Oct. 30, 2010).

86. *See* Deubert, *supra* note 82; *see also* Associated Press, *Report: State Agent Laws Unenforced*, ESPN.com, Aug. 17, 2010, http://sports.espn.go.com/ncaa/news/ story?id=5470067 (stating that more than half of the 42 states with sports agent laws have never revoked or suspended a single license, or invoked a penalty of any sort. "Likewise for the Federal Trade Commission, which in 2004 was given oversight authority by Congress.").

87. *See* Mike Florio, *Marketing Reps Mix It Up in Indy*, NBC SPORTS PRO FOOTBALL TALK, Feb. 27, 2010, http://profootballtalk.nbcsports.com/2010/02/27/marketing-reps- mix-it-up-inindy/; Scott Wolf, *Settlement in Bush's Civil Lawsuit Reached*, DAILY NEWS (LOS Angeles), Apr. 22, 2010, at C7.

88. *See generally* Karcher, *supra* note 83.

89. *See* Rick Alonzo, *Decker Playing Catch-Up: Ex-Gopher Hopes Foot Injury Won't Hurt Draft Stock*, ST. PAUL PIONEER PRESS (Minn.), Feb. 28, 2010, at C3; Tom Kowalski, *Breaking Through Michigan Players Put Talent on Display*, GRAND RAPIDS PRESS, Feb. 28, 2010, at C6; Ian R. Rapoport, *Combine Notebook: McKenzie, Murphy Talk Things Over*, BOSTON HERALD, Mar. 1, 2010, at 66; John Vellante, *Woburn's McLaughlin Gathers Postseason Honors*, BOSTON GLOBE, Jan. 21, 2010, at 5.

90. *See* Albert Breer, *Michael Johnson's Complex Gets Into NFL Draft Game*, DALLAS MORNING NEWS ONLINE, Feb. 28, 2008, http://www.dallasnews.com/sharedcontent/dws/ spt/football/nfl/stories/022808dnspoc ombine.3391566.html; Dale Robertson, *Sports Training is His Business, Danny Arnold's Performance Programs Have a Reputation For Preparing NFL Hopefuls for the Combine, But He'll Work With Anyone Who is Dedicated*, HOUS. CHRON., Feb. 20, 2008, at 1; John Booth, *Training Day NFL Draft Prospects Flock to Duo's Euclid Complex to Prep for the League Combine*, CRAIN'S CLEV. BUS. NEWS, Feb. 20, 2006, at 1; Carter Strickland, *Former Sooners Prepping for Combine, Daily Drills Can Help for Players as They Ready for Draft*, DAILY OKLAHOMAN, Feb. 24, 2005, at 3C.

91. DI MANUAL, *supra* note 14, § 12.1.2.

92. These high school student-athletes need guidance during their discussions with the professional team that has drafted them to properly determine whether or not they want to turn professional or instead enroll in college. However, the use of an agent can jeopardize the eligibility they are considering retaining.

93. The standard practice is for agents to be paid based on a percentage of the contract they negotiated for the player. All union regulations dictate that the agent is to be paid only when the player is paid. It is also important to point out that there can be significant sums of money earned by players pursuant to the collective bargaining agreement, such as performance bonuses and playoff game compensation.

94. From 1990 to 2010, average salaries have risen: 447% in MLB to an average of $3.27 million; 414% in the NFL to an average of $1.8 million; 609% in the NBA to an average of $5.85 million; and 638% in the NHL to an average of $2 million. See GLENN M. WONG, ESSENTIALS OF SPORTS LAW, Ex. 1.2 (4th ed. 2010).

95. See Associated Press, Super Bowl XLIV Mashes M-A-S-H: Saints Victory Over Colts Most-Watched Program in TV History, CHARLESTON GAZETTE & DAILY MAIL (WV), Feb. 9, 2010, at 4B (describing how the 2010 Super Bowl was the most watched program in U.S. television history).

96. The NFLPA limits an agent's compensation to three percent of the player's contract. See NFLPA Agent Regulations, supra note 84, § 4(B). The NBA Players' Association limits an agent's compensation to 4%. Neither the MLBPA or NHLPA limits an agent's compensation, instead, honoring the free market system, they work to obtain on behalf of their constituents. See MLB.com, Major League Baseball Players Association: Frequently Asked Questions, http://mlbplayers.mlb.com/pa/info/faq.jsp#negotiating (last visited July 26, 2010). To view a Standard Representation Agreement between an NFLPA Certified Contract Advisor and player, see NFLPA Agent Regulations, supra note 84, D-1. Other standard agent-player agreements can be viewed as a member of the Sports Lawyers Association at http://www.sportslaw.org, by contacting the respective players association, or contacting the authors of this article.

97. In the NFL, the agent competition is arguably at its fiercest. As of the start of the 2010 NFL season, 773 agents were certified by the NFLPA, but only 338 (43.7%) of them had clients. E-mail from Caitlin Reddinger, Administrative Assistant, Salary Cap & Agent Administration, NFL Players' Association, to Glenn M. Wong, Professor, University of Massachusetts Department of Sport Management (Mar. 23, 2010, 13:57:00 EDT) (on file with author); see also NFLPA Player-Agent Report (on file with NFLPA).

98. The NFLPA Standard Representation Agreement provides a section requiring the agreed upon commission percentage to be checked off, ranging from 1% to 3% in half-percent increments with an "other" option as well. See NFLPA Agent Regulations, supra note 84, D-2.

99. See Mullen, supra note 24.

100. Three days prior to the 2009 Sugar Bowl, featuring sixth-ranked University of Utah versus fourth-ranked University of Alabama, Alabama announced that star left tackle Andre Smith was suspended for the game due to contact with agent Alvin Keels in violation of team rules. See Mr. College Football with Tony Barnhart, Smith's Suspension Will Be Good for Alabama, http://blogs.ajc.com/barnhart-college-football/ (December 30, 2008, 7:05:00 EDT).

101. See, e.g., NCAA, YOUR PATH TO THE STUDENT-ATHLETE EXPERIENCE (2010), available at http://www.ncaapublications.com/p-4193-2010-11-your-path-to-the-student-athlete-experience-pack-of-100-due-late-summerearly-fall-2010.aspx; NCAA, GUIDE TO

THE COLLEGE-BOUND STUDENT-ATHLETE, (2007–2008), *available at* http://www.willamette.edu/athletics/prospective_students/2007-08_cbsa.pdf; NCAA, A CAREER IN PROFESSIONAL ATHLETICS: A GUIDE FOR MAKING THE TRANSITION, (2004), *available at* http://www.ncaapublications.com/p-3957-a-career-in-professional-athletics-a-guide-for-making-the-transition.aspx.

102. However, NFLPA Regulations do not permit agents to talk to student-athletes until after a prospective player's last regular-season college or conference championship game (excluding any post-season bowl game) or December 1, whichever is later, of the college football season immediately prior to the year in which such prospective player would be eligible to apply for the NFL Draft. *See* NFLPA Agent Regulations, *supra* note 84, § 3B(30) (a); Mike Florio, *NFLPA Tweaks Junior Rule, But Doesn't Go Far Enough*, NBC SPORTS, Mar. 18, 2009, http://profootballtalk.nbcsports.com/2009/03/18/nflpa-tweaks-junior-rule-but-doesnt-go-far-enough/; Mike Florio, *Agents Learn of Revision to "Junior Rule,"* NBC SPORTS, Mar. 27, 2009, http://profootballtalk.nbcsports.com/2009/03/27/agents-learn-of-revision-to-junior-rule/. None of the other agent regulations have a rule as to when agents can contact student-athletes.

103. DI MANUAL, *supra* note 14, § 12.3.

104. ROBERT RUXIN, AN ATHLETE'S GUIDE TO AGENTS 160 (4th ed., Jones & Bartlett Publ. 2003).

105. *See* NCAA DI MANUAL § 12.3.4 (1998–99) (citing the section titled "Professional Sports Counseling Panels"); *see also* HOWARD L. GANZ & JEFFREY L. KESSLER, UNDERSTANDING BUSINESS & LEGAL ASPECTS OF THE SPORTS INDUSTRY 161 (Practicing Law Institute 2001).

106. *See* GANZ & KESSLER, *supra* note 105, at 161.

107. *See* DI MANUAL, *supra* note 14, §§ 12.3.4.1, 12.3.4.2.

108. *Id.* § 12.3.4.2.

109. *Id.* § 12.3.4.

110. *See* Albert R. Breer, *Taunton Native Happy to Stay on His Raven Perch*, BOSTON GLOBE, May 23, 2010,http://www.boston.com/sports/football/articles/2010/05/23/taunton_native_happy_to_stay_on_his_raven_perch/?page=4 (noting that Boston College is the only school of its kind offering guidance outside the offices of the individual athletic teams).

111. In 2009, NFL rookies signed contracts with a total value of $1.2 billion, with $600 million in total guaranteed. *See* Liz Mullen & Brandon McClung, *NFL, Union Differ on Rookie Wage Scale*, SPORTS BUS. J., Apr. 26, 2010, www.sportsbusinessjournal.com/article/65536.

112. *See* NCAA's Legislative Services Database, *supra* note 21.

113. *See* Clarett v. Nat'l Football League, 306 F. Supp. 2d 379 (S.D.N.Y. 2004). Clarett argued that the NFL's draft eligibility rule unreasonably restrained trade in violation of Section 1 of the Sherman Act. The district court agreed, finding that because the eligibility rule was in the NFL Bylaws and not the CBA, it was not protected by the non-statutory labor exemption. *Id.* The Court of Appeals for the Second Circuit granted the NFL's motion to stay the district court's decision (which temporarily granted Clarett eligibility) just days before the 2004 draft and eventually reversed the district court, upholding the league's eligibility rules. *See* Clarett v. Nat'l Football League, 369 F.3d 124 (2d Cir. 2004). The Second Circuit Court found that the NFL's eligibility rule fell within the scope of the nonstatutory exemption and the fact that the NFL and the players' union did not bargain

over the rule did not exclude it from the scope of the nonstatutory exemption. *Id.* In the 2006 extension of the NFL CBA, the NFL and NFLPA explicitly negotiated the eligibility clause into the CBA to help prevent any further legal challenges. Clarett was suspended for the 2003 season for receiving improper benefits and then lying about it to NCAA investigators. See *OSU Will Wait Until Spring to Seek Clarett Return,* Cincinnati Post, Sept. 29, 2003, at C6. In the 2005 NFL Draft, he was chosen as the last pick of the third round by the Denver Broncos. Clarett was cut by the Broncos in training camp, failed to sign elsewhere, and has since encountered extensive legal trouble resulting in lengthy periods of incarceration. See Associated Press, *Clarett Agrees to Plea Deal, Will Serive 3½ Years,* Sept. 20, 2006, http://sports.espn.go.com/nfl/news/story?id=2593068.

114. See Jill Painter, *NCAA Turns Away USC's Williams; Top Receiver's Bid to Regain Eligibility Denied; Career Over,* Daily News (L.A.), Aug. 27, 2004, at S1. In the 2005 NFL Draft, Williams was chosen as the 10th overall pick by the Detroit Lions. Williams played three years in the league with three different teams, catching a total of forty-four balls. Former USC head coach and current Seattle Seahawks coach Pete Carroll gave Williams a comeback attempt prior to the 2010 season and Williams successfully made the team. See Arash Markazi, *The Comeback of Mike Williams,* Oct. 23, 2010, http://sports.espn.go.com/los-angeles/nfl/news/story?id=5696566.

115. See John Clay, *Getting Legal Help Not a Good Thing for UK, Morris Case Dragging Out,* Lexington Herald Leader, Nov. 16, 2005, at Cl; The Beat, *Wildcats' Morris Has Penalty Reduced,* Orlando Sentinel, Dec. 16, 2005, at D5. Publicly Morris stated "in exploring my NBA options I made poor choices. Those choices included accepting bad advice while putting distance between me and my coaches and teammates." Jerry Tipton, *Morris Will Be Back on Jan. 10, Confidential Evidence and Fax Change Season,* Lexington Herald-Leader, Dec. 16, 2005, at Al. Morris was deemed to be a free agent by the NBA. Morris eventually returned to Kentucky for his junior year, but in March 2007, five days after his team had lost in the NCAA Men's Basketball Tournament, Morris left school and signed a two-year, $1.6 million dollar contract with the New York Knicks. See *Knicks Sign Kentucky Center Morris to 2-year Deal,* Mar. 24, 2007, http://sports.espn.go.com/nba/news/story?id=2809958.

116. Oliver v. Natl. Collegiate Athletic Assn., 920 N.E.2d 203 (Ohio Com.Pl. 2009).

117. *Id.* at 207.

118. NBA CBA, *supra* note 33, Art. X.

119. See NBA Draft History, www.nbadraft.net/nba_draft_history/index.html (last visited May 4, 2010).

120. There have been some highly publicized attempts to circumvent the rule. First, Brandon Jennings, a California teenager who failed to score sufficiently on his SAT to attend the University of Arizona, played one season of professional basketball in Italy before being drafted 10th overall in the 2010 NBA Draft by the Milwaukee Bucks. See Gary D'Amato, *Bucks' Diminutive Point Guard Brandon Jennings Has Overcome Big Obstacles to Reach the NBA,* Milwaukee J. & Sentinel Online, Nov. 18, 2009, http://www.jsonline.com/sports/bucks/67381447.html. While Jennings had a fantastic rookie season with the Bucks, averaging 20.8 points per game, the story of Jeremy Tyler serves as a cautionary tale. Tyler, also from California, chose to skip his senior year of high school to play at the professional level in Israel. After a lackluster performance, averaging just 2.1 points per game and displaying a disappointing work ethic, Tyler left his team mid-season and returned home to San Diego. Whether he ever plays in the NBA remains to be seen. See

Howard Schneider, *In Israel, Jeremy Tyler's NBA Dreams Come Back Down to Earth*, Wash. Post, Feb. 19, 2010, at D4.

121. *See* NBA Draft History, *supra* note 119. The three #1 overall picks were Greg Oden to the Portland Trailblazers in 2007, Derrick Rose to the Chicago Bulls in 2008, and John Wall to the Washington Wizards in 2010. Thirty-one of the thirty-six players were first round picks and sixteen of them were Top Ten selections.

122. *See* Rick Karcher, *The NCAA's Regulations Related to the Use of Agents in the Sport of Baseball: Are the Rules Detrimental to the Best Interest of the Amateur Athlete?*, 7 Vand. J. Ent. L. & Prac. 215 (2005); Brandon D. Morgan, Oliver v. NCAA: *NCAA's No Agent Rule Called Out, But Remains Safe*, 17 Sports L. J. 303 (2010).

123. *See* Nat'l Collegiate Athletic Ass'n v. Tarkanian, 488 U.S. 179 (1988). *But see* Cohane v. Nat'l Collegiate Athletic Ass'n, 215 Fed. Appx. 13 (2d Cir. 2007). In *Cohane,* the Court of Appeals for the Second Circuit held that the NCAA was a state actor when it conducted an investigation of a state school (the University of Buffalo). The Court differentiated the case from the Supreme Court's 1988 decision in *Tarkanian* in that UNLV had disputed all of the NCAA's charges against Tarkanian such that the NCAA could not have been participating in joint activity with the state. In Cohane's case, Buffalo accepted the NCAA's allegations and immediately forced Cohane's resignation. The Supreme Court of the United States denied the NCAA's petition for review.

124. *See* Bianchi, *supra* note 13; Fitt, *supra* note 13; McCormick, *supra* note 13; Lazaroff, *supra* note 13.

125. A notable example of this problem is legendary Florida quarterback Tim Tebow. *See* Mike Florio, *Urban Feels the Heat On His Failure to Develop Tebow*, NBC Sports Pro Football Talk, Mar. 27, 2010, http://profootballtalk.nbcsports.com/2010/03/27/urban-feels-the-heat-on-his-failure-to-develop-tebow/. During Tim Tebow's first three years, Florida won the BCS National Championship twice (2007 and 2009). Nevertheless, it was a hotly debated topic over whether Tebow possessed the skills to succeed in the NFL. Many felt that Florida coach Urban Meyer, who signed a six-year $24 million contract extension in 2009 despite having four years left on his existing deal, owed it to Tebow to augment his spread offense, which was poorly suited to allow Tebow a chance to improve his professional skill set. This never happened and even though Tebow was ultimately a first-round pick in the 2010 NFL Draft, his professional prospects are highly debatable.

126. *See* Dustin Dow, *Much Pain, No Gain?*, Cincinnati Enquirer, July 1, 2007, at C1 (providing that average NFL career is about 3.5 years); *see also* Rob Hiaasen, *Getting All the Breaks; As Head Trainer, Bill Tessendorf Works to Get Sidelined Ravens Back in the Game*, Baltimore Sun, Dec. 28, 2002, at D1 (emphasizing difficulty in keeping some players on field); Mark Montieth, *NBA Draft—High Hopes*, Indianapolis Star, June 25, 2006, at 1C (explaining that the average NBA career is about four years); David Parkinson, *When the Lights Go Out*, Globe and Mail (Canada), Sept. 18, 2008, at 17 (discussing NHL players' difficulty in finances); *Salary Inflation Caused NHL Troubles*, Buffalo News, Nov. 21, 2004, at C4 (explaining that the average NHL career is about five years); Sam Roberts, *Just How Long Does the Average Career Last?*, N.Y. Times, July 15, 2007, at SP6 (concluding that the average MLB career is about 5.6 years); Desmond Ryan, *Basketball Dreamers Come Up Against Reality*, Philadelphia Inquirer, Dec. 31, 2005, at C1 (discussing reality that NBA careers are often short).

127. *See* Ray Hagar, *Wealth Management Firm Counsels Bighorns Athletes on Fiscal Planning*, RENO-GAZETTE-J. ONLINE, Dec. 30, 2009, http://www.rgj.com/; *see also* Pablo S. Torre, *How (and Why) Athletes Go Broke*, SPORTS ILLUSTRATED, Mar. 23, 2009, http://sportsillustrated.cnn.com/vault/article/magazine/MAG1153364/index.htm.

128. *See* Atwater v. Nat'l Football League Players Ass'n, No. 1:06-CV-1510-JEC, 2009 WL 3254925 (N.D. Ga., Mar. 27, 2009) (providing that six former NFL players unsuccessfully claimed that the NFLPA breached its duty to them by negligently performing background checks on certain financial advisors who participated in the NFLPA's Financial Advisors Program); Timothy Davis, *Regulating the Athlete-Agent Industry: Intended and Unintended Consequences*, 42 WILLAMETTE L. REV. 781, 783 (2006) (discussing several players defrauded by financial advisors, including Scottie Pippen); *see also* Tom Reed, *Jackets Try To Avoid Financial Slipups That Often Beset Athletes*, COLUMBUS DISPATCH (OHIO), Nov. 11, 2009, at 01A (listing players defrauded by financial advisors, including NHL players Sergei Federov and Michael Peca).

129. *See* Reed, *supra* note 128; Hagar, *supra* note 127. The two articles discuss the financial failures of former professional athletes. First, former Boston Celtics player Antoine Walker has been forced to file for bankruptcy as a result of gambling debts despite having earned more than $110 million in a twelve-year career. Additionally, former Knicks and Warriors' star Latrell Sprewell, who made an estimated $50 million to $90 million in a thirteen-year career, lost a $5.4 million mansion and $1.5 million yacht to foreclosure. Lastly, former Celtics star Vin Baker, who made $90 million dollars in a fourteen-year NBA career, saw his home and business go under because foreclosures.

130. *See* Jaramillo, *supra* note 56; Mills, *supra* note 56.

131. *See* Mills, *supra* note 56. Even if a football student-athlete is taking the required number of classes each semester to graduate on time (which is rare), he will rarely attend class during the spring semester of his senior year as he prepares for the NFL Combine. It is then up to the athlete to complete his coursework in the summer or online.

132. For more information on the NCAA's Academic Progress Reports (APR) and Graduation Success Rates (GSR), see NCAA.org, NCAA's Academic Progress Reports (APR) and Graduation Success Rates (GSR), www.ncaa.org (follow "Academics" hyperlink; then follow "How Academic Reform Is Measured" hyperlink) (last visited Oct. 10, 2010).

133. *See* NCAA.org, NCAA Academic Reform, www.ncaa.org/wps/portal (search "Academic Reform"; then follow "NCAA Academic Reform—NCAA.org" hyperlink) (last visited Oct. 10, 2010).

134. *See* NCAA.org, 2009 Graduation Success Rate Report, www.ncaa.org/ (follow "Resources" hyperlink; then follow "Research" hyperlink; then follow "Graduation Rates" hyperlink; then follow "2009 NCAA Division I GSR School Data" hyperlink; then follow "All Division I") (last visited Oct 10, 2010).

135. Letter from Rep. Bill Thomas, Chairman, House Comm. on Ways and Means, to Myles Brand, President, NCAA (Oct. 2, 2006), *available at* www.usatoday.com/sports/college/2006-10-05-congress-ncaa-tax-letter_x.htm.

136. *See* NCAA.org, 2009 Graduation Success Rate Report, www.ncaa.org (follow "Resources" hyperlink; then follow "Research" hyperlink; then follow "Graduation Rates " hyperlink; then follow "Overview of Division I Graduation Success Rate/Division II Academic Success Rate" hyperlink) (last visited Oct 10, 2010). It is also important to note

that the NCAA includes students who transfer from one school and finish at another while the Department of Education does not. *See* Gabriel A. Morgan, *No More Playing Favorites: Reconsidering the Conclusive Congressional Presumption that Intercollegiate Athletics are Substantially Related to Educational Purposes*, 81 S. CAL. L. REV. 149, 175 n. 184 (2007).

137. *See* Jeffrey Isaac, *Professional Athletes and Violent Crime*, THE DAILY TRANSCRIPT (San Diego), Aug. 1, 2006, www.sddt.com/Law/lawyerinbluejeans.cfm?PublicationDate=2006-08-01.

138. 920 N.E. 2d 203 (Ohio Com. Pl. 2009).

139. *See* DI MANUAL, *supra* note 14, § 12.3.2 (permitting student-athletes to secure "advice from a lawyer concerning a proposed professional sports contract.").

140. *Oliver,* 920 N.E. 2d 203.

141. Scott Boras is one of the most successful sports agents ever: his clients have included Greg Maddux, Kevin Brown, Alex Rodriguez, Mark Teixeira, Stephen Strasburg, Bernie Williams, Carlos Beltran, Johnny Damon, Daisuke Matsuzaka, Barry Zito, and many more. He has negotiated approximately $4 billion in guaranteed compensation for his clients. *See* Steve Serby, *Serby's Sunday Q & A With. . . Scott Boras*, N.Y. POST, Dec. 6, 2009, at 82.

142. *Oliver,* 920 N.E. 2d at 207.

143. *See* DI MANUAL, *supra* note 14, § 12.3.2 (permitting student-athletes to "[secure] advice from a lawyer concerning a proposed professional sports contract"). *But see* DI MANUAL, *supra* note 14, § 12.3.2.1 (stating that "[a] lawyer may not be present during discussions of a contract offer with a professional organization or have any direct contact (in person, by telephone or by mail) with a professional sports organization on behalf of the individual. A lawyer's presence during such discussions is considered representation by an agent.").

144. *Oliver,* 920 N.E. 2d at 207.

145. *Id.*

146. *Id.*

147. *Id.*

148. *Id.* at 208.

149. Oliver v. Nat'l Collegiate Athletic Ass'n, 920 N.E. 2d 203, 208 (Ohio Com. Pl. 2009).

150. *Id.*

151. *Id.* at 207.

152. *See* Liz Mullen, *OSU P Andy Oliver Files Suit Against NCAA, Former Advisor*, SPORTS BUS. J., July 2, 2008, www.sportsbusinessdaily.com/article/122046.

153. *Oliver,* 920 N.E. 2d at 215–216.

154. *Id.*

155. *Id.*

156. *See* DI MANUAL, supra note 14, § 19.7.

157. *See* John Seewer, *NCAA, Oliver Settle Out of Court*, DAILY OKLAHOMAN, Oct. 9, 2009, at 3C.

158. Oliver received a $1.495 million signing bonus and a minor league contract. *See* Steve Kornacki, *Tiger Notebook,* SAGINAW NEWS (Mich.), Aug. 20, 2009, at B3.

159. *See* Wong, Skillman & Deubert, *supra* note 21; NCAA's Academic Progress Reports (APR) and Graduation Success Rates (GSR), *supra* note 132.

160. The "death penalty" "is applicable to an institution, if within a five-year period, the following conditions exist: (a) following the announcement of the major case, a major

violation occurs, and (b) the second violation occurred within five years of the starting date of the penalty assessed in the first case. The second major case does not have to be in the same sport as the previous case to affect the second sport." *See* NCAA.org, Frequently Asked Questions about the NCAA Enforcement Process, http://www.ncaa. org/wps/portal/!ut/p/c4/04_SB8K8xLLM9MSSzPy8xBz9CP0os3gjX29   XJydDRwP_ YHcDA08Df89AZwNHQwMLQ_2CbEdFANWftoY!/ (last visited Oct. 10, 2010). The "death penalty" has only been used once, on the Southern Methodist University football program in 1987, though the team didn't actually play again until 1989. *See* Nakia Hogan, *SMU Can't Escape Death Penalty; Twenty Years Later, It Still Has Overwhelming Effect on Program*, TIMES-PICAYUNE (New Orleans), Oct. 19, 2007, at S1.

161. *See* Nakia Hogan, *Bush Probe Results in Big Sanctions for USC, Saints RB Alleged To Have Received Money During College Career*, TIMES-PICAYUNE (New Orleans), June 11, 2010, at D1.

162. *See* NCAA.org, University of Southern California Public Infractions Report, https://webl.ncaa.org/LSDBi/exec/homepage (last visited Oct. 10, 2010); *see also* Brent Schrotenboer, *USC Appeals Penalties It Says Are 'Too Severe'*, SAN DIEGO UNION-TRIB., June 26, 2010, at D5.

163. Between 1980 and 2000, the percentage of Division I institutions that were censured, sanctioned, or put on probation for major violations of the NCAA rules decreased only from 54% to 52%. *See* Morgan, *supra* note 136, at 178 (citing KNIGHT FOUNDATION COMMISSION ON INTERCOLLEGIATE ATHLETICS, A CALL TO ACTION: RECONNECTING COLLEGE SPORTS AND HIGHER EDUCATION 8-9 (2001), *available at* www.knightcommission.org).

164. Thirty-four states and the District of Columbia provide for a cause of action by the institution against a former student-athlete, in addition to the agent. *See* ALA. CODE § 8-26A-16 (2010); ARIZ. REV. STAT. ANN. § 15-1775 (2010); ARK. CODE ANN. § 17-16-116 (2010); COLO. REV. STAT. § 23-16-215 (2010); CONN. GEN. STAT. § 20-5590 (2010); DEL. CODE ANN. tit. 24 § 5416 (2010); D.C. CODE ANN. § 47-2887.15 (2010); GA. CODE ANN. § 43-4A-18 (2010); HAW. REV. STAT. ANN. § 481E-15 (2008); IDAHO CODE ANN. § 54-4816 (2010); 225 ILL. COMP. STAT. ANN. 401/185 (2010); IND. CODE ANN. § 25-5.2-2-13 (2010); IOWA CODE § 9A.116 (2010); KAN. STAT. ANN. § 44-1530 (2010); KY. REV. STAT. ANN. § 164.6929 (2010); MD. CODE ANN., BUS. REG. § 4-415 (2010); MINN. STAT. § 81A.16 (2010); MISS. CODE ANN. § 73-42-31 (2010); MO. REV. STAT. § 436.260 (2010); NEV. REV. STAT. ANN. § 398.490 (2010); N.H. REV. STAT. ANN. § 332-J:14 (2010); N.H. GEN. STAT. § 78C-100 (2010); N.D. CENT. CODE § 9-15.1-15 (2010); OKLA. STAT. ANN. tit. 70 § 821.96 (2010); OR. REV. STAT. § 702.057 (2010); 5 PA. CONS. STAT § 3314 (2010); R.I. GEN.LAWS § 5-74.1-16 (2010); S.C. CODE ANN. § 59-102-160 (2009); S.D. CODIFIED LAWS § 59-10-16 (2010); TENN. CODE ANN. § 49-7-2137 (2010); TEX. OCC. CODE.ANN. § 2051.551 (2010); UTAH CODE ANN. § 15-9-116 (2010); WASH. REV. CODE § 19.225.120 (2010); W. VA. CODE § 30-39-16 (2010); WYO. STAT. ANN § 33-44-113 (2010). Of the thirty-nine states that have adopted the UAAA, only five do not provide for a cause of action against the student-athlete. *See* FLA. STAT. § 468.4562 (2010); LA. REV. STAT. ANN. § 4:426 (2010); N.Y. GEN. BUS. LAW § 899 (2010); OHIO REV. CODE ANN. § 4771.01 (2010); WIS. STAT. § 440.99 (2010). Agent legislation in California and Michigan does not provide for a cause of action against the student-athlete. The remaining states have no legislation concerning athlete-agents. *See, e.g.*, CAL. BUS. & PROF. CODE § 18895 (2010); MICH. COMP. LAWS § 750.411e (2010).

165. For more on the availability of this option, see Tim Epstein, *Show Me the Sanctions!: More Scandals, the Uniform Athlete Agent Act, and an Institution's Cause of Action Against Agents and Former Players*, SPORTS LAW BLOG, http://sports-law.blogspot.com/2010/07/show-mesanctions-more-scandals-uniform.html (July 20, 2010, 16:00:00 EST).

166. *See* Nat'l Collegiate Athletics Ass'n v. Bd. of Regents, 468 U.S. 85, 85 (1984); *see also* Bianchi, *supra* note 13; Fitt, *supra* note 13; Lazaroff, *supra* note 13; McCormick, *supra* note 13.

167. *See* NCAA.org, 2009–2010 NCAA Budgeted Revenues, http://www.ncaa.org/wps/wcm/connect/public/ncaa/answers/nine+points+to+consider_one (follow the "Graphic" hyperlink) (last visited Oct. 10, 2010). Approximately 90% of that total was derived from the CBS contract for the men's basketball tournament. In April of 2010, CBS and the NCAA reached a new fourteen-year, $10.8 billion deal. *See* John Ourand & Michael Smith, *NCAA's Money-Making Matchup, How CBS, Turner Made the Numbers Work in $10.8 Billion Deal*, SPORTS BUS. J., Apr. 26, 2010, www.sportsbusinessjournal.com/article/65533.

168. *See* Letter from Rep. Bill Thomas, *supra* note 135; Morgan, *supra* note 136. *See also* John D. Colombo, *The NCAA, Tax Exemption and College Athletics*, 2010 U. ILL. L. REV. 109 (2010); Brett T. Smith, *The Tax-Exempt Status of the NCAA: Has the IRS Fumbled the Ball?*, 17 SPORTS L. J. 117 (2010).

169. *See* Christian Dennie, *White Out Full Grant-In-Aid: An Antitrust Action the NCAA Cannot Afford to Lose*, 7 VA. SPORTS & ENT. L. J. 97 (2007); Daniel E. Lazaroff, *The NCAA in Its Second Century: Defender of Amateurism or Antitrust Recidivist?*, 86 OR. L. REV. 329 (2007); C. Paul Rogers III, *The Quest for Number One in College Football: The Revised Bowl Championship Series, Antitrust, and the Winner Take All Syndrome*, 18 MARQ. SPORTS L. REV. 285 (2008).

170. *See* Aaron Brooks, *Exploring Student-Athlete Compensation: Why the NCAA Cannot Afford to Leave Athletes Uncompensated*, 34 J. C. & U. L. 747 (2008); Robert A. McCormick & Amy Christian McCormick, *The Myth of the Student-Athlete: The College Athlete as Employee*, 81 WASH. L. REV. 71 (2006); Brian C. Root, *How the Promises of Riches in Collegiate Athletics Lead to Compromised Long-Term Health of Student-Athletes: Why and How the NCAA Should Protect Its Student Athletes' Health*, 19 HEALTH MATRIX 279 (2009).

171. *See generally* NCAA.org, NCAA Budgets and Finances, http://www.ncaa.org/wps/portal/ncaahome?WCM_GLOBAL_CONTEXT=/ncaa/NCAA/About+The+NCAA/Budget+and+Finances/ (last visited Oct. 10, 2010). From this page, you can view the NCAA's budget, revenues, expenses, and revenue distribution amounts. The NCAA gives approximately $103 million in scholarships, $49 million annually in student assistance and $20 million in academic enhancement. Approximately $154 million is distributed to the conferences via the basketball fund. *Id.* (follow the "Current Revenue Distribution Plan" hyperlink).

172. *See* DI MANUAL, *supra* note 14, § 12.01.2.

173. Prior to the NFL Draft, players must take a Wonderlic general intelligence exam and also are interviewed by interesting teams. It has become common practice in the NFL for teams to ask off-beat or even inappropriate questions to test the player's ability to handle adversity. Prior to the 2010 NFL Draft, Miami Dolphins General Manager Jeff Ireland asked Oklahoma State wide receiver Dez Bryant if his mother was a prostitute—for which he later apologized. *See* Gregg Rosenthal, *Jeff Ireland Apologizes To Dez Bryant*, NBC SPORTS PRO FOOTBALL TALK, Apr. 27, 2010, http://profootballtalk.nbcsports.com/2010/04/27/jeff-ireland-apologizes-to-dez-bryant/. Skepticism is raised as to why these

type of pre-employment questions are acceptable in the NFL but not in the general workforce. *See* Mike Florio, *Ken Herock Says No Question Is Off Limits During Pre-Draft Interviews*, NBC SPORTS PRO FOOTBALL TALK, Apr. 29, 2010, http://profootballtalk.nbc-sports.com/2010/04/29/ken-herock-says-no-question-is-off-limits-during-pre-draft-interviews/.

174. The following players have all been given suspensions ranging from six games to a full season or more for various types of illegal and inappropriate conduct: "Michael Vick, Adam 'Pacman' Jones, Tank Johnson, Chris Henry, Donte Stallworth, Ricky Manning, Joey Porter[,] Plaxico Burress and Ben Roethlisberger." *See* D. Orlando Ledbetter, *QB Penalty 'Unprecedented,'* ATLANTA J.–CONST., Apr. 22, 2010, at C1.

175. Under the National Labor Relations Act, certain topics are mandatory subjects of negotiation between employers and employees, including "wages, hours, and other terms and conditions of employment." 29 U.S.C.A. § 158(d) (West 2010). Courts have generally held that disciplinary rules are mandatory subjects of bargaining. *See* Electri-Flex Co. v. NLRB, 570 F. 2d 1327 (7th Cir. 1978); Int'l Bd. of Teamsters, Local No. 320 v. City of Minneapolis, 225 N.W. 2d 254 (Minn. 1975); *see also* Matthew J. Parlow, *Professional Sports League Commissioners' Authority and Collective Bargaining*, 11 TEX. REV. ENT. & SPORTS L. 179, 197–198 (2010).

176. In January 2010, in preparation for negotiations for the CBA set to expire in March 2011, the NFL launched nfllabor.com to disseminate its views on the ongoing labor situation. *See generally* NFLLabor.com, How We Arrived at This Point in NFL Labor, http://nfllabor.com/2010/01/24/81/ (last visited Oct. 10, 2010).

177. *See* Hogan, *supra* note 161.

178. Rose, who led the Memphis Tigers to the NCAA Championship game in 2007–08 (his only season in college), had his SAT score invalidated by the Educational Testing Service. For this and other violations Memphis was forced to vacate its record season and forfeit $615,000 in NCAA Tournament revenue. *See* Dan Wolken, *University of Memphis: NCAA Rules Violation Decision/Not A Banner Day—NCAA Denies Tigers' Appeal as Case Involving Rose Comes to Close*, COMM. APPEAL (Memphis), Mar. 23, 2010, at A1.

179. *See* Wood v. Nat'l Basketball Ass'n, 809 F. 2d 954, 960 (2d Cir. 1987) (citing 29 U.S.C. § 152(3)); *see also* Fibreboard Paper Prod. Corp. v. NLRB, 379 U.S. 203, 210-15 (1964); Time-O-Matic, Inc. v. NLRB, 264 F.2d 96, 99 (7th Cir. 1959); John Hancock Mut. Life Ins. Co. v. NLRB, 191 F.2d 483, 485 (D.C. Cir. 1951).

180. For more information on issues related to this process, see Rick Karcher, *Fundamental Fairness in Union Regulation of Sports Agents*, 40 CONN. L. REV. 355 (2007).

181. *See* NCAA.org, AQ on Uniform Athlete Agencts Act, http://www.ncaa.org/wps/wcm/connect/public/ncaa/resources/latest+news/2010+new s+stories/july+latest+news/faq+on+uniform+athlete+agents+act (last visited Oct. 30, 2010); *see also* GLENN M. WONG, ESSENTIALS OF SPORTS LAW § 12.7 (4th ed. 2010).

182. Sports Agent Responsibility and Trust Act, 15 U.S.C.A. §§ 7801–7807 (West 2004); *see also* Sports Agent Responsibility and Trust Act: Hearing on H.R. 361 Before the Subcomm. on Commercial and Admin. Law of the H. Comm. on the Judiciary, 108th Cong. 4 (2003); John A. Gray, *Sports Agent's Liability After SPARTA?*, 6 VA. SPORTS & ENT. L. J. 141 (2006).

183. The UAAA defines an "athlete agent" as:

an individual who enters into an agency contract with a student-athlete or, directly or indirectly, recruits or solicits a student-athlete to enter into an agency contract.

The term includes an individual who represents to the public that the individual is an athlete agent. The term does not include a spouse, parent, sibling, [or] grandparent[, or guardian] of the student-athlete or an individual acting solely on behalf of a professional sports team or professional sports organization.

UAAA, *supra* note 181, § 2(2). SPARTA uses a substantially similar definition. *See* 15 U.S.C.A. § 7801(2).

184. The UAAA states that:

(a) An athlete agent, with the intent to induce a student-athlete to enter into an agency contract, may not: (1) give any materially false or misleading information or make a materially false promise or representation; (2) furnish anything of value to a student-athlete before the student-athlete enters into the agency contract; or (3) furnish anything of value to any individual other than the student-athlete or another registered athlete agent. (b) An athlete agent may not intentionally: (1) initiate contact with a student-athlete unless registered under this [Act]; (2) refuse or fail to retain or permit inspection of the records required to be retained by Section 13; (3) fail to register when required by Section 4; (4) provide materially false or misleading information in an application for registration or renewal of registration; (5) predate or postdate an agency contract; or (6) fail to notify a student-athlete before the student-athlete signs or otherwise authenticates an agency contract for a particular sport that the signing or authentication may make the student-athlete ineligible to participate as a student-athlete in that sport.

UAAA, *supra* note 181, § 14. SPARTA states that:

It is unlawful for an athlete agent to—(1) directly or indirectly recruit or solicit a student athlete to enter into an agency contract, by—(A) giving any false or misleading information or making a false promise or representation; or (B) providing anything of value to a student athlete or anyone associated with the student athlete before the student athlete enters into an agency contract, including any consideration in the form of a loan, or acting in the capacity of a guarantor or co-guarantor for any debt; (2) enter into an agency contract with a student athlete without providing the student athlete with the disclosure document described in subsection (b) of this section; or (3) predate or postdate an agency contract.

15 U.S.C.A. § 7802.

185. *See generally* UAAA, *supra* note 181, §§ 15–16. For SPARTA, see 15 U.S.C.A. §§ 7803–05.

186. *See* Deubert, *supra* note 82.

187. The BCS is a selection and ranking system designed to create five bowl matchups involving ten of the top ranked teams in the NCAA Division I Football Bowl Subdivision. Six Conferences (Big East, Big Ten, ACC, SEC, Big 12 and Pac-10) are guaranteed to have their regular season champion in a BCS Bowl game. The BCS has no affiliation with the NCAA. For more information, see BCSfootball.org, BCS Selection Procedures, http://www.bcsfootball.org/news/story?id=4819597 (Apr. 26, 2010 13:24:00 EST).

188. *See* Richard Salgado, *A Fiduciary Duty To Teach Those Who Don't Want To Learn: The Potentially Dangerous Oxymoron of "College Sports,"* 17 Seton Hall J. Sports & Ent. L. 135, 145 n. 54 (2007) (citing R. Sellers, et. al., *Life Experiences of African-American Student-Athletes in Revenue Producing Sports: A Descriptive Empirical Analysis,* Acad.

ATHLETIC J. 21 (Fall 1991)); *see also* Christopher M. Parent, *Forward Progress? An Analysis of Whether Student-Athletes Should Be Paid*, 3 VA. SPORTS AND ENT. L. J. 226, 227–228 (2004).

189. *See* NCAA, A CAREER IN PROFESSIONAL ATHLETICS: A GUIDE FOR MAKING THE TRANSITION, app. C at 38 (2004), *available at* http://www.ncaapublications.com/product-downloads/CPAONLINE.pdf (discussed in greater detail later in the article).

190. See sources cited *supra* note 126.

191. *See* Hagar, *supra* note 127; Reed, *supra* note 128.

192. Minor league baseball players make a maximum of $1,100 a month in their first season. *See* Minor League Baseball Frequently Asked Questions, http://web.minorleague-baseball.com/milb/info/faq.jsp?mc=milb_info (last visited Oct. 10, 2010). Players in the National Basketball Developmental League (NBDL) earn between $12,000 and $24,000 for a season. *See* NBA Development League, http://www.insidehoops.com/nbdl.shtml (last visited Oct. 10, 2010). Players on an NFL practice squad can earn $5,200 per week. *See* NFL CBA, *supra* note 31, Art. XXXIV, § 3.

193. Most notably, Josh Childress, a four-year NBA veteran, who averaged 11.8 points per game last season, turned down a five-year $33 million offer from the Atlanta Hawks in 2008 to play in Greece for three years and $32.5 million. *See* Sekou Smith, *Migratory Hawk: Josh Childress Leaves NBA for Greece*, ATLANTA J.–CONST., July 24, 2008, at Cl, *available at* 2008 WLNR 13774417. In addition, several NHL players have returned to their home countries to finish their careers, including Jaromir Jagr, Petr Forsberg and Dominik Hasek. *See, e.g., Czech Goalie Hasek Joins Spartak Moscow,* TIMES OF OMAN, June 9, 2010, *available at* 2010 WLNR 11702788; Jeff Z. Klein, *The Stars of Hockey Play Here, and There,* N.Y. TIMES, Feb. 20, 2010, at D4.

194. List of Professional Sports Leagues, http://en.wikipedia.org/wiki/List_of_professional_sports_leagues (listing professional leagues in all major sports) (Oct. 12, 2010, 10:37:07 PM EDT).

195. *Id.*

196. *Id.*

197. Andrea Cohen, *Young Pros Now Have More Choices After Leaving: Playing Overseas College,* DAILY OKLAHOMAN, July 10, 2008, at 6C.

198. Chris McCosky, *NBA Not Sweating the Euro Lure,* DETROIT NEWS, Oct. 22, 2008, at 2D.

199. Denis Poissant, *Hockey Night in Russia; The NHL Is Still Superior, but It Has Not Faced Competition This Serious Since the Threat from the World Hockey Association,* TORONTO SUN, Jan. 27, 2009, at S10.

200. USBasket.com, Ex-College Basketball Tracker, http://www.usbasket.com/ex-college-basketball-tracker.asp (last visited Oct. 10, 2010).

201. For a list of former University of Massachusetts men's basketball players playing professionally, see *supra* note 200.

202. Following the US Women's dramatic victory in the World Cup Championship in 1999, the Women's United Soccer Association launched in 2000 only to fold three seasons later. In its place, Women's Professional Soccer (WPS) launched in 2009. National Pro Fastpitch (NPF), formerly the Women's Pro Softball League (WPSL), is currently the only professional women's softball league in the United States. The WPSL was founded in 1997 and folded in 2001 but revived in 2004 and currently features six teams. Perhaps the most successful women's league has been the WNBA, which outlasted the three year effort of

the American Basketball League (1996–1998). For more on opportunities for women in sports, see Women's Sports Foundation, http://www.womenssportsfoundation.org (last visited Oct. 10, 2010).

203. *See* Alexander Wolff, *To Russia With Love*, Sports Illustrated, Dec. 15, 2008, *available at* http://vault.sportsillustrated.cnn.com/vault/article/magazine/MAG1149632/index.htm.

204. *See* NCAA, A Career in Professional Athletics: A Guide for Making the Transition 38 (2005), http://www.ncaapublications.com/productdownloads/D108.pdf [hereinafter NCAA, Career Guide].

205. *See id.*

206. *See id.*

207. *See id.*

208. In the six sports considered in the NCAA Career Guide, based on their projections about 1,334 student-athletes turn professional each year in just these sports—the NCAA gives the estimated number of student-athletes per sport per freshmen class year and also the probability of making it professional in that sport: men's basketball (4,500 and 1.3%); women's basketball (4,100 and 1%); football (16,200 and 2%); baseball (7,300 and 10.5%); men's ice hockey (1,100 and 4.1%); and men's soccer (5,200 and 1.9%). *Id.* By multiplying these numbers together, we arrived at the 1,334 figure. However, these calculations would estimate that only 59 men's and 41 women's basketball student-athletes are turning professional ever year—hundreds of athletes short of reality due to international leagues. These estimates also do not include about two dozen other NCAA sports in which athletes may turn professional, such as golf, swimming, tennis, and track & field.

209. *Id.*

210. DI Manual, *supra* note 14, § 2.1.1.

211. The NCAA's Budget for the 2009–2010 Academic Year included over $672 million in expenses. However, how much it spends on compliance is not an available figure and not one to which the NCAA would like to admit. *See* NCAA.org, 2009–2010 NCAA Budget Breakdown, http://www.ncaa.org/wps/wcm/connect/6d3874004e51aadc96e0d-622cf56f2f3/2009-10+Budget+Breakdown_ALL.pdf?MOD=AJPERES&CACHEID=6d3 874004e51aadc96e0d6 22cf56f2f3 (last visited Oct. 10, 2010).

212. *See* DI Manual, *supra* note 14, § 12.01.2.

213. *See* Len Pasquarelli, *Game of Life Important to NFL, Rookie Symposium Furthering League's On-Going Initiative To Enhance Players' Life Skills,* ESPN.com, June 29, 2010, http://sports.espn.go.com/nfl/columns/story?columnist=pasquarelli_len&id=5338948 (discussing the merits and goals of the NFL Rookie Symposium); *see also Former KU Players Embarrass NBA, But There's Still Time For Them To Redeem Themselves,* Kan. City Star, Sept. 4, 2008, at Al (discussing how former Kansas players Darrell Arthur and Mario Chalmers were fined $20,000 each for smoking marijuana in their hotel rooms at the NBA Rookie Symposium in 2008. Both were ordered to attend the Symposium the following year as well).

214. *See* Ledbetter, *supra* note 174.

215. *See* Chris Isidore, *Baseball Close To Catching NFL As Top $ Sport,* CNN.com, Oct. 25, 2007, http://money.cnn.com/2007/10/25/commentary/sportsbiz/index.htm (noting how MLB generates over $6 billion annually); *see also* John Lombardo, *NBA Increases Shared Revenue by 63%,* Sports Bus. J., Apr. 28, 2008, http://www.sportsbusinessjournal.com/art./58828 (discussing annual revenue of NBA as $3.5 billion); Tripp Mickle, *Escrow*

Cash Will Boost NHL, Sports Bus. J., Mar. 2, 2009, http://www.sportsbusinessjournal. com/art./61684 (establishing that NHL generates approximately $2.64 billion annually).

216. *See* Barnhart, *supra* note 100 (discussing the suspension of former Alabama offensive lineman Andre Smith).

217. *See supra* Part II.B.1.a (discussing Oliver v. NCAA).

218. *See* Collins v. Nat'l Basketball Players Ass'n, 976 F.2d 740 (10th Cir. 1992) (*citing* United States v. Hutcheson, 312 U.S. 219 (1941)) (The Court upheld the power of a union to enact regulations governing agents). Generally, parallel conduct, absent evidence of agreement, is insufficient to sustain an antitrust action. *See* Bell Atlantic Corp. v. Twombly, 550 U.S. 544 (2007). Even if an agent could prove that the union and NCAA agreed on certain portions of agent regulations, those agreements would not necessarily unreasonably restrain trade in violation of Section 1 of the Sherman Act.

219. NFLPA Agent Regulations require agents to submit any grievance with a player to arbitration. *See* NFLPA Agent Regulations, *supra* note 84, § 5. Agents may pursue a player in a grievance for commission due on salary paid to the player from a contract negotiated by that agent. In addition, a common grievance occurs when a player fires his agent after the NFL Combine or NFL Draft but before he has signed his rookie contract. As a result, the agent will have already expended $20–$30,000 or more in training and other costs without recouping the benefit. Most agents have players sign an agreement to reimburse the agent for the training expenses should the agent be fired before the rookie contract is negotiated and signed.

220. *See* Cornerstone Sports Consulting, *supra* note 24.

221. *See* UAAA, *supra* note 181.

222. *Id.* § 10.

223. *Id.* § 11.

224. *Id.* § 4.

225. In April of 2010, CBS and the NCAA reached a new 14-year, $10.8 billion deal. *See* Ourand & Smith, *supra* note 167. In July 2010, ESPN and the Atlantic Coast Conference (ACC) reached a 12-year, $1.86 billion deal. Just two years earlier, CBS and ESPN agreed to television deals with the SEC for a total of 15 years and $3.075 billion. *See* Zach Berman, *12-Year Deal With ESPN Means Big Bucks for ACC*, Wash. Post. Online, July 9, 2010, http://www.washingtonpost.com/wpdyn/content/article/2010/07/08/AR2010070803383. html.

226. *See* Dana O'Neil, *Will Agents Get An Invite To The Table?*, ESPN.com, July 20, 2010, http://sports.espn.go.com/ncb/columns/story?columnist=oneil_dana&id=5421033 (referring to "initial discussions [by the NCAA cabinet] regarding current agent and advisor legislations" and "how advisors might assist in providing information to student-athletes who are weighing their options").

227. For more on this viewpoint, see Root, *supra* note 170; *see also* McCormick & McCormick, *supra* note 13; Brooks, *supra* note 170.

228. *See* In re NCAA Student-Athlete Name & Likeness Licensing Litigation, Case No. C 09-01967 CW (N.D. Cal. 2010). In April 2009, former Nebraska quarterback Sam Keller filed a class-action lawsuit against the NCAA and EA Sports for the use of football student-athlete's likenesses in video games. Three months later former UCLA basketball player Ed O'Bannon filed suit alleging that in general the NCAA illegally benefited from the use of student-athlete images and likenesses without permission. In February 2010, a federal district court denied the NCAA's motion to dismiss. In March 2010, the lawsuits

were consolidated as a class action lawsuit. *See* Marlen Garcia, *NCAA Sued Over Player Likenesses*, USA TODAY, July 22, 2009, at 1C; Katie Thomas, *Ex-Players Join Suit vs. NCAA*, N.Y. TIMES, Mar. 11, 2010, at B15.

229. DI MANUAL, *supra* note 14, § 12.01.2.

230. *See* Wong & Deubert, *supra* note 68, at 508. The policy allows for maximum benefits of $20 million with a deductible of $75,000. The NCAA contributes approximately $10 million in annual premiums to the insurance company as part of the program.

231. For the University of Southern California Public Infractions Report (June 10, 2010), Middle Tennessee State University Public Infractions Report (May 22, 2008), Purdue University Public Infractions Report (Aug. 22, 2007), Auburn University Public Infractions Report (Apr. 27, 2004), University of Kentucky Public Infractions Report (Jan. 31, 2002), and others, see NCAA's Legislative Services Database, *supra* note 21.

232. iHoops was created in 2008 to "establish a structure and develop programs to improve the quality of youth basketball in America in order to enhance the athletic, educational, and social experience of the participants." *See* iHoops.com, About iHoops, http://www.ihoops.com/about/ (last visited Oct. 10, 2010). Both the NBA and the NCAA committed to spend up to $15 million on the venture, with another $20 million in shared marketing. The venture is based in Indianapolis and has a 12-member staff. In 2010 it hired highly regarded sports attorney, commentator and former NBA player Len Elmore as its CEO. *See* John Lombardo, *Elmore Scores iHoops Post*, SPORTS BUS. J., May 3, 2010, www.sportsbusinessjournal.com/article/65603.

233. Speakers of Sport, Inc. v. ProServ, Inc., 178 F.3d 862, 864 (7th Cir. 1999).

B. Gender

5 Women in Sport

Gender Relations and Future Perspectives

■ GERTRUD PFISTER

■ INTRODUCTION

The gender of sport in the past was clearly and conspicuously masculine.[1] From the very beginning women in sport were the 'other sex'; they were outsiders, new—or latecomers who, if they were allowed to at all, could take part in 'suitable' forms of exercise and sport. For many years it was commonly believed—and it may still be firmly anchored in popular wisdom today—that certain types of sport and exercise were suitable for women while others were unsuitable, and that the same applied to men. It has always been taken for granted, for example, that men play American football and that women are keen gymnasts and dancers. From the early days of sport in the nineteenth century this assumption, based on the theory of the polarity of gender attributes, seemed to be confirmed not only by everyday convictions and practices but also by scientific knowledge. In 1953, for example, the renowned philosopher Buytendijk commented on the subject of women's football: 'Football as a game is essentially a demonstration of masculinity as we understand it from our traditional view of things and as produced in part by our physical constitution (through hormonal irritation). No one has ever been successful in getting women to play football.'[2]

Since the 1950s female athletes have gained access to more and more sports which were formerly men's domains. But has this changed the situation of women and/or the images and practices of sport? Bodies and physical differences are at the very centre of sport since sport is a system which systematically reveals differences and establishes a ranking based on the individual's performance. Sport, or at least as far as the great majority of sports is concerned, is also a system which, in its competitive and elite forms, is based on a universally valid gender segregation that is scarcely to be found any longer in other areas of western societies. Thus, as a rule, separate competitions are held for men and women, and it is strictly ensured that men do not take part in women's events and vice versa. Frequently, too, different standards and regulations are in operation for the two sexes. Only women, for example, do gymnastics on the asymmetrical bars and balance beam while the rings, pommel horse and parallel bars are reserved for men. Furthermore, in tests or as standards for qualifications, higher levels of performance are generally demanded of men. Frequently, therefore, in discussions on sport and gender the topic quickly turns to the question of the 'real' differences between the sexes. Aren't women's bodies different from men's; aren't men's levels of performance higher than those of the 'weaker sex'? It is impossible here to go into the sex-gender debates that have filled countless pages of feminist literature since the 1960s. Without doubt, the differentiation between sex, the biological aspect, and gender, the cultural aspect of being a women/a man, was important because in broad sections of the population it opened people's eyes not only to the great diversity and multiplicity of gender but also to the socially constructed gender order in our society. Publications and discussions on the construction of gender are currently flourishing. From a constructivist perspective, gender is a structural category (the gender order of society) and an individual practice performed in interactions.[3] This approach emphasizes that gender is not something we have or we are, but something we perform, we do. 'Doing gender' is the construction of gendered identities and images and the enactment of gender in social situations, where we always present ourselves and are perceived as women or men. Sport is an excellent arena for doing gender.

However, gender is not only an issue for the scientific community. Judith Butler's (1990) proposal that we regard gender as process, discourse and performative act has meanwhile reached popular literature as well as the magazines.[4] Information and discussions on homo-, trans- and intersexuality are causing cracks to form in the concept of dual gender, while phenomena like gender play and gender bending illustrate just how gender is constructed and enacted (see, for example, DIE ZEIT dated 28 September 2000). Experimenting with gender characteristics has now become a mainstream trend, the vanguard including sportsmen like David Beckham, with his ever changing hairstyles, nail varnish and shaved chest. He is the idol of both homo- and heterosexuals, and a pioneer of the new 'metrosexual' trend.

Indications that the difference perspective generally seems to have lost currency in the public space are to be found, for example, in the 'men's health movement', which has cast off the myth of the 'stronger sex', or in the success of Natalie Angier's book, 'Woman: An Intimate Geography', which describes women as the very opposite of the 'weaker sex'. In sport the constructivist gender perspective has reinforced demands that women be admitted to 'men's sports' (and vice versa, although men are only excluded from a few sports such as synchronised swimming and rhythmical sport gymnastics).

These tendencies raise the question as to whether this dismantling and/or de-dramatization of gender differences in, as well as outside, sport is a sign pointing towards a new gender order. Or has gender enactment become more subtle? Have gender scripts shifted to other areas, for example to media sport with its focus on (hetero)sexuality? Which course will gender relations in sport and society take in the future?

The discourses of gender have been influenced considerably by the 'linguistic turn' in the social sciences and by post-modern paradigms such as deconstruction, anti-essentialism and differentiation. But how does this relate to sport, which takes the body seriously with its abilities and skills, and its joy and pain, and which only exists with the body's complicity, when it is set in motion, put on show and continually honed?

On this point Lehnert remarks: 'Of course, there are real bodies, but without culture they possess no real significance.'[5] How we perceive our bodies, how we judge their various parts, whether we like our legs or hate our bellies, how we consider changes through pregnancy and ageing, for example, or how we cope with the demands placed on our bodies by factors such as sport—all this depends on our knowledge and experience, and in turn has an effect on our bodies. When we reflect on our bodies, we use language, and language always implies interpretation. Therefore, bodies cannot be 'thought' without culture and as a result cannot exist without culture. In sport, too, the material body, its presentation and its achievements, are given sense and significance through perception, interpretation and evaluation, whereby the aims, the regulations and the evaluations of sporting activities are based on social arrangements.

Cross-cultural comparisons, be it the comparison of different sports cultures in modern times or be it a survey of different eras of the past, clearly reveal that it is not movement itself but the meanings associated with it— along with the social constructions of femininity and masculinity as well as the structural and symbolic gender arrangements in a particular society—that lead to the labelling of sporting activities as either male or female. In what way is this significant, though, for an analysis of gender relationships and the future of (women's) sport?

In answering the questions raised above, I will analyse the present situation and consider future developments with regard to sports participation, media sports and leadership in sport. This choice of foci is related to my theoretical considerations. If sport and different types of sport are social constructs and gender neutral per se, one may assume that men and women show similar patterns of sports participation. Gender differences raise the question as to the causes. These can be explained in terms of gendered scripts and gender arrangements and of individuals 'doing gender'. Likewise, gender enactment in media sports and gender ratios in the executive bodies of sports organizations can be analysed using the theoretical approach described above. The three topics, moreover, are closely interrelated. Men's dominance of sports leadership and their control over the development of sport, for example, may have an adverse effect on women's participation in sport. This is equally true of media sport, whose messages and images provide the scripts for doing gender.

■ FROM A MALE ALLIANCE TO THE WOMEN'S MOVEMENT—THE PARTICIPATION OF WOMEN AND MEN IN GYMNASTICS AND SPORT

Gymnastics, Turnen (German gymnastics) and sport were developed by men and for men from the end of the eighteenth century onwards.[6] It was not until the end of the nineteenth century that, sporadically in Europe and the USA, women started to take part in sporting activities. In spite of frequent and considerable opposition there was a slow but steady increase in the number of women participating in physical activities and of female members of gymnastic and sports clubs.[7] The development of women's sport is reflected in their participation in the Olympic Games. If the founder of the Olympic movement, Baron de Coubertin, had had his way, the women's role would have been merely to marvel at the athletes from the spectators' stands.[8] And so it was that at the first Olympic Games in 1896 women were not admitted to the contests. In 1900, on the initiative of the organizers but without the consent of the International Olympics Committee (IOC), women took part 'officially' in tennis and golf competitions and 'unofficially' in at least eleven sports at the Paris Olympics.[9] Later archery, ice skating and swimming were added to the women's programme. After a lengthy dispute between the IOC, the international amateur athletics federation and the international women's sports association, women were first entered for athletic competitions at the Olympic Games in 1928. In that year the proportion of women among the Olympic contestants was 9.6%. In 2004, the percentage of female athletes had risen to 40.7%.

After the Second World War interest in sport in European countries grew steadily. This is to be seen not only in the successful growth of the sports federations, which in Germany and Denmark, for example, were able to record increasing membership figures year on year but also in surveys in which more and more people reported that they took part in sporting activities.[10] At the same time there was an above-average increase in the number of female club members, as well as of girls and women who were taking up sport outside of the organizations, so that the difference in sports participation between the sexes steadily decreased. In Denmark 46% of the male and 37% of the female adult population is a member of a sports club.[11]

If population surveys are to be believed, the number of women taking part in sporting activities now equals or even surpasses that of men in some European countries. In the Scandinavian countries, as well as in Germany, the Netherlands and Belgium, more than 50% of the male and female population participate in some form of sporting activity.[12] This is only true, however, if one construes sporting activity as a broad and comprehensive term which includes everyday activities such as walking and recreational cycling. If one takes the intensity and frequency of sporting activities into consideration, and if one defines sport as an activity involving competition, men are still ahead of women. According to a study conducted on behalf of the European Commission 18% of men and 12% of women in Europe reported to have been physically active 'a lot' in the last seven days.[13] Men participated on 2.1 days, women on 1.3 days in vigorous physical activities.[14] On days with vigorous activities, men spent an average of 124 minutes, women 61 minutes on their activity.[15] A Danish survey has shown that 31% of the male adult population but only 17% of the female population participate in sport competitions.[16]

Considering present trends in sport and demography, it seems likely that the lead that men have with regard to sports club membership will continue to shorten. This is suggested by, among other things, the increased provision of health sports and seniors' sports in the clubs, the demand for which comes especially from women. In addition, it must be taken into account that the proportion of women in the over-60s age group is rising.

It would not, therefore, appear too far-fetched to forecast a 'women's future' for sport. On the other hand, it must not be forgotten that gender is only one of the factors that determine whether a person takes up sport. Ethnic and social backgrounds, as well as religion, combine to form typical patterns of either participation in, or abstinence from, sport, and these factors influence girls and women more than boys and men. In other words, girls and women from an Islamic cultural background and/or from the lower social strata are marginalized and underrepresented in sport for a great number of reasons.[17]

■ SPORTS HAVE A GENDER

The impression that gender differences in sport are gradually losing their distinct contours must be contradicted, or at least qualified, when one takes a closer look at gender preferences with regard to the sports taken up.

An analysis of the forms and types of sport that men and women participate in reveals an ambivalent picture.[18] What is conspicuous is that women are increasingly taking part in sports that for many years were absolutely taboo for them and which in the last two or three decades have been undergoing a 'sex change'. It is taken for granted today, for example, that women take part in the biathlon (originally a military discipline), water polo, the marathon, the 'iron man', soccer or cycling, all of which were exclusively men's sports until the 1970s. Today female athletes even compete successfully in combat, strength and risk sports such as weightlifting, bodybuilding, ice hockey, boxing, hammer throwing, Sumo wrestling and ski jumping without being stigmatized as freaks. Does this mean that women have conquered men's last strongholds?

For all the discussion of women in 'men's sports', it must be remembered that only a small number of young women take an interest and wish to make their mark in such sports. The great majority of women who take up sporting activities—just like a large number of men—choose so-called 'soft sports' such as cycling, hiking and swimming.[19] Here, a distinct convergence of interests is observable between the sexes.

Largely unnoticed by the mass media, but clearly recognizable if one takes a look at the statistics and results of surveys, is the development of 'women's domains' in sport. Rhythmic dancing and movement classes, as well as health and fitness activities from back pain therapy to relaxation techniques, are almost exclusively sought out by women. Sports associations such as the German Gymnastic Federation or the Danish Gymnastics and Sports Associations (DGI), which provide many health-oriented courses, including all kinds of gymnastics from aerobics to rhythmic gymnastics, now have a 50–70% proportion of women participants.[20] One sport which has become an almost exclusive preserve of girls is horse riding.[21] For girls horses are more than just sports apparatus, but their fascination mostly vanishes when they grow older.

The 'women's sports movement' is part of the current focus on body and health, which is connected with the concern about having or getting the 'right' body, which includes efforts to keep a slim figure, dealing with 'problem zones' and, generally, a more or less rigorous body management.

A much noted trend is the emergence and rise (and sometimes decline) of new types of sport, although it must be added that most trend sports are taken up by only a small minority of the population.[22] Some of the new sports, like inline skating, attract both sexes as well as many age groups, whereas lots of others, from streetball to skateboarding and including one of the latest trends, Parkour (moving through the town or countryside in the most direct way possible), are clearly located in a youth environment oriented to male values.[23] And it is above all risk sports such as ice climbing, adventure races, BMX cycling, base jumping (parachuting from fixed objects), free climbing, etc.—all of them promoted and sponsored by the media—that contribute considerably to the reproduction of gender differences and may be interpreted as the demonstration and enactment of masculinity.[24]

In summary, it can be stated that new—even if perhaps porous—lines of demarcation have developed in sport between the sexes. On the one hand there are very few types of sport today from which one of the two sexes is formally barred (such as men from synchronized swimming). In the light of past developments, which have all been towards opening up different sports for women, it seems likely that any restrictions that still exist for men and women will be removed in all sports. By contrast, men and women's interests in a number of leisure sports appear to be moving increasingly in different directions.

What, then, will be the effects of the inclusion of women or men in sports which are (still) regarded as typical of the opposite sex? First of all, it must be said that the mere authorization to take part in a sport does not mean that gender differences are thus eliminated. On the contrary, in many sports this may lead to new and more subtle forms of gender enactment. In figure skating, for example, masculinity continues to be demonstrated, in spite of—or perhaps even because of—the 'feminization' of the parts of the routine. And gender differences are put on display most impressively in pair skating and ice dancing.[25] Contrary to sports with an objective outcome due to the measurability of performance, in figure skating the presentation and aesthetic value are part of the evaluation. In this way the ruling taste (in Bourdieu's sense of the term), ideas about the 'right' posture and movements, as well as the existing gender arrangements and gender ideals, influence the performances of the athletes, the evaluations of the judges and, as a whole, the image which the media and audiences have of the skaters, of their programmes and of the discipline of the sport itself. 'Doing gender' is an important part of figure skating and the variety of movements and the artistic freedom in this sport allows the athletes, men and women, to do gender in various ways.

Up to the present the deconstruction of gender and the redefinition of 'doing gender' have been studied most intensively in sports which, such as bodybuilding or boxing, are traditionally associated with masculinity and defined as being male sports.[26] Female bodybuilders have to present themselves as women although their muscular bodies signal masculinity. Studies revealed that ideals of body and beauty, along with the prevailing ideas about femininity, undergo radical change when women intrude into the world of sport traditionally occupied by men.[27] However, this does not simply mean the disintegration of gender dichotomies. The results of these studies indicate, instead, that ambivalences emerge in the construction of gender and that conformity and resistance coexist, where women athletes either wish to, or have to, fulfil the traditional ideals of femininity in spite of their 'male' sport. Camilla Obel's study is especially captivating since she states on the one hand that 'bodybuilding is a challenge to categorical ways of thinking about femininity, masculinity and the body'.[28] In her view women bodybuilders cause the disintegration of not only the imagined polarities of femininity and masculinity, but also of nature and culture. On the other hand she inferred from interviews that women bodybuilders do indeed wish to embody bodybuilding, attractive femininity and heterosexuality at the same time.

Changes in body ideals and the images of women athletes are also the topic of a book entitled 'Built to Win'.[29] The two authors describe the phenomenon of how female athletes with strong personalities and lots of self-confidence like the football player, Mia Hamm, are idolized in the United States. Especially in top-level sport, in 'male' domains in particular, a demonstrative enactment of femininity and eroticism increases a sportswoman's 'market value', or even makes her marketable in the first place. Here, one could mention athletes such as 'FloJo', the glamorous and successful runner, or the players of the US soccer team, who presented a very feminine image as winners of the World Championships with make-up and ponytails.[30] Moreover, one must take into consideration that women's integration into 'male' sports is liable to trigger off comparisons between men and women, thus contributing towards cementing a gender dichotomy since in sport differences are 'embodied'. Thus, if men's bodies and performance are considered the standard, then in most athletic disciplines, women must appear as the weaker sex. Finally, it must be borne in mind that women's integration into 'male' sports has so far been accompanied by a large degree of adaptation to, and fitting in with, prevailing sport ideologies, structures and practices. Whether women could succeed in establishing a different kind of everyday sporting practice within traditional 'male' sports in keeping with women's qualities, experience and personal circumstances is debatable, not least because in women's sports, too, there is a trend towards a constant enhancement of performances, which means that techniques and tactics are increasingly being adapted to those of men.

While women now take up men's sports and, in order to integrate, adjust to the norms and values which dominate them, men's interest in 'typical women's' physical activities is negligible. This is just as true of recreational as it is of top-level sports. Men who (wish to) do synchronized swimming or sports aerobics are rare exceptions. Rhythmic sports gymnastics, too, is entirely a women's preserve.

▪ MEDIA SPORTS—HUMAN-INTEREST STORIES, BARE BOSOMS AND FOOTBALL, FOOTBALL, FOOTBALL

Any analysis of either the current sporting landscape or the development of sport is impossible without taking the mass media into account. An event is only real when it surfaces in the media. Even if this sentence may not be accurate in such a drastic form, it is true to say that the mass media have constructed a new reality in sport which is consumed by the public. And for sponsors of sport the only events that count and the only sportsmen and women that exist are those who appear on television. In the sporting reality constructed by the media women are scarcely present. A glance at the sports pages of newspapers shows clearly that nothing, or very little, has changed with regard to the underrepresentation of sportswomen both in newspapers and on television, a fact which was documented in the 1980s already. Now, as before, only 5–15% of mass media sports coverage (whether space in newspapers or time on television) is devoted to women's sports. A study carried out in 2005 of over 10,000 articles in 36 newspapers from nine countries revealed, for example, that only 6% of the articles referred to women's sports.[31]

The way women athletes were and still are depicted today contributes to the marginalization of women's sports due to the emphasis placed on femininity and sexual attraction. Especially in the popular press women athletes continue to be referred to as 'Goldmädel, Rennmiezen und Turnküken' [literally: golden girls, racing pussycats and gymnast chicks], terms which Klein and Pfister chose as the title of their study of the media coverage of women's sport, published in 1985. In past decades the sexualization of women athletes (as well as several male athletes) has gained increasing importance. It cannot be denied, however, that male as well as female athletes are actively involved in the staging of their performances, the construction of their images and their presentation in the media. It simply arouses greater attention and excitement when volleyball players allow themselves to be photographed with bare bosoms or figure skaters appear almost nude in *Playboy* than when a women's handball team wins the German championship. Public attention at (almost) any price seems to guarantee at least financial success.

There are, of course, journalists, both male and female, who report enthusiastically about women's sports. A good example of this is the coverage of the victory of the German team in the women's football World Championship. 'GERMANY WORLD CHAMPIONS: Football Heroines Celebrate Their Historic Triumph' was the headline, for example, of *SpiegelOnline Sport* on 30 September 2007.

It is difficult for journalists, however, to set themselves against the trend and against the alleged interests of readers and viewers. In Germany the lack of interest of journalists in women's sport has always been explained with the need to meet the expectations of consumers. Sports reports are still largely produced by men and for men, while women continue to form a small minority of sports journalists.[32] Those women who venture into the 'lion's den' of sports journalism have to learn to adapt if they do not wish to be 'mauled'. Among the consumers of sport, too, men are in the majority, and it is a fact that women are much less tempted than men to either go to the stadium or sit in front of the television to watch a game of football.[33] Women's interest in media sports coverage depends, among other things, on the type of sport. Thus, when gymnastics or figure skating is shown, the proportion of women viewers increases. Women therefore have nothing against watching sport in general, and, if the appropriate sports are provided, they can indeed be won over as sports consumers. This is especially true of the coverage of major events like the Olympic Games, where women are presented (almost) in relation to their participation in the Games. Here, women make up 40% to 60% of the audience.

In all discussions about media sports it must be taken into account that the media coverage and its consumption, the development of sport, the situation and status of sportswomen as well as the fascination of, and the public interest in, women's sport are all intricately interwoven. The lack of media interest in women's football, for example, leads to the fact that sponsors likewise take no interest in the sport, which in turn has an effect on the game and development, thus contributing generally to its marginalization. Without sponsors or a redistribution of the overall profits generated by football the professionalization of women's football is impossible. And if the players' performance is inadequate and the games are not sufficiently attractive, the prejudice is reinforced that women cannot play football and that it is not worthwhile reporting on their matches. This negative image then has the effect again that few girls show any enthusiasm for the game.[34]

Changes are currently observable in media sports and further changes may be expected in future, not least due to the spread of the new media, above all the internet. The new media not only provide instant and unlimited access to information about sporting events (including those in women's sports) but they also give marginal groups and sports the opportunity of presenting themselves to the public. It is doubtful, however, whether presentations on the internet are able to make up for the marginal role of women's sports in the print media and on television since successful and popular websites on the internet also require ample resources.

The way women competing in men's sports are presented in the mass media may also be described as ambivalent. Generally speaking, there is a wide acceptance of women football players, women wrestlers, women weightlifters and women boxers. Women's boxing especially has now almost gained cult status, as exemplified not only by the film *Million Dollar Baby* but also by the world championship fight of the German boxer Regina Halmich, which took place on 30 November 2007 in a stadium filled to capacity and which was watched by between four and five million television viewers. Another good example of public interest in women playing men's sport is the film *Bend It Like Beckham*. There is generally a perceptible increase in programmes and reports containing aesthetically pleasing images and moving stories, distinctly aimed at a female public. For the media as well as for male consumers of sport, moreover, women athletes who radiate an aura of eroticism in tough men's sports seem to hold a special attraction. Thus, today women who kick a ball are suddenly considered particularly attractive and even sexy.[35]

However, it is questionable whether the focus on female athletes in some articles and programmes indicates a change in media attention. One has to take into consideration the numerous sports magazines and sports channels which focus on men's sports only, explained by their orientation to male target groups that are important for advertisers. It may be assumed that the increased commercialization of sport and the trading of broadcasting rights, along with the growing importance of television for the financing of sport through sponsors, will push typical women's sports like gymnastics, as well as women's sport in general, even further into the margins.[36]

Sports stadiums, and in particular the fans' stands, are still male strongholds, as mentioned above. However, changes appear to be taking place here, too. One new phenomenon, for example, is the fact that girls are beginning to show a growing enthusiasm for ski jumping and football matches, even forming fan communities. In contrast to the male fans, however, the girls' interest in ski jumping or football cannot (only) be explained by their need to identify with the stars of their favourite sport. For the female fans, ski jumpers and football stars seem to play the same role as film stars or music idols, i.e. that of 'love objects'.[37]

▪ THE POWER IN MEN'S HANDS—STRUCTURES OF CONTROL AND LEADERSHIP

The analyses of club and federation boards that are available reveal unanimously that men continue to be in firm control of the sporting world.[38] The higher the positions are, the smaller is the percentage of women who occupy them. Power in sport is still to a high degree in the hands of men. This is true of the leading committees of national as well as international sports federations such as the IOC. In 2003 there were 7,048 senior officials above club level working in an honorary capacity in the Danish sports system. Of these 31% were women. Of the executive committee members of the Danish Sport Federation (DIF) 10% were women; in the Danish Gymnastics and Sports Associations (DGI) the corresponding figure was 33%. This can be contrasted with overall female membership: women represent 39% of DIF members and 47% if DGI members.[39] In Germany, too, women are marginalized in the decision-making committees of sports associations. In 2003, out of a total of 290 executive positions recorded in the leading committees at the DSB (German Sports Confederation) level, 233 were occupied by men and 57 by women, the proportion of positions held by women being 19.7%.[40] In 2003, the IOC had 12 female and 114 male members.[41]

I cannot here go into the complex causes of women's underrepresentation in executive bodies, but I would like to point to the fact that the structures and mechanisms which hinder women's careers in sport are similar to those existing on the labour market.

Looking at the future, one must also pose the question: what will change if and when women have more say? Although it cannot be automatically assumed that women are 'by nature' more cooperative, more empathetic and less aggressive than men, empirical studies on women's leadership styles suggest that, due to their specific experience and the specific circumstances of their lives, women are able to bring about change and provide fresh impetus to the work of political and sports bodies, for example with regard to both aims and strategies.[42] Moreover, they could ensure that, throughout planning and decision-making processes, the actual circumstances of women's lives are given greater consideration in the world of sport than has been the case up to the present. In addition, the greater inclusion of women means the harnessing of hitherto unused abilities and competences which, in view of the complaints about the lack of interest in holding voluntary office, is an aspect that should not be underestimated.

Over the past 30 years there has been a growing discussion about strategies to increase the proportion of women in leadership positions. In the 1970s, with the rise of the new women's movement, the idea of introducing gender quotas was at the centre of heated debates. In the 1980s and the early 1990s there was a shift towards advancement schemes for women and the setting of targets. Today there seems to be a new formula for increasing the presence of women at the senior management levels of politics and industry, a formula which in future can also perhaps be applied to sport. This is the concept of mainstreaming.

Mainstreaming is an approach in women's and gender politics which is being encouraged above all in the European Union. Subsequent to the demands made at the 4th Women's World Congress on 15 September 1995 in Peking, mainstreaming—along with the 4th Campaign for Equal Opportunities—was declared 'a main pillar of European equality policy'.[43] Stiegler describes mainstreaming as the 'permeation of the gender question into hitherto androcentric patterns of thinking, forms of organisation and ways of doing things'.[44] Löffler emphasized that women's politics must not 'remain a tributary of European politics but . . . flow into the "mainstream" of business and industry, growth and cross-border opportunities'.[45] Mainstreaming means the inclusion of both sexes in all industrial, social and political decision making. It is based on the premise that social, industrial and ecological problems can only be solved if the genders of both the decision makers and those affected by the decisions are taken into account. Linked to this is, firstly, the advancement of women, hitherto a discriminated group; secondly, the establishment of framework conditions to ensure equal opportunities; and, thirdly, the creation of gender awareness, particularly among men. One key measure is 'gender controlling', the 'analysis of all political activities from the perspective of the contribution they make to equal opportunities'.[46] This means, for example, that we abandon the ideology of gender neutrality in politics and that we stop regarding gender politics as a women's issue. It is not possible here to go into either the requirements or the problems of mainstreaming. One of the main criticisms of mainstreaming is that this strategy might be used as a pretext for abolishing projects designed exclusively for women. Furthermore, nothing is achieved by simply ensuring a numerical balance of men and women in individual areas or committees. The inclusion of women in management positions, for example, would lead to new kinds of inequality if there was no provision at the same time for the greater involvement of men in child rearing. Moreover, it is not easy to balance the interests and needs of women against those of men (and vice versa) or to implement mainstreaming successfully. This requires not only 'good will' but also knowledge, competence and influence. And in many countries mainstreaming, as well as gender equality in sports organizations, is simply not an issue. In Germany on the other hand a resolution was passed by the German Sports Confederation to introduce gender mainstreaming in 2003.[47] And a survey conducted in 2004 showed that almost 30% of German sports federations had already implemented or wished to implement this strategy, with some federations carrying out pilot projects.[48] The success of these projects remains to be seen, although the relatively large degree of willingness to bring about change in the hierarchical gender relationships existing in sport points to a considerable shift in patterns of thinking towards gender democracy.

INSTEAD OF A RÉSUMÉ: POST-FEMINISM, BACKLASH AND WOMEN'S BOXING

Today the demand for equality between the sexes seems to have been superseded by new trends. Post-feminism has established itself not only in the United States but throughout the world, to a certain degree as a theoretical construct but above all as an attitude and way of life.[49] Young women who combine sexual attractiveness with self-assurance and self-assertiveness accuse their feminist 'mothers' (the members of the 'second wave' of the women's liberation movement) not only of a general hostility towards men, stemming allegedly from a persecution complex and a feeling of victimhood, but also of spirituality and superstition as well as excessive theorizing and an aversion to sex. Even if these reproaches are untenable and in many cases preposterous, they did have an effect. Surveys in the renowned *Time* magazine show, for example, that fewer and fewer women consider themselves feminists.[50] On the other hand an increasing number of women take feminist aims for granted, such as equal rights for men and women. Moreover, celebrities like Madonna or the heroines of the soap series currently being shown on television seem to provide conclusive evidence that women today can achieve everything and especially that, in doing so, they can have lots of fun and be at the centre of attention. Even in cyberspace masculinity and femininity are no longer enacted as the contrast between Superman and the Playboy Bunny. The 'virtual superwoman' is called Lara Croft, an archaeologist who is 'sexy, clever and packs a powerful punch'. An 'amazon with a wasp waist, a silicone bosom and big round eyes', Croft defends herself 'fearlessly against all enemies: animals, monsters and men' during her expeditions.[51] In addition, the question arises whether gender is still of any significance at all in the age of MySpace, 'Second Life' and numerous virtual reality games. In the virtual world everyone can give themselves any identity they like, and in doing so can we also cross gender borders.

Parallel to post-feminist tendencies one can observe a backlash in many areas. Backlash refers here to a political and ideological movement, a response to the threat posed to the hierarchical gender order by feminism: 'Backlash has been constructed as a residual practice that halts or reverses the quest for equality. Triggered by the perception that women are making great strides toward equality, backlash is a reaction to the possibility that women may actually achieve equality.'[52] Backlash tendencies are to be observed, for example, in the decreasing proportions of women in various political decision-making bodies or in the stagnation of the number of women in leadership positions in sports organizations. In the United States opposition is growing to the policy of equal rights in sport guaranteed by Title IX, with the financial backing of women's sport having come under attack, the argument being that the abolition of the privileges granted to men would threaten the existing sport system.[53] Further, the very rejection of the term 'feminism' mentioned above can also be interpreted as a symptom of backlash. And, finally, one could discuss the extent to which post-feminism and backlash are intertwined.

Analyses of the equal opportunities of men and women in different areas of society have revealed namely that the new assertive women of today are 'of course' allowed to take up all kinds of jobs and careers but that promotion and success often end at a 'glass ceiling', a common term used in England and the United States to denote an insuperable, transparent barrier which denies certain groups access to the top levels of power: 'The glass ceiling is not simply a barrier for an individual, based on the person's inability to handle a higher level job. Rather, the glass ceiling applies to women as a group who are kept from advancing higher because they are women.'[54]

Young women's interest in hitherto male sports like bodybuilding and boxing seems to be consistent with post-feminist tendencies found in other areas, for example in popular culture and above all in music. According to Ann Hall 'women's boxing and women's bodybuilding [are] cultural metaphors, barometers if you like, of changes occurring in women's sport generally at the end of the century, as well as changes in feminism'.[55] Few academic studies of women's boxing have so far been undertaken, but it is clear that this sport—whether one likes it or not—has two sides to it as far as women are concerned. On the one hand, boxing could debunk traditional myths about the 'weaker sex'.[56] And, here, the aversion which many people have to women's boxing is quite revealing, showing as it does the prejudices and stereotypes that influence our judgments and, generally, our taste (in Bourdieu's sense of the term). On the other hand, the reports and pictures of women's boxing that appear in the media make sufficiently clear that women boxers are marketed as sex objects and the matches as sensations. Jennifer Hargreaves commented: 'The diversities and representations of the female body in boxing make it difficult to assess the extent to which the sport is a subversive activity for women or an essentially assimilative process with a radical facade.'[57]

The object here is not to discuss the arguments for and against boxing in general, and women's boxing in particular. My purpose, rather, is to show that women's boxing is part of a trend that will alter the way women are seen and judged. The current development seems to point towards men and women being allowed in future to compete in all sports and towards the decline of the myth of the stronger and the weaker sex. Allowing the other sex to take part in types and forms of sport that were previously considered typical of one sex increases the range of sports on offer and thus might lead to a growing interest in sport on the part of both men and women. There is a price to be paid for these developments, however: currently they are linked, among other things, to a sexualization and marketing of the female (and perhaps also male) body. In addition, many of the problems which only men had to face in the past are now harassing women. And so far they have not found any better remedies than the men for dealing with the increasing requirements—and manipulations—of performance, for example.

Sport in the past belonged to men—its future belongs to all human beings! Whether or not this will come about, I do not know. But it would be a good prospect.

▨ NOTES

1. This article was written in 2008. The data and trends are valid in 2010.
2. Buytendijk, cited in Pfister, 'The Future of Football', 100.
3. Lorber, *Paradoxes of Gender*; Connell, *Gender*.
4. No author, 'Intersexualität', 43; Schmidt, 'Tragödie als Schurkenstück', 252–53.
5. Lehnert, *Wenn Frauen Männerkleidung tragen*, 24.
6. German Gymnastics was developed at the beginning of the nineteenth century. It was a political movement and included a broad variety of games and exercises. Gymnastics did not emphasize competition and records but fitness and mass participation (of men).
7. Pfister, 'Olympia nur für Männer?'
8. Ibid.
9. Drevon, *Les Jeux Olympiques Oubliés*.
10. Opaschowski, *Neue Trends im Freizeitsport*; Klages, *Mitgliederentwicklung im Deutschen Sportbund*.
11. Pilgaard, *Danskernes motions—og sportsvaner 2007*.
12. European Commission, *Eurobarometer 2006—Health and Food*. http://ec.europa.eu/health/ph_publication/eb_food_en.pdf, 65ff.
13. Ibid., 66.
14. Ibid., 69.
15. Ibid., 72.
16. Pilgaard, *Danskernes motions—og sportsvaner 2007*.
17. Kleindienst-Cachay, 'Sportengagement muslimischer Mädchen und Frauen in der Bundesrepublik Deutschland'.
18. The term 'sport' is used here for different kinds of body cultures and physical activities.
19. Opaschowski, *Neue Trends im Freizeitsport*.
20. Pfister, *Kvinder på toppen*.
21. Deutscher Olympischer Sportbund. *Bestandserhebung 2007*. http://www.dosb.de/fileadmin/fm-dosb/downloads/2007_DOSB_Bestandserhebung.pdf.
22. Opaschowski, *Neue Trends im Freizeitsport*.
23. Wheaton, *Understanding Lifestyle Sport*; Donnelly, 'Studying Extreme Sport'.
24. Messner, *Taking the Field*.
25. Pfister, 'Doing Gender'.
26. Obel, 'Collapsing Gender'.
27. Heywood and Dworkin, *Built to Win*.
28. Obel, 'Collapsing Gender', 85.
29. Heywood and Dworkin, *Built to Win*.
30. Pfister and Fasting, 'Geschlechterkonstruktionen auf dem Fußballplatz'; Rinehart, 'Babes and Boards'.
31. Schultz Jørgensen. *The International Sports Press*. 2005. http://www.playthegame.org/news/news-articles/2005/international-sports-press-survey-2005.

32. Pfister, 'Frauen in Führungspositionen'.
33. Opaschowski, *Neue Trends im Freizeitsport*; Hedal, 'Motivation og tv-sport'.
34. Pfister, 'The Future of Football'.
35. See among many other sources *Berliner Zeitung*, 11 May 2002, about the new image of women's football. http://www.berlinonline.de/berliner-zeitung/archiv/.bin/dump.fcgi/2002/0511/sport/0299/index.html.
36. Pfister, 'Gender, Sport und Massenmedien'.
37. Fechtig and Janke, 'Ich liebe Lars Riecken'.
38. Pfister, 'Frauen in Führungspositionen des Sports'; Pfister, *Kvinder på toppen*; Hovden, '"Heavyweight" Men'.
39. Pfister, 'Gender Issues'.
40. Pfister and Radtke, 'Biographien von männlichen und weiblichen Führungskräften im feutschen Sport'.
41. Pfister, 'Frauen in Führungspositionen des Sports'.
42. Ibid.
43. Löffler, *Frauenförderung in der Europäischen Union*, 107.
44. Stiegler, *Frauen im Mainstreaming*, 27.
45. Löffler, *Frauenförderung in der Europäischen Union*, 10.
46. Stiegler, *Frauen im Mainstreaming*, 21.
47. Henkel, 'DSB arbeitet nach der Strategie des Gender Mainstreaming'.
48. Haag, 'Zukunftssicherung von Sportvereinen durch Gender Mainstreaming'.
49. Hall, 'Boxers and Bodymakers'. In theoretical discourses post-feminism is based on post-modern notions. Like other theoretical approaches feminism is criticized as being narrative and the concept of gender as being essentialist and ahistoric (Gillis, Howie and Munford, *Third Wave Feminism*).
50. Hall, 'Boxers and Bodymakers', 21.
51. See www.laracroftism.de.
52. Greendorfer, 'Title IX Gender Equity', 82.
53. In the USA the equal rights of men and women in sport are anchored in Title IX, which took effect in 1972. Title IX is part of the Educational Amendments Act and forbids 'sex discrimination in education programs and activities within an institution receiving any type of Federal financial assistance' (Greendorfer, 'Title IX Gender Equity', 82).
54. Morrison, White and Van Velsor, *Breaking the Glass Ceiling*, 13.
55. Hall, 'Boxers and Bodymakers', 31.
56. Hargreaves, 'Women's Boxing'.
57. Quoted in Hall, 'Boxers and Bodymakers', 9.

■ REFERENCES

Angier, Natalie. *Frau: Eine Intime Geographie des Weiblichen Körpers*. München: C. Bertelsmann Verlag, 2000.
Butler, Judith. *Gender Trouble—Feminism and the Subversion of Identity*. London: Routledge, 1990.
Connell, Robert. *Gender*. Cambridge: Polity, 2002.
Donnelly, Michelle. 'Studying Extreme Sport'. *Journal of Sport and Social Issues* 30 (2006): 219–24.
Drevon, A. *Les Jeux Olympiques Oubliés: Paris 1900*. Paris: CNRS, 2000.

Fechtig, Beate, and Klaus Janke. 'Ich liebe Lars Riecken'. In *Mädchen als Fußballfans. Schüler Stars, Idole, Vorbilder*, 10–12. Hannover: Friedrich Verlag, 1997.

Gillis, Stacy, Gillian Howie, and Rebecca Munford, eds. *Third Wave Feminism: A Critical Exploration*. Basingstoke: Palgrave Macmillan, 2005.

Greendorfer, S. L. 'Title IX Gender Equity, Backlash and Ideology'. *Women in Sport and Physical Activity Journal* 7, no. 1 (1998): 69–93.

Haag, Tilla. 'Zukunftssicherung von Sportvereinen durch Gender Mainstreaming'. 2005. http://frauen.dsb.de/fileadmin/fm-frauen-im-sport/downloads/Bericht_Tilla_Haag.pdf.

Hall, Ann. 'Boxers and Bodymakers: Third-Wave Feminism and the Remaking of Women's Sport'. In *Dimensionen und Visionen des Sports*, edited by K. Roth, T. Pauer and K. Reischle, 245–47. Hamburg: Cwalina, 1999.

Hargreaves, Jennifer. 2001. 'Women's Boxing and Related Activities: Introducing Images and Meanings'. *Journal of Alternative Perspectives* 11 (2001). http://epe.lac-bac.gc.ca/100/201/300/ejmas/inyo/2002/11-28/jaltart_hargreaves_0901.htm.

Hedal, Martin. 'Motivation og tv-sport': MA thesis, University of Copenhagen, 2004.

Henkel, Andrea. 'DSB arbeitet nach der Strategie des Gender Mainstreaming'. 2003. http://www.frauenandiespitze.de/documents/best_practices/Erarbeitung_Gender_Meanstreaming_Kon zept_DSB_2003.pdf.

Heywood, Leslie, and Shari L. Dworkin. *Built to Win: The Female Athlete as Cultural Icon*. Minneapolis, MN: University of Minnesota Press, 2003.

Hovden, Jorid. '"Heavyweight" Men and Younger Women. The Gendering of Selection Processes in Norwegian Sports Organizations'. *NORA, Nordic Journal of Women's Studies* 8, no. 1 (2000): 17–32.

Klages,Andreas.*MitgliederentwicklungimDeutschenSportbund*.DeutscherSportbund.2004. http://www.dosb.de/fileadmin/fm-dsb/arbeitsfelder/wiss-ges/Dateien/Mitgliederent wicklung-Jahresmagazin-2004.pdf.

Klein, Marie-Luise, and Gertrud Pfister. *Goldmädel, Rennmiezen und Turnküken. Die Frau in der Sportberichterstattung der BILD-Zeitung*. Berlin: Bartels & Wernitz, 1985.

Kleindienst-Cachay, Christa. 'Sportengagement muslimischer Mädchen und Frauen in der Bundesrepublik Deutschland—Forschungsdesiderate und erste Ergebnisse eines Projekts'. In *Ethnisch-kulturelle Konflikte im Sport*, edited by Klein and Kothy, 113–26. Hamburg: Czwalina, 1998.

Lehnert, Gertrud. *Wenn Frauen Männerkleidung tragen*. München: dtv, 1997.

Lorber, Judith. *Paradoxes of Gender*. New Haven, CT: Yale University Press, 1994.

Löffler, Klaus, ed. *Frauenförderung in der Europäischen Union. 2. Aufl*. Bonn: Europäisches Parlament, 1998.

Messner, Michael A. *Taking the Field: Women, Men, and Sports*. Minneapolis, MN: University of Minnesota Press, 2002.

Morrison, A. M., R. P. White, and E. Van Velsor. *Breaking the Glass Ceiling. Can Women Reach the Top of America's Largest Corporations?* Reading: Addison-Wesley, 1992.

No author. 'Intersexualität: Wenn der kleine Unterschied fehlt'. *Geo Wissen* 26 (2000): 43.

Obel, Camilla. 'Collapsing Gender in Competitive Bodybuilding: Researching Contradictions and Ambiguity in Sport'. *Review for the Sociology of Sport* 31, no. 2 (1996): 185–202.

Opaschowski, Horst W. *Neue Trends im Freizeitsport: Analysen und Prognosen*. Hamburg: BAT, 1995.

Pfister, Gertrud. 'Doing Gender—Die Inszenierung des Geschlechts im Eiskunstlauf und im Kunstturnen'. In *Studier i idrott, historia och samhälle. Tillägnade professor Jan Lindroth pa has 60-arsdag*, edited by Johan Norberg, 170–201. Stockholm: HLS Förlag, 2000.

Pfister, Gertrud. 'Olympia nur für Männer? Auseinandersetzungen über die Beteiligung von Frauen an den Olympischen Spielen'. In *Olympische Spiele: Bilanz und Perspektiven im 21. Jahrhundert*, edited by Michael Krüger, 138–46. LIT Verlag Münster, 2001.

Pfister, Gertrud. 'Frauen in Führungspositionen—Theoretische Überlegungen im Deutschen und Internationalen Diskurs'. In *Hat Führung ein Geschlecht? Genderarrangements in Entscheidungsgremien des deutschen Sports*, edited by Gudrun Doll-Tepper and Gertrud Pfister, 7–48. Köln: Strauß, 2004.

Pfister, Gertrud. 'Frauen in Führungspositionen des Sports—Internationale Tendenzen'. In *Hat Führung ein Geschlecht? Genderarrangements in Entscheidungsgremien des deutschen Sports*, edited by Gudrun Doll-Tepper and Gertrud Pfister, 49–63. Köln: Strauß, 2004.

Pfister, Gertrud. 'Gender, Sport und Massenmedien'. In *Geschlechterforschung im Sport. Differenz und/oder Gleichheit*, edited by Kugelmann, Pfister, and Zipprich, 59–88. Hamburg: Czwalina, 2004.

Pfister, Gertrud. *Kvinder på toppen—om kvinder, idræt og ledelse*. København: Institut for Idræt, Københavns Universitet, 2005.

Pfister, Gertrud. 'The Future of Football is Female!? On the Past and Present of Women's Football in Germany'. In *German Football. History, Culture, Society*, edited by Alan Tomlinson and Christopher Young, 93–126. London: Routledge, 2006.

Pfister, Gertrud. 'Gender Issues in Danish Sports Organizations—Experiences, Attitudes and Evaluations'. *NORA, Nordic Journal of Women's Studies* 14, no. 1 (2006): 27–40.

Pfister, Gertrud, and Kari Fasting. 'Geschlechterkonstruktionen auf dem Fußballplatz'. In *Die lokal-globale Fußballkultur—wissenschaftlich beobachtet*, edited by Dieter Jütting, 137–52. Münster: Waxmann, 2004.

Pfister, Gertrud, and Sabine Radtke. 'Biographien von männlichen und weiblichen Führungskräften im deutschen Sport'. In *Hat Führung ein Geschlecht? Genderarrangements in Entscheidungsgremien des deutschen Sports*, edited by Gudrun Doll-Tepper and Gertrud Pfister, 143–212. Köln: Strauß, 2004.

Pilgaard, Maja. *Danskernes motions—og sportsvaner 2007—nøgletal og tendenser*. København: Idrættens Analyseinstitut, 2008.

Rinehart, Robert. 'Babes and Boards. Opportunities in New Millenium Sport?' *Journal of Sport & Social Issues* 29, no. 3 (2005): 232–55.

Schmidt, Gunter. 'Tragödie als Schurkenstück. Mann ist Mann, Frau is Frau?'. *Der Spiegel* 40 (2000): 252–53.

Stiegler, Barbara. *Frauen im Mainstreaming: politische Strategien und Theorien zur Geschlechterfrage*. Bonn: Friedrich Ebert Stiftung, 1998.

Wheaton, Belinda. *Understanding Lifestyle Sport: Consumption, Identity and Difference*. London: Routledge, 2004.

6 Out of Bounds?

A Critique of the New Policies on Hyperandrogenism

in Elite Female Athletes

KATRINA KARKAZIS, REBECCA
JORDAN-YOUNG, GEORGIANN DAVIS,
AND SILVIA CAMPORESI

This summer, London will capture the world's attention when it hosts the 2012 Olympic Games.[1] At the London Games, more than a decade after the International Association of Athletics Federations (IAAF) and the International Olympic Committee (IOC) abandoned routine sex testing for female athletes, a "sex-testing" policy will once again be in place. The change came in response to the case of Caster Semenya, the South African runner whose sex was first challenged by her competitors and whose spectacular win and powerful physique fueled an international frenzy of speculation about her sex. In the absence of a fair and transparent policy for handling these charges, the IAAF bungled Semenya's case at almost every turn, driving her into hiding to escape scrutiny and humiliation. As a result, the IAAF and the IOC came under intense pressure to rethink how to handle such challenges in the future.

After an 18-month period of review, the IAAF developed a policy that will not return to routine sex testing of all female athletes but that is aimed at systematically responding to questions of eligibility once the sex of a particular female athlete is questioned. In a shift from earlier universal sex testing, the goal is not to determine whether someone is "really" a woman (as previous sex-based exams and tests were meant to do—inevitably failing, as we describe below). Instead, the new policies focus on women with naturally elevated androgen levels (hyperandrogenism). While not disputing that women with hyperandrogenism are female, the new regulations aim to clarify whether women with this condition are "too masculine" to compete with other women (IAAF 2011c, 1). The IOC is expected to release similar policies in time for the 2012 Olympics.

The new policies include a number of rules and regulations, each resting on the assumption that androgenic hormones (such as testosterone and dihydrotestosterone) are the primary components of biological athletic advantage. The policies address hyperandrogenism, a condition in which females produce androgens in excess of the range typical for females. In practice, the policies do not concern all androgens, but focus specifically on testosterone. As such, women with naturally

TABLE 6.1. *Conditions Leading to Hyperandrogenism in Women (First Six Are Intersex Conditions)*

- Congenital adrenal hyperplasia (CAH): 21-hydroxylase or 11β-hydroxylase deficiency.
- 3β-Hydroxysteroid dehydrogenase deficiency.
- 5α-Reductase type 2 deficiency.
- Androgen insensitivity syndrome (AIS).
- Ovotesticular DSD (previously called "true hermaphroditism").
- 17β-Hydroxysteroid dehydrogenase type 3 (17β- HSD3) deficiency.
- Polycystic ovary syndrome (PCOS).
- Adrenal carcinoma.
- Luteoma of pregnancy (IAAF 2011).

high endogenous levels of testosterone, primarily though not exclusively women with intersex traits, or what are also called disorders of sex development (DSD) (see Table 6.1), are presumed to have an advantage over women with lower levels of testosterone. Henceforth, women athletes *known or suspected* to have hyperandrogenism will be allowed to compete only if they agree to medical intervention, or if they are found to be "insensitive" to androgens.

At first glance, the new policies may seem to be an improvement over past approaches by guaranteeing fair competition among female athletes. They do not return to universal sex testing of all female athletes. They also certainly seem like a more systematic response and thus preferable to ad hoc responses to suspicions about the sex of individual female athletes. Finally, they appear to be less invasive and more objective than previous sex testing methods such as routine gynecological exams and chromosomal tests for all female athletes. But questions about the new policies abound. To start, does endogenous testosterone actually confer athletic advantage in a predictable way, as the new regulations suggest? If there *is* advantage from naturally occurring variation in testosterone, is that advantage *unfair*? In other words, elite athletes differ from most people in a wide range of ways (e.g., rare genetic mutations that confer extraordinary aerobic capacity and resistance against fatigue). Why single out testosterone? Will the new policies ensure that athletes are no longer subjected to the sort of inhumane treatment that Caster Semenya endured? Does the policy succeed in balancing the aim of creating a "fair" playing field for women athletes (which is the ostensible goal of sex-segregated sports), judged in relation to the aim of ensuring fairness for individual athletes on the other? What are the broader social implications of the concern about "overly masculine" women competing in sports? More specifically, how might these policies reinforce dominant understandings of sex and gender?

To explore these questions, we begin with a brief discussion of Caster Semenya's case and the new policies that developed in its wake, and then we consider the underlying assumptions concerning the relationship of gender to biology in these regulations. We discuss three broad grounds on which the legitimacy of the new policies can be questioned: the underlying scientific assumptions, the policy-making process, and the potential to achieve fairness for female athletes. On each of these grounds we find that the policies fall seriously short and, for this reason, we conclude they should be rescinded.

■ BACKGROUND

Caster Semenya Debacle

In August 2009, Caster Semenya, a young South African runner, won the women's 800-meter race at the Berlin World Championships in Athletics by a margin of 2.45 seconds and immediately found herself at the center of international controversy amid a frenzy of speculation about whether she was "really" a woman (Clarey 2009). The controversy was sparked by complaints from Semenya's competitors; they pointed not to the large margin of her win, but to what one writer referred to as her "breathtakingly butch" appearance (Levy 2009), remarking, "Just look at her" and "These kinds of people should not run with us. . . .. For me, she is not a woman. She is a man" (Adams 2009; Levy 2009). Shortly after the media reported these comments, a supposedly misdirected fax notified the press that the IAAF had actually required Semenya to undergo "sex testing" shortly *before* her Berlin win (Levy 2009). The IAAF had ordered South African authorities to perform the tests after Semenya broke a national junior record at the African championships in Mauritius. Throughout the testing, Semenya had been under the impression she was undergoing standard doping tests owing to her win (BBC 2009).

In a moment when she might have been celebrating her victory, Semenya endured a cruel and humiliating media spectacle; sports commentators ridiculed her appearance, called her names including "hermaphrodite," and cried out for her medal and prize money to be returned (Levy 2009; D. Smith 2009). Under a typical headline, Time.com trumpeted "Could This Women's World Champ Be a Man?" (Adams 2009). Semenya was reportedly subjected to a two-hour examination during which doctors put her legs in stirrups and photographed her genitalia (Levy 2009; A. D. Smith 2009). Afterward Semenya sent distraught messages to friends and family (Levy 2009; A. D. Smith 2009). Test results purportedly indicated that Semenya had an intersex condition that left her without a uterus or ovaries and with undescended testes producing androgens at three times the typical level for females (known as hyperandrogenism) (Hurst 2009).[2] After these intensely intimate details about Semenya's body became a topic for public debate and scrutiny, she went into hiding; she reportedly required trauma counseling in the wake of claims that sex tests confirmed she was a "hermaphrodite" (Levy 2009; A. D. Smith 2009).

The IAAF banned her from competitions while it completed its investigation. Eventually, after an 11-month investigation—a process that involved 10 months of negotiation with the IAAF involving legal representatives and a high-profile mediator known for his work on international disputes—the IAAF cleared Semenya for competition and her Berlin victory was allowed to stand (Dewey & LeBoeuf 2010).

Although Semenya's Berlin results showed a big improvement over her earlier races in the 800-meter, she nevertheless ranks 26th overall and 7th for "juniors" (she does not rank on either men's list) (IAAF 2011a; 2011b). Semenya had previously not been singled out for such scrutiny, but the combination of her win and her appearance raised suspicion about her sex. Leonard Chuene, then president of Athletics South Africa (ASA), observed, "We took this child to Poland to the junior championship under the IAAF. Why was there no story about it? She was accepted there. No-one said anything there because she did not do anything special. She is the same girl" (Farquhar 2009).

The New Policies

The IAAF came under intense criticism for how they handled Semenya's case and her suffering at the hands of the media and the governing athletics bodies. As a result, the IAAF decided, along with the IOC, to revisit the procedure for when questions are raised about whether a particular athlete should be allowed to compete as a woman.

Following a series of international meetings over 18 months, during which the IAAF and the IOC Medical Commission worked in close coordination, the IAAF announced its policy on hyperandrogenism, which went into effect on May 1, 2011 (IAAF 2011c). At the same time, IOC officials announced that similar rules based on principles almost identical to those in the IAAF guidelines would be released in time for the 2012 Olympic Games in London (IOC 2011).[3]

Although males and females alike produce testosterone, women typically produce about one-tenth the level of males (Braunstein 2011; Longcope 1986; Strauss and Barbieri 1999). The IAAF policy defines the "normal male range" of total testosterone in serum as ≥ 10 nmol/L (IAAF 2011c, 12). Only female athletes who have testosterone levels below the "normal male range," or who have an androgen resistance condition, are permitted to participate in women's competitions (IAAF 2011c).[4]

Under the IAAF policy, female athletes who wish to participate in international competitions come to the attention of the IAAF in one of two ways. If a female athlete already has been diagnosed with hyperandrogenism (or is in the process of being diagnosed), she is required to notify the IAAF and undergo evaluation (as outlined in the policy). A second route to evaluation is that an "IAAF Medical Manager may initiate a confidential investigation of any female athlete if he [sic] has reasonable grounds for believing that a case of hyperandrogenism may exist" (IAAF 2001c, 3). Reasonable grounds can come from "any reliable source," including "information received by the IAAF Medical Delegate or other responsible medical official at a competition" (IAAF 2001c, 3).

Once an athlete has been identified for evaluation, she is required to undergo some combination of three types of exams: (1) clinical exam; (2) endocrine exam (testing urine and blood for hormone levels); and/or (3) full exam (which may include genetic testing, imaging, and psychological evaluation). Following evaluation, a female athlete can only compete if she meets the criteria specified in the policy, specifically, a testosterone level below 10 nmol/L for IAAF competitions (and whatever testosterone level medical examiners deem acceptable for Olympic competitions). If the athlete does not "pass" the evaluation, a final diagnosis and "therapeutic proposal" will be issued to her in writing. She will be banned from competition until she lowers her testosterone levels. If she follows the "prescribed medical treatment" as outlined in the written statement, she may be reassessed for possible participation in future women's competitions. The prescribed treatment will presumably entail either pharmaceutical intervention or gonadectomy, since these are the two ways of lowering testosterone.

Gender and Bodies

We cannot think about the Caster Semenya case or evaluate these new policies without careful attention to common assumptions about gender and its relationship to bodies. For decades now, experts in multiple fields, including medicine, psychology, the social sciences, and the humanities, have distinguished between "sex" (biological and anatomical traits that are used to label a person as female or male) and "gender" (psychological and behavioral traits that are designated as "masculine" or "feminine," that is, traits considered more common for or appropriate to boys and men versus girls and women) (e.g., Kessler and McKenna 1978; Laqueur 1990; Rubin 1975; Russett 1989). Although sex and gender are commonly expected to be concordant in an individual, they are not necessarily so. "Gender verification policies" in elite sports are meant to distinguish competitors on the basis of sex-linked biology—that is, *sex* rather than *gender* (e.g., Wilson 2000).

Sex is commonly thought to be straightforward, consisting of two clear categories of male and female. Yet there are at least six markers of sex—including chromosomes, gonads, hormones, secondary sex characteristics, external genitalia, and internal genitalia—and none of these are binary. For example, it is often assumed that people have either XX or XY chromosomes, but some individuals are born with an extra X chromosome and others have a mosaic karyotype where each cell has one karyotype or the other.

We also often expect the traits of "sex-linked" biology to be concordant in individuals. But development can vary at any point, resulting in various combinations and permutations of sex-linked traits. For centuries, defining sex has required negotiation and has elicited disagreement among scientists and clinicians about which traits or body parts should identify one as male or female (Dreger 1998; Laqueur 1990; Reis 2009; Schiebinger 1989). The breadth of human physical variance is more complex than the categories suggest. Take, for example, women with a condition known as complete androgen insensitivity syndrome

(CAIS), who are born with XY chromosomes, testes, and testosterone levels in the typical range for males. If only taking chromosomal, gonadal, or hormonal factors into account, one would label these individuals male. Yet these women have a completely feminine phenotype, with breast development and female typical genitalia, because their androgen receptors are not responsive to androgens. Designating women with CAIS as male would be inappropriate, given that they are presumed female at birth, are raised as girls, and overwhelmingly identify as female.

Both experts and lay people tend to think of intersex traits as rare aberrations or deviations. And even those experts who understand that sex is complex and its markers are multiple tend, nonetheless, to assert that, as a matter of biology, sex is "objective" (e.g., Wilson 2000). But the demarcation between male and female categories depends on context (Fausto-Sterling 1985; Karkazis 2008; Kessler 1998; Oudshoorn 1994). In the context of reproduction, the presence of a uterus may categorize someone as female. A woman who has undergone a hysterectomy has no uterus in the same way a woman with CAIS has no uterus, yet no one questions whether the former is really still female.

Adding further complexity, sex markers are not binary; each variable contains significant variation, both within and across individuals. For example, women's testosterone levels range widely among women and also by time of day, time of month, and time of life (Haring et al. 2012).[5] Tissue responses also vary across individuals due to differences in hormone receptors that range from subtle to dramatic. Further variations result from interactions with the environment—for example, things like a change in social status or winning or losing a competition (even a "fake" win or loss that is experimentally assigned by a researcher) can stimulate a rise or drop in testosterone (McCaul et al. 1992; Sapolsky 1997).

It is often assumed that people with intersex traits are somehow exceptional because of their complex biologies, but sex is *always* complex. There are many biological markers of sex but none is decisive: that is, none is actually present in *all* people labeled male or female. Sex testing has been and continues to be problematic because there is no single physiological or biological marker that allows for the simple categorization of people as male or female.

Sex Testing and Gender Policing in Elite Sports

Meanwhile, if sex is meant to distinguish females and males depending on *biological* features, gender is used to point to *social* factors (social roles, position, behavior). The "commonsense" view suggests that biological and social features are concordant. Many people regard the outward signs of gender (how someone acts, dresses, behaves) as if they tell us about someone's biology, about their *sex*. And this brings us back to Caster Semenya, whose victory combined with outward signs of gender that many read as "masculine"—her lack of makeup, her impressive musculature, the braids that give the impression of closely cropped hair, and her height—raised suspicion about her sex.

Women first joined the Olympics in 1900 (Drinkwater and International Federation of Sports Medicine 2000; Olympic.org n.d.). From the beginning, only female athletes have been subjected to sex testing because concerns about "fraud" and "fairness" have centered on the possibility that males could unfairly outperform females. Though ad hoc testing had been practiced since at least the 1936 Olympic Games, mass certification of female sex was first implemented by the IAAF in 1946 (Heggie 2010). By 1948, the IOC followed suit and implemented its first formal policy for female sex determination.

Anxiety about women competitors' femininity has plagued the events almost from the beginning (Olsen-Acre 2003; Stephenson 1996). In the earliest iteration of sex testing, female competitors were required to provide medical "certificates of femininity," but the IAAF and IOC provided no standard criteria and exercised no oversight for making this determination (Heggie 2010). Conceivably, these markers could be based entirely on social and cultural criteria of femininity such as hairstyle and dress (Heggie 2010). Thus, outwardly observable feminine characteristics (gender) served as a proxy for biology (sex).

By the 1960s, the IOC and IAAF adopted supposedly standardized tests to verify sex, including compulsory "nude parades" in front of physicians, genital exams, and evaluation of secondary sex characteristics such as hair patterns (Hay 1972; Ritchie et al. 2008; Simpson et al. 1993). Not surprisingly, these exams garnered intense criticism and the IOC and the IAAF adopted chromosomal testing in 1967 to infer an individual's sex chromosomes relying on visualization of Barr bodies in a buccal smear (using cells swabbed from inside a cheek) (de la Chapelle 1986; Heggie 2010).

Adopting this test was based on the assumption that chromosomes are adequate proxies for sex. Using chromosomes to sort individuals into a sex binary, however, leads to peculiar results. The Barr Body Test only detects the presence of X chromosomes. However, the reliance on the presence of X chromosomes as the criterion for female sex excludes women with chromosomal and genetic anomalies: individuals with CAIS who have a 46, XY karyotype and those with Turner syndrome who have a 45, XO karyotype would not be classified as female. Alternatively, it includes men who have more than one X chromosome and thus would incorrectly classify those with Klinefelter syndrome (47, XXY) as females despite their male phenotype. Nevertheless, the Barr Body Test was used throughout the 1970s and 1980s, perhaps because it seemed to be a less invasive and more scientific method of assessing sex.

The problems raised by the exclusive reliance on chromosomes to determine a female athlete's sex reached a head in 1985 when the IOC disqualified Spanish hurdler María José Martínez-Patiño from competitions and withdrew her medals and records because she was "chromosomally male" (Heggie 2010; Martínez-Patiño 2005). Martínez-Patiño, who was born with 46, XY chromosomes and a female phenotype (CAIS), successfully challenged the ruling, arguing that her condition made her completely unresponsive to testosterone and thus gave her no advantage over "normal" XX females (Martínez-Patiño 2005). In response, the IAAF abandoned routine chromosomal and laboratory testing altogether, in favor of returning to a "manual/visual" check for individuals whose femininity was being questioned, and by 1992 had dropped even these exams (Elsas et al. 2000; Heggie 2010, 160).

The IOC, however, turned to a novel technique to detect the presence of the SRY gene—the gene leading to testis development discovered a few years earlier—reasoning that this was the source of male athletic advantage (Dingeon 1993). There was little evidence that this test was useful for sex determination, or any evidence that this gene was linked to athletic advantage. Relying on the presence of the SRY gene for sex determination, however, also classified some women as male. After a round of false positives in the 1996 Olympics—which identified eight women with intersex traits (Genel 2000)—the IOC finally also abandoned all forms of routine sex testing of female athletes (Elsas et al. 2000; Heggie 2010). What followed in the wake of universal sex testing for females was a policy that permitted medical professionals to evaluate on an ad hoc basis individual athletes whose sex has been called into question using a variety of clinical exams and laboratory tests (Genel 2000; Tian et al. 2009).

Despite the longstanding concern about men masquerading as females in elite sports, decades of universal and routine sex testing of female athletes in international sport competitions revealed at best two instances of a man trying to compete fraudulently among women (Cole 2000). Instead, sex testing has mostly "caught" women with intersex traits (Simpson et al. 2000). In fact, while the official rationale for sex testing has been to ferret out men masquerading as females, concerns about possible "unfair advantage" among women with intersex traits go back at least several decades (see Cole 2000). A long-time member of IOC Medical Commission, for example, argued that females with some intersex conditions have "masculine anatomical conditions, [giving them] an unfair and unlawful advantage over the anatomically normal woman athlete" (Hay 1974, 119), and thus "must be barred from competition in order to insure [sic] fair play" (Hay 1972, 998). Justification for "gender verification" has thus intermingled various concerns about unfair advantage created by men impersonating women, performance-enhancing drug use, and women with nonnormative sex and gender traits.

Except for the period when routine biological testing was the policy, perceived gender nonconformity has always played an important role in triggering questions about an athlete's "biological" masculinity. Women athletes are already under a great deal of pressure to appear "feminine" and even "sexy" (Reaney 2011). As the editors of a special issue of Sociological Perspectives devoted to gender and sport observed, "Cultural tensions between athleticism and femininity have long been managed by social control or strong encouragement for women athletes to attend charm schools, to wear long hair, painted nails, or other markers of emphasized femininity, and to emphasize their abilities and willingness to be mothers" (Dworkin and Messner 2002, 348). The cultural equations that link external signs of "femininity" with bodily femaleness also link "normalcy" in gender and sex with heterosexuality (Jordan-Young 2010). In other words, when people see gender nonconformity they often infer homosexuality. Thus, gender policing in sports often takes the form of homophobia (Cyphers and Fagan 2011).

This brief history outlining the failed methods for determining sex shows that the problems with sex testing are not with the tests per se, but with the assumption that any singular marker of sex is adequate to classify people into a two-sex system. It also shows that female athletes have always been under suspicion, and women with intersex traits have often been scapegoats for broad anxiety about the gender contradiction inherent in the very concept of an elite female athlete. From this perspective, the focus on hyperandrogenism might seem to be an improvement because the stated aim is to ensure fairness and not to eliminate athletes who are not "truly" or "fully" women from women's competitions. But the apparently more modest goal of eliminating women whose masculine characteristics confer "unfair advantage" requires a deeper look. Is the new policy based on sound science? Was it developed via a legitimate process? And finally, will it provide "fair" competition for women athletes?

■ CRITIQUE

Scientific Gaps and Flaws

The new policies rest on the notion that the difference in athletic performance between males and females is "predominantly due to higher levels of androgenic hormones in males resulting in increased strength and muscle development" (IAAF 2011c, 1). Both policies rely in particular on testosterone levels as the mark of unfair advantage. Although it may be surprising, given that this is a popular belief and is stated as fact in both IAAF and IOC statements (IAAF 2011c; IOC 2011), the link between athleticism and androgens in general or testosterone in particular has not been proven. Despite the many assumptions about the relationship between testosterone and athletic advantage, *there is no evidence showing that successful athletes have higher testosterone levels than less successful athletes.*

Clinical studies do confirm that testosterone (among many other factors) helps individuals to increase their muscle size, strength, and endurance (Bhasin et al. 1996; Ronnestad et al. 2011; Storer et al. 2003). It may seem logical to infer, then, that a person with more testosterone will have greater athletic advantage than one with less testosterone, but this is not necessarily so. Individuals have dramatically different responses to the same amounts of testosterone, and testosterone is just one element in a complex neuroendocrine feedback system, which is just as likely to be affected by as to affect athletic performance. Studies have shown, for example, that winning a competition raises testosterone—even among fans whose teams prevail, or in experimental subjects randomly assigned to win (McCaul et al. 1992; Oliveira et al. 2009).

Testosterone is far from the decisive factor in athleticism. The most dramatic example is women with CAIS, whose tissues are completely unresponsive to testosterone but who are overrepresented among elite athletes (Tucker and Collins 2010, 138). This fact cannot be readily reconciled with a theory that suggests testosterone is the main source of athletic ability. Moreover, the relationship between testosterone and physique is extremely complex even beyond the issue of receptor variability. Relying on testosterone levels suggests far more certainty than current scientific knowledge allows. Consider women with congenital adrenal hyperplasia (CAH), whose testosterone levels are high. The new policies suggest that these women have a competitive advantage, but women with CAH are disproportionately affected by short stature, obesity, dysregulation of mood hormones, and unpredictable, life-threatening salt-losing crises (Charmandari et al. 2004; Eugster et al. 2001; Meyer-Bahlburg 2011; Speiser and White 2003; Stikkelbroeck et al. 2003; Volkl et al. 2006). Indeed, considering the genital surgery, repeated genital exams, and medical monitoring that women with CAH experience (e.g., Karkazis 2008), athletic competition at an elite level appears "against the odds" for women with CAH.

Because it goes against common wisdom, it is worth repeating that it has not been shown that athletes with higher endogenous testosterone perform better than athletes with lower levels. Furthermore, commentaries sometimes suggest that the psychological aspects of athletic performance, especially competitiveness and willingness to take risks, might be affected by testosterone. Although there is a relationship between testosterone and competitiveness, it is the exact reverse of the usual assumption: Both female and male athletes facing a competition consistently have been shown to experience a rise in testosterone (Bateup et al. 2002; Edwards and O'Neal 2009). Again, however, there are no data to suggest that precompetition testosterone levels predict an athlete's performance on the field.

One of the biggest gaps in current data is that nearly all research on testosterone and athletics has been conducted in men. Direct evidence of the relationship between testosterone and athletic ability in women is limited both by the small number of studies that include women and by the narrow focus of these studies: The few placebo controlled studies of how testosterone affects muscle in women include only severely hypogonadal women with very low estrogen and androgen levels (Dolan et al. 2004; Miller et al. 2006). Although testosterone serves similar physiologic functions in women and men, there are findings that suggest that the specific mechanisms of action might be different (MacLean et al. 2008). Moreover, there is a 10-fold gap in male and female endogenous testosterone levels, but smaller differences (including overlap) in virtually all aspects of athletic strength and performance, suggesting testosterone's effects on athletic ability are likely to be different in men and women. Consider, for example, the eight races ranging between the 100-meter and the marathon at the 2009 Berlin IAAF Championships where Caster Semenya's performance caused such a stir: There was overlap between the male and female times in all but one race (the 10,000-meter) (Tucker and Collins 2010, 136–137). Many aspects of physique or athletic performance differ between males and females, often substantially; however, none of these is close to 10-fold, further underscoring the limitations of a straightforward comparison of average male–female differences in athletic performance to average male–female differences in testosterone levels. There is also no support for knowing the effect of testosterone level on any individual. While females are generally more sensitive to the effects of testosterone than males, curvilinear effects as well as great interindividual differences make extrapolation of the effects of specific amounts in any given individual impossible.

In sum, there is a great deal of mythology about the physical effects of testosterone and other androgens (Fausto-Sterling 1985; Jordan-Young 2010). Likewise, mental effects of androgens are often implied to give an additional boost to athletes, but placebo-controlled studies of testosterone show that increasing testosterone (above minimum functional levels) has no effects on mood, cognitive performance, libido, or aggression (Bhasin et al. 1996; Bhasin et al. 2001; Kvorning et al. 2006). Optimal levels of testosterone is one of many factors that is necessary for athletes to achieve their own "personal best," but comparing testosterone levels across individuals is not of any apparent scientific value.

The Right People to Do the Job?

The shortcomings of the IAAF policy (and perhaps to a lesser degree the IOC policy) derive in part from the process by which it was developed. As the Semenya debacle exploded into the media, the IOC approached the organizers of an upcoming meeting of specialists in intersex to advise the IOC and the IAAF on "how to determine an athlete's eligibility by using better testing modalities as well as clearer definitions of what it means to be a male as well as a female . . . [and to] clarify the medical aspect of these issues" (New and Simpson 2011, vi). Five months later, representatives from the IOC and IAAF met in Miami coincident with the January 2010 "2nd World Conference on Hormonal and Genetic Basis of Sexual Differentiation," a continuing medical education course on DSD (New and Simpson 2011). The conference was not convened for the purpose of developing these policies; rather, that aim was added later. As a consequence, all of the presenters at the conference were medical professionals with expertise not in sports physiology, but in DSD (New and Simpson 2010). An attendee at that public meeting observed that it "failed to produce any clear consensus and only seemed to create confusion about what is now considered fair or allowable so far as sports gender divisions go" (Dreger 2010), perhaps precisely because it was open to those with perspectives other than medical. The day after the CME course the IOC and IAAF representatives met privately with the conference presenters.

In October 2010, the IOC held another closed-door meeting in Lausanne, Switzerland, that included IAAF representatives. Unlike the January meeting that was overwhelmingly populated by experts in DSD, this one included "scientists, sports administrators, sports lawyers (including from the IOC Legal Affairs Department), juridical experts in human rights, experts in medical and sports ethics, female athletes and a representative appointed by the intersex community (Organisation Intersex International)" (IOC 2011; Viloria 2011). Although the IAAF representatives attended the IOC meetings, the IAAF working group consisted of five members all of whom were medical professionals with expertise in endocrinology, gynecology, DSD, or polycystic ovary syndrome (PCOS).

The composition of decision-making bodies affects the content of policies (e.g., Hajer and Wagenaar 2003; Hannagan and Larimer 2010). Although the IOC included a variety of perspectives for the Lausanne meeting, in developing the policies it and the IAAF relied primarily on the expertise of individuals associated with the problematic policies of the last 20 years. Moreover, if the goal was to think about how to assess the role and importance of testosterone in athletic achievement, there were no experts in exercise physiology or the relationship between testosterone and athletic performance involved in the process. Specialists in DSD defined both the problem and the nature of possible solutions, and framed them squarely in biomedical terms. Indeed, the introduction to the published proceedings of January 2010 meeting provides a sealed and self-confident narrative of the important issues in the determination of sex difference and athletic advantage (New and Simpson 2011). The following excerpt is illustrative:

> Those presenting at the conference were world class scientists who achieved high recognition for their work over the years on the biological, genetic, and psychological differences between the sexes. They covered recent advances which could be used to clarify confusions and to address controversies among athletes like the South African track star at the International Amateur Athletic Federation [sic] meet in Berlin in August 2009. Her eligibility to compete as a female athlete brought her international media attention and embarrassment as to what gender [sic] is she. The conference presented an extraordinary amount of data that can help avoid such international attention. The conference taught ways to evaluate, diagnose, and treat those with disorders of sexual differentiation to clinicians who normally do not see these types of patients, may have them in their practice unknowingly, or see them on a regular basis without knowing what to do next. Also, knowing the great importance of modalities such as hormonal assays and psychological tests used along with DNA analysis. (New and Simpson 2011)

And yet, at this meeting and later meetings there were no experts who could answer the pertinent medicoscientific question on which both policies are premised: What does testosterone do to and for the female athlete? (IAAF 2011c; IOC 2011).

Furthermore, the IAAF policy does not engage with the questions that might arise from other relevant perspectives. Should endogenous testosterone levels be viewed as on par with intensive training, the use of hypoxic chambers, or Lasik, which are all accepted ways to enhance an athlete's performance? Under what circumstances, if at all, is it ethical to require individuals to undergo medical intervention in order to compete? What unintended consequences might these policies have for female athletes? For example, how might these new policies re-inforce pressures to adhere to beauty standards that are irrelevant to athletic per-formance? How might the new policies intensify the stigmatization and pressure on lesbian athletes to hide or be especially gender conforming?

The Ethical Principles in Play

The IAAF and IOC outlined several principles on which their policies are based, which form a rubric for helping to determine who is tested, why they are tested, and how they are tested (see Table 6.2) (IAAF 2011c; IOC 2011). The principles outlined under the respective columns for the IOC and IAAF, taken verbatim from the IAAF policy and IOC press release, are predicated on concerns with fairness in female athletic competition, definitions of normal, the health of ath-letes, and protecting privacy and confidentiality.

Fairness

Both policies were constructed based on "respect for the fundamental notion of fairness of competition in female Athletics" (IAAF 2011c). Fairness is, of course, an essential component of athletic competitions. Achieving this fairness, they assert, requires the continued division of athletics into male and female catego-ries.[6] The issue becomes how to determine such divisions.

Current science suggests that any advantage that might be conferred by hy-perandrogenism is so complex that testosterone levels alone are a nearly useless indicator of advantage, and certainly not an appropriate measure for determin-ing eligibility. Furthermore, certain medical conditions give females high levels of testosterone. The new policies ban females with hyperandrogenism on the grounds that they have an unfair advantage. Unlike doping, in hyperandrogen-ism the hormones are not external to the athlete's body and are not added in-tentionally to confer advantage over competitors (i.e., cheating). Women with hyperandrogenism have not introduced any foreign matter into their bodies, nor have they engaged in any unfair practices (Foddy and Savulescu 2011).

Even if some sort of evaluation were available that could decisively link hy-perandrogenism to sporting ability (the traits of which would vary considerably by sport as well), hyperandrogenism should be viewed as no different from other

TABLE 6.2. *Key Principles and Facets of the IAAF and IOC Policies (IAAF 20011c; IOC 2011)* Extracted verbatim from official IAAF and IOC Communications

	IAAF	IOC
Eligibility and compliance	An acknowledgement that females with hyperandrogenism may compete in women's competition in Athletics subject to compliance with IAAF Rules and Regulations. A female with hyperandrogenism who is recognized as a female in law shall be eligible to compete in women's competition in athletics provided that she has androgen levels below the male range (measured by reference to testosterone levels in serum) or, if she has androgen levels within the male range she also has an androgen resistance that means that she derives no competitive advantage from such levels. A female athlete who declines, fails or refuses to comply with the eligibility determination process under the regulations shall not be eligible to compete in women's competition.	A female recognized in law should be eligible to compete in female competitions provided that she has androgen levels below the male range (as shown by the serum concentration of testosterone) or, if within the male range, she has an androgen resistance such that she derives no competitive advantage from such levels. If an athlete fails or refuses to comply with any aspect of the eligibility determination process, while that is her right as an individual, she will not be eligible to participate as a competitor in the chosen sport.
Evaluation	The evaluation of complex cases on an anonymous basis through the use of a panel of independent international medical experts in the field. A pool of international medical experts has been appointed by the IAAF to review cases referred to it under the regulations as an independent expert medical panel and to make recommendations to the IAAF in such cases to decide on the eligibility of female athletes with hyperandrogenism. A three-level medical process under the regulations shall ensure that all potentially relevant data is made available to the expert medical panel for the purposes of evaluating an athlete's eligibility. This medical process may include, where necessary, the expert medical panel referring an athlete with potential hyperandrogenism for full examination and diagnosis in accordance with best medical practice at one of the six IAAF-approved specialist reference centers around the world.	An evaluation with respect to eligibility should be made on an anonymous basis by a panel of independent international experts in the field of hyperandrogenism that would in each case issue a recommendation on eligibility for the sport concerned. In each case, the sport would decide on an athlete's eligibility taking into consideration the panel's recommendation. Should an athlete be considered ineligible to compete, she would be notified of the reasons why and informed of the conditions she would be required to meet should she wish to become eligible again.

(continued)

TABLE 6.2. **Continued**

	IAAF	IOC
Fairness	A respect for the very essence of the male and female classifications in athletics. A respect for the fundamental notion of fairness of competition in female athletics. Competition in athletics will continue to be divided into men's and women's competition recognizing that there is a difference in sporting performance between elite men and women, that is predominantly due to higher levels of androgenic hormones in men.	Rules are needed and . . . these rules should respect the essence of the male/ female classification and also guarantee the fairness and integrity of female competitions for all female athletes. Although rare, some women develop male-like body characteristics due to an overproduction of male sex hormones, so-called "androgens." The androgenic effects on the human body explain why men perform better than women in most sports and are, in fact, the very reason for the distinction between male and female competition in most sports. Consequently, women with hyperandrogenism generally perform better in sport than other women.
Health	The early prevention of problems associated with hyperandrogenism.	In order to protect the health of the athlete, *sports* authorities should have the responsibility to make sure that any case of female hyperandrogenism that arises under their jurisdiction receives adequate medical follow-up.
Privacy and Confidentiality	A respect for confidentiality in the medical process and the need to avoid public exposure of young females with hyperandrogenism who may be psychologically vulnerable. The medical process under the regulations shall be conducted in strict confidentiality and all cases shall be referred to the expert medical panel on an anonymous basis.	The investigation of a particular case should be conducted under strict confidentiality.

biological advantages derived from exceptional biological variation. Numerous biological advantages that everyone accepts are frequently found in groups of elite athletes. Several runners and cyclists have rare mitochondrial variations that give them extraordinary aerobic capacity and exceptional resistance against fatigue (Eynon, Birk, et al. 2011; Eynon, Moran, et al. 2011; Eynon, Ruiz, et al. 2011; Pitsiladis et al. 2011). Basketball players who have acromegaly, a hormonal condition that results in exceptionally large hands and feet, are not banned from competition (Clemmons 2008; Mannix 2007). Perfect vision exists among baseball players at a significantly higher rate than in the general population (Laby et al. 1996). Many have also speculated that Michael Phelps, the record-breaking

Olympian swimmer, has Marfan's syndrome, a rare genetic mutation that results in exceptionally long limbs and flexible joints that help to make him an exceptional swimmer (Foxnews.com 2008). Some elite athletes have variations in the ACE gene (which affects muscle growth and efficiency) and in the NOS gene (which affects blood flow to skeletal muscles) (Ostrander et al. 2009). Elite athletes thus already display myriad types of biological and genetic advantages. Hyperandrogenism is a naturally occurring phenomenon and therefore no different from any other exceptional biological variation in the human body.

Eligibility and Notions of Normal

Both policies state that legally recognized females are eligible to compete in women's competitions provided that they have testosterone levels below the so-called male range (as shown by serum concentration) or "if within the male range, she has an androgen resistance such that she derives no competitive advantage from such levels" (IAAF 2011c; IOC 2011). The policies thus do not exclude female athletes with hyperandrogenism per se, yet they do require that women already diagnosed with these conditions report their condition to the appropriate bodies and undergo evaluation, presumably even if they are already seeing a medical specialist and have no health concerns related to their condition. Moreover, although the policies state that no woman is required to undergo medical intervention, if a woman with hyperandrogenism wants to compete, she must undergo "treatment" as a prerequisite to competition. Treatment would presumably vary on a case-by-case basis and include anything from hormone blockers to gonadectomy. Given that medical intervention is required to compete, we are concerned that compliance with the IOC and IAAF policies may lead to coercion as it relates to treatment, which is especially worrisome if such intervention is medically unnecessary.

Androgen excess is the most common endocrine disorder in women of reproductive age (Abdel-Rahman and Hurd 2010). Using the definition of hyperandrogenism in females as those with testosterone levels "above typical female range"—roughly 1.5–2 nmol/L (averages and ranges for elite female athletes are not known)—females with the diagnoses listed in Table 1 will have hyperandrogenism, but most are unlikely to have endogenous testosterone levels above 10 nmol/L.[7]

The IOC policy, while more flexible, may actually require a much broader group of women to undergo "treatment" in order to compete. It also introduces a high degree of subjectivity: At what point is a woman's testosterone level too high? This could be 3.5 nmol/L for one practitioner and 5.5 nmol/L for another. Of two women with the same levels, one could conceivably be required to lower her levels while the other is not required to. There are yet other problems. When does a difference from the typical female range become meaningful or even problematic and in whose eyes? What is the target level to which a woman must reduce her testosterone? One physician could recommend a woman's level be within the female typical range, whereas another practitioner might simply want it below the male typical range. Given the inconsistent policies discussed earlier, an athlete might be required to undergo intervention according to one policy and not another. Moreover, using testosterone levels alone as a marker of eligibility fails to take into account that some women have androgen resistance that renders their testosterone levels meaningless.

Health, Treatment, and the Question of Medical Need

Both IAAF and IOC policies express concern with health. The IAAF policy aims for "the early prevention of problems associated with hyperandrogenism" and the IOC press release states, "In order to protect the health of the athlete, *sports* authorities should have the responsibility to make sure that any case of female hyperandrogenism that arises under their jurisdiction receives adequate medical follow-up" (IAAF 2011c; IOC 2011, emphasis in original).

Androgens affect various bodily tissues, such as those in the brain, breast, bone, and the cardiovascular system. Some conditions that cause hyperandrogenism present important health issues, and it is certainly possible that the policy will lead some women to a diagnosis they might not otherwise have had available to them (though it must be underscored that there is no provision in the new policy to pay for medical care that the examiners may deem to be necessary). One health concern may be possible malignancy of testicular tissue, often managed with prophylactic gonadectomy. But it is not always clear when removal of the gonads is appropriate: The procedure not only sterilizes individuals but may significantly impair quality of life (e.g., by inducing "hot flashes"). In many cases, however, there is no clear health risk from higher than typical testosterone levels. Yet these policies strongly imply that treatment to lower testosterone levels is medically necessary.

Ironically, though, the anti-androgens used to treat hyperandrogenism can have sequelae that may be particularly problematic for a serious athlete, such as diuretic effects that cause excessive thirst, urination, and electrolyte imbalances; disruption of carbohydrate metabolism (e.g., glucose intolerance, insulin resistance); headache; fatigue; nausea; and liver toxicity (Archer and Chang 2004). Furthermore, testing as proposed in the evaluation can reveal genetic and other medical information that is deeply personal—infertility, mutations, and other conditions that have little bearing on eligibility.

Perhaps some women may derive health benefits from policies on hyperandrogenism. But this is a hypothetical benefit that must be weighed against actual harms of unnecessary medical treatment and stigmatization of women with atypical sex-linked traits. Moreover, the IAAF policy provides for evaluation and recommendation of treatment, but it explicitly states it will not pay for medical intervention creating the potential for financial harm in order to compete. Given the very real documented harms owing to sex testing generally, exclusion of female athletes on the basis of having "male" sex traits, undergoing a gynecological exam under anesthesia, and the mental impact and risk of insensitive and inappropriate discussion and disclosure of information, we suggest that the harms here may be greater than any possible health benefit.

Confidentiality, Leaks, and Whisper Triggers

Another ground on which both policies fall short of their stated principles is the privacy and confidentiality for female athletes, which are undermined by several factors. First, the process of testing, vetting, and treating an athlete takes months, a time during which she is ineligible to compete. As in Semenya's case, the suspension and thus absence of the athlete from competitions not only exacts a psychological toll but also can arouse suspicion; others inevitably notice the "secret" investigation, which violates the athlete's privacy. A recent article co-authored by IOC medical commissioner Arne Ljunqvist and Martínez-Patiño, the Spanish hurdler disqualified years ago, argues that women with DSD "should not be disqualified from competing in elite sports events. Nor should they be stigmatised and their right to privacy should be guaranteed by sports organizations *during the process of gender verification*" (2006, 225–26; emphasis added). We agree that, at the very least, the policies should not suspend female athletes who are being investigated.

Another concern stems from how investigations are brought. The IAAF policy specifically states that females suspected of having hyperandrogenism may be targeted for testing on "reasonable grounds" (IAAF 2011c, 3). It is troubling that more than half of the indicators of hyperandrogenism identified by the IAAF policy to determine which female athletes should undergo sex testing are entangled with deeply subjective and stereotypical Western definitions of femininity: "deep voice, breast atrophy, never menstruation (or loss of menses since several month), increased muscle mass, body hair of male type (vertex alopecia, >17 years), Tanner score low (I/II), F&G score (>6/! minimized by the beauty), no uterus, clitoromegaly [larger than typical clitoris]" [sic] (IAAF 2011c, 20). Moreover, the IAAF notes (without support) that "the individuals concerned often display masculine traits and have an uncommon athletic capacity in relation to their fellow female competitors" (IAAF 2011c, 1). Targeting gender nonconforming female athletes who present as more "masculine" is paradoxical, as the characteristics identified with masculinity—notably, skeletal and muscular development—are also characteristics strongly correlated with athleticism (Heggie 2010, 158).

Outward signs of gender are already triggers that raise suspicion about a female athlete's sex. Indeed, competitors, athletics officials, the media, and the general public began obsessively commenting on Semenya's appearance immediately after her win, asking, "Could she really be a he?" Yet even if outwardly visible markers of gender were not triggers, the manner through which suspicions about sex are reported and acted on will inevitably come to public attention. Indeed, the fact that anyone can make their concerns about an athlete known to an IAAF medical director may mean that leaks of private health information or a whisper campaign about an athlete exists prior to the beginning of an investigation or even triggers an investigation. Confidentiality is an admirable goal, but as long as these testing policies persist, the potential for grave harm to athletes' lives and careers is nearly undeniable and unavoidable.

■ CONCLUSION

A central assumption underlying the IAAF and IOC policies is that atypically high levels of endogenous testosterone in women create an unfair advantage and must therefore be regulated. The current scientific evidence, however, does not support the notion that endogenous testosterone levels confer athletic advantage in any straightforward or predictable way. Even if naturally occurring variation in testosterone conferred advantage, is that advantage unfair? It bears noting that athletes never begin on a fair playing field; if they were not exceptional in one regard or another, they would not have made it to a prestigious international athletic stage. Athletic excellence is the product of a complex entanglement of biological factors and material resources that have the potential to influence athletic advantage. However, the IAAF and IOC target testosterone as the most important factor in contributing to athletic advantage. The policies seek to do the impossible: isolate androgen from other possible biological factors and material resources to determine the impact that it alone, in the form of testosterone, has on athletic advantage. Setting hyperandrogenism apart from other possible biological factors that are not regulated by the IAAF and IOC but that also might influence athletic advantage seems illogical and unfair.

The policies raise troubling concerns about whether they succeed in balancing the aim of creating a "fair" playing field for women athletes against the aim of ensuring fairness for individual athletes. Given the very real documented harms that have come to female athletes who have undergone evaluation and sex testing, these policies are unlikely to protect against breaches of privacy and confidentiality that may arise because they are inconsistent and suspend athletes undergoing evaluation. Furthermore, they require female athletes to undergo treatment that may not be medically necessary and may, in fact, be medically and socially harmful, in order to compete. Finally, beyond those athletes who are directly affected by these investigations, the new policies may intensify the harmful "gender policing" that already plagues women's sports.

Considerations of fairness support an approach that allows all legally recognized females to compete with other females, regardless of their hormonal levels, providing their bodies naturally produce the hormones. While a legal definition of sex opens up a scrutiny of its own, it is currently the single best sex categorization measure we have to rely on. It is true that countries may define sex in different ways, but this variability is not necessarily bad; it also allows countries to do so how they see fit.

The answer to Caster Semenya's case depends on the values that are deemed important in elite sports and competition. Elite sport can value diversity and ensure that all women, including those with intersex traits, have equal opportunity to participate in sports, that they are treated humanely, that they are not forced to undergo what may be unnecessary medical treatment, and that they are not made ineligible based on advantages they may not even have. Performance in sports is both a "celebration of and a challenge posed by our embodiment" (Murray 2009, 236). All bodies, to one degree or another, present functional limitations; "sports provide an opportunity to live fully in those bodies, to test their capabilities and limits, and to integrate them with our will, intellect, and character" (Murray 2009, 237). We need to move beyond policing biologically natural bodies and the resultant exceptional scrutiny of extraordinary women.

▪ NOTES

1. We thank Carole S. Vance for her thoughtful intellectual engagement with an earlier draft of this article and Kirk Neely for answering queries regarding medical aspects of hyperandrogenism. Address correspondence to Katrina Karkazis, Stanford Center for Biomedical Ethics, 1215 Welch Road, Modular A, Palo Alto, CA 94305, USA. E-mail: karkazis@stanford.edu.

2. The testosterone range in adult females is 0.7–2.8 nmol/L and roughly 6.9–34.7 nmol/L in adult males. Roughly 5% of the population does not fall into these ranges (Strauss and Barbieri 1999). If by "three times the *typical level*" it was meant that Semenya had "three times the *most common* level," it is inconceivable that her levels could still be within the usual female range, and well below the typical range for males.

3. Thus, although the IOC rules have not been officially released as of this writing, we expect them to be similar to those adopted by the IAAF.

4. The IAAF policy notes: "The Regulations are of mandatory application to all athletes competing, or seeking to compete, in International Competitions and are recommended as a guide to National Federations in Athletics for the management of any cases that might arise at the national level," suggesting wide implementation especially because this is the only available policy (IAAF 2011c, 2).

5. Measuring testosterone levels is made more complex when one considers that currently available testosterone reference values for women are limited by small and heterogeneous samples, there are various measurement techniques (e.g., conventional immunoas-says and liquid chromatography-tandem mass spectrometry), and laboratories have differing standards and norms (see, e.g., Haring et al. 2011).

6. Notions of women's inferior physical status affect the rules that govern sport, such as female tennis players being limited to three sets in the majors whereas men play five or female speed skaters competing at shorter distances than men. Some sports are not sex

segregated, such as horseracing or car racing, whereas others such as billiards and chess are for reasons that are not clear. Still other sports are not sex segregated at the collegiate level but are at the Olympic level (e.g., riflery and Olympic shooting). Moreover, there are many recent examples of sex integration, such as women in professional golf and girls joining Little League baseball and high school football teams. However, in some sports men will have a distinct advantage whereas in other sports women will tend to excel (e.g., endurance events). We expect the overall value of sex segregation is both sport specific and a moving target, as some differences may diminish as greater numbers of girls play sports at young ages and as opportunities for elite, including professional, competition expand for adult women.

7. A functional adult testis (not a steroidogenic block or PCOS) or tumor could produce testosterone levels above 10 nmol/L; this might include females with partial AIS (PAIS), ovotesticular DSD, and adrenal carcinoma. As a result, the level of 10 is high enough that it would not apply to many women, but these policies will especially target women with intersex traits.

▨ REFERENCES

Abdel-Rahman, M. Y., and W. W. Hurd. 2010. Androgen excess. *MedScape Reference* August 5. Available at: http://emedicine.medscape.com/article/273153-overview

Adams, W. L. 2009. Could this women's world champ be a man? *Time* August 21. Available at: http://www.time.com/time/world/article/0,8599,1917767,00.html—ixzz1hEXnRsSc

Archer, J. S., and R. J. Chang. 2004. Hirsutism and acne in poly-cystic ovary syndrome. *Best Practice & Research Clinical Obstetrics & Gynaecology* 18(5): 737–754.

Bateup, H. S., A. Booth, E. A. Shirtcliff, et al. 2002. Testosterone, cortisol, and women's competition. *Evolution and Human Behavior* 23(3): 181–192.

BBC. 2009. SA chief suspended in Semenya row. *BBC News,* November 5, 2009. Available at: http://news.bbc.co.uk/sport2/hi/athletics/8344591.stm

Bhasin, S., T. W. Storer, N. Berman, et al. 1996. The effects of supraphysiologic doses of testosterone on muscle size and strength in normal men. *New England Journal of Medicine* 335(1): 1–7.

Bhasin, S., L. Woodhouse, R. Casaburi, et al. 2001. Testosterone dose-response relationships in healthy young men. *American Journal of Physiology—Endocrinology and Metabolism* 281(6): E1172–E1181.

Braunstein, G. D. 2011. Testes. In *Greenspan's Basic & Clinical Endocrinology*, chap. 12. Available at: http://www.accessmedicine.com.laneproxy.stanford.edu/content.aspx?aID= 8405050

Charmandari, E., C. G. Brook, P. C. Hindmarsh, et al. 2004. Classic congenital adrenal hyperplasia and puberty. *European Journal of Endocrinology/European Federation of Endocrine Societies* 151(suppl. 3): U77–U82.

Clarey, C. 2009. Gender test after a gold-medal finish. *New York Times* August 19. Available at: http://www.nytimes.com/2009/08/20/sports/20runner.html

Clemmons, A. K. 2008. 7 feet 7 and 360 pounds, with bigger feet than Shaq's. *New York Times* January 9. Available at: http://www.nytimes.com/2008/01/09/sports/ncaabasketball/09asheville.html

Cole, C. L. 2000. One chromosome too many? In *The Olympics at the millennium: Power, politics and the games,* ed. K. Schaffer and S. Smith, 128–146. New Brunswick, NJ: Rutgers University Press.

Cyphers, L., and K. Fagan. 2011. On homophobia and recruiting: Coaches will use a subtle vocabulary to qualify certain programs; It's become pollution. *ESPN* January 26. Available at: http://sports.espn.go.com/ncw/news/story?id = 6060641

de la Chapelle, A. 1986. The use and misuse of sex chromatin screening for "gender identification" of female athletes. *Journal of the American Medical Association* 256(14): 1920–1923.

Dewey & LeBoeuf. 2010. Caster Semenya on track to return to athletics following IAAF settlement. July 6. Available at: http://www.deweyleboeuf.com/en/Firm/MediaCenter/PressReleases/2010/07/CasterSemenyaonTracktoReturntoAthletics.aspx

Dingeon, B. 1993. Gender verification and the next Olympic Games. *Journal of the American Medical Association* 269(3): 357–358.

Dolan, S., S. Wilkie, N. Aliabadi, et al. 2004. Effects of testosterone administration in human immunodeficiency virus-infected women with low weight: A randomized placebo-controlled study. *Archives of Internal Medicine* 164(8): 897–904.

Dreger, A. 1998. *Hermaphrodites and the medical invention of sex*. Cambridge, MA: Harvard University Press.

Dreger, A. 2010. Sex typing for sport. *Hastings Center Report* 40(2): 22–24.

Drinkwater, B. L., and International Federation of Sports Medicine. 2000. *Women in sport*. Malden, MA: Blackwell Science.

Dworkin, S. L., and M. A. Messner. 2002. Introduction: Gender relations in sport. *Sociological Perspectives* 45(4): 347–352.

Edwards, D. A., and J. L. O'Neal. 2009. Oral contraceptives decrease saliva testosterone but do not affect the rise in testosterone associated with athletic competition. *Hormones and Behavior* 56(2): 195–198.

Elsas, L. J., A. Ljungqvist, M. A. Ferguson-Smith, et al. 2000. Gender verification of female athletes. *Genetics in Medicine* 2(4): 249–254.

Eugster, E. A., L. A. Dimeglio, J. C. Wright, et al. 2001. Height outcome in congenital adrenal hyperplasia caused by 21-hydroxylase deficiency: A meta-analysis. *Journal of Pediatrics* 138(1): 26–32.

Eynon, N., R. Birk, Y. Meckel, et al. 2011. Physiological variables and mitochondrial-related genotypes of an athlete who excels in both short and long-distance running. *Mitochondrion* 11(5): 774–777.

Eynon, N., M. Moran, R. Birk, et al. 2011. The champions' mitochondria: Is it genetically determined? A review on mitochondrial DNA and elite athletic performance. *Physiological Genomics* 43(13): 789–798.

Eynon, N., J. R. Ruiz, Y. Meckel, et al. 2011. Mitochondrial biogenesis related endurance genotype score and sports performance in athletes. *Mitochondrion* 11(1): 64–69.

Farquhar, G. 2009. New twist in Semenya gender saga. *BBC News* August 25. Available at: http://news.bbc.co.uk/sport2/hi/athletics/8219937.stm

Fausto-Sterling, A. 1985. *Myths of gender: Biological theories about women and men.* New York: Basic Books.

Foddy, B., and J. Savulescu. 2011. Time to re-evaluate gender segregation in athletics? *British Journal of Sports Medicine* 45(15): 1184–1188.

Foxnews.com. 2008. Michael Phelps unintentionally raises Marfan syndrome awareness. *Foxnews.com* August 21. Available at: http://www.foxnews.com/story/0,2933,408023,00.html

Genel, M. 2000. Gender verification no more? *Medscape Womens Health* 5(3): E2.

Hajer, M. A., and H. Wagenaar, Eds. 2003. *Deliberative policy analysis; Understanding governance in a network society.* Cambridge, UK: Cambridge University Press.

Hannagan, R. J., and C. W. Larimer. 2010. Does gender composition affect group decision outcomes? Evidence from a laboratory experiment. *Political Behavior* 32(1): 51–67.

Haring, R., A. Hannemann, U. John, et al. 2012. Age-specific reference ranges for serum testosterone and androstenedione concentrations in women measured by liquid chromatography-tandem mass spectrometry. *Journal of Clinical Endocrinology and Metabolism* 97(2): 408–415.

Hay, E. 1972. Sex determination in putative female athletes. *Journal of the American Medical Association* 221(9): 998–999.

Hay, E. 1974. Femininity tests at the Olympic Games. *Olympic Review* 76–77(March–April): 119–123.

Heggie, V. 2010. Testing sex and gender in sports; Reinventing, reimagining and reconstructing histories. *Endeavour* 34(4):157–163.

Hurst, M. 2009. Caster Semenya has male sex organs and no womb or ovaries. *Daily Telegraph* September 11. Available at: http://www.dailytelegraph.com.au/sport/Semenya-has-no-womb-or-ovaries/story-e6frexni-1225771672245

IAAF. 2011a. 800 metres all time. August 16. Available at: http://www.iaaf.org/statistics/toplists/inout=o/age=n/season=0/sex=W/all=y/legal=A/disc=800/detail.html

IAAF. 2011b. 800 metres junior all time. August 3. Available at: http://www.iaaf.org/statistics/toplists/inout=o/age=j/season=0/sex=W/all=y/legal=A/disc=800/detail.html

IAAF. 2011c. IAAF regulations governing eligibility of females with hyperandrogenism to compete in women's competitions. Available at: http://www.iaaf.org/mm/Document/AboutIAAF/Publications/05/98/78/20110430054216_httppostedfile_HARegulations(Final)-Appendices-AMG-30.04.2011_24299.pdf

IOC. 2011. IOC addresses eligibility of female athletes with hyperandrogenism. April 5. Available at: http://www.Olympic.org/content/press-release/ioc-addresses-eligibility-of-female-athletes-with-hyperandrogenism

Jordan-Young, R. M. 2010. *Brain storm: The flaws in the science of sex differences*. Cambridge, MA: Harvard University Press.

Karkazis, K. 2008. *Fixing sex: Intersex, medical authority, and lived experience*. Durham, NC: Duke University Press.

Kessler, S. 1998. *Lessons from the intersexed*. New Brunswick, NJ: Rutgers University Press.

Kessler, S., and W. McKenna. 1978. *Gender: An ethnomethodological approach*. New York: John Wiley and Sons.

Kvorning, T., M. Andersen, K. Brixen, et al. 2006. Suppression of endogenous testosterone production attenuates the response to strength training: A randomized, placebo-controlled, and blinded intervention study. *American Journal of Physiology-Endocrinology and Metabolism* 291(6): E1325–1332.

Laby, D. M., A. L. Rosenbaum, D. G. Kirschen, et al. 1996. The visual function of professional baseball players. *American Journal of Ophthalmology* 122(4): 476–485.

Laqueur, T. W. 1990. *Making sex: Body and gender from the Greeks to Freud*. Cambridge, MA: Harvard University Press.

Levy, A. 2009. Either/or: Sports, sex, and the case of Caster Semenya. *New Yorker* November 1: 46–59.

Ljungqvist, A., M. J. Martínez-Patiño, A. Martínez-Vidal, et al. 2006. The history and current policies on gender testing in elite athletes. *International SportMed Journal* 7(3): 225–230.

Longcope, C. 1986. Adrenal and gonadal androgen secretion in normal females. *Clinics in Endocrinology and Metabolism* 15(2): 213–228.

MacLean, H. E., W. S. Chiu, A. J. Notini, et al. 2008. Impaired skeletal muscle development and function in male, but not female, genomic androgen receptor knockout mice. *FASEB Journal* 22(8): 2676–2689.

Mannix, C. 2007. High hopes: He's three inches taller than Yao Ming, but is pro hoops' biggest player ready for the NBA? *Sports Illustrated*. Available at: http://sportsillustrated.cnn.com/vault/article/magazine/MAG1107021/index.htm

Martínez-Patiño, M. J. 2005. Personal account: A woman tried and tested. *Lancet* 366(suppl. 1): S38.

McCaul, K. D., B. A. Gladue, and M. Joppa. 1992. Winning, losing, mood, and testosterone. *Hormones and Behavior* 26(4): 486–504.

Meyer-Bahlburg, H. F. 2011. Brain development and cognitive, psychosocial, and psychiatric functioning in classical 21-hydroxylase deficiency. *Endocrine Development* 20: 88–95.

Miller, K. K., B. M. Biller, C. Beauregard, et al. 2006. Effects of testosterone replacement in androgen-deficient women with hypopituitarism: A randomized, double-blind, placebo-controlled study. *Journal of Clinical Endocrinology and Metabolism* 91(5): 1683–1690.

Murray, T. H. 2009. In search of an ethics of sport: Genetic hierarchies, handicappers general, and embodied excellence. In *Performance-enhancing technologies in sports,* ed. T. H. Murray, K. J. Maschke, and A. A. Wasunna, 225–238. Baltimore, MD: Johns Hopkins University Press.

New, M. I., and J. L. Simpson. 2010. *Program for 2nd World Conference Hormonal and Genetic Basis of Sexual Differentiation Disorders and Hot Topics in Endocrinology,* January 15–17. Available at: http://cme.med.miami.edu/documents/FIUbrochure.pdf

New, M. I., and J. L. Simpson. 2011. Preface. In *Hormonal and genetic basis of sexual differentiation disorders and hot topics in endocrinology: Proceedings of the 2nd world conference,* ed. M. I. New and J. L. Simpson, v–vii. New York: Springer.

Oliveira, T., M. J. Gouveia, and R. F. Oliveira. 2009. Testosterone responsiveness to winning and losing experiences in female soccer players. *Psychoneuroendocrinology* 34(7): 1056–1064.

Olsen-Acre, H. K. 2003. *Sex and gender on the playing field: A feminist critique of drug testing in the Olympic Games.* Undergraduate thesis, Columbia College, New York, NY.

Olympic.org. n.d. When did women first compete in the Olympic Games? Available at: http://registration.Olympic.org/en/faq/detail/id/135

Ostrander, E. A., H. J. Huson, G. K. Ostrander, et al. 2009. Genetics of athletic performance. *Annual Review of Genomics and Human Genetics* 10: 407–429.

Oudshoorn, N. 1994. *Beyond the natural body: An archeology of sex hormones.* New York: Routledge.

Pitsiladis, Y., G. Wang, and B. Wolfarth. 2011. Genomics of aerobic capacity and endurance performance: Clinical implications. In *Exercise genomics,* ed. L. S. Pescatello and S. M. Roth, 179–229. New York: Springer.

Reaney, P. 2011. Female athletes judged by sex appeal. *ABCnews.com* September 13. Available at: http://abcnews.go.com/Technology/story?id=119952&page=1–.TzBv7uNbWG4

Reis, E. 2009. *Bodies in doubt: An American history of intersex.* Baltimore, MD: Johns Hopkins University Press.

Ritchie, R., J. Reynard, and T. Lewis. 2008. Intersex and the Olympic Games. *Journal of the Royal Society of Medicine* 101(8): 395–399.

Ronnestad, B. R., H. Nygaard, and T. Raastad. 2011. Physiological elevation of endogenous hormones results in superior strength training adaptation. *European Journal of Applied Physiology and Occupational Physiology* 111(9): 2249–2259.

Rubin, G. 1975. The traffic in women: Notes on the political economy of sex. In *Toward an anthropology of women,* ed. R. R. Reiter, 157–210. New York: Monthly Review Press.

Russett, C. E. 1989. *Sexual science: The Victorian construction of womanhood.* Cambridge, MA: Harvard University Press.

Sapolsky, R. M. 1997. *The trouble with testosterone: And other essays on the biology of the human predicament.* New York: Scribner.

Schiebinger, L. L. 1989. *The mind has no sex?: Women in the origins of modern science.* Cambridge, MA: Harvard University Press.

Simpson, J. L., A. Ljungqvist, A. de la Chapelle, et al. 1993. Gender verification in competitive sports. *Sports Medicine* 16(5): 305–315.

Simpson, J. L., A. Ljungqvist, M. A. Ferguson-Smith, et al. 2000. Gender verification in the Olympics. *Journal of the American Medical Association* 284(12): 1568–1569.

Smith, A. D. 2009. Fears for Caster Semenya over trauma of test results. *The Guardian* September 12. Available at: http://www.guardian.co.uk/sport/2009/sep/13/caster-emenya-gender-testresults

Smith, D. 2009. Caster Semenya withdraws from race in South Africa. *The Guardian,* September 11, 2009. Available at: http://www.guardian.co.uk/sport/2009/sep/11/caster-emenya-withdrawsrace-south-africa

Speiser, P. W., and P. C. White. 2003. Congenital adrenal hyperplasia. *New England Journal of Medicine* 349(8): 776–788.

Stephenson, J. 1996. Female Olympians' sex tests outmoded. *Journal of the American Medical Association* 276(3): 177–178.

Stikkelbroeck, N. M., A. R. Hermus, D. D. Braat, et al. 2003. Fertility in women with congenital adrenal hyperplasia due to 21-hydroxylase deficiency. *Obstetrical and Gynecological Survey* 58(4): 275–284.

Storer, T. W., L. Magliano, L. Woodhouse, et al. 2003. Testosterone dose-dependently increases maximal voluntary strength and leg power, but does not affect fatigability or specific tension. *Journal of Clinical Endocrinology and Metabolism* 88(4): 1478–1485.

Strauss, J. F., and R. L. Barbieri. 1999. *Yen and Jaffe's reproductive endocrinology: Physiology, pathophysiology, and clinical management.* Philadelphia, PA: Saunders/Elsevier.

Tian, Q., F. He, Y. Zhou, et al. 2009. Gender verification in athletes with disorders of sex development. *Gynecological Endocrinology* 25(2): 117–121.

Tucker, R., and M. Collins. 2010. The science of sex verification and athletic performance. *International Journal of Sports Physiology and Performance* 5(2): 127–139.

Viloria, H. 2011. Opinion: Gender rules in sport—Leveling the playing field, or reversed doping? *Global Herald,* April 11. Available at: http://theglobalherald.com/opinion-gender-rules-in-sport-leveling-the-playing-field-or-reversed-doping/14837

Volkl, T. M., D. Simm, C. Beier, et al. 2006. Obesity among children and adolescents with classic congenital adrenal hyperplasia due to 21-hydroxylase deficiency. *Pediatrics* 117(1): e98–105.

Wilson, D. R. 2000. Gender vs. sex. *Journal of the American Medical Association* 284(23): 2997–2998.

C. Race

7 Race Relations Theories

Implications for Sport Management

■ EARL E. SMITH AND ANGELA HATTERY

▦ RACE AND THE SPORTSWORLD: A LEVEL PLAYING FIELD OR A SEGREGATED INSTITUTION?

Americans (and others) love sports in part because the SportsWorld (i.e., the collective amateur and professional sport industry) is the supposed *level playing field* (Smith, 2009). Structurally, it is purported to consist of equity, equality, fairness, honor, and open access to all spheres of the game. It is presumed to be a venue that offers a diverse array of individuals access to all playing positions and a place somewhere in the larger organizational structure that may include coaching, management, ownership, and access to print and electronic media positions. Certainly when we watch mainstream sports such as football and men's basketball, live or on the television, we see images that seem to confirm our presumptions that the SportsWorld is comprised of a level playing field.[1] Any suggestion that the SportsWorld is actually a mirror representation of the larger society stuns the fans who are not interested in the discussion of the SportsWorld as a site of privilege, race, class, and gender (Smith, 2009).

However, if indeed the SportsWorld was a level playing field as historically purported—with access and opportunity determined through a meritocracy—then the workplace of the SportsWorld would be comprised of trained professionals from different races and ethnicities, cultures, genders, religions, sexualities, national origins, ages, and ability statuses mixing together equally across workplace boundaries using modern technologies to bridge physical distances, exchanging high-quality goods and services, and leveraging capital and human resources for the betterment of the sport organization. This was the SportsWorld envisioned by the former Brooklyn Dodger major league baseball player Jackie Robinson when he retired January 5, 1957 (Robinson, 1972). Unfortunately, long past the 1947 historical occurrence of Robinson's racial integration of professional baseball, his request for full racial integration in sport has yet to be granted and thus, his dream has yet to be realized (Tygiel, 1983).

The reality is that the SportsWorld offers a contrasting reality to a vision of racial harmony. *As an institution,* it continues to perpetuate a lack of integration of cultures (genders, races, nationalities, sexualities, abilities, and so forth). The structure of the management of sport is often elusive, and it perpetuates continual inequality for those who are historically marginalized, resulting in the continuation of workplace conflict and unsatisfactory work opportunities for People of Color, especially when it comes to power positions of management and ownership.[2] Organizational theorists in the world of business (Bell & Nkomo, 2001; Thomas, 2001) have been pounding away at the lack of diversity in the business world. Sociologists have complained that organizations have been "skating around" diversifying. Baron and Pfeffer (1994) put it thus: "Yet remarkably little has been done to bring the firms back into the study of inequality, particularly in ways that are true to the social and relational nature of work organizations" (p. 190). Since sport is a business as well as a social institution, it has also fallen prey to the condition mentioned by Baron and Pfeffer.

The millennium's inaugural decade, concatenated with the three preceding ones, saw the color line of America shift from a society that was predominately composed of only two racial groups—a large White majority and a relatively small Black minority—to a society composed of multiple racial and ethnic groups (Burton et al., 2010). As one-sport scholar put it, "by most accounts, diversity represents one of the most important issues for managers of organizations for sport and physical activity today" (Cunningham, 2010, p. 395). Across the second half of the 20th century and into the beginning of the 21st century, sport has become an increasingly racially diverse institution on the fields and arenas of competition. In fact, in the two most dominant collegiate sports in the United States (football and men's basketball), African American males are not only well represented but are over-represented in these leagues (Lapchick, 2009; Smith 2009). Consequently, African American men make prominent contributions to the financial vitality of the industry and commercial enterprise that sport has become. However, such racial diversity featured on the playing fields is not mirrored in the sport boardrooms, as racial diversity has lagged significantly at every level of sport management, including coaching (Greene, 2008), leadership/administration, marketing, and ownership (Cunningham, 2007; Lapchick, 2009; Smith 2009), where African American men are abysmally absent. For example, using college football as one illustration, the Bowl Championship Series (BCS) consists of 65 colleges and universities. Sixty-three of the head football coaches in the BCS are White males (97%), 2 (or 3%) are African American. The six conference commissioners of the BCS are all White men.

Despite some laudable attempts and organizational management initiatives to create workplace diversity in the SportsWorld, such as: (a) the NASCAR Drive for Diversity—K&N Pro Series which has teamed up with BET TV to promote opening up access for African American drivers into NASCAR; (b) Major League Baseball's "Diverse Business Partners Program," which is designed to increase minority groups and women's access to conduct business with the 30 baseball teams that solicit vendors services; (c) the National Hockey League's initiative to promote hockey in minority neighborhoods under its "Hockey Is for Everyone Initiative"; (d) NCAA initiatives to enhance opportunities for women and minorities in coaching and administration; and (e) a host of similar programs throughout amateur and professional sports that seek to promote diversity and inclusion in the SportsWorld, achieving racial diversity in the management of sport is a feat that has not been successfully accomplished (Greene, 2008; McDowell, Cunningham, & Singer, 2009).

As Lapchick's (2009) *Racial Report Card* also attests, although African Americans play sports, White men run the business of sports. In a very interesting paper, "Minority Issues in Contemporary Sports" law professor Kenneth Shropshire (2004) makes a very poignant observation about accessing the various levels of leadership positions in sport organizations. He put it thus: "Opening up access to power positions is by far the toughest racial hurdle" (p. 199). We agree with the claim made by Shropshire (2004, 1997) about how hard it is to break into top leadership/power positions in sport. To further illustrate the challenges that African Americans face in their quest for sport leadership, we offer the example of Reggie Fowler, an African American male, who put together a proposal in the early 2000s to purchase the Minnesota Vikings professional football team. In a commentary about the failed deal we learn the following:

> Fowler seemed like a perfect fit, his company reported over $300 million in profits in 2004, he'd put together a team of experienced investors and personally convinced McCombs and the citizens of Minnesota that he'd keep the team in the state rather than move to Los Angeles for a new stadium. Seemed like a done deal right? . . . To buy an NFL franchise you have to first put up about 40 percent of the total cost of the team (in the case of the Vikings it was $625 million) then you must prove you have enough money to buy out your next two largest investors if they back out of the deal. After that, the process gets really murky. Even if you have the money and get approved by the team owner, 24 of the 32 NFL franchise owners must vote to let you into their little club. (Johnson, 2009)

NFL owners and members of the finance committee did not even show up for the review of Reggie Fowler's application!

Carrington (2010) argues that "ideas of White intellectual supremacy and Black degeneracy still remain deeply embedded in sports culture."[1] Sport management organizations in the U.S. fall under the rubric that has long been described as sites of contested terrain. What this means is that whereas "big money" sports have become racially diverse on the fields of competition (creating the "product" that yields the revenue), there is tremendous resistance—and we will argue this has resulted in the adoption and implementation of new strategies— that is taking place in the management and business side of the SportsWorld such that the talents of racially diverse individuals are not as actively sought. The sites of contested terrain in sport are deeply embedded in the culture of a (White) racial privilege that will only give up access when it is in their best interest to do so. Consequently, there is an inherent system of race relations that permeates the management of sport, creating racially unlevel and racially segregated boardrooms and front offices. The purpose of the essay is to offer an analysis of the systematic and endemic race relations that may influence the sport management opportunities and experiences of People of Color in general, and African American males in particular.

▪ RACE RELATIONS THEORIES AND SPORT MANAGEMENT

In weaving our arguments about contemporary sport management, we draw on major sociological theories of race relations as viable explanations for the fact that sport management continues to be racialized (Fink & Pastore, 1999). We argue that the new tools used by owners and athletic administrators to maintain a racially segregated workplace (in the boardroom but not on the field) is influenced by social distance and requires the invocation of the new language of symbolic racism (Bonilla-Silva, 2006) and mimics the way segregation remains dominant in American society including in the corporate world, government, on Wall Street, and elsewhere (Thomas 2001; Thomas & Gabarro, 1999; Zweigenhaft & Domhoff, 2006). For example, based on the desire to be politically correct, African American male athletes are no longer discussed as being "too stupid" to quarterback football teams or by extension "lacking the intellectual skills" to coach football (Edwards, 1997). Instead, these athletes (upon retiring from the games they play) are passed over for coaching and administrative positions because they "might not be comfortable" golfing at the country club with alumni and big donors (Smith, 2009).

A superficial analysis of this (and other related scenarios that play out in the SportsWorld) or merely attributing this lack of diversity to discrimination may fail to expose the degree to which racism continues to be a major, if not *the major,* cause of the continued racial segregation in many areas of social life, including the management of the social institution of sport (Feagin, 1991). However, when contemporary theories of race and race relations *frame* the analysis, the role of racism is illuminated. Therefore, this essay seeks to provide a brief overview of some noteworthy race relations concepts and suppositions that may offer insight into the manner in which race resonates and may be operative in creating and maintaining segregated sport management opportunities and experiences.

As stated previously, we frame our analysis in the context provided by scholars of race and race relations. That said, we argue that contemporary race theory does not exist in a vacuum; rather, it is located in a particular historical and social context that was shaped by the theoreticians of the respective eras. It is on their shoulders, as Merton (1972) argues, that contemporary race theory has been built. Because the institution of sport was largely not an institution thought to be worthy of inquiry, and because early race and race relations theory developed during the height of segregation in the SportsWorld, we are not able to provide any examples of ways in which these early theories were applied to the SportsWorld. However, it is our intent to suggest ways in which these early theories could have been applied to sport management and where they may fall short. This discussion is offered primarily to provide a context in which to understand contemporary theories of race and race relations.

Race Relations Cycle

Many would argue that the original theorists of race and race relations in the formal sense come from the University of Chicago during the first half of the 20th Century under the tutelage of Professor Robert E. Park (Lyman, 1968). This "Chicago School of Sociology" systematically created a body of knowledge about minorities but mainly African Americans, defining who they were and describing their place in American society.

Park's 1939 "race relations cycle," with its distinct, linear stages of (1) contact, (2) competition, (3) accommodation, and (4) assimilation, was consolidated as a hegemonic frame to understand the incorporation of racial and ethnic groups into the developing 20th Century. Park's race relation cycle is best understood this way: First, there is contact/competition among social groups. Second, there is racial conflict between the social groups. Third, after the stage of racial conflict, the "losing" group (generally understood as the minority group) is forced to accommodate to the rules of the "victorious" group (generally understood as the majority group). Lastly (the fourth stage), over time there is assimilation to the ruling group's social world, culture, and way of thinking.

One outcome of Park's 1939 theoretical framework (which came to dominate the studies that emerged under his leadership) was the development and adoption of the belief in cultural assimilation, as both a theory and a desirable ideological goal. Park's theoretical contribution of the cycle of race relations continues to serve as a useful guide for understanding the evolutionary as well as the historical aspects of race relations theory, and for explaining race relations in the United States. Park's race relations cycle has proven to be important for American sociologists and others because it provides a structural sequence for viewing the history of race relations between African Americans and White Americans. While it is impossible to say directly that this body of work was *the* defining theoretical thread that shaped race relations theory, it did take hold among many scholars.

With its focus on assimilation and the requirement that the subordinate group accommodate to the beliefs and practices of the dominant group Park's 1939 theory *best explains* the first stage of integration in the SportsWorld: racial integration on the playing fields/arenas. African American athletes Jackie Robinson (baseball), Bill Russell (basketball), and Gayle Sayers (football) all struggled to integrate their respective sports. Although everyone involved had to make accommodations in some ways (see, especially the autobiography by Bill Russell entitled *Second Wind: The Memoirs of an Opinionated Man*, 1979), not surprising it was these pioneers and not their teammates, coaches, owners, or fans who were required to make the greatest accommodations. To further illustrate this concept, professional football players Gayle Sayers (African American) and Brian Piccolo (White) roomed together to challenge segregation in the South—specifically the fact that southern hotels in cities where NFL games were held were still racially segregated. Clearly, the primary requirement for accommodation, and the greatest threat to personal safety, fell on the minority African American athletes like Sayers.

It is important to note that Park's 1939 theory was bound by time and place. Park was writing in a time of Jim Crow segregation and hyper restrictions on immigration, and despite its being bound by time, his theory was useful in shaping the development of the field of race relations theory. Critics of Park's theory (Shills, 1994) argue that he failed to acknowledge the sites of resistance. It was also argued that Park's race relations cycle had an inevitable natural history in that accommodation by minorities and assimilation into the dominant culture were always inevitable; and thus it failed to recognize and acknowledge those places in which minorities *refused* to accommodate to assimilate.

For example, concerning sport management, Park's 1939 theory would struggle to explain the resistance of some African American athletes to the culture of Whiteness with regards to dress and behavior. Both Roger Goodell and David Stern, commissioners of the National Football League (NFL) and the National Basketball Association (NBA), respectively, have struggled to develop policies that force African American athletes to behave according to the standards of "Whiteness." For example, the NBA has imposed dress codes for players such as requiring those seated on the bench to wear a sports jacket, and outlawing chains, pendants, or medallions over the player's clothes while on team or league business. Another example is the NFL-imposed restrictions on end zone celebrations that often involved the display of (African American) gang signs.[2] Although research is scant, it is likely to expect similar examples of racial accommodations and expectations of racial assimilation to be found when examining the process by which sport managers who are racial minorities are immersed in a majority White workplace culture. Although it has some limitations, Park's race relations cycle provides a useful structure and framework for understanding the likely process and potential challenges of integrating racial minorities into the majority culture that pervades sport management.

Social Distance

Looking for conceptual clarity within the theoretical postulations of race relations, and building on the race relations cycle proposed by Park, research by Cornell University Professor Robin M. Williams put forward the hypotheses that it was necessary to subdivide the notion of prejudice into four main components: (a) negative or positive stereotyping of characteristics attributed to outgroups, (b) feelings of personal liking or disliking, (c) attitudes toward public policies (e.g., segregation), and (d) attitudes of social distance (Williams, 1964). These distinctions clarified many problems found in the Park thesis and created pioneering pathways for the subsequent generation of social analysis and theory development.

Consequently, one of the next developments in sociological theories of race was the concept of "social distance," a term coined in the work of Emory Bogardus (1947). He argued that social distance is a function of affective distance between the members of two groups. He put it thus: "in social distance studies the center of attention is on the feeling reactions of persons toward other persons and toward groups of people" (p. 307). Bogardus understood that social distance is essentially a measure of how much or little sympathy the members of a group feel for another group. Bogardus's conceptualization is not the only one used to develop the more contemporary measures of social distance or social distance scales. Several sociologists have pointed out that social distance can also be conceptualized on the basis of other parameters such as the frequency of interaction between different groups or the normative distinctions in a society about who should be considered an "insider" or "outsider" (Merton, 1972).

Building on the work of Bogardus (1947), scholars worked to develop measurement tools that would identify the "modern racism" that developed after the Civil Rights movement of the 1960s. Among these techniques were the revitalization of the social distance theory and the development of more sophisticated scales for measuring intergroup interaction. This research centered on asking Whites and African Americans about their overall attitudes about each other and then comparing these attitudes (which were generally positive) with their preferences for a variety of social interactions that ranged from a relative degree of distance as captured in responses to statements such as: "I would be comfortable having someone of another race work in our office" to very close distance as captured in responses to statements such as: "I would be comfortable having someone of another race move in next door to me" (Schuman et al., 1997). Schuman et al.'s research revealed a steady decline in White's willingness to hold stereotyped beliefs about African Americans—such as that they are less intelligent. However, it simultaneously revealed very little liberalizing in Whites' attitudes and preferences toward or actual experiences having close contact with African Americans. Essentially, it highlighted the presence of a new, modern racism based less on the types of overt prejudice that Bogardus's work measured. Yet, despite the reduction in overall prejudice, there has been very little shift in voluntary integration—i.e., moving into the same neighborhoods, joining the same churches, dating and marrying across racial/ethnic groups, and so forth (Smith & Hattery, 2009a, 2009b).

As applied to sport management, we note that in America especially among fans of college football, the game itself creates a false sense of racial harmony (Carrington, 2010). These same White fans who jump, yell, and scream on Saturday afternoons for African American players like John Clay (Wisconsin), Denard Robinson (Michigan), or Terrell Pryor (Ohio State), all of whom were potential Heisman candidates for 2011, could be the same individuals who slam the doors of access and opportunity for African Americans at work, who resist African Americans moving into their neighborhoods or attending their children's schools, and who socialize their children against forming interracial friendships or dating across racial lines (Carrington, 2010; Feagin & Picca, 2007; Smith, 2009; Smith & Hattery 2009a). Feagin and Picca (2007) refer to this as the difference between the "front stage" and the "back stage." Thus, while African Americans may receive "front stage" treatment as athletes on the playing fields, they receive "back stage" treatment as sport managers.

The theory of social distance is a useful tool for explaining the lack of racial diversity in the leadership of sport. Why? Because sport institutions are close-knit, fraternal communities where intimate interactions are required—precisely the same interactions that Schuman et al. (1997) reveal make Whites uncomfortable. People are often categorized as "in-group" or "out-group" members based on personal characteristics such as their race. In-group members are afforded greater authority, trust, and respect and therefore, are more likely to receive better access to information and resources, more meaningful work assignments, and experience greater job satisfaction (Cunningham, 2007). In-group members are also more likely to celebrate their social closeness. For example, head football coaches socialize with each other in the off-season as well as with the athletic administrators, boosters, and college or university administrators and alumni. These populations are almost exclusively White and male. Just as the research of Schuman et al. (1997) revealed that the same Whites who did not hold overt prejudice were simultaneously resistant to African Americans moving next door, we assert (and Cunningham, 2007, infers) that a similar phenomenon may be present in the SportsWorld. Athletic departments, college and university communities, and alumni are very pleased to have African Americans playing on the fields and in the arenas—especially if this contributes to winning—but they are not particularly comfortable sharing intimate spaces on the golf course, at the annual alumni fundraising dinners, at weekly coaches' breakfasts, or at coaches' conferences. Therefore, they may be reluctant to hire African American men into leadership positions which would ultimately lead to cross-racial intimate contact, and thus, decrease the social distance preferred by many in the White majority.

The notion of social distance is also illustrated in the comments uttered by Fuzzy Zoehler (a professional White male golfer) when Tiger Woods (a professional multiracial male golfer) won his first Masters tournament in 1997. Woods was the first non-White winner of the Masters. The culture of the Masters includes a tradition that the winner determines the banquet menu. Based on

Woods being the winner, Zoeller advised the press to tell Woods "not to serve fried chicken next year" at the Masters annual Champions Dinner. As he left, Zoeller made it even worse by adding, "Or collard greens or whatever the hell they serve" (Dougherty, 2009). His comment intimated that while Zoeller was comfortable competing with Woods on the field (golf course), it was undesirable for him to have dinner with him and be subjected to "his" type of food and sociocultural mores. Therefore, a likely presumption is that the desire for social/racial distance (both among racial minorities and racial majorities) may influence sport management opportunities and experiences for People of Color.

The "Race Project"

Just as definitions and concepts of status groups (race, sexuality, gender) dominate postmodern theories, race and race relations theory is no exception. Contemporary theorists argue that race is a far more complex term than that which is used in everyday language. Rather than simply referring to groups of people who look different from one another (sometimes) and can be distinguished from one another and "grouped" (sometimes), for contemporary scholars of race theory, "race" is a status that is imbued with varying levels of power, privilege, and disadvantage and is expressed in relationship (much as Marx, in the Communist Manifesto, argued class required an acknowledgment of relationship). The contemporary scholars on race, Michael Omi and Howard Winant (1989), propose the following definition of race:

> race is a concept which signifies and symbolizes social conflicts and interests by referring to different types of human bodies. Although the concept of race invokes biologically based human characteristics (so-called "phenotypes"), selection of these particular human features for purposes of racial signification is always and necessarily a historical process. (p. 55)

Omi and Winant (1989) argue further that racial distinctions and boundaries are designed to control the movement of resources. We add to their argument that racial distinctions and boundaries also control *opportunities*. According to Omi and Winant, "A racial project is simultaneously an interpretation, representation, or explanation of racial dynamics, and an effort to reorganize and redistribute resources along particular racial lines" (p. 56). Thus, race and the racial project, as Omi and Winant term it, are constantly shifting in response to politics and power. With regards to sport management, Omi and Winant help us shape the fundamental question we address here: how do race and racial dynamics shape access to leadership positions in the institution of the SportsWorld and how is this related, or not related, to the ways in which race and racial dynamics shape opportunities to play sports at either the intercollegiate or professional levels?

One shortcoming of Omi and Winant's (1989) work is their failure to acknowledge the role of both capitalism and patriarchy in the racialized state

(Bonilla-Silva, 1997, 2006). We argue that race, like class (Marx, 2005), is structured by relationships. Simply put, "races" and all other status groups (class, gender, sexual orientation) are shaped by the relationships within the status group itself. Karl Marx (2005) argued that the *relationships of capitalism* were necessary to define and create the status groups—proletariat and bourgeoisie— just as Franz Fanon (1967) argued that the *relationships of slavery* were necessary to create the status groups—master and slave. When one conceptualizes race as a "transaction" (particularly in situations whereby the transaction has been limited primarily to one type where Whites exploit African Americans) one begins to see the importance of the maintenance and control of the racial boundary— the site where relationships are played out.

With regards to sport management, this perspective illuminates the role that racialized transactions predicated on ideologies play in shaping not only access but also the process by which access to management positions in sport is either gained or denied. For example, Fanon's (1967) "master-slave" rubric can be conceptualized and applied to the SportsWorld and to sport management, where the boundaries between majority White managers and owners and the majority Black players are distinct (see specifically Rhoden's 2006 discussion titled: *Forty Million Dollar Slaves*). Therefore, the sport management may be characterized as what Omi and Winant's (1989) deem the "race project" because racial distinctions and racial boundaries shape the relationship in the SportsWorld (Cunningham, 2007) that subsequently influences the access to opportunities in sport management positions.

Symbolic Racism

Perhaps the most important recent contribution to contemporary race relations theory is the concept of "symbolic racism." Sociologist Bonilla-Silva (2006) argues that symbolic racism represents the new language of racism that has largely developed in response to the climate of political correctness. According to Bonilla-Silva:

> Symbolic racism is a form of racism involving a belief that a minority group (for example African-Americans) no longer face wide-spread discrimination and thus they are deserving of the problems or issues they might face due to the fact that they are lazy or simply do not attempt to resolve their issues. (p. 25)

For example, we see the replacement of the old-fashioned racism of Jim Crow (e.g., segregated White/Colored water fountains) with the shaping of Whites' political attitudes, including Whites' fear of non-White encroachment, even when it does not exist (e.g., opposition to Affirmative Action policies despite the fact that non-Whites remain significantly under-represented in education and most prestigious occupations). It is also expressed in concerns of non-Whites taking over the neighborhood (when in fact housing segregation is as profound as ever), and is conveyed in overall negative feelings about African Americans even if not directed at specific individuals). Bonilla-Silva (2006) also explains that symbolic racism in the post-Civil Rights era is not merely the singular and overt racial events such as public racist comments or hanging nooses from trees but more so a stratified and ingrained system that has material benefits for Whites. For example, the continuation of "steering" in real estate, differential treatment in health care, and the continuation of 'legacy' in education and certain occupations (Hattery & Smith, 2007a). Bonilla-Silva (2006) also demonstrates that people ignore everyday racism because they believe racism exists only in the explicit forms it did before the modern Civil Rights revolution of the 1960s. In addition, Bonilla-Silva points out the inherent dissonance in the belief of accomplishing equality (despite the mounds of evidence that structured discrimination continues to exist), and thus blaming minorities for their own "failings" such as higher rates of unemployment, lower rates of high school graduation, and higher rates of poverty and reliance on social safety net programs. This new style of discrimination comes in many forms, from denying access to housing in certain neighborhoods, to the blocking of financial transactions such as bank loans and even to judicial discrimination that produces racialized differentials in sentencing for similarly situated crimes (Bonilla-Silva 2006; Hattery & Smith, 2010). This type of discrimination could also be functioning in the SportsWorld where racial minorities are denied access to job announcements and opportunities, information, resources, access to promotions, and so forth (Cunningham, 2007).

Bonilla-Silva (2006) also notes that the idea of *colorblindness* allows current racist trends to continue unchallenged in America. He likens colorblindness to a modern-day racial Trojan Horse—a strategy that allows Whites to believe that race no longer matters because they have the privilege of being oblivious to or dismissive of data that suggests the contrary. Colorblind racism is the most significant political tool available for Whites to explain and ultimately justify the racial status quo, which is to keep things as they are (Bonilla-Silva, 1997). "Whites rationalize minorities' contemporary status as the product of market dynamics, naturally occurring phenomena, and Black imputed cultural limitations" (Bonilla-Silva, 2006, p. 2). When applied to the SportsWorld, Whites may conclude that if there are no (or few) African American men in sport leadership (such as head football coaches, athletic directors, or professional team owners) this must be simply the result of the market or a lack of interest among these men for this particular position. Symbolic racism, as reflected in colorblind attitudes, is the ultimate belief among Whites in a level playing field.

Symbolic racism theory also provides the lens for interrogating shifts in the language that Whites use to talk about race issues. For example, few Whites may be willing to indicate or admit that they think African Americans are "less intelligent," though evidence from studies of both hiring practices and college admissions suggest the persistence of just this kind of belief (Wise, 2004). For example, Whites developed a new way to talk about race in that they no longer touted a belief in segregated schools but instead argued and voted for "neighborhood" schools. This neighborhood school movement was ostensibly about the sensibility of keeping children in their own neighborhoods and creating the opportunity for them to walk to school—thus cutting down on transportations costs. Yet, in the South, where this movement thrives, the neighborhood school movement is built largely on the reality that neighborhoods remain racially segregated (Hattery & Smith, 2007b) and thus "neighborhood" schools would reflect the racial composition of neighborhoods and be similarly segregated. As a result of this movement, which on the surface has nothing to do with race, today's children attend schools that are less racially diverse and more racially segregated than those attended by their parents (Boger & Orfield, 2005). This "race neutral" language continues to perpetuate structural and symbolic racism.

Applied to the SportsWorld, this new race neutral language of symbolic racism allows college athletic directors to maintain a segregated pool of head football coaches and athletic administrators while using the language that some candidates (read African Americans) simply don't "fit in." And, this language of "fit" is highly connected to the notion of social distance as we articulated it in the previous discussion. This scenario of "fit" speaks from the new language of symbolic racism, and yet it also yields a logical knitting of the fears expressed in the tenets of social distance theory.

Symbolic racism also reflects the belief held by many Whites, including those who consider themselves to be very liberal on race issues, that overt discrimination has largely ended and that the playing field is more or less level. This belief in effect releases them *personally* from being associated with or being blamed for any persistent racial gaps in health, education, and wealth (Bonilla-Silva, 2006) on which there is substantial evidence (Hattery & Smith, 2007a). For example, a poll conducted by the *Wall Street Journal* and *NBC* in January 2010 reported:

> While 72% of whites now say that race relations are good, a slightly smaller percentage of African Americans—64%—say the same thing. On affirmative action, 49% believe that it is needed to counteract past discrimination against minorities, versus 43% who think affirmative action programs have gone too far. Not surprisingly, African Americans (81%) and Hispanics (69%) support affirmative action more than whites (41%) do.[3]

These types of poll data reveal much more than the racial gap in attitudes about the racial climate and policies like affirmative action; they also underscore Bonilla-Silva's (2006) point that Whites largely believe that racial problems and discrimination are a thing of the past and thus they are not responsible for making changes in their own lives, or (for those with power) attempting to make changes in the organizations in which they work. This shift in racial attitudes from believing African Americans are "less intelligent" to the belief that racial discrimination has largely disappeared (and racial gaps in education or wealth are the result of individual inadequacies), though more palatable, continues to place the "blame" on African Americans' failure to attain the American Dream (Hattery & Smith, 2007a) squarely on their individual shoulders without recognizing the continued role that structural inequality plays in shaping racialized access to the opportunity structure (Bonilla-Silva, 2006; Hattery & Smith, 2007a).

Applying symbolic racism theory to sport management helps us to understand the dangers of the likely perceptions in sport that the playing field is level, and there must simply not be any "qualified" African American men who can serve as head coaches, athletic directors, managers, owners, etc., or they simply do not want these type of positions. The danger in this shifted attitude is that it: (a) shifts the responsibility of repairing the hidden ills, (b) masks the identification of the "real" problems, and (c) dismisses the need for systemic changes. Sport leadership positions are deeply rooted in a system of racial stratification that is effectively illuminated through the lens of symbolic racism (Carrington, 2010; Smith, 2009).

Theories of Power

Inherent in the race relations theories previously discussed is the undercurrent of power (or lack thereof). As Marx (2005), Fanon (1967), and others have articulated, power is an essential element in the particular shapes and contours that race relations take. For more than 150 years theorists have been developing structural models—as opposed to the individual explanations that are so popular among individual actors—to explain inequalities of race, but also class, gender and geography (e.g., patterns of colonization). Göran Therborn (1999) argues in *The Ideology of Power and the Power of Ideology* that the state establishes dominant or hegemonic ideologies that dictate specific terms for behavior. This includes the defining of: (a) what is, (b) what is good, and (c) what is possible. In addition, Therborn argues that social change will only occur when such change advances the interests of the ruling class. Thus, when we think about the shift in Whites' racial attitudes across the 20th Century, it is apparent that Whites' attitudes only begin to change or shift when there is a social cost *for not doing so.*

At the height of the Civil Rights movement, as images of water cannons and police dogs circulated in newspapers around the globe, the reputation of Whites in America was threatened. How could Americans (read White Americans) agitate globally for democracy when they prevented their own citizens (read Black Americans) from full participation, full citizenship rights (Kerber, 1997)? In this light, many Whites, especially outside of the South, identified a self-interest in modifying their racial attitudes. Similarly, in the early years of the 21st Century we argued that our understanding of shifts in ideologies can be best explained by coupling theories of modern racism and theories of power, which suggests that structural racism will only be addressed if and when it is conceptualized as a threat to the ruling class. For example, as applied to collegiate sports, the Black Coaches Association attempts to use techniques of shaming and embarrassment to highlight the lack of racial diversity in the leadership of college football. To the degree that they can link diversity initiatives in business to the realm of college football, and thus create embarrassment on the part of (White) athletic directors, college presidents, and alumni, the pressure to become more racially diverse may bear fruit. Or, following the example of *Brown v. Board of Education*, if a ruling body such as the NCAA demands racial diversity among its member institutions, and can punish the lack of it, such diversity is a likely outcome. Therefore, fully understanding the likely impact of the previous race relations concepts (race relations cycle, social distance, and symbolic racism) requires a requisite understanding of the institutional power dynamics at play.

Theories of Segregation

One last concept related to race relations that warrants discussion here is the notion of segregation. Segregation—in a variety of forms—is a widely used strategy for maintaining status boundaries, limiting and controlling access to the opportunity structure, and enforcing second-class citizenship (see, for example, Epstein, 2007). Epstein explores the importance of boundaries in maintaining social hierarchies for patriarchy:

> The enforcement of the distinction [based on sex/gender] is achieved through cultural and ideological means that justify the differentiation. This is despite the fact that, unlike every other dichotomous category of people, females and males are necessarily bound together, sharing the same domiciles and most often the same racial and social class statuses. . . . I am convinced that societies and strategic subgroups within them, such as political and work institutions, *maintain their boundaries*—their very social organization—through the use of invidious distinctions made between males and females. (p. 4; emphasis added)

This framework helps us to distill the unique nature of racial segregation as it has been structured in the United States and contributes to our ability to advance our thinking about the roles boundary maintenance and segregation have played in structuring access to opportunities in the management of intercollegiate and professional sport. In particular, we argue that Epstein's understanding of the way in which the intimacy of gender relations *requires* the enforcement of distinctions can be applied to understanding intimate relations between Whites and African Americans in the SportsWorld. In short, the greater the intimacy, the greater the need to maintain the boundary and to enforce the second-class status of the oppressed group. Or as C. Vann Woodward (2001) argued in *The Strange Career of Jim Crow*, segregation pushed "Negroes" further and further into the margins.

The SportsWorld, especially the fields and arenas of competition, is an environment of intense intimacy both physically and emotionally. Physical and emotional intimacy arises from a variety of sources including the intimacy of the locker room—a setting in which men parade around naked—rooming together on road trips, sharing meals, and so forth. However, the situation on the fields of competition contrasts the notion argued by Epstein (i.e., the greater the intimacy, the greater the need to maintain boundary). Instead, the greater the physical contact and emotional intimacy between athletes, the greater the trust for successful competition.

We illustrate this point by recalling the historic case of Brian Piccolo and Gayle Sayers that we alluded to earlier. In a bold move that he hoped would ease the transition to integration, then Chicago Bears coach George Halas assigned Brian Piccolo, who is White, to room with Gayle Sayers, who is African American. Though it had the intended impact on these two men—they became great friends whose families spent time together at each other's homes and in restaurants, etc.—it shook both the team and the public, who were aghast that a hotel room would be integrated! This was during the same time when hotel rooms were not only *not integrated* but hotels, especially across the South, remained segregated, a burden on teams from the North that traveled with integrated squads. In a more contemporary example, a high degree of trust is required between a quarterback and his wide receiver in football or between a point guard and his center in basketball. Based on that trust, passes on both field and court may be made in a "racially blind" manner (as they are targeted to a position and not to a "raced" person). In such cases, racial segregation would not benefit the team, the organization, and ultimately the opportunity for the "system" to produce revenue.

However, based on the racial composition of the managers and leaders of the SportsWorld (Cunningham, 2007; Lapchick, 2009) the notion of segregation is pronounced. In looking at the business side of the sport it becomes clear, as Herb Snitzer (1991) demonstrates, that the dominant group in American society fails to see African Americans in any other light except as *participants* (not managers or owners) of the vast sport and entertainment enterprise. While one can argue with this pronouncement, it becomes difficult to do so in light of evidence demonstrating the persistence of a negative stereotype of African Americans (as well as African American athletes) as being intellectually inferior yet "naturally" gifted for athletics (Bobo, 2001; Jones, 1964; Smith, 2009).

We would never support rigid quota rules, for example, that require that if 50% of a team is African American, then at minimum 50% of the staff should be African American. Yet, when it comes down to the hard facts of access to opportunities (and not just after the playing days are over), it remains clear that African Americans are not being weaved into the business side of sports. Even where one might assume that African Americans are being accepted as full members of the team—for example, in intercollegiate athletics—the research by McDowell, Cunningham, and Singer (2009) shows that in the area of student support services they are not:

One area in which intercollegiate athletics does mirror general societal trends is in the clustering of racial minorities in certain positions, an occurrence known as occupational segregation. Occupational segregation is said to exist when racial groups are distributed inconsistently across occupations or are allocated to certain positions, as compared to being equally represented in all available positions. This phenomenon becomes evident in the intercollegiate athletic context, as close examination of NCAA data reveals a skewed racial minority composition, in that racial minorities are disproportionately concentrated in a few administrative and coaching positions. (p. 432)

While segregation on the fields of competition in sport is slowly dissipating, and may have completely dissipated in the high-profile sports of football and men's basketball, such is not the case for the racial segregation of the management of sport, where racial boundaries are maintained, where race limits and controls access to leadership opportunities, and where a second-class citizenship is enforced. Therefore, it is important that sport management scholars and practitioners continue their understanding of how the race relations concepts previously discussed (particularly social distance and symbolic racism) contribute to the maintenance of racially segregated boundaries in sport management.

▪ CONTRIBUTIONS OF RACE RELATIONS THEORIES TO SPORT MANAGEMENT RESEARCH

As demonstrated in this essay thus far, elements of the race relation cycle, social distance, symbolic racism, power, and segregation create, perpetuate, and sustain a racial dominance, hierarchy, and thus social (dis)order in sport management. Such racial dominance also shapes sport management research methods. However, few scholars have focused their research on race relations in sport management, and even fewer have examined how race relations in the institution of sport may have contributed to the incredibly low rate of participation of African American men in sports leadership.

In relation to the theoretical approaches to understand the impact of race relations on the access, opportunities, and experiences in sport management, one has to consider the methodological approaches to the research in question. For instance, scholars who have begun to carefully look into issues surrounding methods of social and behavioral science research have also begun to question mainstream approaches that are now used to answer a variety of research questions. Zuberi and Bonilla-Silva (2008) raise several important questions in this regard that directly apply to our ability to better understand the racial composition of intercollegiate and professional sport personnel: (a) Who defines the research questions? (b) Which lens is used during the analysis? and (c) Who establishes the assumptions of any area of research?

Standpoint theory argues that one's standpoint, or social location, is extremely powerful in shaping who defines the research questions and which lens is used during the analysis (Hawkesworth, 2006). With regards to sport management, there is a dearth of research in sport management defined and framed by the conceptual standpoint of race relations theories. Consequently, there is a void in research on the manner in which "rules" of contact, conflict, accommodation of the dominant group, and assimilation, as well as structures of sequence (illuminated by Park's race relations cycle), may influence the ideologies that undergird research on race in sport management. Regarding the lens used to analyze race in sport management, we are struck by the fact that despite the wealth of research "counting" diversity and cataloging those African American men who are hired as head football coaches, little research exists on how the processes of social distance and symbolic racism may contribute to the continued racial segregation and lack of racial presence and power in leadership positions in sport management. While "general" descriptive research may allow for an accurate depiction of the racial gap in the management of sport, research through the lens of race relations theories allows for a better understanding of what shaped and contributed to the racial gap. Lastly, elements of the race relations cycle, social distance, and elements of symbolic racism may challenge the longstanding assumptions that have historically framed research about race and the perceived "readiness" or "appropriateness" of African American men for leadership in a manner that offers new insight. Therefore, regarding research about race and sport management, it is our contention that race relations theories appropriately allow for the proper definition of the research problem, lens for the analyses, and contextualization of the underlying assumptions.

◼ SUGGESTIONS FOR PROMOTING RACIAL DIVERSITY IN SPORT MANAGEMENT

We argue that if there is a desire for the racial gap to be closed in the leadership of sport, then the principles that have been operating, which parallel those identified in the race relations theories previously discussed, must be replaced with systematic processes that are transparent and that adhere to the same hiring practices required of the majority of other jobs on college and university campuses and in Corporate America. Specifically:

(a) Searches for sport management positions must be conducted nationally and even internationally.
(b) Racially diverse pools of applicants for sport management positions must be developed as the part of any major hiring.
(c) Recruiting for sport management positions should be conducted in racially diverse environments including at high schools, at coaching clinics, and at seminars rather than limiting recruiting to the ranks of college assistant coaches. This approach would likely reduce the powerful "legacy" rules that currently dominate hiring practices, a system African Americans have been generally left out of.

That said, we offer several practices that would lead the way toward recognizing the race relations governing the management of sport and addressing some of the problems previously discussed:

(a) Systematic reviews of the process and outcomes of sport management hiring should be conducted every 3–5 years by a governing body, perhaps the NCAA or NCAA conferences.
(b) Evidence that universities are continuing to operate under the principles of nepotism should result in sanctions.
(c) Human Resource "Monitors" must be trained in decoding the language of symbolic racism so that they can combat it when it occurs.
(d) Based on the need for assimilation and accommodation by racial majorities and racial minorities in a given setting, Human Resources Personnel should offer guidelines and suggestions for creating a racially inclusive workplace culture.

■ CONCLUSION

During the majority of the 20th Century the "simple" explanation of discrimination was used to explain the lack racial diversity in the management of sport. We contend that this explanation is unsuited for the complexities of the 21st Century. Rather than taking a strictly discrimination approach, and also moving beyond simply *counting* the number of African American men in leadership positions, we have analyzed and sought to *explain* this under-representation using a theoretical lens drawn from the long history of race relations theory that pervades North American sociology. As illustrated in this essay, race relations cycle, social distance theory, symbolic racism, segregation, and power can be combined and interwoven to explain various aspects of the process by which leadership in the SportsWorld has remained racially segregated. Independently and collectively, these concepts help us understand the continuation of a system of racial stratification in the SportsWorld. Unless the SportsWorld embraces the types of policies and practices we have suggested that are sensitive to the race relations that permeate sport, it will find itself in a crisis from which it may not be able to emerge; and the business of sport will remain a world that is closed and highly racially segregated.

■ NOTES

1. Interview with B. Carrington. September 8, 2010. Retrieved September 27, 2010, from: http://www.utexas.edu/know/2010/09/08/ben_carrington_book/.
2. Harry Edwards, personal communication, October 2009.
3. See: http://firstread.msnbc.msn. com/archive/2010/01/18/2176748.aspx.

■ REFERENCES

Baron, J., & Pfeffer, J. (1994). The social psychology of organizations and inequality. *Social Psychology Quarterly, 57*(3), 190–209.

Bell, E., & Nkomo, S. (2001). *Business Week.* Retrieved June 25, 2010, from http://www.businessweek.com/careers/content/aug2001/ca2001087_306.htm

Bobo, L. (2009). Post-racial America looks pretty racial to me. *Atlanta Journal Constitution,* July 22, Retrieved July 10, 2010, from http://www.ajc.com/opinion/post-racial-america-looks-98280.html

Bobo, L. (2001). Racial attitudes and relations at the close of the Twentieth Century. In N. Smelser & W. Wilson (Eds.), *America becoming: Racial trends and their consequences* (Vol. 1, pp. 244–301). Washington, DC: National Academy Press.

Bogardus, E. (1947). Measurement of personal-group relations. *Sociometry, 10*(4), 306–311.

Boger, J. C., & Orfield, G. (2005). *School resegregation: Must the South turn back?* Chapel Hill: University of North Carolina Press.

Bonilla-Silva, E. (2006). *Racism without racists: Color-blind racism and the persistence of racial inequality in the United States.* Lanham, MD: Rowman & Littlefield.

Bonilla-Silva, E. (1997). Rethinking racism: Toward a structural interpretation. *American Sociological Review, 62*(3), 465–480.

Burton, L., Bonilla-Silva, E., Ray, V., Buckelew, R., & Freeman, E. (2010). Critical race theories, colorism, and the decade's research on families of Color. *Journal of Marriage and the Family, 72,* 440–459.

Carrington, B. (2010). *Race, sport and politics.* Thousand Oaks, CA: Sage.

Cunningham, G. B. (2010). Understanding the under-representation of African American coaches: A multilevel perspective. *Sport Management Review, 13,* 395–406.

Cunningham, G. B. (2007). *Diversity in sport organizations.* Scottsdale, AZ: Holcomb Hathaway.

Dougherty, R. (2009). Fuzzy Zoeller racist Tiger Woods comments overshadow 30 years at Augusta. *Associated Content,* Lifestyle Section, April 11. Accessed September 27, 2010, from http://www.associatedcontent.com/article/1641441/fuzzy_zoeller_racist_tiger_woods_comments.html?cat=22.

Edwards, H. (1997). The end of the 'Golden Age' of Black sports participation? *South Texas Law Review, 38,* 1007–1027.

Ely, R. J., & Thomas, D. (2001). Cultural diversity at work: The effects of diversity perspectives on work group processes and outcomes. *Administrative Science Quarterly, 46,* 229–273.

Epstein, C. F. (2007). Great divides: The cultural, cognitive, and social bases of the global subordination of Women. *American Sociological Review, 72,* 1–22.

Fanon, F. (1967). *Black skin, White masks.* New York: Grove Press.

Feagin, J. (1991). The continuing significance of race: Antiblack discrimination in public places. *American Sociological Review, 56*(1), 101–116.

Feagin, J., & Picca, L. (2007). *Two-faced racism: Whites in the backstage and frontstage.* New York: Routledge.

Fink, J. S., & Pastore, D. L. (1999). Diversity in sport? Utilizing the business literature to devise a comprehensive framework of diversity initiatives. *Quest, 51,* 310–327.

Greene, L. (2008). Football coach contracts: What does the student-athlete have to do with it? *University of Missouri Kansas City Law Review, 76,* 665–696.

Hattery, A., & Smith, E. (2010). *Prisoner re-entry and social capital: The long road to reintegration.* Latham, MD: Lexington Books.

Hattery, A. J., & Smith, E. (2007a). *African American families.* Thousand Oaks, CA: Sage.

Hattery, A. J., & Smith, E. (2007b). Social stratification in the New/Old South: The influences of racial segregation on social class in the Deep South. *Journal of Property Research, 11*(1), 55–81.

Hawkesworth, M. E. (2006). *Feminist inquiry: From political conviction to methodological innovation.* New Brunswick, NJ: Rutgers University Press.

Johnson, J. (2009). Rush Limbaugh meets Reggie Fowler. *Pittsburg Courier,* October 22. Retrieved September 25, 2010, from http://www.newpittsburghcourieronline.com/index.php?option=com_content&view=article&id=604:rush-limbaugh-meetsreggie-fowler&catid=40:opinion&Itemid=54.

Jones, R. (1964). Proving Blacks inferior: The sociology of knowledge. In J. Ladner (Ed.), *The death of White sociology* (pp. 124–135). New York: Random House.

Kerber, L. K. (1997). The meanings of citizenship. *Journal of American History, 84*(3), 833–854.

Lapchick, R. (2009). The Racial and Gender Report Card. *The Institute for Diversity and Ethics in Sport.* Retrieved April 07, 2016, from http://www.tidesport.org/reports.html

Lapchick, R., & McMechan, D. (2009). *The buck stops here: Assessing diversity among campus and conference leaders for Football Bowl Subdivision (FBS) schools in the 2009-10 academic year.* Orlando, FL: The Institute for Diversity and Ethics in Sport, College of Business Administration, University of Central Florida.

Lyman, S. (1968). The race relations cycle of Robert E. Park. *Pacific Sociological Review, 1*(1), 16–22.

Marx, K. (2005). *The communist manifesto and other writings.* New York: Barnes and Noble Classics.

Merton, R. K. (1972). Insiders and outsiders: A chapter in the sociology of knowledge. *American Journal of Sociology, 78*(1), 9–47.

McDowell, J., Cunningham, G., & Singer, J. (2009). The supply and demand side of occupational segregation: The case of an intercollegiate athletic department. *Journal of African American Studies, 13,* 431–454.

Omi, M., & Winant, H. (1986). 1989. *Racial formation in the United States: From the 1960s to the 1980s.* New York: Routledge & Kegan Paul.

Robinson, J. (1972). *I never had it made.* New York: Harper Collins.

Schuman, H., Steeh, C., Bobo, L., & Krysan, M. (1997). *Racial attitudes in America: Trends and interpretations* (Rev. Ed.). Cambridge, MA: Harvard University Press.

Shils, E. (1994). The sociology of Robert E. Park. In R. Gubert & L. Tomasi (eds.), *Robert E. Park and the Melting Pot Theory* (pp. 20–27). Italy: Reverdito Edizioni, University of Trento Publications.

Shropshire, K. (2004). Minority issues in contemporary sports. *Stanford Law & Policy Review, 15,* 189–215.

Shropshire, K. (1997). Merit, ol' boy networks, and the Black-bottomed pyramid. *Hastings Law Review, 47,* 455–472.

Smith, E. (2009). *Race, sport and the American dream.* Durham, NC: Carolina Academic Press.

Smith, E., & Hattery, A. J. (2009a). *Interracial relationships in the 21st Century.* Durham, NC: Carolina Academic Press.

Smith, E., & Hattery, A. J. (2009b). *Interracial intimacies: An examination of powerful men and their relationships across the color line.* Durham, NC: Carolina Academic Press.

Snitzer, H. (1991). The Realities of Cultural Change. *Reconstruction, 1*(3), 33.

Therborn, G. (1999). *The Ideology of Power and the Power of Ideology.* London: Verso.

Thomas, D. (2001). They go with John Jones, Caucasian male. An interview with David Thomas by Pamela Mendels. *Business Week,* May 30. Retrieved June 25, 2010, from http://www.businessweek.com/careers/content/may2001ca20010530_003.htm

Thomas, D., & Gabarro, J. (1999). *Breaking through: The making of minority executives in corporate America.* Cambridge, MA: Harvard Business Press.

Tygiel, J. (1983). *Baseball's great experiment: Jackie Robinson and his legacy.* New York: Oxford University Press.

Williams, R. (1964). *Strangers next door: Ethnic relations in American communities.* Englewood, NJ: Prentice-Hall.

Wise, T. (2004). *White like me: Reflections on race from a privileged Son.* New York: Soft Skull Press.

Woodward, C. V. (2001). *The strange career of Jim Crow.* New York: Oxford University Press.

Zuberi, T., & Bonilla-Silva, E. (Eds.). (2008). *White logic, white methods: Racism and methodology.* Lanham: Rowman & Littlefield Publishers.

Zweigenhaft, R., & Domhoff, W. (2006). *Diversity in the power elite: How it happened, why it matters.* New York: Rowman & Littlefield.

8 'Black Athletes in White Men's Games'

Race, Sport and American National Pastimes

■ DAVID K. WIGGINS

African Americans have fought for many years to become full participants in their nation's most popular sporting pastimes. Like other groups, including white ethnics such as Irish Americans, Jewish Americans and Italian Americans, African Americans have always desired to participate in sports at the highest levels of competition, in those sports with national followings and in those sports that could potentially bring large financial rewards. This desire was stimulated as much as anything else by the need to achieve success in the common American experience of sport and as a way to realise the elusive dream of full citizenship and acceptance. From pugilist Bill Richmond and Tom Molineaux in the early nineteenth century to track and field's Jesse Owens and baseball's Jackie Robinson in the early to mid-twentieth century to boxing's Muhammad Ali, basketball's Michael Jordan, football's Jerry Rice and golf's Tiger Woods in the late twentieth and early twenty-first centuries, African Americans have sought entry into America's most popular sports through dogged determination—or with an unhealthy 'fixation' as one noted scholar puts it—and hard work.[1]

Unfortunately, while African Americans have achieved much success in an institution referred to by English literature and Afro-American studies scholar Gerald Early as the 'ultimate meritocracy', they have always struggled to become full participants in sport because of the racism and accompanying structural differences in the USA.[2] The pattern of African American participation in sport extends back to slavery and has remained remarkably similar ever since. Although I do not agree with the assertions by some writers and scholars that contemporary sport is another form of slavery, I do believe a legacy from slavery was the development of two decidedly different patterns of sport that must be acknowledged if we are to understand the complex role of sport in the lives of African Americans.[3] It is true that slaves were on occasion able to transcend the horrendous conditions of the institution and participate in various types of cultural activities, recreations and sports among themselves and out of view of the planter and his family.[4] These activities in the slavequarter community allowed slaves a much needed sense of independence, some degree of control over their own lives, an opportunity to satisfy their competitive impulses and a chance to exhibit their unique style of physical movement and gift for improvisation. All of these were perhaps most visible in the dancing and hunting activities of slaves. This pattern, sport behind segregated walls as I have always called it, would continue unabated following emancipation and through most of the first half of the twentieth century and beyond.[5]

It is also true, however, that some of the more physically gifted, trustworthy and perhaps even more malleable slaves were involved in the sporting life of the planter. A class of men enthralled with sports, southern planters used slaves in a number of different ways in their own recreations and sports activities.[6] Evidence makes clear that these slaves were different from the ordinary field hands and even house slaves, because they often had more freedom of movement, special privileges and closer relationships with their owners. Evidence also indicates that some slaves earned their freedom as a result of their good behaviour and athletic successes. This pattern, in which athletically gifted blacks were able to exhibit their physical skills and realise material benefits, yet were ultimately never able to exert any significant individual or institutional control over the activities they participated in, has continued to the present day and is why the title of the late historian Manning Marable's 1973 essay 'Black Athletes in White Men's Games' is still an accurate description of sports in the USA.[7]

Two of the most significant sports for both slaves and their owners were hunting and horse racing. According to historian Ted Ownby, hunting had 'roots deep in southern history' and no group was more enthusiastic about it than plantation owners who used their slaves in an assortment of ways as they pursued small animals and large game.[8] Before the sport took on its modern trappings with game commissions and elaborate rules, plantation owners roamed the countryside searching for deer and other animals with their slaves who were often responsible for the training and handling of dogs used in the hunt.[9]

The participation of slaves in horse racing brought them far more attention than did the more solitary sport of hunting.[10] Although impossible to pinpoint exactly when slaves began to participate in what would become America's first national spectator sport, it is probable that they started serving as trainers, groomers and riders of horses in significant numbers by the latter stages of the eighteenth century in mostly southern states. These slaves realised an elevated status in the slavequarter and were treated with some care by slave owners who wanted to ensure the health of one of their most important commodities.[11] Freed from the intensive labour on plantations, these slaves travelled the south and were sometimes even paid for their services.

One of the most famous of these slaves was Austin Curtis, a talented trainer, groomer and jockey who helped manage the racing stable of Willie Jones in Roanoke, Virginia. Referred to as 'America's first truly great professional athlete' by historian Edward Hotaling, Curtis led the Jones stable to numerous victories and became one of the top riders in the sport. In 1791, because of 'his fidelity to his master' and 'his honesty and good behaviour on all occasions' Curtis was officially freed by Jones.[12] Austin Curtis aside, slave riders were largely objectified, mere bodies not adequately acknowledged for their humanity, let alone their successes. Slave jockeys were, after all, still slaves. They were property like the horses they rode, only far less valuable. Often they were not even given the respect of a surname, riding anonymously under impersonal designations such as Abe, Charlie, Cato, Frank, Richard, John or Tom.[13]

Edward Hotaling may be right about Austin Curtis's prominence among African American athletes of his time. But the two African American athletes who have garnered more attention from historians and perhaps tell us more about national pastimes and the interconnection between race and sport from an international perspective at the turn of the nineteenth century are the boxers Bill Richmond and Tom Molineaux.[14] The two men were skilled fighters who successfully plied their skills in a sport that had yet to become a national pastime in the USA. Evidence of this, as pointed out by historian Elliott Gorn, is that everything we know about Molineaux—and for that matter Richmond as well—came from English sources, a clear sign that during this period 'boxing was socially and culturally meaningless on these shores, and so it went largely ignored'.[15] Regardless, Richmond and Molineaux were important trans-national figures who were the first of several outstanding African American athletes to travel overseas to seek fame and fortune. They were also, as historian Theresa Runstedtler has recently noted about other black boxers in the nineteenth century, athletes who led 'migratory lives, often overlapping with those of sailors, itinerant labourers, and travelling performers'.[16]

Richmond, who is sometimes described as either a free man or slave by historians, was born in either 1763 or 1765 on Staten Island, New York. At some point, British general Hugh Percy, who was in charge of British forces during the War of Independence, made Richmond his servant and took him to England where he first became a journeyman cabinetmaker, then a successful boxer and later the owner of the Horse and Dolphin Tavern in London. Not only did Richmond serve the fancy at the Horse and Dolphin Tavern, but he trained young boxers intent on gaining glory in the sport.[17]

The most famous of the boxers who trained under the tutelage of Richmond was Molineaux. It has long been held that Molineaux, who was born in either Virginia or Maryland in 1784, was a slave who won his freedom after winning money for his master in several boxing matches. As inspirational as the story sounds, there is no evidence to indicate whether Molineaux was born a slave or a free man. What is certain is that at some point Molineaux made his way to New York City where he worked as a porter and dock worker while also engaging in informal boxing matches with visiting seamen and fellow workers. In 1809, he sailed for England to seek matches with the greatest boxers in the world. After honing his boxing skills under the watchful eyes of Richmond at the Horse and Dolphin Tavern, Molineaux fought a number of important bouts, including two championship fights with the great Tom Cribb in 1810 and 1811, neither of which he won.[18]

For some 60 years after Molineaux's death, African Americans participated in sport in relative obscurity. By the mid to latter stages of the 1870s, however, a select number of outstanding African American athletes would begin to distinguish themselves in the ever expanding and increasingly more structured world of white-organised sport and even establish national and sometimes international reputations for their athletic exploits. At the college level, the largest number of African Americans participated in 'king football', while a smaller number competed in track and field and an even smaller number played baseball.[19] Coming largely from upper middle class families who placed a great deal of emphasis on education and career achievements, these student-athletes competed at some of the most prestigious universities in the country.[20] At the professional level, an indeterminate number of African Americans continued to compete as jockeys and boxers as well as baseball players, cyclists and pedestrians.[21]

Historians must be careful not to oversimplify the experiences of African American athletes during this period, but one pattern becomes clear when considering their lives. Although realising success by virtue of their outstanding physical talents and work ethic, all of them had to depend on white coaches, managers and benefactors to negotiate the complex relationship among race, sport and American culture if they wanted to establish and maintain productive athletic careers. Knowing racism could suddenly raise its ugly head and jeopardise their careers required that African American athletes cater to and strengthen ties with the white sport establishment. Their vulnerability did not prevent them from occasionally speaking out about racial discrimination, although white benefactors sometimes voiced louder complaints about inequitable treatment directed at African American athletes in which they had so much invested. Isaac Murphy, the great jockey who captured three Kentucky Derbys, could not have realised such enormous success on the track without patrons such as horse owners J. W. Hunt Reynolds and Elias 'Lucky' Baldwin. Australia's Peter Jackson's great boxing career was made possible partly because of the friendship and support of his long time personal manager Charles 'Parson' Davies, a Chicago entrepreneur who was both a promoter of pedestrian races and handler of fighters. Indianapolis's Marshall 'Major' Taylor's success as a bicyclist was largely a result of Louis D. Munger who became, in the words of historian Andrew Ritchie, 'Taylor's boss and employer, his advisor and protector, he was also his friend, his father-figure and his athletic coach'. Boston's Frank 'black Dan' Hart's outstanding career as a pedestrian was financed by Daniel O'Leary, an Irish immigrant and sports entrepreneur who had been a champion 6-day runner himself and promoter of races.[22]

Unfortunately, any dreams about the unlimited possibilities of colour-blind sports would be shattered by the turn of the twentieth century as a variety of factors contributed to the deterioration of black rights in this country, hardening of racial lines and the widespread belief in the inferiority of African Americans.[23] As a result, African American athletes were barred from playing some white-organised sports and experienced greater difficulty in gaining access to others.[24] The rate, level and degree of exclusion of African American athletes from white-organised sport, however, were dependent on the status and prominence of the particular sports in question as well as the social relevance and context in which they were held.[25] During this period, a highly select number of African American athletes continued to participate in intercollegiate sport at predominately white universities in the north. These schools were willing to play black athletes in an effort to realise much desired victories and national prestige.[26] Importantly, by 1904 some of these athletes, many of whom were banned from competing in sports at the professional level, began representing the USA in the Olympic Games. Experiencing racial discrimination on a daily basis at home, these athletes competed for US Olympic teams whose officials were more interested in realising international prestige through sport than in ameliorating the living conditions of black Americans.[27]

While a select number of African American athletes would find success in predominantly white college sport and the Olympic Games after the turn of the century, black jockeys were virtually eliminated from a profession they once dominated. The underlying reason for this exodus was the hardening of racial lines in the USA. But it also had to do with the elevated status of jockeys and the resulting increase in pay for their services as well as the northern migration of southern blacks, which, ironically enough, had the effect of decreasing the number of black riders who had always been trained on southern farms and plantations.[28]

To some extent, African American athletes would suffer the same fate in baseball. No African American would play Major League Baseball from the time of Moses Fleetwood Walker's 1-year stint with the Toledo Mudhens in 1884 until Jackie Robinson's inaugural season with the Brooklyn Dodgers in 1947.[29] The power brokers in the sport would for years deny entry to African Americans. Questioning publicly whether black players had the requisite skills to play the game yet in reality more concerned about keeping the sport lily white, Commissioner Kenesaw Mountain Landis and club owners kept African Americans out of baseball while at the same time effectively fostering the imaginary notion that baseball was the national pastime that most vividly represented this country's commitment to equality and democratic values.[30]

Unlike the jockey profession and baseball, African Americans would continue to participate in boxing, but not without difficulty in navigating the slippery and cruel nature of racism and racialist thinking. A sport that was of monumental importance to African Americans and many white ethnic groups during the first half of the twentieth century, boxing was always about masculinity and fraught with racial symbolism that fascinated audiences who were both enthralled and ambivalent about the bloody contests in the ring.[31] African Americans took special delight in the sport, even black leaders who promulgated racial uplift by holding tight to Victorian notions of propriety, because it provided opportunities, in the words of Tiger Flowers' biographer Andrew Kaye, 'where a Black man could openly strike a White man with impunity'.[32] Indications of the pride and euphoria that resulted from victories in the ring by African Americans were made clear from the writings of distinguished black literary figures such as James Weldon Johnson, Richard Wright, Ralph Ellison, James Baldwin and Maya Angelou.[33] One boxer who garnered an extraordinary amount of attention from black writers, poets and song writers was Joe Louis, the hard-punching fighter who became an iconic figure in black America because of his racially symbolic triumphs in the ring over Primo Camera and Max Schmeling, among others.[34]

The triumphs of black boxers were especially unsettling to whites because to them those triumphs disrupted the natural social order and challenged the belief in their own racial superiority and true manhood. This fact led to the search for 'white hopes', which meant finding boxers who could confirm white America's belief in racial superiority by triumphing over black boxers in the squared circle. It was also why white boxers were sometimes reluctant to enter the ring against black opponents, especially in the heavyweight division, which was imbued with far more racial meaning than the lighter divisions because of the size of the fighters.[35] The result was that some of the great black heavyweights of the early twentieth century fought each other on multiple occasions. For example, Sam Langford, the great boxer from Nova Scotia, Canada, who was never able to fight for the heavyweight championship in spite of his enormous ring skills, fought Sam McVey, Joe Jeanette and Harry Wills a combined 52 times. Jack Johnson, America's first black heavyweight champion who caused enormous controversy across racial lines for insisting on living life on his own terms and refusal to acquiesce to the white power structure, fought Jeannette five times in 1907 alone.[36]

The African American athletes who participated in predominately white-organised sport during the first half of the twentieth century were obviously a select group, but the largest majority of African American athletes were forced to pursue other opportunities in sport by the beginning of the twentieth century. Several of the greatest African American athletes at the turn of the twentieth century did what Tom Molineaux and Bill Richmond had done many years before and travelled to other lands to pursue fame and fortune in their respective sports. Marshall 'Major' Taylor became an international celebrity in bicycling, realising many important victories in France, Australia and other foreign countries.[37] Willie Simms rode in several horse races in England and his fellow rider Jimmy Winkfield rode to victories in faraway places such as Poland and Russia.[38]

These athletes, who were seemingly motivated to travel to foreign countries to make more money and prolong their careers as much as they wanted to escape the racism in the USA, were truly exceptional individuals and should not be lumped together with most African American athletes who responded to their exclusion from predominantly white-organised sports by establishing their own separate sports teams and leagues. Set up at both the amateur and professional levels of competition in a variety of different sports and within and outside of educational institutions, these separate—or parallel—teams and leagues were remarkably similar to those in predominantly white-organised sport, yet reflected distinctive aspects of black culture. They were particularly important because they provided physically gifted athletes an opportunity to compete at high levels of competition and realise much needed respect, adulation and money. They were also important because it offered the opportunity to exhibit race pride, black self-help, organisational skills and business acumen. Scholars interested in the black experience in sport are familiar with teams and organisations such as the Homestead Grays, New York Renaissance Five, Harlem Globetrotters, New York Brown Bombers, Washington Bears, National Negro Bowling Association, American Tennis Association, Colored Intercollegiate Athletic Association, United Golfers Association and Colored Speedway Association.[39]

Importantly, African American women were participants and sometimes stars on these separate teams and leagues. Prime examples were their involvement in bowling and track and field. From the very beginning of the organisation in 1939, black women were involved as players and leaders in the National Negro Bowling Association. Two African American women were original founders of the organisation that came about because of the racially exclusionary policies of the American Bowling Congress, and scores of others were provided an opportunity to participate in the traditionally working class sport marked by its inexpensiveness, sociability and emphasis on skill and techniques rather than brute strength and power. Although the exact figures are not available, there is little question that African American women made up a significant portion of the estimated six to eight million women bowlers in the USA in the 1950s. Historian Susan Cahn wrote that bowling 'gained acceptance as a "feminine" sport by successfully associating itself with notions of middle-class feminine respectability and heterosexual leisure'.[40] The national pastime for women of all colours might be the most apt descriptor.

African American women also distinguished themselves in track and field behind segregated walls. A decidedly different sport from bowling because of its mannish image, skimpy uniforms, and emphasis on speed, strength and power, it was Tuskegee Institute then later at Tennesse State where African American women realised national acclaim in track and field. The two institutions had enormously talented women's track and field teams that garnered multiple titles and championships made possible by the great performances of athletes such as Alice Coachman, Barbara Jones, Mae Faggs, Martha Hudson, Willy White and Wilma Rudolph. Not unexpectedly, African American educators, coaches and social commentators did their best to overcome the mannish image of women track and field competitors. Edward Temple, the long-time track and field coach at Tennessee State, once noted that 'None of my girls have any trouble getting boyfriends. I tell them that they are young ladies first, track girls second'.[41]

Although all of the parallel teams and leagues could be deemed historically important in their own way, it was high school basketball, college football and professional baseball that perhaps provide the most insight into the pattern of sport behind segregated walls. At the beginning of the twentieth century, Edwin B. Henderson, the great civil rights activist, educator and historian of the black athlete, introduced 'Basket Ball' to black students in Washington, DC's segregated public schools. The sport spread rapidly among segregated institutions, with African American high schoolers enthusiastically embracing basketball through their participation in tournaments sponsored by state interscholastic athletic associations across much of the south and mid-west and the prestigious National Interscholastic Basketball Tournament for black High Schools. For much of the first half of the twentieth century, basketball was like so many other sports in the African American community in that it helped build race pride and fostered collective ties and important networks among different groups. It was also a tool to make visible the seriousness with which blacks approached formal learning and a way to provide physically talented but disadvantaged youth the opportunity to receive a college education.[42] In essence, basketball for many African Americans was a means to develop character and model citizenship. By the late 1930s, however, basketball in the African American community at both the interscholastic and intercollegiate levels was transitioning from what historian Pamela Grundy terms a 'character-building exercise into a major spectator event'.[43] This transition, evidenced more broadly by the introduction of basketball at the Berlin Olympics in 1936 and creation of the National Invitational Tournament in 1938 and National Collegiate Athletic Association tournament the following year, would produce even more enthusiasm for the sport, lead to new rules and accompany changes in playing styles and foreshadow the modern era in which education among black males was superseded by the singular pursuit of athletic glory and professional contracts.[44]

Black college football was equally important in generating enthusiasm behind segregated walls. By the decade of the 1920s, historically black colleges and universities (HBCUs), particularly in the mid-Atlantic and southern states, took to the game with great enthusiasm. Although a number of reasons account for its enormous popularity among HBCUs, football among these institutions was to a great extent about measuring, as historian Raymond Schmidt points out in *Shaping College Football*, 'their educational and athletic products against the standards of white college society'.[45] Using the predominantly white institutions of Harvard, Yale and Princeton—the 'Big Three'—as an important barometer, HBCUs sought through football much desired respect and appreciation. This desire to measure up was perhaps most visible in the annual rivalry football games, often held on Thanksgiving Day, played between prestigious black institutions.[46]

One of the earliest and most significant of these games was played between Howard and Lincoln Universities. At their most popular between 1919 and 1929, the Howard-Lincoln Thanksgiving Day football games, which were accompanied by a variety of elaborate social activities, was a way for these two famous schools to make visible their sense of racial pride and self-determination while simultaneously gauging their games against the more nationally known predominantly white university football teams and their concomitant rituals.[47] The Howard and Lincoln Thanksgiving Day games, the annual 'classic' as it was known, did not just mimic those of the 'Big Three' and other predominantly white universities. They were racially distinctive events that reflected the black aesthetic experience and culture in Philadelphia and Washington, DC, and the USA more generally. The most creative aspect of the 'classic' was the 'rabbles', an improvisational dance by students from both Howard and Lincoln who walked in irregular formation around the field playing their musical instruments and singing songs honouring their own schools and disparaging their adversaries.[48]

The innovation, spontaneity and improvisational style characteristic of 'rabbles' and other celebrations were also evident among African American athletes themselves. Reacting to racism in American culture and knowing that they had to be superior to their white counterparts just to compete, African American athletes spent countless hours honing their talents and playing with a distinctive black style that would revolutionise virtually every sport in which they competed. Whether it was Bill Richmond's black Atlantic fighting style or the dancing of 'Cool Papa' Bell on the baseball paths or R. C. Owens's alley-oops or Willie Mays's one-handed catches or Julius Erving's wildly acrobatic dunks or Billy 'white shoes' Johnson's end-zone celebrations, African American athletes have exhibited a flashy and unique style that set them apart from other athletes and fascinated fans of all races. Educator Richard Majors has termed this performance style 'Cool Pose', contending that it is most evident among black men in sport and designed to exhibit their masculinity in a society that has marginalised them.[49] This distinctive performance style would be commoditised by the mainstream sports establishment, which recognised that money could be made from the popularity and fascination with physically gifted African American athletes.[50]

Rivalling high school basketball and college football for popularity behind segregated walls was Negro League Baseball. The most written about and well known of all the separate sport institutions in the African American community, Negro League Baseball was remarkably similar to Major League Baseball with regard to rules, regulations and code of ethics. For instance, both leagues sponsored a World Series and East–West All-Star Game, the latter event being one of the most important social-athletic spectacles in the African American community. The essential differences of the Negro leagues were the relatively low salaries, playing styles, inadequate transportation and facilities, poor housing accommodations, lack of legally binding player contracts and keeping of accurate statistics and records.[51]

Negro League Baseball was also different from other sports behind segregated walls. In contrast to high school basketball and college football, two sports which at the time offered limited opportunities at the professional level of competition, the Negro Leagues were never 'meant to be ends in themselves'.[52] They were considered temporary, intended to display independence and self-organisation, and showcase great African American athletes who desired to play against whites in America's national pastime. This does not mean there was ever any unanimity of opinion or no feelings of ambivalence among African Americans about the prospects of blacks participating in Major League Baseball. The owners in Negro League Baseball, while just as horrified as anyone in the African American community about racial discrimination, were able to own teams only because of the 'Gentleman's Agreement' among the leaders of Major League Baseball.[53] Although owners in Negro League Baseball, with the notable exceptions of Effa Manley of the Newark Eagles and Andrew 'Rube' Foster of the Chicago American Giants, were reluctant to voice opposition to the campaign to integrate Major League Baseball for fear of being branded racially disloyal, they were certainly aware that desegregation of the sport would put their enterprises at serious risk, and the best they could hope for was that entire teams from the Negro Leagues rather than individual players would be allowed entry into the national pastime. This was a serious dilemma for many African Americans during the age of racial segregation, faced with a pluralism that necessitated choices among individual success, group loyalty and integrationist ambitions.[54]

With that said, it is important to note that some separate black sports organisations were led by whites, a factor that ran counter to the need for African Americans to express their skills of self-organisation and independence. The owner of Negro League Baseball's Kansas City Monarchs was the white J. L. Wilkinson, who signed Jackie Robinson to his first professional contract. Oscar Schilling and Harry Earl, two white employers of the Cincinnati, Indianapolis and Western Railway, were founding members of the Colored Speedway Association, which sponsored the famous Gold and Glory Sweepstakes race among African Americans in Indianapolis. The Jewish promoter and businessman Abe Saperstein founded and ran the Harlem Globetrotters, the legendary black basketball team that eventually transitioned from a serious club to a comedic one that fits neatly into the historic minstrel tradition in the USA. Adopting the style of play from the Negro Leagues that had always been characterised by clowning and racialised humour, the Saperstein-led Globetrotters were showcased on State Department tours during the Cold War—as were individual African American athletes such as Althea Gibson, Mal Whitfield, Jackie Robinson, Rafer Johnson, Mae Faggs and Jesse Owens—in an effort to counteract the negative perceptions of race relations in the USA.[55]

In 1947 history was made when Jackie Robinson became the first African American to play modern Major League Baseball. Partly a result of the vigorous campaigns waged against lily-white baseball by black and white sportswriters and a newfound militancy among African Americans stimulated by the democratic ideology of the Second World War, Robinson's entry into the Major Leagues with the Brooklyn Dodgers was of great symbolic importance to the black community since it was one indication that the national pastime perhaps really did stand for equality and freedom of opportunity.[56] Not lost on the serious observers of sport is the fact that desegregation of the National Football League just a year earlier brought none of the attention and level of enthusiasm generated by Robinson's debut with the Dodgers. Although Woody Strode and Kenny Washington were extraordinarily gifted athletes who, ironically enough, had been teammates of Robinson's at University of California, Los Angeles, their opening season with the Los Angeles Rams resulted in little fanfare, and there was no representational significance attached to the event mainly because of the relatively minor status of professional football at the time.[57]

Robinson's entry into Major League Baseball also had important practical implications since it helped lead to the desegregation of the national pastime and other sports. This process, however, would be slow and uneven, with not every team in Major League Baseball having an African American on its roster until 1959, and the National Football League not completely desegregating until the Washington Redskins were pressured to add Bobby Mitchell to its roster in 1962.[58] Southern intercollegiate athletic conferences were even slower to integrate, with the desegregation of different sports taking place in different conferences throughout the late 1960s and early 1970s.[59]

The slow rate of integration was largely, besides the advanced age of some players and limited black talent pool in baseball and vigilance in maintaining racial quotas, a result of the deliberate approach of the leaders in intercollegiate and professional sport who were searching for, in the parlance of historian Damion Thomas, 'The Good Negroes' to desegregate their teams. Like Branch Rickey before them, the leaders in predominantly white-organised sport spent much time selecting talented African American athletes who had the requisite intelligence, personality and non-threatening character to both cope with and handle appropriately the racial hostility they were likely to encounter in a largely white environment. Darryl Hill, the University of Maryland wide receiver who became the first African American to integrate the Atlantic Coast Conference in 1963, recalled 50 years after his historic milestone that

> they [Maryland] needed someone who was a good student, who had a good attitude and good temperament. They needed the right guy, so to speak, because they were taking a risk. If they got the wrong guy you wouldn't have seen another [African American player] at Maryland for a long time.[60]

Irrespective of the rate of integration, the entry of African Americans into predominantly white sport would ultimately have a deleterious effect on separate black sports organisations. It led to the demise of Negro League Baseball and gradually drained the best athletic talent out of HBCUs. Sport sociologist and activist Harry Edwards offered an insightful explanation of why black sport organisations were so negatively impacted. He pointed out that it was the method of integration, not integration itself, that put many parallel black sports organisations out of business. Motivated by 'business and politics' rather than 'brotherhood', the leaders in white-organised sport took a 'one-way and selective' approach, instead of 'two-way and structural' approach, to integration. The result was that leaders in white-organised sport went about cherry picking the most talented athletes from separate black sports organisations with no intention of permitting the heads of those organisations to discuss, let alone become, equal partners in the post-Jackie Robinson era.[61] This approach confirmed the fears of Effa Manley and Andrew Rube Foster and cemented in place the long-held pattern extending back to slavery in which African Americans were largely relegated to positions as athletes while whites filled multiple positions as athletes, managers, executives and owners.[62]

The method of integration, while helping to cement the power relations in sport, would have relatively little to do with the participation patterns of African American athletes. Which sports they participated in and at what level of competition would result from a variety of other economic, social, political and cultural factors—all of which would play a role as more African Americans made their way into baseball following Robinson historic debut with the Dodgers. Larry Doby broke the colour barrier in the American League some 11 weeks after Robinson's first appearance with the Dodgers when he signed a contract with the Cleveland Indians.[63] Following Robinson and Doby into Major League Baseball over the next decade were great African American players such as Roy Campanella, Don Newcombe, Ernie Banks, Frank Robinson, Elston Howard, Willie Mays and Hank Aaron.[64] In 1959, when the Boston Red Sox signed outfielder Pumpsie Green, thus becoming the last team to desegregate, there were 69 African Americans in Major League Baseball, which constituted 17% of all players. In 1968 African Americans represented 18%, and by 1975 they constituted 27%, their highest total ever.[65]

After 1975, the percentage of African American ballplayers began to drop rather dramatically in Major League Baseball. By 1983 they represented 19%. In 1999 it was down to 13%. Four years later, the percentage had declined an additional four points. By 2011 the percentage of African American players was just 8.5%.[66] The decline in the number of African Americans in Major League Baseball, and in the sport more generally, has garnered much attention from baseball observers who have offered a variety of reasons explaining the phenomenon. A commonly held belief is that African Americans simply do not have the financial resources or the space necessary to develop the skills required to achieve success in the sport. Others have argued that African Americans, unlike their Latin American counterparts who currently make up 24.2% of all Major League players, do not have the necessary family and community support that leads to participation in the sport.[67] Sports columnist Chris Isidore contends that the limited number of African Americans in baseball has more to do with the smaller number of college baseball scholarships now available and the changing nature of the Major League draft. Typically possessing far fewer financial resources, only a relatively small number of African Americans compete in college baseball because of the limited availability of scholarships, which, in turn, means fewer African American players are available for the Major League draft.[68] Finally, Gerald Early contends that African Americans have not taken up baseball in greater numbers because they have less affection for the sport than do whites. 'Baseball has little hold on the Black American imagination' wrote Early on the eve of the 60th anniversary of Jackie Robinson's entry into Major League Baseball. 'Relatively few Blacks watch the game. The game is not passed on from father to son or father to daughter. Lacking that, the game simply will not have much resonance with African Americans'.[69]

While the various reasons given for the declining number of African Americans in baseball are interesting to contemplate, far more important is why so many people are concerned with the declining numbers to begin with? The leaders in Major League Baseball are concerned because in theory, the addition of more African American players means more African American fans. This is the same reasoning that motivated Branch Rickey and the other owners involved in the initial desegregation of the sport.[70] For Major League Baseball, however, the decline in the number of African American players is about more than just the bottom line. The dearth of African American players in Major League Baseball runs counter to its romanticised version of the past and the belief that more than any other institution it continues to reflect the commitment to democratic principles and freedom of opportunity regardless of race, creed or colour.[71] This idealised view is best reflected in the commemorative events Major League Baseball sponsors each year paying homage to Negro League Baseball and the civil rights struggle. Among these events are the Negro League Weekend, Jackie Robinson Day, Civil Rights Game and various Negro League Tribute Games.[72]

This idealised view does not resonate so strongly with African Americans, who need no reminding of a brand of baseball that was forced on them because of racial segregation, and who have now moved on to great success in football and basketball. Of these two sports, it is basketball in which African Americans have been so dominant and garnered so much attention and publicity and fame.[73] Basketball can now legitimately lay claim as a national pastime and African Americans are enormously passionate about it and integral to its success and popularity. 'Heaven is a playground for African Americans', they are the 'Asphalt Gods' and the best when it comes to playing the 'City Game'.[74] African Americans comprise some 75% of all players in the National Basketball Association (NBA). All but one member of the US Olympic men's basketball team in 2012 were African Americans, while nine players on the Olympic women's basketball team in 2012 were African Americans.[75]

The possible reasons for the high percentage of African Americans in basketball are many and varied. Some observers of the sport contend that African Americans, many of whom have come from impoverished urban settings, have turned to basketball because it requires limited financial resources and relatively small physical space.[76] Other observers of the sport have argued that African

Americans are perfectly suited to the game because it allows them to experience and exhibit the 'feint', 'deception' and 'improvisation' that is integral to black cultural style. In his frequently cited book *The Joy of Sports,* Michael Novak claims that basketball represents the black experience more than any other sport and will become 'more black with every passing year'. The sport is now, writes Novak, played with the 'style of the city: sophisticated, cool, deceptive, swift, spectacular, flashy and smooth. But the mythos became more than urban. It became in a symbolic and ritual way uniquely black'.[77]

Another explanation is that the sport, much like boxing during the era when it had such a hold on the public imagination in the USA, was a way to escape the ghetto and climb up the socio-economic ladder.[78] Still other observers argue that African Americans have realised particular success in basketball because of the support received from educational institutions, an argument that is very plausible and has much merit.[79] Not always having the financial backing from family members or easy access to 'country club' sports such as golf or tennis, African Americans have found success in basketball largely through the support and organisational structure of schools, which I and many others, ironically enough, have chided for their academic neglect of black student-athletes. The dependence on schools for their success in basketball, and football for that matter, will probably continue to exist for African Americans because of the increased privatisation of youth sports in the USA which effectively disadvantages children from low-income families. The decline in publicly supported youth sport programmes, concomitant rise in private sport clubs and leagues for children that typically require participation fees and purchase of expensive equipment, coaching fees and exorbitant travel costs, will continue to delimit the opportunities for African American athletes who often come from single-parent households with lower overall wealth and resources.[80]

Regardless of why African Americans have found success and identify most closely with the sport, basketball is extraordinarily important in understanding the interconnection between race and sport in the USA. It encapsulates very vividly the role that African Americans have always played in sport and how they have been judged and categorised and portrayed in a country where racialist thinking continues to take place and still matters.[81] As a sport with enormous media popularity and entertainment value, basketball possesses a visibility and intimacy that makes clear the simultaneous attraction and fear of the black body that has been evident since at least the late nineteenth century.[82]

Basketball also makes apparent the continual concern that leaders in sport have with maintaining a proper numerical balance between black and white athletes. While those in Major League Baseball have lamented the lack of African American players in the sport for fear of losing out on black fans and in an attempt to hold on to its nostalgic image of the past, those in basketball have had to find ways to make their increasingly black sport more palatable to the American public. The decision of Texas Western's Don Haskins to start five black players against Adolf Rupp's University of Kentucky Wildcats in the 1966 NCAA title game was a watershed event in that it was the first time an all-black team had started a major championship in any sport. Basketball great Bill Russell made clear the seriousness in which people considered the racial composition of teams when he famously noted that the rule for playing blacks 'was two at home, three on the road, four if you're behind, and five if you need to win the playoffs'. The debate about quotas has never completely subsided as evidenced by the recent remarks of Tyrone Terrell, Chairman of the African American Leadership Council in St. Paul, Minnesota, who suggested that the Minnesota Timberwolves intentionally stacked its roster with white players so as to attract more white fans.[83]

Now that the NBA is predominantly black, questions have also turned to how to deal with the 'edgy culture' and ghetto image portrayed in the league so as not to alienate white audiences and corporate sponsors. The level of concern about projecting a negative image in the NBA was reflected most visibly by Commissioner David Stern's decision to implement a league-wide dress code. This has taken place, ironically enough, while African Americans continue to discuss 'daily around dinner tables, in barber shops, on basketball courts—wherever black folks gather and share thoughts on our race', which members of the black community are 'keeping it real' and not being 'sellouts'. Some African Americans, writes *Washington Post* sportswriter Jason Reid, 'become uneasy when the most successful among us', including athletes who have always served as important symbols of possibility and achievement, 'make any mention of shedding "blackness" or do not possess the supposed "street cred" resulting from being reared in south central Los Angeles, the south side of Chicago, or any number of such areas in the United States'.[84]

In addition to concerns about numerical representation and alienation of influential stakeholders, basketball helps illustrate the continued 'Dilemma of the Double Burden' faced by African American women with regard to finding their way in the larger women's sport movement. Although nearly a third of the women participating in Division I college basketball are African Americans, just 2.7% of women on scholarship in all other collegiate sports are African Americans. Equally troubling is the fact that African Americans hold only 1.5% of all coaching positions in women's college sports.[85]

These numbers reflect the failure to provide the same opportunities for African American women athletes that were given to their white counterparts in the post-Title IX era.[86] This failure has ensured the near invisibility of African American women athletes and made clear the lasting difficulties in overcoming racial and gender discrimination. What is visible, then, is the languishing of African American women athletes vis-à-vis their white counterparts, a circumstance that also has never been adequately addressed by African American male athletes who have concentrated on their own racial struggles in an effort to exert the sense of masculinity traditionally denied them by white America. This lack of cooperation between black male and female athletes has always been the norm, but it has been strained by the integration of American mainstream sports, a process that has encouraged a focus on individual accomplishments rather than group solidarity.[87]

The lack of cooperation between African American female and male athletes seems not to matter in stock car racing, the distinctive southern pastime that now has a national following as evidenced by the fact it is America's number one spectator sport.[88] Having its origin among whites on the red clay in the south and always closely associated with bootlegging, stock car racing has had very few black drivers on the circuit during its some 65-year history. The only African American who realised any sustained success on the National Association for Stock Car Auto Racing (NASCAR) circuit was Wendell Scott, the light-skinned Danville, Virginia native who had 147 top 10 finishes in 495 career starts in Grand National Races.[89]

The dearth of African Americans in stock car racing should not come as a surprise since the sport helps define how white men, especially lower-class white men, in the south think of themselves and that it is a relatively new pastime that provides important connections to the southern past. NASCAR, which is supported by 114 Fortune 500 companies, has established programmes to attract more minority drivers and fans to the sport. These programmes, however, have realised just a modicum of success. Although there are a few promising African American drivers on the horizon, most notably Darrell Wallace, Jr., who signed with Joe Gibbs Racing, sponsors are reluctant to cast their lot with black drivers for fear of losing support from predominantly white fans.[90]

It is now clear that African American athletes continually negotiate covert rather than more overt forms of racism as they strive to realise success in an institution still dominated by a white power structure. Unfortunately, this quest has required contemporary African American athletes, like their athletic forebears, to often take neutral positions on racial issues so as not to jeopardise their careers in sport. The quest for college scholarships, promise of professional contracts and allegiance to powerful coaches and owners have made them reluctant to speak out on larger racial issues and problems still encountered by African Americans. The fact of the matter, however, is that white America has always been less tolerant of black athletes who did speak out on racial issues and took political stances. Many of those African American athletes of yesteryear who are now being celebrated— such as legendary performers Curt Flood, Muhammad Ali, Tommie Smith, John Carlos and Bill Russell—suffered a great deal for their activism and protests they lodged against racial discrimination. Ethnic studies scholars David Leonard and Richard King make the compelling argument that the media in the USA have romanticised the courageous stands taken by the aforementioned athletes against racial injustice while downplaying or even ignoring contemporary struggles for racial equality as a way to 'ridicule and demonise' today's black athletes.[91]

Irrespective of these claims, overt forms of racism are now taboo in the USA and racial issues are seldom discussed publicly. Unlike many other parts of the world where racist songs, slogans and taunts are common at football matches and other sporting venues, open racism is not tolerated by players and fans in the USA, and racialist discourse typically takes place privately in segregated rather than integrated settings. When this standard mode of operation is violated, the perpetrators are usually roundly criticised and draw the wrath of individuals both within and outside of sport. In 1987, Al Campanis, long-time general manager of the Los Angeles Dodgers, told Ted Kopple on ABC's programme *Niteline* coinciding with the 40th anniversary of Jackie Robinson's entry into Major League Baseball that blacks 'may not have some of the necessities to be let's say, a field manager, or perhaps a general manager' in the sport. The backlash to these comments was so intense that Campanis was forced to resign his position two days later. In 1988, Jimmy 'The Greek' Snyder, a long-time reporter on the CBS show *The NFL Today*, told an interviewer in Washington, DC, that blacks were better athletes than their white counterparts because they were 'bred to be that way since the days of slavery' when the 'slave owner would breed his big black with his big woman so that he could have a big black kid'. Snyder was fired from CBS for these comments. In 2009, Don Imus, a member of the National Broadcaster Hall of Fame, was fired by CBS for calling the members of the Rutger's women's basketball team 'nappy-headed hos'. Michael Johnson, the legendary African American sprinter who won multiple gold medals at the 1992, 1996 and 2000 Olympic Games, caused enormous debate when he predicted prior to the 2012 Olympics in London that black American and Caribbean runners would dominate the sprints because they possessed a superior athletic gene that had been bred during slavery. Most recently golfer Sergio Garcia, when asked by Golf Channel's Steve Sands whether he would be inviting Tiger Woods to dinner during the upcoming US Open, remarked that 'we will have him round every night. We will serve fried chicken'. Garcia suffered a seemingly insurmountable public backlash and was forced to issue an apology for his racially insensitive comments.[92]

The above comments by Michael Johnson, while not costing him his position as an announcer with the BBC, are important because it reminds us that the belief in biological determinism with regard to sport performance is still prevalent. Although this way of thinking fits neatly into the deep-seated stereotypical notions about blacks, it can, ironically enough, be a psychological advantage. Like so many young black men, Johnson grew up believing in the superiority of the black body and that it was his fate as well as other members of his race to realise success in sport. Sport sociologist Jay Coakley refers to this way of thinking as a 'collective sense of biological cultural destiny' and, when combined with the belief that opportunities to realise fame and fortune in other professions are severely limited, has inspired black athletes to strive for success at record-setting levels in sport.[93]

Johnson's comments are also a reminder that perhaps no sport, with the possible exception of basketball because of the phenomenon of the Dream Team and the growth of the game internationally, has been more important than track and field in introducing African Americans to the rest of the world. Although the sport has garnered relatively little scholarly attention and realised more popularity elsewhere, the hopes and dreams of the USA in international sport have often rested on the shoulders of talented African Americans in track and field. Even during the days of racial segregation, African American athletes represented the USA in global competitions. The world watched with much admiration as African American athletes dominated track and field in important international contests such as the USA and USSR track meets, the Olympic Games and World Championships.[94]

If viewed with an uncritical eye, it appeared that by the dawn of the twenty-first century African Americans athletes had reached the Promised Land. If viewed with a more critical eye, it is clear that these athletes were, to use the terminology of the German press in describing Jesse Owens and his teammates on the 1936 Olympic track and field team, 'Black Auxiliaries' who returned home to face continuing racial and economic discrimination.[95] If viewed with a more critical eye and in the totality of their sport experiences, including participation in various national pastimes, it is also clear that these African American athletes and those who followed them had realised athletic success without any promise of gaining control of an activity they helped to build and sustain and one that holds out such enormous importance for so many people in the USA. In all, from the time they were slaves living on southern farms and plantations to the present day, African Americans have made continual efforts to compete with and against their white counterparts on an equal basis in highly organised sport. These efforts have resulted in a relatively large number of African Americans participating in selected sports during different periods of time and having very limited involvement and virtually no control over many other sports throughout the history of the USA.

This pattern of participation should be a reminder to us all about the true status of black athletes in the USA. Unlike Jewish, Italian, Irish and other European ethnics whose accomplishments in sport ultimately coincided with improved economic conditions and social mobility, African Americans have been unable to realise the same results because of historical context and racism in a capitalist society. This fact has only served to fuel the desire for success in sport among impoverished young African American males, in particular who see it as the only alternative to welfare, crime and life on the streets.[96] Unfortunately, with major shifts in a post-industrial economy and simultaneous privatisation of youth athletic programmes and other factors, sport is providing fewer opportunities for African Americans and deferring realisation of the American dream. There is a whitening of national pastimes in the USA that the racially privileged and economically powerful perpetuate, but fail to acknowledge.

■ **NOTES**

1. Hoberman, *Darwin's Athletes*.
2. Early, *Level Playing Field*.
3. Edwards, 'Black Athletes', 43–52; Rhoden, *Forty Million Dollar Slaves*; and Hawkins, *New Plantation*.
4. Wiggins, 'Play of Slave Children', 21–39; and Wiggins, 'Sport and Popular Pastimes', 61–88.
5. See note 4 above.
6. Breen, 'Horses and Gentlemen', 239–257.
7. Marable, 'Black Athletes in White Men's Games', 143–149. See the chapter 'Performing for "Old Massa"' in David K. Wiggins, 'Sport and Popular Pastimes in the Plantation Community: The Slave Experience'. Ph.D. dissertation, University of Maryland, 1979, 202–247.
8. Ownby, 'Manhood, Memory, and White Men's Sports', 103–118.
9. Wiggins, 'Sport and Popular Pastimes in the Plantation Community', 235–238.
10. While it would never be considered a national pastime, corn shuckings were extraordinarily important and enjoyable activities that held out special cultural meanings to slaves. See Wiggins 'Sport and Popular Pastimes in the Plantation Community', 203–213; and Abrahams, *Singing the Master*.
11. Hotaling, *Great Black Jockeys*; and Boulware, 'Unworthy of Modern Refinement', 429–448.
12. Hotaling, *Great Black Jockeys*, 30.
13. Additional information on Curtis can be found in Mackay-Smith, *Colonial Quarter Race Horse*; and Davie, 'Quarter Racing', 450–452.
14. Gorn, *Manly Art*; Obi, 'Black Terror', 99–114; Brailsford, *Bareknuckles*, Chap. 6; and Smith, *Black Genesis*, Chaps. 2 and 3.
15. Gorn, *Manly Art*, 36.
16. Runstedtler, *Jack Johnson, Rebel Sojourner*, 8.
17. Brailsford, *Bareknuckles*, Chap. 6; and Smith, *Black Genesis*, Chap. 3.
18. Brailsford, *Bareknuckles*, Chap. 6; and Smith, *Black Genesis*, Chap. 3.
19. Demas, *Integrating the Gridiron*; Berryman, 'Early Black Leadership', 17–28; Wiggins, 'Prized Performers', 164–177; and Wiggins, 'Strange Mix of Entitlement and Exploitation', 95–113.
20. See note 19 above.
21. Hotaling, *Great Black Jockeys*; Hotaling, *Wink*; Wiggins, 'Isaac Murphy', 15–33; Wiggins, 'Peter Jackson', 143–163; Peterson, *Peter Jackson*; Tygiel, *Baseball's Great Experiment*; Zang, *Fleet Walker's Divided Heart*; Ritchie, *Major Taylor*; Balf, *Major*; Lucas and Smith, *Saga of American Sport*, 276.
22. Wiggins, 'Peter Jackson', 143–163; Wiggins, 'Isaac Murphy', 15–32; Ritchie, *Major Taylor*; and Lucas and Smith, *Saga of American Sport*, 276.
23. Woodward, *Strange Career of Jim Crow*; Logan, *Betrayal of the Negro*; and Litwack, *Trouble in Mind*.
24. For an early essay on black athletes, see Zuckerman, Stull, and Eyler, 'Black Athlete', 142–146.
25. Wiggins, 'Notion of Double Consciousness', 133–155.

26. Demas, *Integrating the Gridiron*; Berryman, 'Early Black Leadership'; Wiggins, 'Prized Performers' and Wiggins, 'Strange Mix of Entitlement and Exploitation'.

27. George Poage was the first African American to compete and capture medals in Olympic competition, winning bronze medals in the 220 m and 440 m hurdle races in the 1904 Games in St. Louis. See Bunch and Robinson, *Black Olympians*.

28. Hotaling, *Great Black Jockeys*, 311–340.

29. Zang, *Fleet Walker's Divided Heart*.

30. For a one-volume survey on baseball that includes good information on black players, see Rader, *Baseball*.

31. Gorn, *Manly Art*, esp. Chap. 4; Early, *Tuxedo Junction*, esp. 115–195; Early, *Culture of Bruising*, 5–109; and Bederman, *Manliness and Civilization*, 1–5, 8, 41–42.

32. Kaye, *Pussycat of Prize Fighting*, 8.

33. Johnson, *Black Manhattan*; Wright, *Black Boy*; Richard Wright, 'High Times in Harlem: Joe Louis as a Symbol of Freedom', *New Masses*, July 5, 1938, 18–20; Richard Wright, 'Joe Louis Uncovers Dynamite', *New Masses*, October 8, 1935, 18, 19; Ellison, *Invisible Man*; Baldwin, *Fire Next Time*; and Angelou, *I Know Why the Caged Bird Sings*.

34. See note 33 above.

35. The search for a 'white hope' was perhaps never so intense than when white Americans tried to find a boxer to enter the ring against the great yet controversial black heavyweight Jack Johnson. See Roberts, *Papa Jack*; and Ward, *Unforgivable Blackness*.

36. See in particular Roberts, *Papa Jack*, Chap. 6.

37. Ritchie, *Major Taylor*; and Balf, *Major*.

38. Hotaling, *Great Black Jockeys*, 295–301, 311–322; and Hotaling, *Wink*.

39. For examples of the literature on separate sports teams, leagues and organisations, see the 'bibliographic essay and list' in Wiggins and Miller, *Unlevel Playing Field*, 447–477; and Grundy, *Learning to Win*.

40. Cahn, *Coming on Strong*, 220.

41. Quoted in Cahn, *Coming on Strong*, 133.

42. Wiggins, 'Edwin Bancroft Henderson', 91–112; and George, *Elevating the Game*, 15, 26, 28, 29, 32.

43. Grundy, *Learning to Win*, 176.

44. Isaacs, *All the Moves*.

45. Schmidt, *Shaping College Football*, 131.

46. See, for example, Aiello, *Bayou Classic*.

47. Wiggins, 'Biggest Classic of Them All'.

48. Miller, 'To Bring the Race Along Rapidly', 119; and Oriard, *King Football*, 321–323.

49. Majors, 'Cool Pose', 184, 185.

50. See in particular Obi, 'Black Terror', 99–114; Rhoden, *Forty Million Dollar Slaves*, esp. Chap. 6; George, *Elevating the Game*, esp. 52–55, 59, 60, 74–77; Tygiel, *Baseball's Great Experiment*, esp. 19–21, 84, 191, 257, 336; Oriard, *King Football*, 319–327; and Houck, 'Attacking the Rim', 151–169.

51. See Lester, *Black Baseball's National Showcase*.

52. Early, *Level Playing Field*, 174.

53. For a nice analysis of one Negro League baseball team, see Snyder, *Beyond the Shadow of the Senators*.

54. Gerald Early makes this point very well in his *Level Playing Field*.

55. Thomas, *Globetrotting*; Thomas, 'Around the World', 778–791; Bruce, *Kansas City Monarchs,* esp. 14, 15, 18–22; and Gould, *For Gold and Glory,* 37–41, 143–146, 148, 149.

56. The best known work on Robinson is Tygiel, *Baseball's Great Experiment.*

57. Information on Strode, Washington, and the integration of professional football, can be gleaned from Kaliss, *Men's College Athletics*; Demas, *Integrating the Gridiron*; Strode and Young, *Goal Dust*; and Ross, *Outside the Lines.*

58. Smith, *Showdown.*

59. Martin, *Benching Jim Crow.*

60. Thomas, *Globetrotting.* The slow pace of integration is made very clear in Martin, *Benching Jim Crow.* For the Hill quote, see Jason Reid, 'A Wide Receiver Whose Route Went Well Beyond the Football Field', *Washington Post,* October 16, 2012.

61. Edwards, 'Transformational Developments', 19.

62. Powell, *Souled Out?,* Chap. 10.

63. Moore, *Pride Against Prejudice.*

64. More scholarly work needs to be done on this first wave of African American baseball players.

65. Comeaux and Harrison, 'Labels of African American Ballers', 4.

66. Ibid.; Deron Snyder, 'Decline in Black Players Should Concern All Who Love Baseball', *Washington Times,* August 18, 2011. Retrieved April 19, 2012 from http://www. was hingtontimes.com/news/2011/Aug/18/Snyder.

67. Ruck, *Raceball.*

68. Chris Isidore, 'Green Behind Decline of Blacks in Badeball', *CNN Money,* April 13, 2007. Retrieved April 19, 2012 from http://money.cnn.com/2007/04/13/commentary/ sportsbiz/index.htm).

69. Gerald Early, 'Where Have We Gone, Mr. Robinson?', *Time,* April 12, 2007, 1. Retrieved April 20, 2012 from http://www.time.com/time/magazine/article/0,9171,1609796,00. html; and Gerry Everding, 'Blacks Aren't Playing Baseball Simply Because They Don't Want to Says Gerald Early', *Newsroom,* Washington University in St. Louis, April 12, 2007, 1. Retrieved April 19, 2012 from http://news.wustl.edu/news/pages/9233.aspx.

70. Tygiel, *Baseball's Great Experiment,* 51–54.

71. Black sportswriters were fond of pointing out the hypocrisy that Major League Baseball best represented America's commitment to democratic principles. Wiggins, 'Wendell Smith', 5–29; and Rieslar, *Black Writers/Black Baseball,* 33–55.

72. Ruck, *Raceball.*

73. George, *Elevating the Game*; Boyd and Shropshire, *Basketball Jones*; and Boyd, *Young, Black, Rich, and Famous.*

74. These titles are taken from Telander, *Heaven is a Playground*; Mallozzi, *Asphalt Gods*; and Axthelm, *City Game.*

75. Coakley, *Sports in Society,* 310.

76. Powell, *Souled Out?,* 252.

77. Novak, *Joy of Sports,* 105.

78. For an interesting study that examines how black boxers cope with rather than escape the ghetto, see Wacquant, 'Social Logic of Boxing', 221–254.

79. Early provides the clearest statement of this argument. See Early, *Level Playing Field,* 202–204.

80. Coakley, *Sports in Society,* 127–129.

81. Boyd and Shropshire, *Basketball Jones,* 1–11.

82. Ibid.

83. For information on the Texas Western and University of Kentucky game, see Fitzpatrick, *And the Walls came Tumbling Down.* The Russell quote is taken from Novak, *Joy of Sports,* 110. The comments by Terrell are discussed in Phil Taylor's 'Too White, or All Right?', *Sports Illustrated,* November 12, 2012, 108.

84. Jason Reid, 'No Shades of Blackness', *Washington Post,* December 15, 2012. For a discussion of the NBA and its image, see Powell, *Souled Out?,* Chap. 5.

85. The phrase 'The Dilemma of the Double Burden' was used by William Rhoden in Chap. 9 of his *Forty Million Dollar Slaves.* He provides these statistics on p. 225 of the book.

86. Welch Suggs, 'Left Behind', *Chronicle of Higher Education,* November 30, 2001; Fields, 'Title IX', 126–145; and Craig T. Greenlee, 'Title IX: Does Help for Women Come at the Expense of African Americans?', *Black Issues in Higher Education,* April 17, 1997, 24–26.

87. Wiggins, 'Notion of Double-Consciousness'; Rhoden, *Forty Million Dollar Slaves,* 197–218; and Wiggins, 'With all Deliberate Speed', 329–346.

88. For information on NASCAR, see Ownby, 'Manhood, Memory, and White Men's Sports', 103–118; Rybacki and Rybacki, 'King, the Young Prince', 294–325; and Pierce, *Real NASCAR.*

89. Donovan, *Hard Driving.*

90. Viv Bernstein, 'Driver's Seat Elusive for Black Racers', *New York Times,* May 19, 2012. Retrieved October 7, 2012 from http://www.nytimes.com/2012/05/20/sports/autoracing/nascar-struggles-with-diversity-as-drivers-seat-eludes-black-drivers; and Bob Pockrass, 'Drive for Diversity: NASCAR's Push to Develop Minority Drivers Moving Slowly', *Sporting News,* June 4, 2012. Retrieved October 7, 2012 from http://aol.sportingnews.com/nascar/story/2012-06-04/nascar-drive-for-diversity-program-darrell-wallace-jr.-brian-france.

91. Leonard and King, 'Revolting Black Athletes'.

92. Graham L. Jones, 'Dodgers Fire Campanis Over Racial Remarks', *Los Angeles Times,* April 9, 1987. Retrieved November 24, 2012 from http://articles.latimes.com/1987-04-09/news/mn-366_1_black-leaders; Jonathan Rowe, 'The Greek Chorus: Jimmy the Greek Got It Wrong But So Did His Critics', *Washington Monthly,* April 20, 1988, 31–34; 'CBS Fires Don Imus Over Racial Slur', *CBS News,* February 11, 2009. Retrieved June 7, 2013 from http://www.cbsnews.com/2.00_201_162.2675273.html; Chris Chase, 'Michael Johnson Says Slavery Descendants Run Faster because of "Superior Athletic Gene"', *Yahoo Sports,* July 5, 2012. Retrieved September 1, 2012 from http://sports.yahoo.com/blogs/olympics-fourth-place-medal/michaeljohnson-says-slavery-descendants; and Cindy Boren, 'Sergio Garcia Apologizes for "Fried Chicken" Remark About Tiger Woods (updated)', *Washington Post,* May 22, 2013. Retrieved June 7, 2013 from http://www.washingtonpost.com/blogs/early-lead/wp/2013/05/22.

93. Coakley, *Sports in Society,* 286. Discussions regarding the relationship between race and athletic performance are covered in Wiggins, 'Great Speed but Little Stamina', 158–185; Miller, 'Anatomy of Scientific Racism', 119–151; Dyreson, 'American Ideas About Race', 173–215; and Sammons, '"Race" and Sport', 203–298.

94. See Turrini, *End of Amateurism.*

95. Baker, *Jesse Owens.*

96. Levine, *Ellis Island to Ebbets Field,* esp. 281–285.

▪ REFERENCES

Abrahams, Roger D. *Singing the Master: The Emergence of African American Culture in the Plantation South.* New York: Penguin, 1992.

Aiello, Thomas. *Bayou Classic: The Grambling-Southern Football Rivalry.* Baton Rouge: Louisiana State University Press, 2010.

Angelou, Maya. *I Know Why the Caged Bird Sings.* New York: Ballantine Books, 2009.

Axthelm, Pete. *The City Game.* New York: Harper and Row, 1970.

Baker, William J. *Jesse Owens: An American Life.* New York: Free Press, 1986.

Baldwin, James. *The Fire Next Time.* London: Penguin, 1964.

Balf, Todd. *Major: A Black Athlete, a White Era, and the Fight to be the World's Fastest Human Being.* New York: Crown Publishers, 2008.

Bederman, Gail. *Manliness and Civilization: A Cultural History of Gender and Race in the United States.* Chicago: University of Chicago Press, 1995.

Berryman, Jack W. 'Early Black Leadership in Collegiate Football: Massachusetts as a Pioneer'. *Historical Journal of Massachusetts* 9, no. 2 (June 1981): 17–28.

Boulware, Hunt. 'Unworthy of Modern Refinement: The Evolution of Sport and Recreation in the Early South Carolina and Georgia Lowcountry'. *Journal of Sport History* 35, no. 3 (fall 2008): 421–448.

Boyd, Todd. *Young, Black, Rich, and Famous: The Rise of the NBA, the Hip Hop Invasion, and the Transformation of American Culture.* New York: Doubleday, 2003.

Boyd, Todd, and Kenneth L. Shropshire, eds. *Basketball Jones: America Above the Rim.* New York: New York University Press, 2000.

Brailsford, Dennis. *Bareknuckles: A Social History of Prize-Fighting.* Cambridge, MA: Lutterworth, 1988.

Breen, T. H. 'Horses and Gentlemen: The Cultural Significance of Gambling Among the Gentry of Virginia'. *William and Mary Quarterly* (3rd series) 34, no. 2 (April 1977): 239–257.

Bruce, Janet. *The Kansas City Monarchs: Champions of Black Baseball.* Lawrence: University Press of Kansas, 1985.

Bunch, Lonnie G., and Louie Robinson. *The Black Olympians: 1904–1984.* Los Angeles: California Afro-American Museum, 1985.

Cahn, Susan K. *Coming on Strong: Gender and Sexuality in Twentieth-Century Women's Sport.* New York: Free Press, 1994.

Coakley, Jay. *Sports in Society: Issues and Controversies,* 10th ed. New York: McGraw-Hill, 2009.

Comeaux, Eddie, and C. Keith Harrison. 'Labels of African American Ballers: A Historical and Contemporary Investigation of African American Male Youth's Depletion From America's Favorite Pastime, 1885–2000'. *Journal of American Culture* 27, no. 1 (March 2004): 67–80.

Davie, Allen Jones. 'Quarter Racing of the Olden Time'. *American Turf Register* 3 (1832): 450–452.

Demas, Lane. *Integrating the Gridiron: Black Civil Rights and American College Football.* Brunswick, NJ: University Press, 2010.

Donovan, Brian. *Hard Driving: The Wendell Scott Story, The American Odyssey of NASCAR's First Black Driver.* Hanover, NH: Steerforth Press, 2008.

Dyreson, Mark. 'American Ideas About Race and Olympic Races from the 1890s to the 1950s: Shattering Myths or Reinforcing Scientific Racism?' *Journal of Sport History* 28, no. 2 (summer 2001): 173–215.

Early, Gerald. *A Level Playing Field: African American Athletes and the Republic of Sports.* Cambridge, MA: Harvard University Press, 2011.

Early, Gerald. *The Culture of Bruising: Essays on Prize Fighting, Literature, and Modern American Culture.* New York: Ecco Press, 1994.

Early, Gerald. *Tuxedo Junction: Essays on American Culture.* New York: Ecco Press, 1989.

Edwards, Harry. 'The Black Athletes: 20th Century Gladiators for White America'. *Psychology Today* 7 (1973): 43–48.

Edwards, Harry. 'Transformational Developments at the Interface of Race, Sport, and the Collegiate Athletic Arms Race in the Age of Globalization'. *Journal of Intercollegiate Sport* 4, no. 1 (June 2011): 18–31.

Ellison, Ralph. *Invisible Man.* New York: Modern Library, 1992.

Fields, Sarah K. 'Title IX and African American Female Athletics'. In *Sports and the Racial Divide: African American and Latino Experience in an Era of Change,* edited by Michael Lomax, 126–145. Jackson: University Press of Mississippi, 2008.

Fitzpatrick, Frank. *And the Walls Came Tumbling Down: Kentucky, Texas Western, and the Game that Changed American Sports.* New York: Simon and Schuster, 1999.

George, Nelson. *Elevating the Game: The History and Aesthetics of Black Men in Basketball.* New York: Simon and Schuster, 1992.

Gorn, Elliott J. *The Manly Art: Bareknuckle Prize Fighting in America.* Ithaca, NY: Cornell University Press, 1986.

Gould, Todd. *For Gold and Glory: Charlie Wiggins and the African American Racing Car Circuit.* Bloomington: Indiana University Press, 2007.

Grundy, Pamela. *Learning to Win: Sports, Education, and Social Change in Twentieth-Century North Carolina.* Chapel Hill: University of North Carolina Press, 2001.

Hawkins, Billy. *The New Plantation: Black Athletes, College Sports, and Predominantly White NCAA Institutions.* New York: Palgrave MacMillan, 2010.

Hoberman, John. *Darwin's Athletes: How Sport has Damaged Black America and Preserved the Myth of Race.* Boston: Houghton Mifflin, 1997.

Hotaling, Edward. *The Great Black Jockeys: The Lives and Times of the Men Who Dominated America's First National Sport.* Rocklin, CA: Prima, 1999.

Hotaling, Edward. *Wink: The Incredible Life and Epic Journal of Jimmy Winkfield.* New York: McGraw-Hill, 2005.

Houck, Davis W. 'Attacking the Rim: The Cultural Politics of Dunking, in Basketball Jones: America Above the Rim'. In *Todd Boyd and Kenneth Shropshire,* edited by Todd Boyd, and Kenneth Shropshire, 151–169. New York: New York University Press, 2000.

Isaacs, Neil D. *All the Moves: A History of College Basketball.* New York: Harper and Row, 1984.

Johnson, James Weldon. *Black Manhattan.* New York: Arno Press, 1968.

Kaliss, Gregory J. *Men's College Athletics and the Politics of Racial Equality: Five Pioneer Stories of Black Manliness, White Citizenship, and American Democracy.* Philadelphia: Temple University Press, 2012.

Kaye, Andrew M. *The Pussycat of Prize Fighting: Tiger Flowers and the Politics of Black Celebrity.* Athens: University of Georgia Press, 2004.

Leonard, David J., and C. Richard King. 'Revolting Black Athletes: Sport, New Racism, and the Politics of Dis/identification'. *Journal for the Study of Sports and Athletes in Education* 3, no. 2 (July 2009): 215–234.

Lester, Larry. *Black Baseball's National Showcase: The East-West All-Star Game, 1933–1953.* Lincoln: University of Nebraska Press, 2001.

Levine, Peter. *Ellis Island to Ebbets Field: Sport and the American Jewish Experience.* New York: Oxford University Press, 1992.

Litwack, Leon. *Trouble in Mind: Black Southerners in the Age of Jim Crow.* New York: Vintage Books, 1998.

Logan, Rayford W. *The Betrayal of the Negro from Rutherford B. Hayes to Woodrow Wilson.* New York: Collier Books, 1965.

Lucas, John A., and Ronald A. Smith. *Saga of American Sport.* Philadelphia: Lea & Febiger, 1978.

Mackay-Smith, Alexander. *Colonial Quarter Race Horse.* Richmond, VA: Helen Kleberg Groves, 1983.

Majors, Richard. 'Cool Pose: The Proud Signature of Black Survival'. *Changing Men: Issues in Gender, Sex and Politics* 17 (winter 1986): 184–185.

Mallozzi, Vincent M. *Asphalt Gods: An Oral History of the Rucker Tournament.* New York: Doubleday, 2003.

Marable, Manning. 'Black Athletes in White Men's Games, 1880–1920'. *Maryland Historian* 4, no. 2 (fall 1973): 143–149.

Martin, Charles H. *Benching Jim Crow: The Rise and Fall of the Color Line in Southern College Sports, 1890–1980.* Urbana: University of Illinois Press, 2010.

Miller, Patrick B. 'The Anatomy of Scientific Racism: Racialist Responses to Black Athletic Achievement'. *Journal of Sport History* 25, no. 1 (spring 1998): 119–151.

Miller, Patrick B. 'To Bring the Race Along Rapidly: Sport, Student Culture, and Educational Mission at Historically Black Colleges During the Interwar Years'. *History of Education Quarterly* 35, no. 2 (summer 1995): 111–133.

Moore, Joseph T. *Pride Against Prejudice: The Biography of Larry Doby.* Westport, CT: Greenwood Press, 1988.

Novak, Michael. *The Joy of Sports: End Zones, Baskets, Balls, and the Consecration of the American Spirit.* New York: Harper Collins, 1976.

Obi, T. J. Desch. 'Black Terror: Bill Richmond's Revolutionary Boxing'. *Journal of Sport History* 36, no. 1 (spring 2009): 99–114.

Oriard, Michael. *King Football: Sport and Spectacle in the Golden Age of Radio and Newsreels, Movies and Magazines, the Weeklies and the Daily Press.* Chapel Hill: University of North Carolina Press, 2001.

Ownby, Ted. 'Manhood, Memory, and White Men's Sports in the American South'. *The International Journal of the History of Sport* 15, no. 2 (August 1998): 103–118.

Peterson, Bob. *Peter Jackson: A Biography of the Australian Heavyweight Champion, 1860–1901.* Sydney: Croydon, 2005.

Pierce, Daniel S. *Real NASCAR: White Lightening, Red Clay, and Big Bill France.* Chapel Hill: University of North Carolina Press, 2010.

Powell, Shaun. *Souled Out? How Blacks are Winning and Losing in Sports.* Champaign, IL: Human Kinetics, 2008.

Rader, Benjamin G. *Baseball: A History of America's Game.* Urbana: University of Illinois Press, 1992.

Rhoden, William C. *Forty Million Dollar Slaves: The Rise, Fall, and Redemption of the Black Athlete.* New York: Crown Publishers, 2006.

Rieslar, Jim. *Black Writers/Black Baseball: An Anthology of Articles from Black Sportswriters who Covered the Negro Leagues.* Jefferson, NC: McFarland and Company, 1994.

Ritchie, Andrew. *Major Taylor: The Extraordinary Career of a Champion Bicycle Racer.* San Francisco: Bicycle Books, 1988.

Roberts, Randy. *Papa Jack: Jack Johnson and the Era of White Hopes.* New York: Free Press, 1983.

Ross, Charles K. *Outside the Lines: African Americans and the Integration of the National Football League.* New York: New York University Press, 1999.

Ruck, Rob. *Raceball: How the Major Leagues Colonized the Black and Latin Game.* Boston: Beacon Press, 2011.

Runstedtler, Theresa. *Jack Johnson, Rebel Sojourner: Boxing in the Shadow of the Global Color Line.* Berkeley: University of California Press, 2012.

Rybacki, Karyn Charles, and Donald Jay Rybacki. 'The King, the Young Prince, and the Last Confederate Soldier: NASCAR on the Cusp'. In *The Sporting World of the Modern South,* edited by Patrick B. Miller, 294–325. Urbana: University of Illinois Press, 2002.

Sammons, Jeffrey T. '"Race" and Sport: A Critical Historical Examination'. *Journal of Sport History* 21, no. 3 (fall 1994): 203–298.

Schmidt, Raymond. *Shaping College Football: The Transformation of an American Sport, 1919–1930.* Syracuse, New York: Syracuse University, 2007.

Smith, Kevin R. *Black Genesis: The History of the Black Prize Fighter, 1760–1870.* New York: iUniverse, 2003.

Smith, Thomas G. *Showdown: JFK and the Integration of the Washington Redskins.* Boston: Beacon Press, 2011.

Snyder, Brad. *Beyond the Shadow of the Senators: The Untold Story of the Homestead Grays and the Integration of Baseball.* New York: McGraw-Hill, 2003.

Strode, Woody, and Sam Young. *Goal Dust.* New York: Madison Books, 1990.

Telander, Rick. *Heaven is a Playground.* Lincoln: University of Nebraska Press, 1995.

Thomas, Damion. 'Around the World: Problematizing the Harlem Globetrotters as Cold War Warriors'. *Sport in Society* 14, no. 6 (August 2011): 778–791.

Thomas, Damion. *Globetrotting: African American Athletes, and Cold War Politics.* Urbana: University of Illinois Press, 2012.

Turrini, Joseph M. *The End of Amateurism in American Track and Field.* Urbana: University of Illinois Press, 2010.

Tygiel, Jules. *Baseball's Great Experiment: Jackie Robinson and His Legacy.* New York: Oxford University Press, 1983.

Wacquant, Loïc J. D. 'The Social Logic of Boxing in Black Chicago: Toward a Sociology of Pugilism'. *Sociology of Sport Journal* 9, no. 3 (September 1992): 221–254.

Ward, Geoffrey C. *Unforgivable Blackness: The Rise and Fall of Jack Johnson.* New York: Alfred A. Knopf, 2004.

Wiggins, David K. 'The Biggest Classic of Them All: The Howard and Lincoln Thanksgiving Day Football Games, 1919–1929'. In *Rooting for the Home Team: Sport Community and Identity,* edited by Daniel A. Nathan, 36–53. Urbana: University of Illinois Press, 2013.

Wiggins, David K. 'Edwin Bancroft Henderson: Physical Educator, Civil Rights Activist, and Chronicler of African American Athletes'. *Research Quarterly for Exercise and Sport* 70, no. 2 (June 1999): 91–112.

Wiggins, David K. 'Great Speed but Little Stamina: The Historical Debate Over Black Athletic Superiority'. *Journal of Sport History* 16, no. 2 (summer 1989): 158–185.

Wiggins, David K. 'Isaac Murphy: Black Hero in Nineteenth Century American Sport'. *Canadian Journal of History of Sport and Physical Education* 10, no. 1 (May 1979): 15–33.

Wiggins, David K. 'The Notion of Double-Consciousness and the Involvement of Black Athletes in American Sport'. In *Ethnicity and Sport in North American History and Culture,* edited by George Eisen, and David K. Wiggins, 133–153. Westport, CT: Praeger, 1994.

Wiggins, David K. 'Peter Jackson and the Elusive Heavyweight Championship: A Black Athlete's Struggle Against the Late Nineteenth Century Color-Line'. *Journal of Sport History* 12, no. 2 (summer 1985): 143–163.

Wiggins, David K. 'The Play of Slave Children in the Plantation Communities of the Old South, 1820–1860'. *Journal of Sport History* 7, no. 2 (summer 1980): 21–39.

Wiggins, David K. 'Prized Performers, But Frequently Overlooked Students: The Involvement of Black Athletes in Intercollegiate Sport on Predominantly White University Campuses, 1890–1972'. *Research Quarterly for Exercise and Sport* 62, no. 2 (June 1991): 164–177.

Wiggins, David K. 'Sport and Popular Pastimes: The Shadow of the Slavequarter'. *Canadian Journal of History of Sport and Physical Education* 11, no. 1 (May 1980): 61–88.

Wiggins, David K. 'Strange Mix of Entitlement and Exploitation: The African American Experience in Predominantly White College Sport'. *Wake Forest Journal of Law and Policy* 2, no. 1 (May 2012): 95–113.

Wiggins, David K. 'Wendell Smith, The Pittsburgh Courier-Journal and the Campaign to Include Blacks in Organized Baseball, 1933–1945'. *Journal of Sport History* 10, no. 2 (summer 1985): 5–29.

Wiggins, David K. 'With All Deliberate Speed: High School Sport, Race and Brown v. Board of Education'. *Journal of Sport History* 37, no. 3 (fall 2010): 329–346.

Wiggins, David K., and Patrick B. Miller. *The Unlevel Playing Field: A Documentary History of the African American Experience in Sport.* Urbana: University of Illinois Press, 2003.

Woodward, C. Vann. *The Strange Career of Jim Crow.* New York: Oxford University Press, 1966.

Wright, Richard. *Black Boy (American Hunger): A Record of Childhood and Youth.* New York: Harper Collins, 1993.

Zang, David W. *Fleet Walker's Divided Heart: The Life of Baseball's First Black Major Leaguer.* Lincoln: University of Nebraska Press, 1995.

Zuckerman, Jerome, G. Alan Stull, and Marvin H. Eyler. 'The Black Athlete in Post-Bellum Nineteenth Century'. *Physical Educator* 29, no. 3 (October 1972): 142–146.

D. Disability

9 The "Second Place" Problem

Assistive Technology in Sports and

(Re) Constructing Normal

■ DENISE A. BAKER

■ **INTRODUCTION**

Suppose that several months before an athletic event a sprinter's leg strength and metabolic capabilities are quantified and judged to be at or below the same range of function as that of his past or present athletic peers. During the time leading up to the competition our sprinter is not permitted to strengthen his legs, and in fact must ensure that his legs remain *at* or *below* the same range of function they were at the time they were initially measured. While our runner's legs, which are arguably the most critical component in a running competition, must stay in the same condition, his competitors may actively work to strengthen their legs beyond that same range of function in an attempt to break existing records of human performance. This restriction would seem inequitable, but this is the case, whether explicit or implicit, for athletes who need[1] to use one or more prosthetic limbs to participate in athletic competitions against individuals who do not need assistive technologies to compete.

It is at the core of competitive sports that one person be allowed to have certain kinds of advantages over another competitor without being disqualified (e.g., stronger muscle, better training, better genetics, more drive), otherwise every truly "fair" competition is likely to end in a tie. And there are certain types of technologies considered to be "equipment" that can be used to achieved an advantage for one player over another, such as the cutting-edge ski suit designed by US Ski and Snowboard Association to reduced drag (and race time) for US Olympic skiers competing in the 2014 winter games (Westly 2014; Polyana 2014). However, in the discourse about the use of assistive technologies (AT) in competition, in particular prosthetic limbs, an advantage that can be attributed in some way to that technology is treated as a distinctly different type of advantage (an unfair one). Perhaps one of the most salient examples of this perceived distinction occurred in 2008 when sprinter Oscar Pistorius was barred from competing in the Beijing Summer Olympics because the two prosthetic legs (called Cheetahs) he was using at the time were deemed to afford him an unfair advantage over the other "able bodied" sprinters he would be competing against

(International Association of Athletics Federation 2008). Another high-profile case occurred in the late 90's, when pro-golfer Casey Martin was barred from using a golf cart between holes in the PGA Tour. A degenerative circulatory disorder in Martin's right leg made it essentially impossible for him to walk the 18 hole course, however golf carts were explicitly banned during the tournament and the PGA Tour argued that use of one was would threaten the "purity" of the sport and provide Martin with an "unfair advantage" over other golfers (Cherney 2003). In 2001, Martin successfully sued the PGA Tour under Title III of The Americans with Disabilities Act which mandates equal access to public places, and won the right to use the golf cart (US Supreme Court 2001). More recently, long-jumper and Paralympic gold medalist Markus Rehm of Germany was banned from competing in the European Athletics Championship. Using a carbon fiber prosthetic leg, Rehm was competing against "able-bodied" athletes for a spot on Germany's track and field team, but despite his qualifying performance, the German Athletics Association (Deutscher Luftsport-verband) did not permit him to join the team because they deemed his prosthetic leg to be an unfair advantage (Borden 2014; Zaccardi 2014).

Objections to AT use in sports are generally raised when (1) the AT being used is perceived to afford the user a potentially "unfair advantage," (2) when it is perceived to threaten the purity of the sport, and/or (3) when the use of the AT is perceived as a precursor to a slippery slope with some morally dreadful end. While these objections have been explored and rebutted extensively in existing literature (Corrigan et al. 2008; Edwards 2008; Wolbring 2008), the broader implications for individuals with disabilities using AT have been neglected. This paper argues that the underlying assumption that undergirds all of these objections to AT use in sports is that quantified standards of "normal" human performance exist and are implicitly canonical, and that this assumption disproportionately restricts individuals with disabilities from the same opportunities to achieve greatness as individuals without disabilities. This paper uses the Olympics as a framework to understand how these three objections hold some individuals with disabilities accountable to "normal standards" (NS) that cap achievement opportunities to a status quo, while individuals without disabilities are able to push beyond the boundaries of these normal standards without moral scrutiny.[2]

▪ CHALLENGES IN DEVELOPING A NORMAL STANDARD

While Casey Martin's petition to use a golf cart during the PGA tour serves as an excellent example of objections to the use of AT in elite sports as a threat to fair play, Oscar Pistorius's petition to compete in the 2008 Summer Olympic as a sprinter using two prosthetic legs ignited a feverish debate about not only fairness in sports but how we understand the notion of a "normal" human body. In the Martin case, the debate was not focused on whether riding a golf cart was an advantage over walking (because it clearly has advantages in covering long distances), but whether walking between holes was a substantive part of the game (i.e., whether it mattered to the act of "golfing"; Cherney 2003). In the Pistorius case however, there was no question that the prosthetic legs were an essential component in the act of running and so the debate was necessarily focused on quantifying whether the technology itself would provide an unfair advantage in the act of running. In order to make this determination the International Association of Athletics Federations (IAAF), which is recognized by the International Olympic Committee as the primary governing body for athletics, determined that the prosthetic legs would have to be compared to some standard measure that defined what a natural human leg "should" be able to do. They assembled a team of scientist to conduct biometric analysis of Pistorius as well as five "able-bodied athletes at the same level of 400 m sprint performance," to be used as the comparison group (Brüggemann et al. 2007). Tests included VO2 (maximal oxygen uptake), lactate levels, ground force measurements, observational measure of sprinting motions such as stride length, vertical movement, and swing position, as well as materials analysis of the prosthetic (Brüggemann et al. 2007). The summary findings were used by the IAAF to ultimately classify Pistorius's prosthetics legs as "technical aids,"[3] which are contravened in Olympic competition, and subsequently Pistorius was declared ineligible to participate. The rational for classifying the prosthetic legs as technical aids is summarized in the IAAF's report abstract:

The metabolic tests indicated a lower aerobic capacity of the amputee than of the controls. In the 400 m race the handicapped athlete's VO2 uptake was 25% lower than the oxygen consumption of the sound controls, which achieved about the same final time. The joint kinetics of the ankle joints of the sound legs and the "artificial ankle joint" of the prosthesis were found to be significantly different. Energy return was clearly higher in the prostheses than in the human ankle joints. The kinetics of knee and hip joints were also affected by the prostheses during stance. The swing phase did not demonstrate any advantages for the natural legs in relation to the artificial limbs. In total the double transtibial amputee received significant biomechanical advantages by the prostheses in comparison to sprinting with natural human legs. (Brüggemann et al. 2007)

Pistorius immediately and successfully appealed the IAAF's decision through the Court of Arbitration for Sport (CAS).[4] CAS ruled that the interpretation of the test results were highly subjective and a review of the findings by a different group of scientists concluded the results showed no *clear* advantage for Pistorius[5] (Hunter et al. 2008). While the ruling allowed Pistorius to compete in the Olympics and other IAAF-sponsored venues, the issue of holding him accountable to a normal standard was actually reinforced. When considering the question of "whether the IAAF Council's Decision to ban Pistorius from IAAF sanctioned events unlawfully discriminatory," the CAS report stated:

> ... disability laws only require that an athlete such as Mr Pistorius be permitted to compete on the same footing as others. This is precisely the issue to be decided by this Panel: that is, whether or not Mr Pistorius is competing on an equal basis with other athletes not using *Cheetah Flex-Foot* prostheses. As counsel for the IAAF rightly mentioned, if this Panel finds that Mr Pistorius' Cheetah Flex-Foot prostheses provide no advantage to Mr Pistorius, he will be able to compete on an equal basis with other athletes. If the Panel concludes that Mr Pistorius does gain an advantage, the Convention would not assist his case. (Hunter et al. 2008)

What is critical here is that, although the stated requirement is that Pistorius "be permitted to compete on the same footing as others," the counsel interprets this requirement to mean he will only be allowed to compete if he is found to perform at or below some set of performance standards based on a group of his peers, which is not a restriction that "able-bodied" athletes are held accountable to. The counsel also stated that the central part of their evaluation was to determine whether Pistorius had an *overall* net advantage or disadvantage and to focus "on the overall effect of the prosthesis and not on whether Mr Pistorius had an advantage at only one point in the race" (Hunter et al. 2008). In effect this restricts Pistorius even further; for example, should his metabolism be naturally better than other athletes any potential advantage this might afford would also be a factor in the overall net advantage being attributed to the prosthetic use. In which case, even if the Cheetah could objectively be classified as inferior to a natural human leg in every way, Pistorius could still be barred from competing if he were to significantly outperform his peers while using it. CAS also qualified their decision by adding that Pistorius could not change or alter his prosthetic legs for future competitions and that "with future advances in scientific knowledge, and a testing regime designed and carried out to the satisfaction of both parties, the IAAF might in the future be in a position to prove that the existing *Cheetah Flex-Foot* model provides Mr Pistorius with an overall net advantage over other athletes" (Hunter et al. 2008). Essentially the CAS report allowed Pistorius to compete because they could not *prove* that his prosthetic legs afforded an unfair advantage, but the emphasis on comparing and restricting Pistorius (and presumably other athletes in a similar situation) to remain at or below a normal standard of performance was reinforced.

In an ironic decision by the German Athletics Association, long-jumper Markus Rehm was permitted to compete for a spot on the country's track and field team while using his prosthetic leg; however, after qualifying with an 8.24 m jump the Association announced publicly that Rehm would, nonetheless, not be selected for the team. The Association cited undisclosed (at the time this paper was written) biometric data that they felt cast "significant doubt" about whether Rehm's use of his prosthetic leg would be fair to other "able-bodied" competitors as it may provide an unfair advantage (Borden 2014). This example reinforces the precedent set by CAS's ruling about Pistorius by again using biological normal standards to compare and restrict an athlete using AT to either perform at or below the norm or be barred from competition.

▪ AN UNFAIR ADVANTAGE

New York Times sports writer Selena Roberts defended Oscar Pistorius's right to compete in the 2008 Olympics: "If research proves a competitive edge for Cheetahs, track's caretakers can look for ways to modify Pistorius's advantage" (Roberts 2007). However, assuming that the "modification" Roberts refers to does not mean to amplify the advantage, there is an implicit assumption that the prosthetic legs should be measured against some NS and that they should be reconfigured to fall at (or below) that NS in order for Pistorius to compete fairly. However, it is unlikely that this would require other competitors with no limb absence(s) to go through a similar process to ensure that their legs are at or below that NS. Edwards (2008) defends Pistorius's right to compete with his prosthetic legs, even if they are found to provide an "unfair advantage" of some kind. While he does not specifically address the issue of NSs, he points out that the international nature of the Olympic Games undoubtedly brings together many athletes who have "unfair advantages" over other athletes simply by the nature of the economic and geographic circumstance they were born into. Indeed, athletes who are considered able-bodied have been permitted to compete in elite sports with known potentially unfair advantages numerous times in the Olympics and other elite sports. For example, professional cyclist Miguel Indurain won an Olympic gold medal and five consecutive Tour de France races with his success partially attributed to his natural physical attributes that afforded him abnormally high cardiac output (twice as much as other cyclists at the time), abnormally low resting pulse, and an abnormally high lung capacity (Roberts 2007). Indurain was not required to "modify" his physiology to bring these functions within the NS that existed at the time. Olympic middle-distance runner Caster Semenya faced scrutiny from the IAAF because the association had concerns that her overly masculine physique posed an unfair advantage (Fox 1995). Semenya was required to undergo a gender test and was eventually cleared for future competition, presumably because she was found to indeed be a woman. In this case, any unfair advantage over other women Semenya garnered from her masculine physique was not actually problematic, but rather it was her perceived gender that caused the IAAF concern. Once the gender issue was settled the athlete was free to use her perceived abnormalities to gain a competitive edge (Thomas 2012); she was not required to feminize her appearance or weaken her muscles to bring them back to a level at or below a NS.

There are certainly existing restrictions that limit the type of enhancements athletes identified as able-bodied (as well as those identified as disabled) can engage in. Performance enhancing drug (PED) use is a particularly powerful example of employing technology to gain a competitive advantage, and numerous restrictions are placed on the use of such drugs in competitive sports. However, the arguments used to support the ban of PEDs are by no means indisputable and in many ways are plagued with the same moral dilemmas posed by the use of AT in competitive sports. For example, the argument that PEDs create a situation in which players can gain an unfair advantage can also be said of any number of training and nutrition approaches, socioeconomic factors, equipment choices, elective surgeries, and genetic differences between players. And as with AT, to identify an "unfair advantage," some method of objectively measuring "normal" performance must be agreed upon. Yet, even if such a method exists, it is possible that the use of a PED might result in an unfair advantage for one player, while allowing another player to barely reach the NS, in which case the latter player's use of PED might be considered completely fair.

Another argument used to support a ban on PEDs is that they pose an unnecessary health risk to players. This argument seems ironic when the sports they are used for (such as football or luge) are often unnecessarily far more dangerous than the drugs themselves (when used under a Doctor's supervision) and in some cases drugs classified as PEDs are also used on non-athletes to prevent injury, speed up recovery time, and improve healing (Murray 2008). This argument is illustrative of at least one way in which PED and AT restrictions are differently motivated. AT use in competitive sports is not a health concern for competitors at large, while one could argue it is a health concern if an able-bodied athlete feels compelled to seek a voluntary amputation in order to use a prosthetic limb that could give him/her a significant advantage; the act of using a prosthetic limb is not a health risk in the same way that the act of using PEDs can be.

Objections to PED use are highly complex, incongruent, and morally and ethically charged, and it is notable that there are numerous ways in which the debates about AT and PED use in elite sports are similar. There are arguments to support the ban of PEDs that could be used to support a ban or restriction on AT use; and likewise, there are arguments to support the use AT that could easily be mapped onto the legalization of PED. However, as a global community we have agreed that individuals with disabilities should have the same opportunities to compete in athletics as those who do not have disabilities, and as a global community we have decided to endorse the use of AT for that purpose. The issue at hand is not whether AT should or should not be used, but how it is regulated in certain sporting events. Various sporting organizations (and fans) have come to an agreement to ban steroid use, just as the baseball community came to agree that first base should be 90 feet instead of 50 feet from home plate, that football players can no longer horse-collar an opposing team's player, and that Olympic swimmers can only wear certain swimsuits. The rules that govern sports are arbitrary in the sense that they are not set forth by an omnipotent and unbending power; rather, they are constructed and reconstructed by arbiters, such as judges or oversight committees, as they see fit or necessary according to new safety concerns, changing social norms, and/or commercialization goals. As such, questions of purity and fairness are necessarily measured against these "arbitrary" rules. Athletes who use PEDs are criticized and/or punished because they are breaking established rules; however, the criticism that athletes using AT face is much more nuanced in that the "established" rule is a NS that is not clearly defined.

Interestingly, there are athletes identified as having a disability who have used AT in elite sports to compete against individuals identified as "able-bodied," in which there has been little or no controversy. Competing in parallel bars, vault, and rope climbing, American gymnast George Eyser won six medals (including three gold) in the 1904 Summer Olympics while using a prosthetic leg made of wood (Madrigal 2012). Eyser's accomplishments are highly celebrated, including pop culture references such as a third place ranking in *Rolling Stone* magazine's "Top 100 Greatest Olympians" (Reilly 2014). Likewise, professional archers Neroli Fairhill of New Zealand and Paola Fantato of Italy each competed in Olympic archery events from a seated position while using a wheelchair and neither faced notable public scrutiny or sanction (Tributes 2006; Paola 2014). Similarly uncontroversial are examples of athletes identified as disabled who choose not to use available AT to compete against athletes identified as able-bodied. For example, Natalie du Toit of South Africa competed in the 2008 Olympics open water 10 km swim with a left leg absence and without the use of a prosthetic; her accomplishments in both "able-bodied" and "disabled" swimming competitions have branded her as "an inspiring model for thousands of disabled as well as able-bodied people" (Hawthorne 2006, p. 208). Natalia Partyka, also of South Africa, is a well-respected Olympic (and Paralymbic) table tennis player who has a right forearm and hand absence; she too competes without AT and without notable controversy (Lakhani 2012). In contrast to Pistorius and Martin, all of these athletes were/are arguably more likely to be at a disadvantage than to harness any substantial enhancement from the nature of their AT use or impairment. This may contribute to an understanding of why they were/are not criticized for violating the purity of their sport, or for garnishing some sort of unfair advantage, but rather were/are embraced and lauded as "heroic," "role models," and "perseverant" (Hawthorne 2006, p. 208; Lakhani 2012; Madrigal 2012; Reilly 2014). And though it might seem intuitive that any athlete who is compelled to compete with a perceived disadvantage (e.g., limited mobility from a seated position, swimming with one leg, losing a shoe part way through a race, losing a loved one shortly before a competition, etc.) may be exalted in this way simply for persevering through "adversity," the broader point is to highlight that competition between those perceived as disabled and those perceived as able-bodied is not inherently viewed as "unfair," nor is the use of AT in such competition. If an individual is not perceived to use his/her AT or disability to get ahead of the game, there is little or no controversy; however, as with the cases of Pistorius, Rehm, and Martin, performance that is potentially enhanced by AT or disability is quite objectionable. This is evidenced in implicit and explicit rules that fix individuals using AT to a NS meant to objectively identify and prevent that line from being crossed.

Arguably, competing with the use of an AT could serve to be such an advantage that it changes the nature of the action the user is performing. For example, Edwards suggests that the arguments surrounding Oscar Pistorius's right to compete in the Olympics should not focus on whether he has an unfair advantage but, rather, whether the prosthetics enable him to run or to do something else, such as bounce. If it's the latter, Edwards argues that Pistorius would no longer be competing in the same sport and therefore should not be permitted to compete in the running event (Edwards 2008). The type of advantages afforded by enlarged lungs or abnormally high muscle mass would not likely result in a fundamental change in the action being performed in competition and so might be considered a more acceptable form of advantage than the kind afforded by such an AT. However, if, for example, Pistorius's Cheetah legs were indeed found to facilitate running rather than something else, it is unlikely that the runner's prosthesis would no longer be held to a NS.

The issue of holding people with perceived disabilities who use AT accountable to a NS is, whether explicitly or implicitly, ubiquitous inside and outside of sports. While it may be in the form of a high school basketball team protesting an opposing team player's participation because her prosthetic legs seem to allow her to jump higher than all other players, it may also be in the form of an insurance policy that only covers the cost of an AT that enables an individual to achieve a recognized NS of function while excluding a superior technology that might allow the person to perform beyond that NS. Perhaps the most prevailing example of restricting individuals with disabilities to a NS occurs within the medical and legal fields, in which decision makers resolve which AT should be considered therapeutic and which should be deemed enhancements. In the simplest terms, a therapeutic technology may be defined as one that allows an individual to perform a task(s) at some level above his current limitations, but at or below some predetermined NS. On the other hand, an enhancing technology may be defined as one that allows an individual to perform above that predetermined NS. Problematically, the quantified values of the NSs used in these types of classifications are not universally held, and instead may be quite adaptable.

In competitive sports, NS are measured in a number of ways and are known to change over time, such as when existing records are broken, when competition is opened up to a new group of competitors, or when new equipment is introduced. So far, NSs of athletic performance for "able-bodied" competition are, not surprisingly, based on the performance of individuals without perceived disabilities. What is particularly relevant here is that these same individuals are not morally or ethically bound to those NSs while individuals with perceived disabilities using AT may be. That is to say the individuals without disabilities are not restricted to perform within those NSs in the future and so can push beyond the NS by changing their training, nutrition, medication (which could include legal steroids such as an asthma inhaler, or performance enhancing drugs that have not yet been banned), essential/nonessential surgery (such as Lasik surgery for an archer), body modification (such as shaving body hair), or by upgrading equipment (Westly 2014; Guttmann 2002). If successful, these athletes are likely applauded and, in turn, a new NS can be created based on their latest performance. Individuals with disabilities who use or make changes to their AT to compete are not similarly located; rather, performing above the NS may be morally scrutinized and perceived as "cheating" or "suspect." Essentially, this adaptability in the NS of athletic performance sets up a model in which athletes using an AT to compete against "able-bodied" athletes can only achieve a fixed rank of second place at best; first place is simply not available. This is not to suggest that there should be a moral obligation to allow individuals using assistive technologies to compete in organized competitive events without technological restrictions but, rather, it is meant to draw attention to this particular problem of trying to shackle "fairness" to a constrained measurement for some competitors but not others.

■ PURITY

Elio Locatelli, a representative of the International Association of Athletics Federations, was involved with the 2007 technical assessment of Pistorius's prosthetics. After the initial decision was made to ban Pistorius from competing with his prosthetic legs, Locatelli is reported to have explained "it affects the purity of sport. . . . [N]ext will be another device where people can fly with something on their back" (Roberts 2007). Locatelli draws on two objections here, one related to "purity" and the other related to a slippery slope argument which will be discussed in the next section.

The link between purity and the running competition that Locatelli makes not only applies to the procedural rules (e.g., staying in one's own lane) but also intimates purity of the body. Body purity, or at least an absence of external technologies, was indeed the model used in the original Olympic Games when participants competed in the nude, but cultural, economic, geographic, and technological influences have resulted in numerous changes in this interpretation over time (Guttmann 2002). Sports once conducted in the nude now allow (or require) high-tech items such as running shoes, specialized clothing, and other equipment that has dramatically changed athletic performance. If the use of a prosthetic limb is objected to on the grounds that it violates the purity of a sport, this implies that sport in its current state has a purity to violate, in which case the standards of purity have changed to include some forms of technology. It seems likely that the purity of a sport is centrally linked to fairness, so by integrating technology into a sport in such a way that the changes have applied to all competitors at once, the purity is preserved by maintaining fairness. In this respect, although differences in various socioeconomic factors between competing countries mean that some competitors will have access to more effective forms of approved technologies than others, because the *potential* advantages afforded by these technologies exist for all, it is not viewed as a violation of the purity of the sport (Guttmann 2002). It would seem, then, that the standard of purity in Olympic sports today is related to equal *potential access* to the advantages afforded by an approved technology, not equal distribution of those advantages.

In order to maintain this form of "technological purity," guidelines are constructed that require technologies be restricted to particular dimension regarding size, shape, tensile strength, springiness, etc. (XIII Olympic Congress 2009). However, the athlete's "body purity" is not restricted in this same manner; legs are not required to remain within a particular length range, muscle mass does not need to fall at or below a particular level, etc. With the exception of sports such as wrestling and boxing, in which a physical characteristic like weight might impact how a competition is organized, if the biological characteristics of an individual body part could facilitate a significant advantage, generally this would not restrict one's right to compete.[6] Rather, biological characteristics that facilitate a significant advantage are more likely to be admired and valued rather than morally scrutinized (Fox 1995). Further, as Bostrom and Sandberg (2009) note, there are numerous rules and norms "to protect and improve cognitive function," so too are there such rules and norms to protect and improve the physical body. For example, myriad federal and state laws protect employees and the general public from physical harms, employers and health insurance companies often offer employees free gym memberships, and individuals who are perceived as having physical impairments are often treated as having a medical problem that should be treated and rectified. In contrast, Bostrom points out that public policy to limit or reduce cognitive capacity do not currently exist, and again the same can be said of policies to limit or diminish the physical body. This helps explain why Miguel Indurain was not banned from elite competitions for having abnormally high lung capacity and heart strength (Fox 1995). These two notions of purity have a direct impact on the perceptions and rights of individuals using prosthetic technology in athletic competition. If a prosthetic is viewed as a piece of equipment, technological purity would dictate that a competitor could not use it unless all other competitors had potential access to use the technology as well. Although rules could be instituted to ensure all competitors could use a prosthetic(sis) to replace an absent limb(s), it is unrealistic to argue that this falls within the spirit of the definition of equal potential access since a competitor would be compelled to have a limb removed to make the access meaningful. On the other hand, if a prosthetic is viewed as a replacement for an absent body part, it is then an extension of the body and, with respect to the notion of body purity, should not be subject to restrictions in design and performance. However, when an athlete is using a prosthetic it is both a technology and an extension of the body. As a result the current use of a prosthetic technology in Olympic sports violates both notions of purity; it is not available to all athletes unless they have a limb loss, and it must adhere to certain restrictions in design and performance (i.e., adherence to a normal standard; International Association of Athletics Federation 2008).

There are also claims that support a different purity argument, one that refers to the purity of human nature. In his book *Beyond Therapy*, Leon Kass (2003) stops short of characterizing the use of biotechnology as good or bad, but defends a position of caution and scopic contemplation about how we understand and define human nature, and how biotechnological answers to perceived human deficiency change that understanding. Kass argues that "superior performance" is central to human nature, and through the mechanization of performance, either through steroids or genetics for example, we risk dehumanizing the competitors and threatening the purity of the sport. He also argues that the use of biotechnologies in competitive sports may threaten the validity of the competitive outcomes.

> . . . when is the alienation of biological process from active experience dehumanizing, compromising the lived humanity of our efforts and thus making our superior performance in some way false—not simply our own, not fully human?" (p. 131)

Although Kass is not addressing the issue of whether to allow athletes using AT to compete against athletes who do not, this argument would suggest that if they were to compete their accomplishments could be perceived as "not simply (their) own, not fully human" (assuming a device such as a prosthetic limb is not considered part of human biological processes). In this case athletes using AT would be compelled to question whether what they do is fully human and whether they ought to participate. This is disquieting to say the least, given the individual and collective struggles that many people with impairments have endured to secure equal rights and opportunities. However, within the discourse surrounding transhumanism and technology, the idea that incorporating technology into our bodies will change what it means to be human and what it means to interact with other humans is familiar moral quagmire. This particular notion of purity has not been expressed by the athletic community at large however, and for now, athletes using AT are welcomed to pursue the Olympic dream regardless of how their particular technology changes their human nature. Which brings us back to the issue at hand here, which is how this can be brought about ethically and meaningfully.

To create equal opportunity for individuals using a prosthesis in competitive sports our notions of technological or body purity must change. Technological purity would need to allow some individuals to use technologies not available to others, or body-purity must change to include prosthetic technology as a true extension of the physical body and therefore only be restricted in the same way as for individuals not using a prosthetic. Both understandings of purity rely on standards that exclude individuals who use prosthetics from being part of their ongoing construction. While new technologies designed for able-bodied competitors can be used to continually reshape a sport's standards of technological purity, prosthetic technologies are currently excluded from this standard, and while able-bodied competitors reshape the standards of body-purity through genetic anomalies, nutritional changes, or advanced training, improvements in an individual's prosthetic body are also excluded from consideration in this process. Currently, individuals using AT in competitive sports could only conform to these existing notions of purity by abandoning their technology, which in many cases would then prevent the athlete from performing critical functions needed to participate, effectively excluding the individual from competition altogether.

▪ SLIPPERY SLOPE

If the use of AT in sports could be done is such a way as to ensure at least technological purity (i.e., providing able-bodied competitors with some alternative, compensatory technology), this would still not address the accountability to a NS that athletes using AT are confronted with. A prosthetic is not merely an auxiliary piece of equipment; it is also a body part, and it is this latter conceptualization that has proved most problematic in determining how prosthetics can be used in competition. The intuitive response is that fairness can be achieved by ensuring that replacement body parts be equal in form and function to the "species typical" body parts they are intended to replace. However, as discussed earlier, this restricts an individual using a prosthetic to a NS that other competitors are not subject to. The suggestion that an athlete should be permitted to use prosthetic technology designed to provide an advantage over other competitors is antithetical to notions of purity, and generates objections similar to Locatelli's second point that "next will be another device where people can fly with something on their back" (Roberts 2007). This is the familiar slippery slope argument that dogged Pistorius and his supporters, as well as other athletes wishing to use AT in competitive sports (Caplan 2008). The objection is that allowing an individual to use a prosthetic device to gain advantage over an individual not using such a device would result in a technological arms race (no pun intended) that would end with individuals amputating healthy limbs in order to replace them with high-tech prosthetics (Longman 2007; McNamee and Edwards 2006; Roberts 2007). The argument makes a number of assumptions including: (1) retaining one's healthy limbs is a better state of the human condition than having prosthetic replacements, (2) policies or cultural norms would sanction this behavior, (3) individuals would be willing to engage in this behavior, and (4) a NS exists upon which an "advantage" can be defined from. The focus here is not whether these assumptions are correct or whether the inevitability of the slippery slope argument is valid,[7] but, rather, to highlight how individuals using prosthetics are left out of the process of determining where the slope is currently located. In other words, a NS has to be set in order to determine when a step toward the slope is being taken, and these NSs are based on the performance measures of able-bodied individuals, not using prosthetic technologies. To obtain a level of performance above that NS by use of assistive technology is viewed as not only an unfair advantage but a step toward doom (Edwards 2008; Longman 2007; McNamee and Edwards 2006). On the other hand, performance levels that are increased because of other forms of technological advancements, such as changes in equipment, are generally only scrutinized when the changes are dramatic. This was the case during the 2008 Olympics when record-smashing swim times were attributed to a new type of swimsuits, with 94% of the new records set by athletes wearing the full-body technology (Crouse 2008). Athletes and trainers protested that the suits should be considered "technical aids" and therefore banned because of their ability to trap air for added buoyancy, and because the teams using them were violating the purity of the sport (Crouse 2008). The suits were subsequently banned by the Federation Internationale de Nation (FINA, the world governing board of elite swimming) and new regulations were put in place to govern future swimsuit designs; however, the original suits were not reclassified as technical aids and previous records set using the now banned suits were not impacted (Crouse 2008; Wilson 2009).

That the previous swimming records were not invalidated after the suits were banned means that subsequent athletes must compete against these new times. This is significant here for four reasons: first, it demonstrates that it is permissible that a piece of technology be used to push well beyond the existing NS of human performance even if only for a short time; second, it is permissible that a technology can facilitate an unfair advantage over other competitors; third, it is permissible to violate technological purity of the games (subsequent competitors will not have the opportunity to use the high-tech suits); and finally, that a leap in performance enhancing technology does not necessarily result in subsequent steps down a slippery slope.

■ DISCUSSION

The question of limiting individuals using AT to a NS may not seem particularly pressing given there are still very few examples of these athletes crossing over to "able-bodied" events. The reason for this is unclear, but the existence of organizations such as the Paralympics and Special Olympics where athletes using AT only compete against other athletes using AT is certainly a contributing factor. No doubt the state of AT development has also been critical in motivating athletes using AT to competing in traditionally "able-bodied" venues. While AT might have been a deterrent in the past, the development of lighter, more functional, and more sophisticated AT is closing potential performance gaps and in so doing, allows more athletes to compete in both arenas. For example, developments in lower limb technology have enabled some student athletes to participate and excel in team sports alongside players who do not use AT. Such is the case with Austrian teen Martin Hofbauer, who recently became the first soccer player using a prosthetic leg to be officially endorsed to play by FIFA (2013). Although there are relatively few athletes in this position, this number will no doubt increase in the coming years. For this reason, the need to ensure that athletes using AT to compete against "able-bodied" athletes have equal access to achieve excellence is all the more pressing. And, while Hofbauer's case serves as a positive example, based on existing rulings (such as CAS's ruling that Pistorius could only compete if his prostheses were found to provide NO advantage and the German Athletics Association's passing over of Markus Rehm to avoid controversy) and based on the past behavior of the IAAF, athletes using AT to compete in *individual* sports still face an uphill battle if they wish to compete in IAAF-sponsored events such as the Olympics, and an even steeper hill stands in the way of moving beyond second place.

Allhoff et al. (2011) note that within the broader discourse surrounding human enhancement "there are passionate and opposing forces engaged in this international struggle for clarity and policy." While fairness, purity, and the slippery slope argument figure centrally in these conversations, they are primarily focused on enhancements to species typical bodies and cognitive states—species non-typical bodies are considered as an afterthought (if they are considered at all). Within competitive sports, this second-place consideration is evident both in the way governing bodies have had difficulty applying existing rules to accommodate individuals using AT to compete and in the way that the current system ensures that these same individuals are literally bound to "second place" performance if they are to avoid moral scrutiny.

To address this problem, determination of fair versus unfair advantage in competitive sports should focus on factors that are less dependent on the types of bodies athletes have. One approach builds off a question posed by Edwards (2008) as to whether Oscar Pistorius is actually running, as opposed to bouncing, when he competes using his Cheetah legs. This would require the creation of an international, interdisciplinary organization to include representatives from (at least) engineering, ethics, and sports governance, whose role would be to define, quantify, and regulate the mechanical actions that constitute the defining components of a sport, moving away from trying to define and then standardize the human body. For example, agreements could be reached about what mechanical principles or thresholds indicate that running becomes bouncing, swimming becomes floating, throwing becomes launching, jumping becomes catapulting, etc. Measures of human performance might still be used in defining the mechanical actions that constitute the critical components of a sport, however, if based on negotiated properties of a motion that apply to athletes of any level and if the measures are then made static for all competitors moving forward. This approach could be a more just way of handling AT in sports. In this case identifying unfair advantages would not be determined by comparing certain individuals' performance to a group of their peers but, rather, by comparing individuals' performance to pre-established objective measures. These measures would apply to all athletes; for example, if a technological device such a specialized ankle brace provides more bounce than is allowable by the pre-determined standard, the brace would be banned from use in a running competition. Likewise, if a prosthetic leg exceeds this maximum bounce, it too would be banned and a compliant brace or prosthetic would need to be used in its place. This suggestion would be complex and undoubtedly difficult to implement; however, the current system (using biological NS's) is arguably more complex and difficult to implement and, as discussed in this paper, treats athletes using AT unfairly.

Admittedly this approach would be not only difficult but also impossible in some sports or aspects of a sport. In this case, when biological performance standards must be used, the theoretical boundaries of human performance should be considered rather than what is typical or average at the time the standards are devised, even if no human has been able to yet reach those theoretical limits. For example, in archery if a limit was set for the amount of human grip force that can be exerted on the bow handle, this limit should be set according to the theoretical limits of human grip strength rather than the typical grip strength of a "representative" group of archers. In this respect an individual using a prosthetic hand to grip the bow would have the same opportunity and the same compulsion to stay within the same grip strength limits that his/her competitors were held to. However, this raises a new concern: Couldn't athletes using AT immediately, and perhaps simply, adjust their devices to reach these theoretical limits, while athletes not using AT would be forced to exert great physical and emotional effort just to approach these limits? Maybe. But, this may or may not matter; it would depend entirely on how the "theoretical limits" and "objective measures" defined for the sport interact with one another to influence actual performance. It would most certainly need to be a significant factor in deciding how to define a sport by the sum of its parts, but it need not be a factor that derails the entire exploration of such an approach. Interestingly, many of the arguments presented throughout this paper would suggest that creating an opportunity for AT users to jump ahead to some pre-established theoretical limit of human performance would actually be more fair than the current system that has evolved. Although it could be argued that for athletes using AT, the race to the top would become a race to find the best engineer, this is what "able-bodied" athletes have done for centuries in elite sports. They are matched with coaches that can devise the best technology solutions (through physical, nutritional, and psychological training regimes) to engineer a body that can beat all other competitors; that opportunity, as argued in this paper, is not afforded to athletes using AT in elite sports. Suggesting that sporting competitions would be more just if athletes using AT were allowed to jump ahead in this way is problematic to say the least, but it is an interesting exercise in table-turning.

Of course, these two particular methodologies would be socially disruptive and no doubt controversial, but they are mentioned here to act, at least, as a starting point to a broader discussion about uncoupling the (often unsettled) body as the measuring stick of "normal" from many of the ways in which issues of fairness and equity for individuals with physical impairments are decided. Organizations such as the IAAF need time to evaluate how new technology affects the integrity of a sport, and this process may involve a trial-and-error approach. The existence of such a process helps strengthen the falsification of the "Purity" argument and the "Slippery Slope" argument laid out in this paper by demonstrating that sports can and do change over time. However, in its current form, the process of evaluating new technology against NSs tied to biological performance to substantiate an "Unfair Advantage" will continue to leave athletes using AT in second place at the podium and equal opportunity more broadly.

■ CONCLUSION

The aim of this paper has been to highlight some of the problems that exist with the current conceptualizations of "fairness" for athletes using assistive technologies in integrated sports. Athletes who use AT that is suspected to give them an unfair advantage are at risk of being perceived as cheating or otherwise violating the purity of the sport. But the standards on which an unfair advantage is judged are problematic. An athlete's AT is generally restricted (whether implicitly or explicitly) to engineering standards that correlate with the typical capabilities of athletic peers (i.e., a prosthetic leg should be about the same as a "normal" leg). However, "able-bodied" athletes are not restricted to these types of standards and therefore have the opportunity to push beyond the typical; athletes using ATs do not have this same opportunity. This paper does not argue that AT use in sports should not be limited in some way but, rather, that ensuring equal access and opportunity to individuals using AT requires a new approach to the way in which those limits are established. In particular, governing bodies such as IAAF and CAS should recognize that the methods and language they currently use surrounding the use of AT equates "unfair" advantage with "any" advantage and so the net result inevitably discriminates against athletes using AT.

■ ACKNOWLEDGMENTS

I am grateful to Nick Schweitzer, Joe Herkert, Jay Klein, and Troy McDaniel (Arizona State University) for helpful comments on an earlier version of this paper. No funding was used to complete this research. Portions of this paper were presented at the 2014 IEEE International Symposium on Ethics in Engineering, Science, and Technology, May 2014.

▪ NOTES

1. I use the term "need" here, but it is should be noted that not all athletes with limb absence use a prosthetic limb(s) to compete in organized sports. For example, Anthony Robles won the 2010–2011 NCAA individual wrestling championship with a left leg absence, but never used a prosthetic leg to compete. Ironically, critics complained that Robles's limb absence gave him an unfair advantage over other wrestlers (Merrill 2013).

2. In some cases "able-bodied" athletes (as well as athletes using AT) do experience moral scrutiny when they employ the use of certain drugs or supplements that may or may not afford an unfair advantage. The differences and similarities to AT use are discussed in the context of performance enhancing drugs in the section "An Unfair Advantage."

3. Technical aids are defined in Rule 144.2(e) of the IAAF competition rules "as technical device that incorporates springs, wheels or any other element that provides the user with an advantage over valid athletes" (International Association of Athletics Federation 2008).

4. After Pistorius's successful appeal, he was unable to make the qualifying time required for entry into the 2008 Beijing Summer Olympics, but was able to compete in the 2012 London Summer Olympics.

5. CAS also noted that the lead scientist, Prof. Peter Bruggemann, had not been given access to all the information IAAF had regarding the case, and that the IAAF had put certain restriction on Prof. Bruggemann that prevented him from evaluating all aspects of Pistorius's athletic performance, such as Pistorius's slower performance when sprinting around curves.

6. Unless perhaps these physical characteristics are achieved through the use of banned PEDs, but even then, records set by able-bodied athletes who have used illegal PEDs to change the physical characteristics of their body to facilitate a significant advantage, though criticized, are not always refuted after the fact. This was the case for numerous German swimmers in the 1976 Summer Olympics when it was revealed 15 years later that the swimmers had been using illegal PED at the time; the International Olympic Committee ruled that the medals would not be stripped and the records would not be removed (Clarey 1998).

7. For further analysis of technology and the slippery slope argument more broadly, see (Tributes flow for archery legend Fairhall 2006; Paola Fantato Bio et al. 2014).

▪ REFERENCES

Allhoff, F., Lin, P., & Steinberg, J. (2011). Ethics of human enhancement: An executive summary. *Science and Engineering Ethics, 17*(2), 201–212. doi:10.1007/s11948-009-9191-9.

Borden, B. S. A. M. (2014, August 18). For jumper, renewed debate over athletic versus prosthetic. *New York Times,* D1. Retrieved October 10, 2014, from http://www.nytimes.com/2014/08/18/sports/for-a-jumper-with-one-leg-debate-is-athletic-vs-prosthetic.html.

Bostrom, N., & Sandberg, A. (2009). Cognitive enhancement: methods, ethics, regulatory challenges. *Science and Engineering Ethics*, *15*(3), 311–341. doi:10.1007/s11948-009-9142-5.

Brüggemann, G., Arampatzis, A., & Emrich, F. (2007). Report 1512/2007 biomechanical and metabolic analysis of long sprint running of the double transtibial amputee athlete O. Pistorius using cheetah sprint prostheses—comparison with able-bodied athletes at the same level of 400 m sprint performance. Institute of Biomechanics and Orthopaedics German Sport University Cologne. A study performed on the request of the IAAF. Retrieved April 11, 2016, from http://www.udel.edu/biology/rosewc/kaap427627/reserve/run/Pistorius_Final_Report_bruggerman2007.pdf.

Caplan, A. (2008, May 22). "Blade Runner" ruling subverts nature of sport. *NBC News*. Retrieved December 12, 2014, from http://www.nbcnews.com/id/24758518/ns/health-health_care/t/blade-runner-ruling-subverts-nature-sport/#.Ux4aS_1dU08.

Cherney, J. L. (2003). Sport, (dis)ability, and public controversy: Ableist rhetoric and Casey Martin v. PGA Tour, Inc. In R. S. Brown & D. J. O'Rourke III (Eds.), *Case studies in sport communication* (pp. 81–104). Westport, CT: Praeger.

Clarey, C. (1998, December 16). Despite doping, olympic medals stand. *International Herald Tribune*, 22.

Corrigan, T. F., Paton, J., Holt, E., & Hardin, M. (2008). Discourses of the "Too Abled": Contested body hierarchies and the Oscar Pistorius case. *International Journal of Sport Communication*, *3*, 288–307.

Crouse, K. (2008, July 24). High-tech era in final days as swimming bans suits. *New York Times*, D1.

Edwards, S. D. (2008). Should Oscar Pistorius be excluded from the 2008 Olympic Games? *Sports, Ethics and Philosophy*, *2*(2), 112–125.

FIFA gives green light for prostheses player Martin Hofbauer. (2013, May 12). *Sportal. de*. Retrieved April 21, 2014, from http://www.sportal.de/fifa-gibt-gruenes-licht-fuer-prothesen-spieler-martin-hofbauer-1-2013051227033700000.

Fox, N. (1995, June 25). A giant in the saddle; profile; Miguel Indurain. *The Independent*. Retrieved March 01, 2014, from http://www.independent.co.uk/sport/a-giant-in-the-saddle-profile-miguel-indurain-1588209.html.

Guttmann, A. (2002). *The Olympics: A history of the modern games* (2nd ed.). Champaign: University of Illinois Press.

Hawthorne, T. (2006). Natalie Du Toit: Tumble turn. Cape Town, South Africa: *Oshun Books*. Retrieved from http://books.google.com/books?id=_DVPeKm7TZwC&pgis=1.

Hunter, M., Rivkin, D., & Rochat, J. P. (2008). Arbitration CAS 2008/A/1480 Pistorius v/IAAF, award of 16 May 2008 (Vol. 2008, pp. 1–14). Retrieved April 11, 2016, from http://jurisprudence.tas-cas.org/sites/CaseLaw/Shared%20Documents/1480.pdf.

International Association of Athletics Federation. (2008, January 14). Oscar Pistorius—independent scientific study concludes that cheetah prosthetics offer clear mechanical advantages. *IAAF org*. Retrieved November 10, 2013, from http://www.iaaf.org/news/news/oscar-pistorius-independent-scientific-stud-1.

Kass, L. (2003). *Beyond therapy: Biotechnology and the pursuit of happiness*. Washington, DC: President's Council on Bioethics.

Lakhani, N. (2012, August 25). Paralympic profile: Natalia Partyka, table tennis. *The Independent*. Retrieved from http://www.independent.co.uk/sport/olympics/paralympics/paralympic-profile-natalia-partyka-table-tennis-8079380.html.

Longman, J. (2007, May 15). An amputee sprinter: Is he disabled or too-abled? *New York Times*. Retrieved from http://www.nytimes.com/2007/05/15/sports/othersports/15runner.html?pagewanted=all.

Madrigal, A. C. (2012, August 10). How a guy with a wooden leg won 6 Olympic medals. *The Atlantic*. Retrieved from http://www.theatlantic.com/technology/archive/2012/08/how-a-guy-with-a-wooden-leg-won-6-olympic-medals/260988/.

McNamee, M. J., & Edwards, S. D. (2006). Transhumanism, medical technology and slippery slopes. *Journal of Medical Ethics, 32*(9), 513–518. doi:10.1136/jme.2005.013789.

Merrill, D. (2013, March 18). The one-legged wrestler who conquered his sport, then left it behind. *Deadspin*. Retrieved from http://deadspin.com/the-one-legged-wrestler-who-conquered-his-sport-then-1-452888181.

Murray, T. H. (2008). Sports enhancement. In M. Crowley (Ed.), *Birth to death and bench to clinic: The Hastings Center bioethics briefing book for journalists, policymakers, and campaigns* (pp. 153–158). New York: Hastings Center. Retrieved from http://www.thehastingscenter.org/Publications/BriefingBook/Detail.aspx?id=2206.

Paola Fantato Bio, Stats, and Results. Sports reference, Olympic sports. Retrieved November 14, 2014, from http://www.sports-reference.com/olympics/athletes/fa/paola-fantato-1.html.

Polyana, K. (2014, February 13). Science, not muscle, driving many Olympic wins. *Associated Press*. Retrieved October 12, 2013, from http://bigstory.ap.org/article/science-not-muscle-driving-many-olympic-wins.

Reilly, D. (2014, February 7). 100 greatest US Olympians, higher, faster and stronger. *Rolling Stone*. Retrieved April 21, 2014, from http://www.rollingstone.com/culture/pictures/100-greatest-us-olympians-20140207.

Roberts, S. (2007, July 18). Fear of disability the same on a course or a track. *New York Times*. Retrieved February 24, 2014, from http://www.nytimes.com/2007/07/18/sports/othersports/18roberts.html?_r=0.

Thomas, J. (2012, August 11). Caster Semenya 2012 Olympics: Did the South African runner lose the women's 800 meters on purpose? *Slate*. Retrieved March 01, 2014, from http://www.slate.com/blogs/five_ring_circus/2012/08/11/caster_semenya_2012_olympics_did_the_south_african_runner_lose_the_women_s_800_meters_on_purpose_.html.

Tributes flow for archery legend Fairhall. (2006, June 13). *New Zealand Herald*. Retrieved April 25, 2014, from http://www.nzherald.co.nz/nz/news/article.cfm?c_id=1&objectid=10386306.

US Supreme Court, N.C. PGA Tour, Inc. v. Martin (2001). Retrieved from http://supremecourtobserver.com/cases/US/532/532US661/532us661.pdf.

Westly, E. (2014). Engineering the ideal Olympian five technologies that will give US athletes an edge. *Popular Science, 284*(2), 35–47.

Wilson, S. (2009, July 24). FINA bans hi-tech swimsuits with only textile suits allowed from 2010. *The Telegraph*. Retrieved January 10, 2014, from http://www.telegraph.co.uk/sport/olympics/swimming/5900497/Fina-bans-hi-tech-swimsuits-with-only-textile-suits-allowed-from-2010.html.

Wolbring, G. (2008). Oscar Pistorius and the future nature of Olympic, Paralympic and other sports. *ScriptEd, 5*(1), 139–160. doi:10.2966/scrip.050108.139.

XIII Olympic Congress. (2009). 121st IOC Session & XIII Olympic Congress, Copenhagen, Denmark 2009. In *XIII Olympic Congress*. Copenhagen: International Olympic Committee.

Zaccardi, N. (2014, July 31). German amputee long-jumper won't fight European championships exclusion. *OlympicTalk, NBC Sports*. Retrieved August 3, 2014, from http://olympictalk.nbcsports.com/2014/07/31/markus-rehm-germany-amputee-long-jump-european-championships-track-and-field/.

10 More Similar Than Different

The Psychological Environment of Paralympic Sport

■ KRISTEN D. DIEFFENBACH
AND TRACI A. STATLER

Over the last few decades, advances in cultural attitudes, improved legal support, and advancements in assistive technologies and medicine have combined to help both level and expand the playing fields for individuals with disabilities. As opportunities for novice through top tier athletes in both disability and inclusive sport continue to grow, more and more individuals with disabilities are getting involved, increasing the demand for professionals prepared to assist and support these efforts. An emerging body of work has begun exploring the disability sport experience supplementing the mental skills and sport psychology research focused on able-bodied athletes. This research indicates that athletes with disabilities, regardless of the environment, and particularly at the elite level, share many more similarities with their able-bodied counterparts than differences. This paper is designed to provide an understanding of the unique elements of disability sport and to highlight the "common" experience of elite athletes with disabilities.

■ DISABILITY AND SPORT: A BRIEF HISTORY

The foundation for modern disability sport is commonly credited to Sir Ludwig Guttmann and his creation of the Stoke Mandeville Games in England in 1948 (Brittain, 2010). Originally designed as a rehabilitation activity for injured military veterans, Sir Guttmann's vision grew into the modern Paralympic Games. Today, just like the Olympic Games, the Paralympics Games bring together top competitors from around the globe to compete in a wide range of team and individual summer and winter sports. And just like the Olympics, Paralympic participants are elite athletes who require specialized training, dedication, and resources in the pursuit of the Olympic dream.

From the first official Paralympic Games held in Rome in 1960 with 400 participants from 23 different countries (Brittain, 2010), the arena for athletes with disabilities has grown exponentially. Most recently over 4,000 athletes from 148 countries competed in 20 sports at the 2008 Summer Games in Beijing (2008 Summer Paralympics, n.d.) and another 500 winter sport athletes representing

44 countries took part in 5 sports at the 2010 Vancouver Games (Paralympic Games Vancouver 2010, n.d.). It has been estimated that over 4,200 will take part in the 480 events comprising the London Paralympic Games in 2012 (Brittain, 2010). For those interested in the full history of the Paralympic Games, Ian Brittain's *The Paralympic Games Explained* (2010) provides an excellent review of the birth and growth of the Paralympic movement through the preparation for the London-based Games in 2012.

The growing number of elite Paralympians presents only the tip of the athlete development iceberg in disability sport. For every athlete named to a Paralympic squad or who meets a qualification standard, there are many talented hopefuls training and preparing in anticipation of earning the next spot on the team. Recognizing this growth potential and increasing interest, many countries are fostering the development of Paralympic sports by creating partnerships between able-bodied sport governing bodies and their Paralympic sport counterparts and encouraging grass-roots and community disability sport programs.

From a sport performance standpoint, talent development, across all performance domains including disability sport, is instrumental to peak athlete development. Current theories of talent development highlight the importance of deliberate practice (Ericsson & Charness, 1994) and systematic, linear, and intentional physical, psychological, technical, and tactical knowledge and skills development (Farrow, Baker, & MacMahon, 2007).

Although several models of intentional development in sport exist, the Canadian Long Term Athlete Development (LTAD) model is one of the most comprehensive and holistic to date. It provides a framework that works for the traditional youth through adulthood talent development concept, as well as for the acquired disability model. Highlighting acknowledgement that athletes are athletes, with similar development needs, the disability sport LTAD model parallels the able-bodied sport pathway by providing a seven-stage road map of sport developmental to guide the training of the beginner through elite performer (Higgs, Balyi, Norris, & Way, 2010). While the disability sport LTAD model does have two additional stages (awareness and first contact) that are not found in the able-bodied LTAD model, these occur only at the foundational level, with the remaining categories emphasizing the similarities in athlete preparation across situations.

◼ DISABILITY AND SPORT TODAY

It has been estimated that 1 in 200 Americans uses a wheelchair (Goosey-Tolfrey, 2010) and, according to the U.S. Census Bureau (2010), 29% of Americans have some degree of disability that interferes with daily living activities and/or learning. Furthermore, the Census Bureau also indicates that there are currently 5.5 million military veterans with a service-related disability. An increasing number of these individuals are discovering or rediscovering sport, with many beginning their journey towards Paralympic competition. Yet, service providers involved in sport environments such as recreational directors, coaches, sport educators, athletic trainers, and sport psychology consultants remain unfamiliar with the opportunities available to individuals with a disability and the opportunities to work with this athlete population.

Due to the depth of possible conditions that might impact how an individual participates in sport, ranging from visual impairment to limb amputation, disability sport utilizes a series of categorization and classification procedures to provide a fair competitive setting (Sherrill, 1999). Similar to the concept of weight classes in wrestling, the type and severity of an athlete's disability is the key factor in determining competitive category to ensure they will compete against others with similar disabilities. The Paralympic Games have five different disability categories including amputee, cerebral palsy, wheelchair, visual impairment, and les autres (a broad category for disabilities that do not fall into another category). In 2010, a sixth category, intellectual disabilities, was reinstated for the London 2012 Games.

In addition to the category of disability, the severity of an athlete's disability, or classification, is an important factor in determining competitive placement. Athlete classification has evolved from systematic assessment of an individual's handicap to a far more positive and performance-focused determination of ability level (Thomas & Smith, 2009). While the classification procedures are dynamic and undergo refinement as needed (Beckman, 2009), the disability sport governing bodies have been striving to develop a uniform and consistent set of procedures that is in the best interests of both the athletes and the fairness of the sporting competition. A detailed explanation of the current classification criteria and procedures can be found on the International Paralympic Movement Website (http://www.paralympic.org/Classification/Introduction).

■ UNDERSTANDING THE ATHLETE

In working with any population, an appreciation and understanding of individual uniqueness is a top priority for developing an effective relationship. Ideally this partnership is neither overshadowed nor influenced by pre-determined notions or by expectations based on a group classification (e.g., age, gender, or disability). This does not mean, however, that generalized knowledge about a group is not valuable. Such information can provide cultural insight, a foundation for realistic expectations, a starting point for understanding, and guidance in problem solving. In the case of high-performance athletes with disabilities, while some studies suggest both similarities and difference between elite able-bodied and disabled athletes (e.g., Martin, 1999; Martin & McCaughtry, 2004), the preponderance of the research to date indicates that the needs and characteristics of Paralympic athletes have not been found to differ significantly from those of their Olympic counterparts (e.g., Dieffenbach, Statler, & Moffett, 2009; Martin, 2010; Page, O'Connor, & Wayda, 2000). Most notably the reasons for participating and the mental approach necessary for pursuing elite competition found among athletes with disabilities are analogous to the findings in the able-bodied sport literature.

In prior explorations into why individuals with disabilities participate in sport, athletes cited a wide range of positive participation benefits, such as improved physical well-being and increased social opportunities, to a positive impact on personal empowerment and self-understanding (e.g., Huang & Brittain, 2006; Martin, Adams-Mushett, & Smith, 1995; Wu & Williams, 2001). Studies examining performance strategies, mood states, and motivation have also reported that both able bodied and disabled athlete groups demonstrate more similarities than differences (e.g., Henschen, Horvat, & Roswal, 1992; Perreault & Vallerand, 2007).

However, while their reasons for participating have been found to be similar to those of their able-bodied counterparts, there is some indication that athletes with disabilities may have a unique perspective regarding their motivation to compete. A 1999 study by Pensgaard and colleagues (1999) examining elite skiers with and without disabilities reported the two groups had similar motivational profiles, although the athletes with disabilities were found to have higher levels of satisfaction with their results and efforts. Another notable motivational difference from the able-bodied sport research reported by this population has been participation to help with post-injury transition (Asken, 1991; Wheeler, Malone, VanVlack, Nelson, & Steadard, 1996).

Researchers have also examined the perceptions of athletes with disabilities in other areas commonly studied in able-bodied sport. These studies have found that athletes with and without disabilities have comparable levels of self-esteem and body image scores (Martin, 2002, 2006a, 2006b, 2008) and levels of athletic identity (Groff & Zabriskie, 2006). Therefore prior research clearly lends credence to the idea that despite the more obvious environmental circumstances, able-bodied and disabled athletes share similar performance needs, characteristics, and benefits.

■ MENTAL SKILLS TRAINING AND PEAK PERFORMANCE

In competition and training at the Paralympic level of sport, both coaches and athletes indicated high value in the use of mental skills, as well as the benefit of working with a sport psychology consultant in preparation for the Paralympic Games (Dieffenbach et al., 2009). Although research suggests that many athletes with disabilities may already be using mental training skills (Perreault &

TABLE 10.1. *Paralympic Coach and Athlete Rankings of Importance of Mental Skills*

Coach Top 12	Athlete Top 12
Confidence	Confidence
Concentration/Focus	Concentration/Focus
Communication Skills	Motivation
Motivation	Strategies to Stay Positive
Strategies to Stay Positive	Relaxation
Team Cohesion	Communication Skills
Imagery/Visualization	Ways to Cope with Adversity
Ways to Cope with Adversity	Team Cohesion
Relaxation	Arousal/Emotional Control
Arousal/Emotional Control	Stress Management Techniques
Stress Management Techniques	Imagery/Visualization
Media Training	Media Training

Vallerand, 2007), research also indicates athletes are interested in learning more about the field and how to apply the skills effectively (e.g., Dieffenbach et al., 2009; Kirkby, 1995). Of the commonly taught mental skill areas, confidence and focus/concentration are consistently ranked as the most important two skills by both coaches and athletes (see Table 10.1), with a multitude of other skills being closely ranked behind them (Dieffenbach et al., 2009). Unfortunately, although both coaches and athletes participating in the 2008 Paralympic Games indicated an interest in working with a sport psychology consultant to learn and improve mental skills in preparation for the Games, not all athletes reported having access to a SPC (Dieffenbach et al., 2009), suggesting that service providers may need to actively seek ways to better connect with these athletes.

■ **COACHES AND PARALYMPIC ATHLETES**

Across all sport outlets, Hanrahan (2007) points out that acknowledgement and understanding of the athlete is central to an effective coach–athlete relationship. In able-bodied sport studies, poor, negative, or improper coach–athlete relationships have been linked to negative athlete experiences as well as poor performance (e.g., Jowett, 2003; Poczwardowski, Barot, & Henschen, 2002). Similarly, negative coaching styles, behaviors, and relationship issues were found to cause stress and inhibit performances among wheelchair basketball players (Campbell & Jones, 1997, 2002) indicating that athletes with disabilities are also like able-bodied athletes with regard to elements that potentially negatively impact performance.

Another area of concern negatively impacting performance and the sport experience for athletes with disabilities is the lack of qualified coaches (e.g., DePauw & Gavron, 1991; DePauw & Gavron, 2005; Martin, 2010). DePauw and Gavron (1991) reported that only 16% of the disability sport coaches they assessed had a disability themselves and, although it is not necessary to have a disability to understand disability, the majority of coaches reported limited exposure to and minimal training with athletes with disabilities prior to working with this population. These findings were echoed in a recent study of elite disability sport which found the majority of Paralympic coaches had little to no disability sport specific training or personal participation experience prior to working with disability based sport. (Dieffenbach et al., 2009). Moreover, limited coaching experience with and knowledge of athletes with disabilities have consistently been identified as factors having detrimental effects on performance (e.g., DePauw, 1994; DePauw & Gavron, 1991; DePauw & Gavron, 2005). Studies exploring how coaches work with athletes with disabilities have suggested that they need to learn strategies to both help athletes build and maintain confidence (Ferreira, Chatzisarantis, Caspar, & Campos, 2007) and to develop coping skills within the sport context (Campbell & Jones, 2002). Based on their research in disability sport, Cregan and colleagues (2007) note the importance of coach–athlete communication for a positive and productive sport collaboration.

▪ BARRIERS TO PARALYMPIC PERFORMANCE

Despite the findings explained above indicating more similarities than differences between able-bodied and disabled athletes, the very nature of performing at an elite level with a disability requires some understanding of potential barriers. Despite the growth of modern disability sport opportunities and increased visibility of athletes with disabilities, one of the largest potential road blocks for talent development among athletes with disabilities is the lack of knowledge among coaches, athletes, and the community at large regarding the opportunities for sport participation (Williams 1994; Rudell & Shinew, 2006). Another major barrier involves lack of adequate resources. Even with the passing of the Americans with Disabilities Act over 20 years ago and the many subsequent legal and cultural "wins" related to increased access, at the elite level, Paralympic athletes and coaches have reported concerns regarding facility accessibility, transportation, and affordable equipment necessary to sustain and facilitate the level of preparation necessary to compete on the elite stage (e.g., Dieffenbach et al., 2009). Ultimately, while "pockets" of disability accessible training environments exist for elite athletes, unlike their able-bodied fellow athletes, many elite training sites remain inaccessible, limiting the access to both top training facilities and support services.

▪ CONCLUSION

Working with high-performance athletes in pursuit of their competitive goals can be a demanding and often high-pressure pursuit. It can be both professionally challenging and rewarding. In the world of elite disability sport and the

Paralympics, athletes have similar motivational sources, and face many of the same preparation needs and skill demands as any other elite athlete. Based on the parallels between these groups, professionals seeking to work with and support athletes with disabilities are advised to use an elite athlete paradigm as a foundation.

Having emphasized the fact that more similarities than differences have been found between disabled and able-bodied athletes, the fact remains that there are a few notable areas unique to disability sport. The areas of difference with the greatest potential for negative impact on performance center on the lack of access. This includes access to important elements for competitive preparation, such as coaches knowledgeable about disability sport in general, as well as training modifications for those with disabilities, and accessible training facilities. While progress is being made, these barriers still present a sizeable problem. Working with these athletes to brainstorm strategies for handling barriers, expanding the pool of knowledgeable coaches, and improving access are key steps forward in working with this population.

■ REFERENCES

2008 Summer Paralympics. (n.d.). 2008 Summer Paralympics Website. Retrieved from www.disabled-world.com/sports/paralympics/2008

Asken, M. J. (1991). The challenge of the physically challenged: Delivering sport psychology services to physically disabled athletes. *Sport Psychologist, 5*, 370–381.

Beckman, E. M. (2009). Towards evidence-based classification in Paralympic athletics: Evaluating the validity of activity limitation tests for use in classification of Paralympic running events. *British Journal of Sports Medicine, 43*, 1067–1072.

Brittain, I. (2010). *The Paralympic Games explained.* London, UK: Routledge.

Campbell, E., & Jones, G. (2002). Sources of stress experienced by elite male wheelchair basketball players. *Adapted Physical Activity Quarterly, 19*, 82–99.

Campbell, E., & Jones, G. (1997). Pre-competition anxiety and self-confidence in wheelchair sport participants. *Adapted Physical Activity Quarterly, 14*, 96–107.

Cregan, K., Bloom, G., & Reid, G. (2007). Career evolution and knowledge of elite coaches of swimmers with a physical disability. *Research Quarterly for Exercise & Sport, 78*, 339–350.

DePauw, K. P. (1994). A feminist perspective on sport and sports organizations for persons with disabilities. In R. D. Steadward, E. R. Nelson, & G. D. Wheeler (Eds.), *VISTA 93—The outlook* (pp. 457–477). Edmonton, AB, Canada: Rick Hansen Centre.

DePauw, K. P., & Gavron, S. J. (2005). *Disability sport* (2nd ed.). Champaign, IL: Human Kinetics.

DePauw, K. P., & Gavron, S. J. (1991). Coaches of athletes with disabilities. *Physical Educator, 48*, 33–40.

Dieffenbach, K., Statler, T., & Moffett, A. (2009). *Pre and post Games perceptions of factors influencing coach and athlete performance at the Beijing Paralympics.* Final report. Colorado Springs, CO: USOC and Paralympic Program.

Ericcson, K. A., & Charness, N. (1994). Expert performance: Its structure and acquisition. *American Psychologist, 49*, 725–747.

Farrow, D., Baker, J., & MacMahon, C. (2007). *Developing sport expertise: Researchers and coaching put theory into practice.* London, UK: Routledge.

Ferreira, J. P., Chatzisarantis N., Caspar, P. M., & Campos, M. J. (2007). Precompetitive anxiety and self-confidence in athletes with disability. *Perceptual Motor Skills, 105,* 339–346.

Goosey-Tolfrey, V. (2010). *Wheelchair sport: A complete guide for athletes, coaches and teachers.* Champaign, IL: Human Kinetics.

Groff, D., & Zabriskie, R. (2006). An exploratory study of athletic identity among elite alpine skiers with physical disabilities: Issues of measurement and design. *Journal of Sport Behavior, 29,* 126–141.

Hanrahan, S. J. (2007). Athletes with disabilities. In G. Tenenbaum & R. C. Eklund (Eds.), *Handbook of sport psychology* (3rd ed., pp. 845–858). Hoboken, NJ: John Wiley.

Henschen, K., Horvat, M., & Roswal, G. (1992). Psychological profiles of the United States wheelchair basketball team. *International Journal of Sport Psychology, 23,* 128–137.

Higgs, C., Balyi, I., Norris, S., & Way, R. (2010). No accidental champions: Long term athlete development for athletes with disabilities. Vancouver, BC, Canada: Canadian Sport Centres.

Huang, C., & Brittain, I. (2006). Negotiating identities through disability sport. *Sociology of Sport Journal, 23,* 352–375.

Jowett, S. (2003). When the honeymoon is over: A case study of a coach–athlete dyad in crisis. *The Sport Psychologist, 17,* 446–462.

Kirkby, R. J. (1995). Wheelchair netball: Motives and attitudes of competitors with and without disabilities. *Australian Psychologist, 30,* 109–112.

Martin, J. J. (2010). Athletes with disabilities. In S. J. Hanrahan & M. B. Anderson (Eds.), *Routledge handbook of applied sport psychology: A comprehensive guide for students and practitioners* (pp. 432–440). London, UK: Routledge.

Martin, J. (2008). Multidimensional self-efficacy and affect in wheelchair basketball players. *Adapted Physical Activity Quarterly, 25,* 275–288.

Martin, J. (2006a). Psychosocial aspects of youth disability sport. *Adapted Physical Activity Quarterly, 23,* 65–77.

Martin, J. (2006b). The self in disability sport and physical activity. In A. P. Prescott (Ed.), *The concept of self in education, family and sports* (pp. 75–89). Hauppauge, NY: Nova Science.

Martin, J. (2002). Training and performance self-efficacy, affect, and performance in wheelchair road racers. *Sport Psychologist, 16,* 384.

Martin, J. (1999). A personal development model of sport psychology for athletes with disabilities. *Journal of Applied Sport Psychology, 11,* 181–193.

Martin, J. J., Adams-Mushett, C., & Smith, K. L. (1995). Athletic identity and sport orientation of adolescent swimmers with disabilities. *Adapted Physical Activity Quarterly, 12,* 113–123.

Martin, J., & McCaughtry, N. (2004). Coping and emotion in disability sport. In D. Lavalle, J. Thatcher, & M. V. Jones (Eds.), *Coping and emotion in sport* (pp. 225–238). Hauppauge, NY: Nova Science.

Page, S., O'Connor, E., & Wayda, V. (2000). Exploring competitive orientation in a group of athletes participating in the 1996 Paralympic trials. *Perceptual and Motor Skills, 91,* 491–502.

Paralympic Games Vancouver. 2010. (n.d.). Official Website of the Paralympic movement. Paralympic Games. Retrieved from https://www.paralympic.org/vancouver-2010

Pensgaard, A., Roberts, G., & Ursin, H. (1999). Motivational factors and coping strategies of Norwegian Paralympic and Olympic winter sport athletes. *Adapted Physical Activity Quarterly, 16,* 238–250.

Perreault, S., & Vallerand, R. (2007). A test of self-determination theory with wheelchair basketball players with and without disability. *Adapted Physical Activity Quarterly, 24,* 305–316.

Poczwardowski, A., Barot, J. E., & Henschen, K. P. (2002). The athlete and coach: Their relationship and its meaning. *International Journal of Sport Psychology, 33,* 116–140.

Rudell, J., & Shinew, K. (2006). The socialization process for women with physical disabilities: The impact of agents and agencies in the introduction to elite sport. *Journal of Leisure Research, 38,* 421–444.

Sherrill, C. (1999). Disability sport and classification theory: A new era. *Adapted Physical Activity Quarterly, 16,* 206–215.

Thomas, N., & Smith, A. (2009). *Disability, sport and society: An introduction.* London, UK: Routledge.

U.S. Census Bureau. (2010). U.S. Census 2010 Website. Retrieved from http://2010.census.gov/2010census

Wheeler, G. D., Malone, L. A., VanVlack, S., Nelson, E. R., & Steadward, R. D. (1996). Retirement from disability sport: A pilot study. *Adapted Physical Activity Quarterly, 13,* 382–399.

Williams, T. (1994). Disability sport socialization and identity construction. *Adapted Physical Activity Quarterly, 11,* 14–31.

Wu, S., & Williams, T. (2001). Factors influencing sport participation among athletes with spinal cord injury. *Medicine & Science in Sports & Exercise, 33,* 177–182.

PART III

Athletes as Role Models

Athletes are role models, whether they like it or not. They are the highly visible pinnacles of success in their field. Unlike accounting or waste management—fields that likely have their own superstars—sports have champions who speak to an incredible number of hearts and minds. Many of us play sports. We have lived our own sagas of glory and defeat, which are made quaint by the epic battles we see on TV. We attempt to mimic the styles and strategies that are only partly responsible for the incredible feats of star athletes. Even those of us who do not play sports recognize that the best athletes are equal parts artist and machine. We all aspire to, or at least appreciate, their greatness. But how best can athletes bear the role-model burden?

As discussed in Part I, the bounds separating the playing field from the rest of life are not solid. The combination of natural talent and effort that an athlete embodies on the field is inextricably part of that person who exists off the field. Psychologically, young fans are not the best at separating the athlete from the person. Can we blame them? Many of the qualities that help make an athlete great—discipline, teamwork, communication, courage, leadership, mental toughness—also help make a great person. In the same way that children and adolescents have difficulty understanding that good parents make mistakes, young people assume the good in-game qualities of athletes imply off-the-field goodness as well. Superstars who make inhuman shots, and are rewarded by society with millions of dollars, understandably become the poster people for acceptable life behavior. Athletes who react to bad calls by cursing at the ref, or who bite the ears of aggressive opponents, or get arrested for DUIs or domestic violence calibrate these choices to the "OK" range of the youth moral barometer.

Just because athletes have this power, does this morally obligate them to use it responsibly? Some who say no to that question argue that parents, and not athletes, are responsible for instilling moral beliefs in their children. Are parents the only ones with this job? What about siblings, teachers, pastors, or politicians? Where do we draw the line? Some also say that athletes are only responsible for excelling in their sports. Are brilliant plays and helping your team win the only requirements for sports stars? What about exhibiting respect and tolerance? Abusive and dangerous behavior either on the field or off it is morally problematic because these actions directly harm people. But these behaviors may also influence others to act in similarly harmful ways. Do we have an ethical duty to prevent negative influence? When athletes sign their first professional contracts, should there be a written or verbal clause that explains they are signing up to be role models?

As Lynch, Adair, and Jonson point out in chaper 11, being a positive role model might be a uniquely difficult task for some professional athletes. It is hard to understand how athletes who participate in aggressive sports can compartmentalize the brutal behaviors sanctioned on the field, isolating them from the rest of life where these behaviors are unacceptable. While we cannot forgive football players or MMA fighters when they abuse other people off the field or outside the ring, some say it is logical and likely that they would transgress in this way. However, not all or even most aggressive sport athletes make bad life choices, and there are certainly some athletes from less aggressive sports who do. If we decide that athletes have a responsibility to be good role models, it does not appear impossible for athletes from any sport to take up the mantle.

Parents and other direct influences have the greatest responsibility for shaping the attitudes and behaviors of their children. Athletes who impress questionable ideas of right and wrong on young fans make those parents' jobs harder. Athletes are on the values-imparting team. It is likely that the most efficient and effective path to virtuous young people, and to a future of both respectful players and astonishing plays, is carved by an upstanding team that includes both parents and pro athletes.

11 Professional Athletes and Their Duty to Be Role Models

■ SANDRA LYNCH, DARYL ADAIR, AND PAUL JONSON

■ INTRODUCTION

It is widely claimed or assumed that professional athletes are (or should be) role models for sports fans (particularly young people who look up to them). These expectations involve questions of athlete responsibility that are underpinned by ethical principles and associated with assumptions about the conduct of public sporting figures. These are complex issues, partly because the concepts of athleticism, sport and play are interrelated within a network of meanings; in some respects they share meanings and in other respects their meanings differ. As we shall argue, variance in their meanings draws attention to different and somewhat contradictory values that complicate ethical reasoning in the context of sport, and create confusion or ambivalence in relation to what can be expected of professional athletes, both 'on and off the field'. Player codes of conduct attempt to ensure that professional athletes do not behave in ways that bring the game they play into disrepute, but the language used in these codes is typically very general and consequently the clauses of these codes are open to interpretation.

This chapter explores a set of factors relevant to a consideration of the intuition or demand that professional athletes have a duty to be role models both 'on and off the field'. It begins by exploring responses to the expectations associated with this demand and then investigates tensions implicit in requirements that professional athletes accept the designation of role model. The second section of the chapter considers understandings of sport from an ethical perspective and its relationship to professionalism. Its aim is to examine the extent to which the ethical imperatives associated with sport can be upheld or undermined within the context of professional sport. Finally, the third section explores a complex range of issues to be taken into account in any attempt to justify the idea that professional athletes should accept the designation of role model.

■ ROLE MODELLING: EXPECTATIONS AND INTUITIONS

Both the media and the academic literature (Wilson, Stavros, & Westberg, 2008) regularly alert us to the transgressions of professional athletes on and off the field and to the negative repercussions of such behaviour for players, their colleagues, clubs, organisations or other stakeholders. A recent weekend newspaper report provides a typical illustration referring to the previous week as one in which 'yet another slew of NRL [National Rugby League] footballers' misadventures with alcohol seeped through the headlines'; and in which 'the players' role model status and their apparent habitual problems with alcohol' focus attention on concerns about the players' personal irresponsibility (Murphy, 2013). However, calls to professional athletes to recognise their alleged obligations as role models for younger players within their sports are sometimes rebuffed by the athletes themselves. For example, in 1993 Charles Barkley, a US National Basketball Association player, famously said: 'I'm not a role model. . . . [T]he ability to run and dunk a basketball should not make you God Almighty. There are a million guys in jail who can play ball. Should they be role models? Of course not; . . . Just because I dunk a basketball doesn't mean I should raise your kids' (Wellman, 2003, p. 332).

This is a somewhat hyperbolic position, given that the suggestion is that Barkley ought to accept the designation of role model, rather than that he ought to take on the rearing of other people's children. However, he is not alone in his view. Phil Gould, the General Manager of an Australian Rugby League Football Club and a former professional coach and player, recently commented in the following terms about the responsibility of those involved in the professional game.

> What about parents taking responsibility for the education of their own kids, instead of demanding rugby league set the standard for socially acceptable behaviour? If the school principal doesn't like what he sees on TV, then he should tell the students why he won't tolerate it in his school. What makes you think the game should have to pull in its horns to educate your students? And why do our game's leaders so meekly give in to these complaints? (Gould, 2013)

Gould's comments appear to reject the notion that professional football players should be expected to be role models; moreover, Barkley's statement identifies an uncontentious minimalist approach which implies that role models ought to be chosen from among the cohort of law-abiding citizens. The implication, therefore, is that a person's athletic talent is distinct from his/her status as a law-abiding citizen as illustrated by the fact that convicted felons ought not be seen as role models regardless of their competence on a basketball court.

In making a distinction between being a talented athlete and being a law-abiding citizen or failing to be a law-abiding citizen, Barkley misses the main point motivating the common intuition that professional athletes have a responsibility to behave as role models for their young fans—if not for the community in general. That point is not contingent on the fact of Barkley's talent—although such talent and the dedication necessary to develop it are admirable and inspiring. Rather, the point underpinning the common intuition relies on the fact of what Barkley's talent has made possible for him. His talent has enabled him to play basketball professionally, to make his living in this way and to gain public attention. The response of Karl Malone (an NBA colleague of Barkley's) to Barkley's claim deals with these issues, associating the call to be a role model with notions of choice and responsibility.

> Charles, you can deny being a role model all you want, but I don't think it's your decision to make. We don't choose to be role models, we are chosen. Our only choice is whether to be a good role model or a bad one. I don't think we can accept all the glory and the money that comes with being a famous athlete and not accept the responsibility of being a role model, of knowing that kids and even some adults are watching us and looking for us to set an example. I mean, why do we get endorsements in the first place? Because there are people who will follow our lead and buy a certain sneaker or cereal because we use it. (Malone, 1993)

Christopher Wellman's response to Barkley's claims supports Malone's approach. Wellman argues that our responsibilities towards others fall into at least three categories: the first identifies presumed social responsibilities to others generally, for example normative responsibilities not to lie, cheat or harm others; the second identifies our special responsibilities to those others with whom we are in particular relationships (e.g. our children, our clients, our employers, our patients or our students); and the third deals with responsibilities we acquire by virtue of our capacities. Wellman appears to assume that because of their 'on-field' capacities professional athletes also acquire responsibilities to take the moral 'high road' by comparison with the average person who lacks these capacities. However, this point does not take account of the necessary connection between the professional athletes' capacities and their high public profiles. Wellman argues that many of those who admire professional athletes' talents and capacities are likely to take their cues from those athletes in contexts other than sport (Wellman, 2003). We might challenge the claim that professional athletes are obliged to act as role models solely because their admirers take behavioural cues from them; that challenge might be made on the basis of the (admittedly contentious) assumption that fans have a choice as to whether or not they do this. But the broader question, of whether professional athletes have an obligation to act as role models because others have that expectation of them, remains. Karl Malone's position is simply to acknowledge that it is a matter of fact that 'there are people who will follow our [the professional athletes'] lead and buy a certain sneaker or cereal because we use it'; and then to argue that if a professional athlete accepts the glory and the money associated with being a famous athlete, endorsements being one aspect of this fame, then that athlete must accept the responsibility for being a role model.

Malone's position raises questions for the individual professional athlete of fairness and responsibility in relation to the benefits associated with role of professional athlete and the connection with social expectations to be a role model.

The extant scholarly literature is ambivalent as to conclusions on the question of the nature, scope and relevance of professional athletes as role models, especially in terms of their lives off the field (Fleming, Hardman, Jones, & Sheridan, 2005; Hahn, 2010; Lines, 2001). But there are evident tensions between the values definitive of living the life of a professional athlete and the values we associate with living an ethically defensible and virtuous life in general. There is evidence that some professional sportspeople attempt to quarantine the values implicit in living life well—the set of values that we take to be shared by members of a civilised society and which theorists such as Mary Gentile identify as honesty, respect, responsibility, fairness and compassion (Gentile, 2010)—from their lives as professional athletes. US heavy weight boxing champion Larry Holmes claimed in a *60 Minutes* interview that 'to be good in sports, you have to be bad'. Holmes claims that he deliberately adopts an aggressive attitude towards his opponent when he enters the ring, one which is at odds with his usual behaviour. 'I have to change, I have to leave the goodness out and bring out all the bad ... like Dr. Jekyll and Mr. Hyde' (Boxhill, 2003, p. 217). Bredemeier, Shields, and Horn (2003) discuss other examples of competing moralities in sport by comparison with everyday life. Comments such as that made by Steve Finnane, an Australian Rugby Union prop who broke the jaw of an opponent in a match against Wales in 1978, also suggest the adoption of an 'on-field' attitude which is at odds with 'off-field' behaviour: 'I regret breaking his jaw. Terrible. But I don't regret hitting him. I think anyone regrets hurting someone in a match. Afterwards *you like to think* it's all over' (Fishman, 1985, emphasis added).

On the face of it, we might question whether the acceptance of what might appear to be aggressive 'on-field' or 'in-the-ring' behaviour is consistent with the notion of the professional athlete as a role model in wider society. The comments of Holmes and Finnane suggest that attitudes to aggression in sport are ambivalent or at least unclear. Accidents do occur during robust physical contact as players legitimately attempt to assert their dominance over one another; at the same time, aggression is regarded by some as an integral part of professional sport. Holmes' comments suggest this, as do further comments made by Phil Gould:

> How can anyone think that sanitising a product built on all-out aggression will improve its appeal? This is poor analysis. I don't know where we draw the line. I just fear that the rugby league game our administrators are leading us towards could become a game that eventually loses its appeal. (Gould, 2013)

Aggression's role in sport will be discussed below, but this discussion will firstly focus on the ambivalence or confusion about morality which is manifest within the context of play and sport, and which attitudes to aggression illustrate. Some theorists attribute the source of this confusion to a failure to distinguish between sport, play and ancient notions of athleticism and the consequent (mistaken) assumption that a single set of ethical imperatives relating to sport might apply in different contexts (Keating, 2003). It is our view that there are ambiguities about values and ethical imperatives within sport, which when investigated have implications for our understanding of the concept of the role model. In particular, these ambiguities have implications for codes of ethics and sporting contracts which attempt to enforce a code of behaviour for professional athletes that applies to 'off-field' behaviour, while also addressing the constitutive and regulatory rules associated with 'on-field' behaviour.

■ THE VALUES IMPLICIT IN SPORT AND ATHLETICS

This section explores the meanings that have been and are attached to the terms 'sport' and 'athletics' and examines the connections between sport and play in order to establish how the expectations associated with these activities interact with one another and how they might affect our expectations of professional athletes. The *Oxford English Dictionary* defines sport as a 'diversion, entertainment, or fun; a pastime', although it recognises that this definition is somewhat archaic (OED online, 2013a). Sport is also defined as 'an activity involving physical exertion and skill in which an individual or team competes against another or others for entertainment.' These definitions encompass notions of fun, play and recreation as well as notions of competition and physical exertion. However, the Australian Sports Foundation specifically precludes from its definition of sport activities which are purely recreational or whose purpose relates primarily to social activity or entertainment; rather, sport is defined as 'a human activity capable of achieving a result requiring physical exertion and/or physical skill, which, by its nature and organisation, is competitive' (Australian Sports Foundation [ASF], 2013). Keating (2003) points out that the moral attitude appropriate to sport—that of sportsmanship (or sports-womanship)—is often broadened to a notion of moral excellence more generally (an all-encompassing moral category). He acknowledges that the notion is sometimes associated with a moral minimum which includes the detailing of penalties for assaults or threats to officials by players or fans. But he emphasises that sport in some contexts is also associated with a kind of diversion (from the serious side of life) and is dominated by a spirit of moderation and generosity. Keating appears to have in mind parklands sport or sport dominated by Corinthian ideals, rather than professional, competitive sport. When compared with the comments of Holmes, Kinnane and Gould (above) making a connection between sport and characteristics or social values applicable to living well generally indicates a disparity in the use of the term 'sport' in these different contexts due to the ambivalence or ambiguity to which this chapter draws attention.

By comparison, athletics is defined in the *Oxford English Dictionary* as 'the practice of physical exercises by which muscular strength is called into play and increased' (OED online, 2013b); the athlete is defined as 'a competitor in the physical exercises—such as running, leaping, boxing, wrestling'—[exercises] that formed part of the public games in ancient Greece and Rome' (OED online, 2013c). Keating argues for a clear distinction between athletics as a competitive activity for which the prize awarded to the victor is the *raison d'être* of the activity, and sport as an activity engaged in for pleasure (Keating, 2003, pp. 65–66)—if not for its own sake. Certainly, Keating's comments generally reflect historical understandings of the athletic ideal which centre upon assumptions about manliness, physicality and aggressive competition (Dunning, 1990). The Ancient Greek athlete as exemplar was an avowedly masculine figure and the feats of athletes at the early Olympics exemplified male power and the subjugation of women. Athletes competed at the Olympic Games in the hope of pleasing the Gods (the most powerful of whom were male) and of bringing glory to themselves and the towns they represented. They also participated in the hope of financial or in-kind rewards. Thus on the ancient conception, athletics is essentially a competitive activity with religious overtones, aimed at victory in a contest between men and characterised by values of perseverance and self-sacrifice (Kidd, 2013; Young, 1984).

However, the notion of the prizes for achievement is at stark odds with the so-called revival of the modern Olympic Games, which were devoted to the 19th century code of amateurism, to its rejection of pecuniary interest, any extrinsic reward and religiosity (Kidd, 2013; Young, 1984). The modern or 19th-century Olympic ideal regarded amateur sport as a form of play; financial reward for taking part in sport was rejected since it made the playing field a type of workplace. Fundamentally, an amateur athlete was thought to have a strong sense of fair play and, since he (*sic*) competed in sport for its own sake rather than for material reward, he represented the ideal of an athletic gentleman (Allison, 2001; Vamplew, 1988b). Nonetheless, a common misconception of the congruence between the ancient and modern Olympic ideals persists, despite the fact that '[t]he true aims of the athletes in ancient Greece were rewards and life-long appointments to various positions in the military or the city administration' (Menenakos et al., 2005, p. 1348).

Menenakos et al. (2005) go on to argue that the Olympic idealism dominating modern athletic culture is in fact a myth and the interaction between that myth and the rise of professional sport conceals a process that begins to undermine the distinction between athletics and sport which Keating defends. In Victorian England when sports like rugby and rowing were first codified, they were taken to have a civilising and character building effect on young boys and were associated with a wider movement referred to as 'muscular Christianity'. This movement valued the development through sport of both a strong body and a powerful mind for young men who were to become leaders (Mangan, 1981). However, the adoption of various organised sports in the Victorian era had unintended consequences; sports became popularised—particularly among the working classes— and were sometimes associated with payment of players and with wagering.

Since both professionalism and gambling were deemed to contradict the intrinsic character-building purposes of the sports, their emergence in sport was challenged by the force of the amateur ideology (Holt, 1989; Vamplew, 1988a). From the perspective of the amateur code, if a player could be paid to win he could also be paid to lose. However, the last quarter of the 20th century clearly illustrated the challenge that professionalism and gambling presented as they escalated the decline of the power of the amateur ideal in elite-level sport. Professionalism and gambling in modern sport in fact suggest that professional sport has more in common with the ancient ideal of athletics—given the fierce competition and financial reward involved—than it has with the modern Olympic ideal or with Keating's notions of sport as an activity engaged in for pleasure and for its own sake. The pervasiveness of aggression in much professional sport is one point of similarity. It is also worth noting that competition for rewards in some ancient athletic events (e.g. boxing, wrestling and pankration) involved significant aggression and violence leading to physical trauma and, on some occasions, death. Again, this is in profound contrast to the modern Olympic Games, where physical clashes in contact sports have undergone what Elias and Dunning have described as a 'civilising process' (Elias & Dunning, 1986). Our argument here is that it is worth noting the similarities between professional sport and ancient athleticism firstly in relation to the place of competition, material reward and aggression; and secondly in relation to the appeal and force of athletic excellence which leads to public admiration and adulation of athletes.

Rules against professionalism were removed from the Olympic charter in 1986, though some sports—such as boxing—chose to quarantine the Olympic Games for amateur boxers. Tennis had already gone 'open' in the late 1960s, international cricketers were full-time professionals by the mid-1970s, and rugby union eventually succumbed to professionalism in the mid-1990s (Allison, 2001). This coincided with the expansion of television and, crucially, with live broadcasting—all of which added to exposure and to the commercial value of the sports as products. Athletes were now paid handsomely as both sports performers and media entertainers (Whannel, 1992) and their appeal to the general public was obvious. Ideals of 'civilising' participation in sport for its own sake became overshadowed by the quest for excellence and its associated rewards (Strenk, 1979); and this helps to explain Keating's claims (2003) that the essential distinction between sport and athletics is invariably ignored today. Professional sports-people have much in common with ancient athletes and the features of both begin to affect or 'infect' modern notions of sport in general.

Like Keating, Reid (2002) challenges this kind of infection by emphasising notions of sport as play, as a diversion from the demands of the serious, practical pursuits of everyday life and as entirely distinct from any form of professional-ism. Reid argues that:

> In fact, sport is only possible as long as the contestants decide to *view* it as play. We create sport and attribute meaning to otherwise meaningless activities. Why else jump things you could go around, why flip on a balance beam . . . why flip at all?
>
> We even create sports like mountain-climbing, in which participants purposely risk their lives. It's hard for many to see anything playful about that. But just as sport may be a metaphor for life, so it may be a way to confront death – to tap it on the forehead and run back to life – before the game is truly over. There's a sense in which risking life forces us to take responsibility for our lives. (2002, p. 78)

Clearly, as Reid's comments emphasise, this definition of sport cannot be applied to professional sports people. Sport may well be best understood by analogy with Wittgenstein's notion of a 'family resemblance' concept. Such concepts, as Davis (2002) explains, 'are like equilibria that contain discordant elements' (pp. 139–140); their generality is produced out of the overlapping and criss-crossing senses in which that concept has come to be used in society, so that no single or essential meaning is shared by all uses of the concept. On this view, sport can be seen as a phenomenon created to serve different social pur-poses and involving different expectations. The use of the term 'sport' in the professional arena differs from its use in recreational and other contexts because it serves different purposes. Suits (1988) appears to take a Wittgensteinian ap-proach when he distinguishes between the concepts of play, game and sport by means of using three overlapping circles. Professional athletes cannot view their careers as play. This is partly, as Reid's comments imply, because play requires a particular kind of intentionality—a recognition that when we are playing our activity is non-serious, that it is purposeful but also without particular pur-pose (Bateson, 1972; Huizinga, 1950). Twenty-first century professional athletes survive—in terms of their value—by what they achieve in the sporting arena and to the extent that they satisfy their professional and contractual obligations. Their activity is serious for them and has a definite and particular purpose. At the same time, cultural assumptions persist about the intrinsic value of sport from an ethical perspective, about its contribution to the development of traits and virtues that are constitutive of living life well and about its connections with play. Interplay inevitably occurs between these cultural assumptions about sport and understandings of professional sport. This interplay leads to confu-sion or ambivalence about the ethical values which ought to guide the profes-sional athlete. Given the demand that the goal of the professional athlete is to win and to achieve the extrinsic rewards associated with winning, ambivalence about the role of aggression in professional sport should not be unexpected. Consequently, disagreement about the expectations of professional athletes as role models is also to be expected.

■ ETHICAL REASONING IN SPORT

The difficulty of distinguishing the ethical ideals associated with sport from the ideals of athleticism and the characteristics and dispositions regarded as necessary to the professional athlete has led some theorists to investigate the kind of reasoning which is typical within the sporting arena. Bredemeier and Shields (1994) argue that a transformed notion of reasoning—what they refer to as 'game reasoning'—occurs in sport. Their research compared the performance of 50 US college students, both athletes (basketball players) and non-athletes, in relation to reasoning about standard moral dilemmas. They found discrepancies in performance in that the non-athletes' moral reasoning was evaluated as more mature than that of the athletes; and further, the athletes' reasoning in response to sport-specific dilemmas was less mature or adequate than their corresponding reasoning about everyday life (1994). On the view of Bredemeier and Shields (1994), mature moral action is marked by a focus on relational responsibility—that is, on equalising the obligations and benefits in one's various relationships. By comparison, sport is generally characterised by a greater degree of personal freedom, by a lessening of relational responsibility and by more egocentric moral thinking. The researchers explain these discrepancies by arguing that sport is somehow 'set apart' or bracketed from everyday life; the concept of 'bracketed morality' in reasoning within sport has been supported in previous research by Bredemeier and Shields (1986a, 1986b). Bredemeier and Shields argue that unlike everyday life, sport allows participants to focus narrowly on performance and to largely set aside other concerns. Moral issues do arise in sport, but participants are appropriately and legitimately acting egocentrically in this context. Sport is taken to involve a transformation of cognition and affect and hence the egoistic change that moral reasoning undergoes when one moves from everyday life into sport is generally regarded as legitimate by players and observers.

The researchers argue that this change occurs partly because moral authority in sport is by design externalised and placed in the hands of officials; and partly because moral issues of fairness and protection are already presupposed within the concept of sport. But they also argue that the morality of sport is inevitably characterised by a certain leniency. Reid notes that 'it's hard to imagine sports without deception, fouls, and incessant attempts to get away with something' (2002, p. 186) and this may explain the attribution of leniency; but as Reid also points out, sports consist of rules and hence there is a quandary here as to how we discern when rule-breaking actually threatens the game and when leniency is appropriate on the field.

While one might reasonably challenge the extent to which data about competent college athletes can be applied to professional athletes, the comments of Holmes, Kinnane and Gould (above) might recommend consideration of the applicability of the data to professional athletes. The focus of this chapter is not on the nature of moral reasoning in sport; however, the research of Bredemeier and Shields suggests that defending the intuition that professional athletes have a duty to be role models both within and beyond the sporting context will be a more complex matter than distinguishing the nature of various types of ethical responsibility, as Wellman (above) has done. The 'on-field' context is itself the site of moral dilemmas, while both 'on and off-field' contexts are complicated by the interplay we have identified in understandings of sport and ideals of athleticism. The consequent confusion that arises in relation to our expectations of professional athletes gives some support to two related claims: firstly, that competing moralities exist in sport in general and in the professional context; and secondly, that given these competing moralities, explaining the relationship between the values attached to living well 'off-field' in everyday life and the values attached to living well as a professional athlete is not a straightforward process.

The question of articulating the ethical responsibilities of professional footballers as role models 'off-field' is particularly problematic, given that the contracts of employment they are required to sign can unrealistically imply that those responsibilities need not be limited. Such contracts usually require the athlete to behave in a manner that will not bring the sport into disrepute and to observe the association's code of conduct. The code will include rules of behaviour that the athlete must observe both on the field (the constitutive and regulatory rules of the sport) and off the field. It will also contain reference to the sanctions that will ensue if there is proven breach.

A typical example of such contractual rules and codes is that of the arrangements made with Australian Rugby Union (ARU) in consultation with the Rugby Union Players Association (RUPA) and that form part of the Collective Bargaining Agreement between the ARU and RUPA. ARU contracts generally require that all participants in the game are bound:

> to promote the reputation of the game and to take all reasonable steps to prevent the game from being brought into disrepute . . . not to conduct themselves in any manner, or engage in any activity, whether on or off the field, that would impair public confidence in the honest and orderly conduct of matches and competitions or in the integrity and good character of participants . . . and not to do anything which adversely affects or reflects on or discredits the game, the ARU, any Member Union or Affiliated Union of the ARU, or any squad, team, competition, tournament, sponsor, official supplier or licensee, including, but not limited to, any illegal act or any act of dishonesty or fraud. (Australian Rugby Union [ARU], 2013)

What is immediately evident is the generality of the language in these clauses, which refer to '*anything* which adversely affects or reflects on or discredits the game, the ARU . . .'; to taking '*all reasonable* steps to prevent the game from being brought into disrepute'; and to protecting 'the *integrity and good character* of participants'.

These legal devices are powerful because of both their generality and their breadth of scope. What is of particular interest is that they not only relate to 'off-field' behaviour but they in effect allow a sporting association (the ARU in this case) to sanction *all* behaviour by an athlete, whether or not it is illegal and whether or not it relates to the sport. The ARU is no doubt justifiably concerned with the extent to which infringement of these clauses might cause reputational damage to the game and impact upon its viability as a sport and as a commercial enterprise. However, from the perspective of the professional athlete bound by this contract, the demand would suggest not that the professional Rugby Union players have an ethical responsibility to behave as moral exemplars, but that they have a contractual obligation to do so. Of course, there is an ethical imperative to honour a contract. But the ARU contract measures the reality of the threat which the action of a particular footballer might pose to the game in terms of the perception of loss to the sporting association and the sport, rather than in terms of a commitment to particular ethical standards or to what can realistically be expected of professional athletes from an ethical perspective.

In fact, competing ethical imperatives might suggest that a professional athlete's right to free agency is limited by extremely general but restrictive contracts. This is so despite the fact that athletes are (theoretically) free to refuse to sign such contracts; and despite the fact that sporting associations and the community in general are right to be critical of unethical behaviour on the part of revered and well-remunerated professional athletes. However, there is room for questioning the reasonableness of some of the demands made of professional athletes, for recognition of the complexity of ethical decision-making in the context of sport and for attention to be focussed on alerting professional athletes to that complexity. Part of that process ought to involve providing training to assist professional athletes developing an appreciation of the contentious nature of ethical responsibility in the context of sport; secondly, in critically reflecting on their own patterns of ethical reasoning and thirdly, in learning to defend, articulate and act on their own values. This is an area for further research, as are the questions of the genesis and reasonableness of the demands made of professional athletes to act as role models.

■ CONCLUSION

The literature and media commentary indicate some confusion or ambiguity about the nature of the ethical demands which attach to sport, given the different contexts in which sport is played, its association with play and the different ways in which the concept of 'sport' is used and has been used in the past. As a consequence the claim that professional athletes have a special obligation to act as role models for their fans and the community more generally is a matter of debate and disagreement. This chapter argues that disagreement is to be expected because the meanings attached to sport overlap and interconnect, and in some cases conflict. Deciding whether or not professional athletes should accept and respond to the designation of role model, both within the sporting arena but beyond it, requires a recognition of the complex nature of sport and of the obligations that can be taken to attach to its different forms. Further research to examine claims in the literature that competing imperatives might have an impact on the nature of athletes' capacity for ethical reasoning would provide clarity. Effective ethical decision-making in this context must be founded on recognising the competing imperatives associated with sport in different contexts; but it must also recognise the rights of professional athletes, their preparedness to respond to ethical demands and the responsibilities of those who contract them to play in assisting them.

▪ REFERENCES

Allison, L. (2001). *Amateurism in sport: An analysis and a defence.* London: Frank Cass.

Australian Rugby Union. (2013). *Code of conduct by-laws.* Retrieved from http://www.rugby.com.au/LinkClick.aspx?fileticket=3cJMoqgJdXg%3d&tabid=1968

Australian Sports Foundation. (2013). *Definition of sport.* Retrieved from http://asf.org.au/who/definition_of_sport

Bateson, G. (1972). *Steps to an ecology of mind: Collected essays in anthropology, psychiatry, evolution, and epistemology.* San Francisco, CA: Chandler Publishing Company.

Boxhill, J. (Ed.). (2003). *Sports ethics: An anthology.* Malden, MA: Blackwell Publishing.

Bredemeier, B. J. L., & Shields, D. L. L. (1994). Applied ethics and moral reasoning in sport. In J. R. Rest & D. Narváez (Eds.), *Moral development in the professions: Psychology and applied ethics* (pp. 173–188). Hillsdale, NJ: Lawrence Erlbaum Associates.

Bredemeier, B. J., & Shields, D. L. (1986a). Game reasoning and interactional morality. *The Journal of Genetic Psychology, 147,* 257–275. doi:10.1080/00221325.1986.9914499

Bredemeier, B. J., & Shields, D. L. (1986b). Athletic aggression: An issue of contextual morality. *Sociology of Sport Journal, 3,* 15–28.

Bredemeier, B. J., Shields, D. L., & Horn, J. C. (2003). Values and violence in sports today: The moral reasoning athletes use in their games and in their lives. In J. Boxhill (Ed.), *Sports ethics: An anthology* (pp. 217–220). Malden, MA: Blackwell Publishing.

Davis, J. (2002). A Marxist influence on Wittgenstein via Sraffa. In G. Kitching & N. Pleasants (Eds.), *Marx and Wittgenstein* (pp. 131–143). New York: Routledge.

Dunning, E. (1990). Sociological reflections on sport, violence and civilization. *International Review for the Sociology of Sport, 25*(1), 65–81.

Elias, N., & Dunning, E. (1986). *Quest for excitement: Sport and leisure in the civilizing process.* Oxford: Blackwell.

Fishman, R. (1985, October 24). Organised mayhem: It's all in the game. *Sydney Morning Herald.* Retrieved from http://news.google.com/newspapers?nid=1301&dat=1985102 4&id=eDZWAAAAIBAJ&sjid=KugDAAAAIBAJ&pg=3858,6192462

Fleming, S., Hardman, A., Jones, C., & Sheridan, H. (2005). 'Role models' among elite young male rugby league players in Britain. *European Physical Education Review, 11*(1), 51–70.

Gentile, M. (2010). *Giving voice to values: How to speak your mind when you know what's right.* New Haven, CT: Yale University Press.

Gould, P. (2013). Gould: Rugby League likely to take a big hit. Retrieved from http://www. stuff.co.nz/sport/opinion/8915933/Gould-Rugby-league-likely-to-take-a-big-hit

Hahn, K. L. (2010). *Are athletes good role models?* Detroit, MI: Greenhaven Press.

Holt, R. (1989). *Sport and the British: A modern history.* Oxford: Oxford University Press.

Huizinga, J. (1950[1938]). *Homo ludens: A study of the play-element in culture.* London: Routledge & Kegan Paul.

Keating, J. (2003). Sportsmanship as a moral category. In J. Boxhill (Ed.), *Sports ethics: An Anthology* (pp. 63–71). Malden, MA: Blackwell Publishing.

Kidd, B. (2013). The myth of the ancient games. *Sport in Society, 16*(4), 416–424.

Lines, G. (2001). Villains, fools or heroes? Sports stars as role models for young people. *Leisure Studies, 20*(4), 285–303.

Malone, K. (1993, June 14). One role model to another. *Sports Illustrated.* Retrieved from http://sportsillustrated.cnn.com/vault/article/magazine/MAG1138690/

Mangan, J. A. (1981). *Athleticism in the Victorian and Edwardian public school: The emergence and consolidation of an educational ideology.* Cambridge: Cambridge University Press.

Menenakos, E., Alexakis, N., Leandros, E., Laskaratos, G., Nikiteas, N., Bramis, J., & Fingerhut, A. (2005). Fatal chest injury with lung evisceration during athletic games in Ancient Greece. *World Journal of Surgery, 29*(10), 1348–1351.

Murphy, D. (2013, June 22–23). News review. *Sydney Morning Herald.*

OED online. (2013a). *Sport.* Oxford: Oxford University Press. Retrieved from http://www. oed.com/view/Entry/187476?rskey=IqdWFA&result=1&isAdvanced=false#eid

OED online. (2013b). *Athletics.* Oxford: Oxford University Press. Retrieved from http:// www.oed.com/view/Entry/12495?redirectedFrom=Athletics#eid

OED online. (2013c). *Athlete.* Oxford: Oxford University Press. Retrieved from http:// www.oed.com/view/Entry/12489?redirectedFrom=athlete#eid

Reid, H. L. (2002). *The philosophical athlete.* Durham, NC: Carolina Academic Press.

Strenk, A. (1979). What price victory? The world of international sports and politics. *The ANNALS of the American Academy of Political and Social Science, 445*(1), 128–140.

Suits, B. (1988). Tricky triad: Games, play, and sport. *Journal of the Philosophy of Sport, 15*(1), 1–9.

Vamplew, W. (1988a). Sport and industrialisation: An economic interpretation of the changes in popular sport in nineteenth-century England. In J. A. Mangan (Ed.), *Pleasure, profit, proselytism: British culture and sport at home and abroad, 1700–1914* (pp. 7–20). London: Routledge.

Vamplew, W. (1988b). *Pay up and play the game: Professional sport in Britain, 1875–1914.* Cambridge: Cambridge University Press.

Wellman, C. (2003). Do celebrated athletes have special responsibilities to be good role models? An imagined dialog between Charles Barkley and Karl Malone. In J. Boxill (Ed.), *Sports ethics: An Anthology* (pp. 333–336). Malden, MA: Blackwell Publishing.

Whannel, G. (1992). *Fields in vision: Television sport and cultural transformation.* London: Routledge.

Wilson, B., Stavros, C., & Westberg, K. (2008). Player transgressions and the management of the sport sponsor relationship. *Public Relations Review, 34,* 99–107.

Young, D. (1984). *The Olympic myth of Greek amateur athletics.* Philadelphia, PA: Ares.

12 An Exploratory Study of Professional Black Male Athletes' Individual Social Responsibility (ISR)

■ KWAME AGYEMANG AND
JOHN N. SINGER

■ INTRODUCTION

Present-day professional Black male athletes in the American context, in comparison to their predecessors of the Civil Rights Movement, do not confront, for the most part, the harsh realities that Black people faced on a daily basis during that time period. For instance, overt forms of racism, including physical and verbal abuse and outright denial of resources and opportunities (Agyemang, Singer, & DeLorme, 2010). In contrast, today's professional Black male athlete (due in large part to the efforts of their predecessors) enjoys multimillion dollar contracts with sport organizations and sponsors, the media spotlight, a comfortable standard of living, and celebrity status (Powell, 2008). Speaking on the ascent of professional Black male athletes, Rhoden (2006) typified the current status of this once overtly marginalized group with the following assertion:

> Black faces and black bodies are used to sell everything from clothing to deodorant and soft drinks. Their gestures, colorful language, and overall style are used by Madison Avenue to project the feel and fashion of inner-city America to an eager global marketplace—they're the stealth of ambassadors of hip-hop culture and capitalism, bridges between the "street" and the mainstream. (p. 1)

This is a lush life that many others would arguably covet, perhaps, but there are certainly other aspects and responsibilities that envious parties may not be so keen to uphold. For instance, while it may appear present-day professional Black male athletes have little to no responsibility outside the context of their sport; the current era subjects these individuals to intense media scrutiny and extensive pressure to act in a socially responsible manner, which most likely results from their current idol-like status. Furthermore, stakeholder cynicism is arguably at its peak, with transgressions involving Kobe Bryant (alleged sexual assault), Ron Artest and Ben Wallace ("Malice at the Palace" fight), Plaxico Burress (shooting himself in nightclub), and Michael Vick (imprisoned for dog fighting), among others, tainting the image of all professional Black male athletes. One commentator even went as far as describing professional Black male athletes as "high-salaried, drug-sniffing black guys" (Hughes, 2004, p. 164).

More recently, a few well-known, prominent Black journalists and authors called on professional Black male athletes to respond to the scrutiny and heightened pressure by illustrating socially responsible behavior (e.g., Powell, 2008; Rhoden, 2006; Roach, 2002). In view of this, these authors argue that professional Black male athletes have failed at being responsible. There is also the presumption that Black male athletes immensely shape the minds of younger generations of Blacks (Sailes, 1986), thus providing more impetus for this population of men to be socially responsible. It begets the question as to what a socially responsible role entails and if they owe a responsibility to society (e.g., Charles Barkley once said he was not a role model). From a research perspective, this issue remains unexplored. This led us to the following research question: (1) how does one view the individual social responsibility (ISR) of professional Black male athletes as a social group? To that end, the purpose of this study was to qualitatively explore the notion of ISR of professional Black male athletes by giving voice to Black male employees of a National Basketball Association (NBA) organization. More specifically, the perspectives of the actual athletes themselves, as well as other employees of the NBA organization, are highlighted.

We believe the significance in this work is that, to date, there is not an ISR framework (general business or sport), thus providing us the opportunity to commence dialogue on this timely issue. However, given the absence of an ISR framework and literature, it should be noted that our theoretical musings were influenced by corporate social responsibility (CSR). However, CSR research takes a macro-level approach, investigating the social responsibility of large-scale corporations and businesses as a whole, whereas ISR is geared toward the micro-level (i.e., the individual). Given our focus on professional Black male athletes, the following provides further rationale as to why we have chosen to center our attention on this population and an overview of CSR.

▨ LITERATURE REVIEW

The Black Male Athlete

As scholars who are interested in American chattel slavery and the legacy of racism that emerged from it, it is our contention that we should pay attention to the deleterious influence and residual effects this "peculiar institution" (Stampp, 1957) has had on the Black community, particularly on Black males. Reese (2000) described the Black male in American society as an emasculated individual, defining emasculation as "the active undermining of the cultural integrity of the Black community by limiting the opportunity and ability of Black men to assume their natural positions within their families and communities" (p. 192).

According to Jenkins (2006), this particular subpopulation of the Black community has experienced "underachievement, lack of inclusion, and backward progression" (p. 127) within most sectors of American society. However, sport has grown into one of the few sectors where Black males (particularly as athletes) tend to be embraced and supported and is "one of the few places where an African American man can be a man" (Harrison, Harrison, & Moore, 2002, p. 131).

In this regard, the professional Black male athlete provides an excellent illustration for studying ISR. Agyemang and Singer (2011) argued that, in the aftermath of the Civil Rights Movement of the 1950s and 1960s, athletic competition became one social institution in the American context in which Black males, resulting from their athletic prowess, were afforded a number of opportunities (as athletes). Concerned with their financial bottom lines and seeing the economic benefit Black male athletes could potentially bring to their organization, White power brokers soon acknowledged that the continued exclusion of the Black male athletic body from participation was not in their best interests (Sage, 2007). In this regard, Black male athletes' complete amalgamation into competition once solely dominated by Whites has helped grow sport into a multi-billion dollar industry and healthy commercial enterprise (Agyemang & Singer, 2011).

The healthy status of the sport industry has enabled professional athletes in the current era to be looked on as brands in their own right (Chadwick & Burton, 2008; Milligan, 2009). Accompanied by this status though is notoriety and fame. However, with notoriety and fame come expectations from society and some believe these have not been met. For instance, Rhoden (2006) asserted, "Black athletes have abdicated their responsibility to the community with treasonous vigor" (p. 8). Moreover, in an interview with *Color Lines* magazine, Harry Edwards (architect of the 1968 Olympic boycott and author of *The Revolt of the Black Athlete*) added the following about the current Black male athlete:

> Today's black athlete is very different. If you asked them about the history of the black athlete, many couldn't tell you much. They don't find that history relevant to their world. Some even get angry when you ask them about it. One up-and-coming NBA star was asked about Oscar Robertson and he said, "Don't know, don't care, and don't take me there." They don't care about whose shoulders they stand on. They have no idea about who set the table at which they are feasting. And the worse part about it is not that they are ignorant of this history, but they are militantly ignorant. The sad part about it is that when people forget how things came about, they are almost certainly doomed to see them go. (as cited in Leonard, 1998, p. 3)

While athletes from other races and ethnicities most certainly have expectations from society, the pressure put on professional Black male athletes arguably exceeds their counterparts, especially given the history of racism and the central role Black males play in the commercial success of the American sport industry. Given this, professional Black male athletes were pinpointed to begin studying

ISR. Lastly, it is worth noting that we do recognize there are concerns pertaining to the ISR of Black male athletes outside the borders of the USA (see Vecsey, 2003; Wade, 2004). However, our endeavor to focus on this social group is embedded in our experiences working with professional Black male athletes in the U.S. (as mentors, advisors, and former instructors) and understanding that this population plays a potentially crucial role in social changes and impacting future generations.

Corporate Social Responsibility (CSR): A Broad Overview

Scholars have long debated the CSR construct and what it involves. Dating back to the 19th century, CSR was equated with philanthropic donations (Godfrey, 2009). Fast-forward to the 20th century and Howard Bowen's (1953) *Social Responsibilities of the Businessman,* which presented the business community with the first modern definition of CSR (Carroll, 1999). Based on the premise that businesses have the ability to affect the lives of citizens, he defined CSR as the following: "It refers to the obligation of businessmen to pursue those policies, to make those decisions, or to follow those lines of action which are desirable in terms of the objectives and values of our society" (p. 6). Howard Johnson's (1971) *Business in Contemporary Society: Framework and Issues* presented a number of definitions and views of CSR, such as businesses implementing social programs to maximize their profits. Finally, Drucker (1984) contended the purpose of "social responsibility of business is to tame the dragon, that is to turn a social problem into economic opportunity and economic benefit, into productive capacity, into human competence, into well-paid jobs, and into wealth" (p. 62). A proliferation of definitions, indeed; however, Carroll's (1979) is arguably the most cited: "The social responsibility of business encompasses the economic, legal, ethical, and discretionary expectations that society has of organizations at a given point in time" (p. 500). Despite the scholarly output, however, it is only recently that CSR has come to the forefront from a practical perspective. This is due to consumer distrust emanating from the transgressions of Enron, British Petroleum, Arthur Anderson, and Merrill Lynch, among others (Walker & Kent, 2009).

CSR in the Sport Industry

As societal expectations of corporations have risen, more attention has been given to CSR in sport from scholars and practitioners. From a research perspective, there are ample studies detailing the CSR phenomena in sport (e.g., Babiak & Wolfe, 2006, 2009; Breitbarth & Harris, 2008; Smith & Westerbeek, 2007; Walker, Kent, & Rudd, 2007). These scholars have noted that sport, unlike other industries, is unique due to the high level of commitment from its consumers and its employees are deemed influential members of the community (Walker

& Kent, 2009). To demonstrate this, Babiak and Wolfe (2009) asked the following: "Can we imagine the type of passion one sees at a World Cup soccer game, or a Yankees-Red Sox playoff game, exhibited by devotees of Harley Davidson or any traditional product?" (p. 722). Also distinguishing sport is how its organizations can strategically utilize their athletes' celebrity status and deploy them to engage in socially responsible acts (e.g., NBA Cares and Basketball without Borders).

From a practical standpoint, there are numerous examples of sport organizations engaging in CSR initiatives. For instance, Fédération Internationale de Football Association (FIFA) has engaged in a "Say No to Racism" campaign to fight against discrimination in soccer (Jindela, 2010). This was demonstrated in the 2010 World Cup pre-match festivities, as both teams held up a banner with the embroidered slogan. Furthermore, shoemaker Adidas launched a CSR campaign to encourage South African children concerning school and HIV/AIDS education (AIDS, a concern for FIFA, 2011). In the American context, the Philadelphia Eagles of the National Football League (NFL) instituted a "Go Green" environmental campaign with the goal of providing a clean community for Philadelphia residents (Walker & Kent, 2009). Speaking on behalf of the NFL, former commissioner Paul Tagliabue stated the following: "the NFL is becoming progressively more invested in corporate social responsibility (CSR) initiatives in an effort to establish itself as a socially conscious organization. . ." (as cited in Babiak & Wolfe, 2006, p. 214).

While it is apparent CSR has been given much attention from scholars and practitioners, a great majority have focused on the macro-level. That is, little attention has been given to the micro-level or the individuals who carry out socially responsible acts. It is important to give voice to those engaging in these activities, which this study set out to accomplish.

▪ METHODOLOGY: BASIC INTERPRETIVE QUALITATIVE STUDY

Scholars who carry out qualitative research are interested in understanding the multiple constructions and interpretations of reality that people in various social contexts have at particular points in time. For this particular study, we employed a basic, interpretive qualitative study design with the goal of understanding how our participants made meaning of and interpreted professional Black male athletes' ISR. This interpretation and meaning-making "is mediated through the researcher as instrument, the strategy is inductive, and the outcome is inductive" (Merriam, 2002, p. 6). The first author of this study took the lead as we sought to discover and understand our participants' perspectives on social responsibility. In the sections to follow, we discuss issues related to access, the sampling of our participants, and the collection and analysis of our data.

Gaining Access

Initial access was acquired via an individual who was employed as the content manager of the NBA organization, which served as the case for this study. The lead researcher had an established relationship with the content manager through their attendance at the same undergraduate institution; consequently, initial access was less problematic. This was particularly significant since gaining access to conduct research with elite populations, i.e., those pockets of society that are commonly not easily available through normal means (e.g., celebrities) can be time consuming and complex. Conducting research with such populations can cause a researcher to "go through hoops" to gather the information they need. For instance, the gatekeepers of these organizations value their own time, as well as that of their employees. As a result, it is probable that they may require some type of convincing for a researcher to begin their investigation (Altinay & Wang, 2009; Okumus, Altinay, & Roper, 2007).

The content manager put the lead researcher into contact with the organization's director of communications and was also contributory in that he identified likely participants for the study. Upon being put into contact with the director of communications, a research prospectus was sent via email, inquiring about the possibility of interviewing stakeholders of the organization. Approval was given to do interviews in the facility where the organization operates, such as in the media room, courtside of the playing floor, as well as the players' locker room.

Sampling of Participants

In sampling participants, we employed what Patton (2002) referred to as purposeful sampling, particularly criterion sampling, a process in which all participants must meet predetermined set criteria. To that end, all participants had to either be Black male athletes competing for the NBA team or stakeholders employed by the organization. Snowball sampling was also utilized, which Groenewald (2004) defined as "a method of expanding the sample by asking one informant or participant to recommend others for interviewing" (p. 46). During the interview process, participants were asked if they knew other individuals who they felt could contribute to the study. Purposeful and snowball sampling was also utilized out of convenience, in that the participants were obtainable due to the lead researcher's relationship with the content manager, which Berg (2001) avowed is acceptable in situations where the researchers desire preliminary information.

The final sample consisted of three professional Black male athletes and five stakeholders of the NBA organization (see Table 12.1). While we originally planned to have more athletes in the study, the nature of their schedules did not

TABLE 12.1

Pseudonym	Age	Race/ethnicity	Gender	Profession	# of years in profession
LeMichael	34	Black/African American	Male	NBA Athlete	12 years
Pierre	23	Black Caribbean/ French	Male	NBA Athlete	5 years
Dietrick	31	Black/African American	Male	NBA Athlete	10 years
Watson	27	Black/African American	Male	Content Manager	2 years
Marques	45	Black/African American	Male	Advanced Scout	15 years
Coach Cecil	43	Black/African American	Male	Assistant Coach	18 years as a player/3 as coach
MM	39	Black/African American	Male	Sales Executive	N/A
Mo	25	Black/African American	Male	ESPN Radio Broadcasting/ Advertising	5 years

permit this to occur. The five stakeholders held the following roles within the organization: content manager, advanced scout, assistant coach, sales executive, and reporter for the local ESPN radio station. All participants characterized themselves as Black and were asked to choose pseudonyms for themselves.

Data Collection and Analysis

We employed three data collecting techniques: (a) demographic questionnaires, (b) individual in-depth, semi-structured interviews, and (c) analysis of relevant documents. Demographic questionnaires were used to generate preliminary information about the participants. Interviews began by inquiring about this information and provided gender, race, ethnicity, age, profession, and any other information relevant to the participants, which assisted with getting to know them (see Table 12.1). Individual in-depth, semi-structured interviews were utilized as the main data gathering technique. Interviewing is known to be synonymous with qualitative inquiry and has become a common way in which we as humans come to know others (Fontana & Frey, 2005). In the case that in-person interviews could not take place, telephone interviews occurred. For example, telephone interviews took place with the advanced scout and sales executive because arrangements were unable to be made to meet in person due to traveling schedules and other duties related to their employment with the sport organization. In sum, interviews lasted a minimum of 35 minutes and went as long as an hour.

The analysis process began after the first interview was conducted. Interviews were listened to in order to gain first impressions. Lincoln (personal communication, October 6, 2009) stated the implementation of this process is significant in that it supplies the researcher with questions for future interviews with participants. In regards to this study, participants were contacted afterward to gather their opinions on any question they did not receive. Furthermore, throughout the interviewing process, the recorded interviews were listened to regularly. This paved the way for a better understanding of the participants or, as Maykut and Morehouse (1994) put it, "understanding the person's point of view" (p. 25). Marshall and Rossman (1995) also mentioned the significance of this process, asserting it allows the researcher to have a better grasp on participants' responses.

Open coding was employed to determine initial themes. Schwandt (2001) defined coding as "a procedure that disaggregates the data, breaks it down into manageable segments, and identifies or names those segments" (p. 26). In regards to coding, we utilized what Corbin and Strauss (2008) have characterized as open coding, which they define as "Breaking data apart and delineating concepts to stand for blocks of raw data" (p. 195). In doing so, we read the transcripts and field notes of the observations continuously until we felt we encompassed a good understanding of the data. This process allowed us to forge initial themes for the study and axial coding (Corbin & Strauss, 2008), then permitted us to crosscut or relate initial themes to one another. In other words, we broke down the initial themes into more concrete themes. For instance, this possibly involves collapsing themes together into one theme. From this process emanated our themes from the study, which are elaborated on below in the results.

The lead researcher also emailed copies of the transcripts to all the study participants to ensure trustworthiness and to allow participants to correct and/or clarify any of their statements. Furthermore, participants were asked to offer comments regarding the initial interpretations of the data. Feedback was asked to be sent back via email, which a majority of the participants accomplished. Also, peer-debriefing sessions were utilized to further confirm trustworthiness. This involved outsiders (to the research project) familiar with qualitative inquiry offering the researchers insight and feedback on their initial interpretations. An outsider's perspective may be able to point out something in the data the researcher(s) are unable to capture (Lincoln & Guba, 1985).

▪ RESULTS

The participants revealed that (a) owing a social responsibility to self, (b) being a role model, (c) responsibility to the Black community, and (d) engaging in genuine activity were the most salient issues concerning the ISR of Black male athletes. Figure 12.1 depicts each theme, accompanied by key buzzwords. Below, we report each of the themes with expressive quotations from the participants.

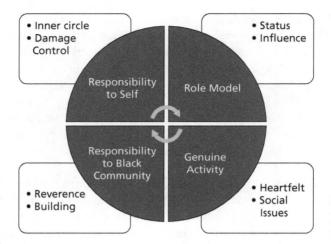

Figure 12.1

Responsibility to Self

Centered on past misdeeds of Black male athletes (e.g., Michael Vick, Dante Stallworth, Plaxico Burress), the participants regarded their social responsibility to themselves as a priority. MM stated the following:

> I think a lot of athletes have this mindset, I'm an athlete, I'm untouchable, but you've actually seen a couple of athletes where they've actually been sent to jail. Plaxico Burress. Michel Vick. If it can happen to a superstar like Michael Vick, it can happen to anybody.

They rated this as a priority because they argued that by keeping themselves out of trouble, they would be better equipped to be socially responsible to outside stakeholders. Dietrick referred to his responsibility to self by stating, "My whole thing is, there's a small amount of people in my huddle and I try to stay away from people who can get me into trouble." Mo then added, "If you're an athlete, basically you can't be a jackass. You can't be a Pacman Jones. Like just be a decent human being. Do what you're supposed to do. Go about your business in an adult fashion and everything should be okay." Mo was very candid when speaking on this topic and made this statement after a discussion of how some Black male athletes keep bad company, which then leads to not being responsible to themselves. It was in this light that he mentioned Pacman Jones, who had a host of problems involving nightclubs. LeMichael also commented on this:

> For me, I have first-hand experience where I had a situation where some people around me were doing negative things that could have portrayed my image to be negative. I did some damage control, continued to stay positive within the community, so it never really got broadcasted in the media.

While LeMichael had the wherewithal to employ "damage control" for his circumstance, other Black male athletes have not been so successful in years past. Coach Cecil, an assistant coach for the team, provided further commentary:

And another thing is they roll with boys now. And the responsibility to me as an athlete with your boys is to let them know, look, if something goes down and y'all get into it at the club, even if I don't do nothing, everything is going to fall on me. When we go out, the responsibility is to chill and relax and have a good time. If anything goes down, we need to get out of here or walk away. And a lot of times, that's where a lot of the Black male athletes get into trouble with their boys—not thinking, having attitudes, thinking I'm this person instead of thinking I'm your friend, I'm your boy, I'm going to make sure you don't get into trouble. Some guys don't know how to handle success. Hopefully guys understand that your boys can get you into trouble as we saw with Michael Vick, sadly to say. But I think that's the responsibility of the athlete to let the boys know, hey, we're going out to have a good time; we're not looking for any drama. If anything happens, walk away because at the end of the day, it's going to be on me, not you.

Speaking with passion and conviction, Marques added the following about the company Black male athletes keep:

At the same time, you've got to look at yourself in the mirror as an athlete and make a decision. Do I go left or do I go right? Some just don't get it. Some will never get it. And a lot of it, again, starts back in the way they came up, their upbringing, and of course, who they have in their circle. That's one of the biggest problems, who they have in their circle. At some point, you've got to cut June Bug and Ray Ray and them loose. Love them from a distance because they're bringing you down and they're going to cost you at some point. . ..

And sometimes, athletes they just really don't think. Some of them just don't get it. They don't get the fact that they are really blessed to have what they have and to do what they do. You get paid to play sports. How hard is it to carry yourself in a respectable manner? I mean, sure you can have fun. Have fun at home. Who said you have to be out in the clubs, driving drunk or carrying pistols? You can have fun at home. You got enough money to do that. Bring the people to your house and you can determine who comes in and out of your home.

These statements provide insight on the general perception of the Black male athlete in the American context and illustrate the importance of behaving in a socially responsible manner.

Role Models

Being seen as role models was very important for the participants. As stated previously, Black youth are immensely shaped by Black sports heroes (Sailes, 1986), thus necessitating Black male athletes to be role models. Below, Marques commenced the discussion by differentiating between Black male athletes and Black males. In doing so, he verbalized a reality that many Black male athletes may not realize:

> We are looked upon differently than the average Black male because we can run faster, we can shoot the ball better, we can go out and throw a football better than the average Blackman. So we're held to a higher regard than the average Black person. We are Black no matter how much better we are than everybody else. But again, I do think that Black male athletes are held at a higher regard just because they are athletes and because of what they bring to the so-called powers that be as far as finances are concerned.

Because they are held in a higher regard, Coach Cecil commented on the multiple eyes watching the every step of these athletes:

> You're on top of the world. And when I say on top of the world, a lot of people view you different because you're on TV, you play basketball, you're doing something that kids would love to do or not only kids, but what adults would love to do.

Marques then went on to voice his opinion on whether or not this characterization is fair:

> Black male athletes are in the spotlight; they're held at a higher regard. I mean, our Black kids look up to them and treat them as if they are elite. And they are elite. But they're looked upon as if they are better than everyone else. And is it fair? No, not really. It's not fair but as a man, you've got to think about it, think about who you're affecting, what lives you're affecting, how many lives you're affecting, especially the ones who look like you, day in, day out.

As witnessed above, the participants in this study felt it was significant that Black male athletes portray themselves in a positive light, keeping in mind the influence they have on the values of Black youth. Illustrated below, Coach Cecil describes an instance that typifies the influence Black male athletes can have on society:

> And it's amazing the way they look up to us. They might listen to things we say more than they listen to their parents. So I think we do have a responsibility of what we do and how we say it. You look around the world today, and I don't know who started the thing of wearing your pants below their tail, but you see kids catch on to that, especially the Black kids. I was riding down the street the other day and me and my personal assistant—I don't like to call him a personal assistant—but my business partner who is with me and he said, "look at that." And I look over there and it's a kid with his pants down almost down to basically his thigh. A lot of times these kids see that athletes and the Black male athletes wearing their pants like that. They're going to think it's right to wear their pants like that as well. . . .

It could affect a lot of things if our Black male athletes get arrested, especially if they let them off. I think that's a bad way of showing things to the community and to young kids. They look at us, we got money, and that means if we can break the law or do something, which means we got power, especially when you can get away with it. But I think it hurts a lot of our youth because they do see us getting arrested or they do see this on TV as a TI who just got out of jail and now he's right back going to jail. [They] could influence the youth in the Black neighborhoods and things like that so they can stay out of trouble because all they have to do is say they drinking some Crystal [liquor] and then everyone else start picking up Crystal when they go to the clubs. It's a trend; it really is.

Mo gave his opinion on Black male athletes as role models by stating that "it comes with the territory" and quoting Holy Scripture:

It's one of those things, "to who much is given, much is required," you know. And a lot of them aren't necessarily comfortable with being role models, but if you're blessed to be in the position they're in, there's certain sacrifices you have to make. And you got to carry yourself a certain way, you know. Sure they're adults, and we're humans, we all make mistakes, but I feel there are certain things you just shouldn't be involved in.

Here, as well, Mo referenced athletes committing transgressions (see Wilson, Stavros, & Westberg, 2008) and how this is a way not to carry oneself. He followed this up with suggesting what Black male athletes can do to positively affect Black communities:

They can show kids that you don't have to be content with your current circumstances and that there is a way out. If you work hard and you do what you're supposed to do, and you actually go to school and get an education, there's more than just what you see down the corner and the block. There's more than that and you know, there's more in life than the newest pair of Jordans that come out. There's more to life than that. Half the time, you see kids who come from impoverished backgrounds or whatever you want to call it, half the time, the reason they never make it out is because nobody else has shown them any other way, that you can be better if you strive to be better. Nobody has ever showed them, "hey there is something different out there." So it's like, if you don't know any better, you're not going to do any better. And if you're one of those guys made out of that background then shame on you for not coming back and showing kids that you can do better. And I'm not just saying making commercials, you know, and marketing your shoes. You need to go back to those communities and those types of schools and set up programs to where it's like, you know what, if you follow these steps [pause]. Like give these kids a blueprint or some kind of guideline or plan saying, if I follow this certain criteria, I can better my situation and the generations coming behind me, and they keep passing it forward.

The participants also felt it was especially important to be role models for Black youth, given that many of them may have parent(s) absent from the home working multiple jobs. Watson spoke of this scenario and how Black male athletes must be knowledgeable of the influence they could potentially have on Black youth:

It should be parents, but a lot of times; parents are having to work two, three jobs just to put food on the table. They might not be there. He's [child] seeing how LeBron James holds himself, so he might want to be a basketball player, but at the same time those figures, entertainers, athletes, all of them, have to hold themselves accountable knowing that people are watching them, knowing that kids are watching them. So you're not going to raise the children, but you can be a role model for them without even knowing them.

As a current athlete, Pierre provided further commentary on being a role model:

A lot of people are looking at you, especially media or other guys are looking at you like you're someone. They know that you play in the NBA and when you play in the NBA, you got to show the people a good image of the NBA, even if you go into a mall. So you can't do stupid stuff. Some stuff may have happened in the past, but you got to be careful what you're doing and show the people respect for the game and respect for other people.

When speaking of role models, the participants cited Charles Barkley's Nike commercial during the 1990s, when he expressed his views on role models. As Watson stated, "It goes back to something Charles Barkley said a couple of decades ago. He was like, I'm not a role model." Participants did not disagree with Barkley when he stated that parents should be role models; however, they did disagree with him stating that he was not a role model and implying other Black male athletes were not either. When asked whether he thought it was fair for Black male athletes to be looked on as role models, MM expressed the following:

Personally, I do think it's fair because they're in the public eye. It's part of their job. I may not like it all of the time, but in a way, I do think it's fair more times than not just because of what they do.

He then went on to articulate his thoughts on Charles Barkley's commercial:

Well, I agree that parents should be role models, but I disagree with Charles that he's not a role model because as an adult, we're all role models whether it's negative or positive. So I would disagree with him in that sense. Again, you're in the public eye and when you're in the public eye, people want to emulate you for whatever reason. A lot of it is what a lot of people perceive athletes to be about, money and the fame. So I think you are a role model whether you want to be or not.

Responsibility to Black Communities

Participants regarded the responsibility to Black communities as vital. Included in this was their responsibility to Black male athletes past and future. For instance, Dietrick pointed out, "Black male athletes such as Muhammad Ali and Jim Brown paved the way and laid the foundation so today's athletes can be successful and accepted the way that they are." He then added the following:

> I think so many people have done so much to get us in this situation as far as from Rosa Parks, MLK, to people like you said, Jim Brown and Jackie Robinson. They sacrificed so much for us to get us to this level that I feel that when you put yourself in position to shine negatively on other BMA, it's criminal.

Coach Cecil also noted the sacrifices made by these early pioneers and stated that current Black male athletes must "continue to make it better for the athletes who are coming up today and in the future." LeMichael additionally provided commentary related to this notion, noting how individuals such as Magic Johnson took the baton from those who came before them and paved the way for Michael Jordan and athletes thereafter. Speaking about the future, he asserted, "I can tell you the only best way to go forward is our future."

Furthermore, a number of the participants stated that because many Black male athletes come from lower socioeconomic status neighborhoods, they should be willing to serve Black communities. In reference to this, Marques stated, "If you talk about how bad the hood was or how bad this place was for you where you came up, why don't you do something to help it or build it up? Yeah I think they're responsible for helping because if they don't, who will?" In view of the backgrounds from which many Black male athletes come, Mo explained that these individuals must go back to these communities to lend a helping hand:

> I feel like, if you're a kid and you came from one of those less than fortunate backgrounds, I feel like it's almost, it is, it's not almost, it's imperative that you reach out. When you see kids who are just like you were when you were a kid growing up, I feel like shame on you for not reaching out and giving them opportunities that you didn't have. Now you're in a position where you can create opportunities for those kids where they do have a better shot at making whatever dreams come true. Whether or not they want to go to college, become a lawyer, doctor, whatever it is. But if you're in a position to help out those kids, shame on you for not helping them out at this point, especially when it's nothing for you; it's no sweat off your back.

Marques's elaborate commentary below summarizes the sentiments of all the participants:

> Anytime you can educate a young mind, you're doing something positive because so many of us are falling by the wayside; so many of us are dropping out of high school. We're quick to give up. I just think that in our communities, they need to

see our faces more; they need to see that we care more and not just by flashing a couple of dollars or driving through to see what I've done, "this is what I am, you can do it too." But okay, "how can I do it?" Tell me how to get there. Just like my position, for example, when I talk to kids, I always let them know the reality is that most of you, or all of you, are probably not going to be pro athletes, but there are so many other avenues in pro sports that you can take. I mean, I didn't know this position existed when I first started. I didn't start out doing this. I walked in with merchandising. That was my way in the door. So I like to tell them that story and let them know there are other avenues and I'm not here to dash your dreams, but the reality is, everybody cannot make it. So building things in the community to educate young people and maybe put up a community center that's just not sports based, but educationally based and teaching social responsibility. How to be a man. How to treat women. How to respect each other. How to work with one another. These are things that are lacking in the home because there are parents absent. So many kids growing up pretty much raising themselves. These are things that need to be done.

Genuine Activity

The participants suggested Black male athletes be involved with certain causes in which they have a genuine interest. They also felt that the activity should be genuine. For instance, Coach Cecil inquired, "are you doing it out of your heart or are you doing it because you want to help someone? Or, are you doing it for the exposure to just get your name out there?" Marques added:

> You shouldn't do anything for glory, for a public gratification or to be applauded and be looked upon as this pillar in society. You should do it because you enjoy doing it. You should do it because you want to do it. You should do it because you want to help somebody that looks like you.

Pierre spoke of discretionary activity in which he took part that he also felt passionate about:

> We do a lot of stuff. For Christmas, we're going out to give some presents to kids. It's a lot of different stuff. Sometimes we just do a little camp. We do it with all the kids or we go to the hospital to go see the kids and sick people. And I think it's important. I think the kids love it. And we love it too so that's why it's important.

LeMichael also referred to a foundation he started that hosts basketball camps and gives scholarships, for which he received a community assist award. According to the foundation's website, its aim is to assist youth pursue their dreams. To complement this, his personal website alluded to how he delivered turkeys during Thanksgiving to communities in need. In addition, Dietrick provided these comments on his own discretionary activities:

I'm starting my fund right now for single parent mothers. And umm, I also do some stuff back at my high school as far as scholarship things and giving basketball camps, and giving back to the program and helping them out just because I understand how hard it is to get funding at a 95% Black school.

Document analysis, i.e., reviewing relevant documents from this individual's personal webpage, provided information on Coach Cecil's foundation as well, which he started when he was a player in the NBA. Furthermore, the lead researcher was able to observe discretionary activity while attending practice and a preseason game where players signed autographs and took pictures with fans. They seemed to interact well with the fans and appeared as if they enjoyed doing so.

Participants were adamant that Black male athletes speak on social issues as part of their discretionary duties. For example, Watson verbalized:

If you see injustices, and you see it all the time even now days you see lynchings or some type of racial issue or something like that, don't be afraid to say that's not right. Athletes don't realize that by saying that it doesn't make you look bad, it makes you look like you're concerned. And so they don't, they're too busy trying not to look bad and not to have a stance on something as opposed to just saying, we all know that's not right and if it takes me saying that's not right it will probably make the situation better than by not saying anything at all.

Seeming displeased with the amount of activism that currently takes place among Black male athletes, Marques added:

It's okay for an athlete, a Black male athlete anyway, to state his stance on politics because it's only going to encourage people that look up to him and follow him. I mean, if he believes in Barack, then speak up and don't be quiet about it. If you believe in Barack's stance on insurance or Medicare, then say that.

■ DISCUSSION

The purpose of this study was to qualitatively explore the notion of the ISR of professional Black male athletes by giving voice to Black male employees of a National Basketball Association (NBA) organization. The themes delineated illustrate the participants' thoughts on this timely subject matter. Although tentative, the findings from this study offer some preliminary implications that we discuss below.

The first theme, responsibility of the self, is noteworthy in that participants spoke of keeping good company around them and exercising "damage control." In regard to the Black male athlete, transgressions on the part of a few Black male athletes have arguably tainted the image of this population. While these individuals represent merely a minority and should not be considered a representative sample of all professional Black male athletes, such transgressions by a few may in fact cast a negative light on most, if not all, Black male athletes. For one, as the participants alluded, these individuals are in the public eye; people are watching their every move. Hutchinson (1996) suggested the media has assassinated the image of Black males. For this reason alone, it is imperative that they safeguard themselves and make sound personal decisions.

In comparison to CSR, this theme was especially noteworthy and is the closest to the economic responsibility of a corporation. Firstly, consider the history of CSR. It was not until the transgressions of a few companies that demands for it came to the forefront (Walker & Kent, 2009). It was interesting to hear the participants allude to the transgressions of other athletes as even more reason to engage in ISR. Furthermore, essential components of CSR are following the legal mandates of the society in which one does business while also practicing sound ethics. This can also apply to professional athletes, considering the scrutiny they face. Of Carroll's four components of CSR, he stated organizations have a responsibility to make a profit. While the participants did not say they had a responsibility to do so, by being responsible to themselves, they are arguably increasing their economic responsibility (e.g., garnering contracts with teams and sponsors).

The participants' thoughts on the second theme, role models, were very consistent with previous literature in this area. For instance, a study done by Melnick and Jackson (2002) found that the influence of sports icons "extended well beyond simple admiration for some respondents to include impacts on beliefs, values, self-appraisals, and behaviors" (p. 429). Likewise, Williams (1994) noted that Michael Jordan was deemed the most likely celebrity to influence adolescent values. More recently, Buksa and Mitsis (2011) discussed how Generation Y perceives athletes as role models. In regard to professional Black male athletes, Sailes (1986) emphasized that they immensely shape Black youth. Sharp (2009) added, prominent Black male athletes "remain the most accessible examples of deliverance from childhood economic hardships because they'll remain the most familiar" (p. 1). Considering this, professional Black male athletes should utilize their status to their advantage and positively influence those who look up to them (Agyemang, 2012). One potential area to which they could lend a helping hand is assisting with the high school dropout rate of Black youth. Recently, LeBron James of the NBA collaborated with State Farm Insurance to release a commercial advocating for children to stay in school. As alluded to earlier, what these athletes do is heavily scrutinized. Consequently, they should utilize their role model status, take advantage of this, and pave the way for positive change. Doing so is very similar to how organizations are expected to be "corporate citizens" (Walters & Chadwick, 2009), undertaking activities that meet social demands. Agyemang (2014) applied this term to professional athletes, coining the term "athlete citizens." This pertains to the manner in which professional athletes conduct themselves and make a positive impact on society. Fulfilling athlete citizen responsibilities would certainly showcase a professional athlete as a role model.

The third theme detailed the ISR of professional Black male athletes to Black communities. Firstly, the participants felt that they owe a responsibility to Black male athletes who paved the way for them as well as to those who will come after them. These comments are especially interesting in view of past negative pronouncements concerning current Black male athletes (see Leonard, 1998; Powell, 2008; Rhoden, 2006; Roach, 2002). Participants acknowledged that current Black male athletes must act responsibility as a "thank you" to those who paved the way for them, in addition to leading the way for future Black male athletes to build off of their success.

Participants also thought Black male athletes should be involved in Black communities as a means to facilitate development. Authors such as Powell (2008), Rhoden (2006), and others have stated that current professional Black male athletes have not lived up to their duty to serving these populations. While the participants neither necessarily agreed nor disagreed with these sentiments, their comments certainly illustrate a need for Black male athletes to be involved with Black communities. Along these same lines, the participants also touched on the need for these individuals to be more involved in light of realities in Black communities. The participants were quick to point out single-parent homes, school dropouts, and other factors. Given the love and adoration Black communities have for Black male athletes (Sailes, 1986), they have the potential to have a large impact, which is very similar to early definitions of CSR (e.g., affecting the lives of citizens).

A survey recently conducted by ESPN and Hart Research Association touched on Black male athletes' social responsibility to Black communities. Surveying 100 Black professional athletes, 81% of the participants advocated Black male athletes take more of an active role in the Black community (Fainaru-Wada, 2011). One of the participants in the survey stated the following:

> You need more black athletes doing more positive things. A lot of people in the ghetto, in poor neighborhoods like where I grew up, don't believe there's life outside of the city, outside what they know. We need to be in there showing them, telling them, that there is. (Fainaru-Wada, 2011)

The statement not only reaffirms what was stated in this study, but also illustrates the need for Black male athletes to get more involved.

The last theme was related to professional Black male athletes involving themselves with genuine causes. Participants asserted these activities must be something for which the athlete has passion and be heartfelt, such as causes concerning the Black community or other general causes. For instance, one participant mentioned how he helped out his former high school that had a predominately Black population, while others hosted basketball clinics. In one case, Marques spoke of a time he held a camp and how the community wanted the Black athletes to be more visible. Another example of these activities is educational initiatives (e.g., athlete funded scholarships and facilitating big brother/big sister programs).

From a CSR perspective, the way participants regarded genuine causes was fairly similar to the manner in which Carroll (1979) expressed the last component of his CSR definition (i.e., discretionary responsibility): roles left to the judgment and choice of the business. However, while Carroll stated society has no specific message as to what discretionary activity requires, from the sentiments of the participants, it was almost as if society demanded that Black male athletes carry out discretionary initiatives. While Carroll gave donations as an example, what the participants described as genuine causes are similar to what scholars have identified as cause-related sports marketing (see Irwin, Lachowetz, Cornwell, & Clark, 2003), i.e., when a sport team works with a charitable organization to engage in CSR activity. In this case, a professional athlete could utilize their stardom to accomplish similar acts and bring awareness to a social cause. The professional athletes in this study illustrated the desire to engage in this type of activity, while all participants felt it is necessary.

■ CONCLUSION AND FUTURE RESEARCH DIRECTIONS

Despite the (de)limited nature of the study, in that it contained single interviews with a small sample of three professional Black male athletes and five other stakeholders of one sport organization, it supplies a noteworthy first step for studying the broader concept of ISR. Because we focused our attention on professional Black male athletes, we acknowledge that the present study is only directly generalizable to the current sample. However, because the goal of qualitative research is to present thick description of the findings and allow the reader to determine if the results are transferrable to other similar participants and social contexts, our primary concern was not with generalizability. We do recognize that future work related to this important topic should be conducted to come to a better understanding of ISR more broadly. For one, future research can examine stakeholders' (e.g., media, fans, community members, etc.) opinions of CSR and could gather information on how to better serve the needs of these groups. One such study could utilize a participatory action research (PAR) (see Kemmis & McTaggart, 2005) approach involving athletes and community members, which would give participants a sense of ownership. Athletes and community members could potentially describe how they can assist each other in building the community.

Furthermore, researchers may want to continue to employ qualitative techniques to further gauge professional Black male athletes' responsibility to Black communities. To do so, scholars may consider taking a phenomenological approach, which would match Black male athletes with individuals in the Black community. The sample of Black male athletes could comprise those who already play an active role in the Black community, as well as those who may have not realized this responsibility. Furthermore, participants within the community could be those who advocate and/or wish to work alongside these athletes to foster change within these communities as it relates to a number of issues.

Related to the above notion, a PAR approach could also be used to explore professional Black male athletes' responsibility to Black communities. Via this approach, the sampled groups would be able to have ownership of what comes from the research. Thus, the academic researcher would be working in collaboration with the individuals in the community. This effort could potentially lead to additional emancipatory knowledge, while also serving as discretionary responsibilities depending on what comes from the research. For instance, the research may inspire the Black athletes to either donate to the community or commence a scholarship for youth.

Also utilizing a qualitative approach, researchers could garner perceptions on how respective leagues assist with athlete social responsibility. Individual athletes could be interviewed as well as communication directors, community relations representatives, and other groups who have a vested interest in social responsibility. This study could elicit preliminary perceptions on current initiatives that are in place to facilitate ISR (e.g., Basketball without Borders and NBA Cares) from the athletes. Researchers could investigate if enough is being done in this regard.

Lastly, as it stands, CSR is more or less a strategic resource to benefit the image of an organization (e.g., Fitzpatrick, 2000; Sheth & Babiak, 2010; Walters & Chadwick, 2009). In fact, many organizations now mention CSR initiatives on their websites. Given the purpose of a business, there are logical reasons for this. With such a focus, however, it is a concern that organizations are focusing entirely too much on CSR from a strategic standpoint rather than placing more emphasis on the individuals and the decisions they make as agents of an organization. After all, "Corporations do not make decisions; they simply set the milieu in which individuals make choices" (Devinney, 2012). If the individuals in your organization are not engaging in socially responsible acts, the corporation cannot be socially responsible. Considering that calls for CSR originated from the indiscretions of individuals working for large corporations, it could be argued that there is a need to shift from CSR to ISR in regard to research. That is, more attention needs to be put on the actions of the individual (in the workplace) and not solely on the organization as a whole.

■ REFERENCES

Agyemang, K. J. A. (2012). Black male athlete activism and the link to Michael Jordan: A transformational leadership and social cognitive theory analysis. *International Review for the Sociology of Sport, 47*(4), 433–445.

Agyemang, K. J. A. (2014). Toward a framework of "athlete citizenship" in professional sport through authentic community stakeholder engagement. *Sport, Business, Management: An International Journal, 4*(1), 26–37.

Agyemang, K. J. A., & Singer, J. N. (2011). Toward a framework for understanding Black male athlete social responsibility (BMASR) in big-time American sports. *International Journal of Sport Management and Marketing, 10*(1/2), 46–60.

Agyemang, K. J. A., Singer, J. N., & DeLorme, J. (2010). An exploratory study of Black male college athletes' perceptions on race on athlete activism. *International Review for the Sociology of Sport, 45*(4), 419–435.

AIDS, a concern for FIFA. (2011, December 1). FIFA website. Retrieved from http://www. fifa.com/aboutfifa/socialresponsibility/news/newsid=1550443/index.html

Altinay, L., & Wang, C. L. (2009). Facilitating and maintaining research access into ethnic minority firms. *Qualitative Market Research: An International Journal, 12*(4), 367–390.

Babiak, K., & Wolfe, R. (2006). More than just a game? Corporate social responsibility and Super Bowl XL. *Sport Marketing Quarterly, 15*, 214–222.

Babiak, K., & Wolfe, R. (2009). Determinants of corporate social responsibility in professional sport: Internal and external forces. *Journal of Sport Management, 23*, 717–742.

Berg, B. L. (2001). *Qualitative research methods for the social sciences.* Boston, MA: Allyn and Bacon.

Bowen, H. R. (1953). *Social responsibilities of the businessman.* New York, NY: Harper & Row.

Breitbarth, T., & Harris, P. (2008). The role of corporate social responsibility in the football business: Towards the development of a conceptual model. *European Sport Management Quarterly, 8*(2), 179–206.

Buksa, I., & Mitsis, A. (2011). Generation Y's athlete role model perceptions on PWOM behaviour. *Young Consumers, 12*(4), 337–347.

Carroll, A. (1979). A three dimensional conceptual model of corporate social performance. *Academy of Management Review, 4*(4), 497–505.

Carroll, A. (1999). Corporate social responsibility: Evolution of a definitional construct. *Business & Society, 38*(3), 268–295.

Chadwick, S., & Burton, N. (2008). From Beckham to Ronaldo—assessing the nature of football player brands. *Journal of Sponsorship, 1*(4), 307–317.

Corbin, J., & Strauss, A. (2008). *Basics of qualitative research: Techniques and procedures for developing grounded theory* (3rd ed.). London, UK: Sage.

Devinney, T.M. (2012). *Individual social responsibility.* Retrieved from http://www. modern-cynic.org/2012/03/18/individual-social-responsibility/

Drucker, P. F. (1984). The new meaning of corporate social responsibility. *California Management Review, 26*, 53–63.

Fainaru-Wada, M. (2011). Survey shows split on racial opportunity. *ESPN News.* Retrieved from http://sports.espn.go.com/espn/otl/news/story?id=6006813

Fitzpatrick, K. (2000). CEO views on corporate social responsibility. *Corporate Reputation Review, 3*, 292–301.

Fontana, A., & Frey, J. H. (2005). The interview from natural science to political involvement. In N. K. Denzin & Y. S. Lincoln (Eds.), *The Sage handbook of qualitative research* (pp. 695–727). Thousand Oaks, CA: Sage.

Godfrey, P. (2009). Corporate social responsibility in sport: An overview and key issues. *Journal of Sport Management, 23*(6), 698–716.

Groenewald, T. (2004). A phenomenological research design illustrated. *International Journal of Qualitative Methods, 3*(1), 42–55.

Harrison, L., Harrison, C. K., & Moore, L. N. (2002). African American racial identity and sport. *Sport, Education, and Society, 7*(2), 121–133.

Hughes, G. (2004). Managing Black guys: Representation, corporate culture, and the NBA. *Sociology of Sport Journal, 21*(2), 163–184.

Hutchinson, E. O. (1996). *The assassination of the Black male image.* New York, NY: Simon & Schuster Paperbacks.

Irwin, R. L., Lachowetz, T., Cornwell, T. B., & Clark, J. S. (2003). Cause-related sport sponsorship: An assessment of spectator beliefs, attitudes, and behavioral intentions. *Sport Marketing Quarterly, 12*(3), 131–139.

Jenkins, T. S. (2006). Mr. Nigger: The challenges of educating Black males within American society. *Journal of Black Studies, 37*(1), 127–155.

Jindela, I. T. (2010). World Cup quarter-finalists "Say no to racism." Retrieved from http://africabusiness.com/2010/07/01/world-cup/

Johnson, H. L. (1971). *Business in contemporary society: Framework and issues.* Belmont, CA: Wadsworth.

Kemmis, S., & McTaggart, R. (2005). Participatory action research: Communicative action and the public sphere. In N. K. Denzin & Y. S. Lincoln (Eds.), *The Sage handbook of qualitative research* (3rd ed.) (pp. 559–603). Thousand Oaks, CA: Sage.

Leonard, D. (1998). What happened to the revolt of the Black athlete? *Color Lines.* Retrieved from http://colorlines.com/archives/1998/06/what_happened_to_the_revolt_of_the_black_athlete.html

Lincoln, Y. S., & Guba, E. G. (1985). *Naturalistic inquiry.* New York, NY: Sage.

Marshall, C., & Rossman, G. B. (1995). *Designing qualitative research* (2nd ed.). Thousand Oaks, CA: Sage.

Maykut, P., & Morehouse, R. (1994). The qualitative posture: Indwelling. In P. Maykut & R. Morehouse (Eds.), *Beginning qualitative research: Aphilosophic and practical guide* (pp. 25–40). London, UK: Falmer Press.

Melnick, M. J., & Jackson, S. J. (2002). Globalization American-style and reference idol selection. *International Review for the Sociology of Sport, 37*(3/4), 429–448.

Merriam, S. B. (2002). Introduction to qualitative research. In S. B. Merriam (Ed.), *Qualitative research in practice: Examples for discussion and analysis* (pp. 3–17). San Francisco, CA: Wiley, John & Sons, Inc.

Milligan, A. (2009). Building a sports brand. *Journal of Sponsorship, 2*(3), 231–242.

Okumus, F., Altinay, L., & Roper, A. (2007). Gaining access for research. *Annals of Tourism Research, 34*(1), 7–26.

Patton, M. (2002). *Qualitative evaluation and research* (3rd ed.). London, UK: Sage.

Powell, S. (2008). *Souled out? An evolutionary crossroads for Blacks in sport.* Champaign, IL: Human Kinetics.

Reese, L. E. (2000). The impact of American social systems on African American men. In L. Jones (Ed.), *Brothers of the academy: Up and coming Black scholars earning our way in higher education* (pp. 191–196). Sterling, VA: Stylus Publishing.

Rhoden, W. C. (2006). *Forty million dollar slaves.* New York, NY: Three Rivers Press.

Roach, R. (2002). What ever happened to the conscientious black athlete? *Black Issues in Higher Education, 19*(4), 20–21.

Sage, G. H. (2007). Introduction. In D. Brooks & R. Althouse (Eds.), *Diversity and social justice in college sports: Sport management and the student athlete* (pp. 1–17). Morgantown, WV: Fitness Information Technology.

Sailes, G. A. (1986). The exploitation of the Black athlete: Some alternative solutions. *Journal of Negro Education, 55*(4), 439–442.

Schwandt, T. A. (2001). *Dictionary of qualitative inquiry.* Thousand Oaks, CA: Sage.

Sharp, D. (2009). With Obama's success, more than the ball is in kids' court. *USA Today.* Retrieved from http://usatoday30.usatoday.com/sports/columnist/sharp/2009-01-20-obama-success-on-kids_N.htm

Sheth, H., & Babiak, K. (2010). Beyond the game: Perceptions and practices of corporate social responsibility in the professional sport industry. *Journal of Business Ethics, 91*(3), 433–450.

Smith, A. C. T., & Westerbeek, H. M. (2007). Sport as a vehicle for deploying social responsibility. *Journal of Corporate Citizenship, 25,* 43–54.

Stake, R. E. (2005). Case studies. In N. K. Denzin & Y. S. Lincoln (Eds.), *The Sage handbook of qualitative research* (3rd ed.) (pp. 443–466). Thousand Oaks, CA: Sage.

Stampp, K. M. (1957). *The peculiar institution: Slavery in the ante-bellum South.* New York, NY: Knopf.

Vecsey, G. (2003, February 2). SOCCER; England battles the racism infesting soccer. *The New York Times.* Retrieved from http://www.nytimes.com/2003/02/02/sports/soccer-england-battles-the-racism-infesting-soccer. html?pagewanted=all&src=pm.

Wade, S. (2004, November 28). Racism in soccer still prevalent. *ESPN News.* Retrieved from http://espnfc.com/feature?id=317756&cc=5901.

Walker, M., & Kent, A. (2009). Do fans care? Assessing the influence of corporate social responsibility on consumer attitudes in the sport industry. *Journal of Sport Management, 23,* 743–769.

Walker, M. B., Kent, A., & Rudd, A. (2007) Consumer reactions to strategic philanthropy in the sport industry. *Business Research Yearbook: Global Business Perspectives, 14*(2), 926–932.

Walters, G., & Chadwick, S. (2009). Corporate citizenship in football: Delivering strategic benefits through stakeholder engagement. *Management Decisions, 47*(1), 51–66.

Williams, J. (1994). The local and the global in English soccer and the rise of satellite television. *Sociology of Sport Journal, 11,* 376–397.

Wilson, B., Stavros, C., & Westberg, K. (2008). Player transgressions and the management of the sport sponsor relationship. *Public Relations Review, 43,* 99–107.

PART IV
Power and Corruption

Do money and power make it harder to make good decisions? Or just easier to make bad decisions? Sports comprise one of the largest global multi-billion-dollar industries. Those who control sports carry immense social influence. The International Olympics Committee (IOC) and the Fédération Internationale de Football Association (FIFA) regularly compel cities to spend hundreds of millions on transforming their landscapes to increase their chances of hosting the Games or the World Cup. Big Division I football and basketball programs bring hundreds of millions of dollars to their schools, and spend a good bit of it on themselves. The self-aggrandizing practices of powerful sports entities enable competitions around which many of us schedule our social lives, but at what cost? Many championships bring in their wake sex trafficking, hooliganism, traffic congestion, and other problems to these cities. Some employ heinous labor practices and displace poor residents to build stadiums. Many big sport colleges deprive their athletes of meaningful educations, and some protect and support abusive coaches. Are these evils inevitable in high-powered, major sports?

Hosting games, and being part of a winning team, generates money, respect, and power. Those responsible for leading a bid or helping a team win, including city politicians, team managers, coaches, and athletes, are under immense pressure and are given low thresholds for failure. Losing a bid or a few games can jeopardize job security. Approaching the owners and operators of elite teams, programs, and leagues with a bribe might mean gaining an edge that could lead to a renewed contract, personal profit, and opportunities for future wealth for a coach, company, or politician. Owners and sponsors are tempted by countless offers for a piece of control, and these executives have the resources and leverage to take advantage without being caught. Sometimes they have the power to continue presiding after being caught. Sepp Blatter, ex-FIFA president, was called out for receiving secret bonuses and accepting bribes for many years, before the U.S. FBI gave him a persuasive reason to resign.

Unpredictability of outcome is perhaps the primary source of a sport's power. Sports are stories whose endings we are obsessed with guessing. When we are right, we feel validated. When we are wrong, we come back to guess again. Gambling on the outcome of sports intensifies the feelings of validation and defeat. Putting a wager on a game directly connects one's livelihood to the story. If your team is favored, you take pride in their superiority. If your team is an underdog, you are inspired by the possibility of miraculously earning the pedestal.

Although the odds of winning a sports bet are greater than in many casino games or lotteries, the vast majority of sports bettors still lose. An ethical question remains whether we ought to allow bookmakers with superior knowledge of probability to take advantage of fans fueled by mathless hope.

But it is not just the bookmakers who take advantage. While many fans strip their wallets to become more connected to the game, athletes and coaches sometimes strip their own game to fill their wallets. Since shortly after the inception of sports betting, there have been teams "fixing" match outcomes to take part in the winning bet. Why would players who gave everything to reach the pinnacle of their sport then cheat the sport of its core unpredictability?

As explained by Declan Hill, in chapter 15, many players involved in match-fixing are nearing the end of their careers. They have lost much of their physical endurance, strength, and speed. No matter how much they condition and practice, biological degradation prevents them from achieving the same athletic feats to which they were accustomed at their peak. Meanwhile, they are surrounded by the new crop of fresh young superstars in their physical prime. How does one in this position stay competitive? The game is all they know, most if not all of what they love. As opportunities for intrinsic reward, like the thrill of being a successful player, diminish, it makes sense that they turn more to extrinsic rewards like money. But they no longer have the big contracts concomitant with being high-goal scorers or brilliant defenders. So, when aging athletes are pressured by their peers or friends to help fix a match and can make a lot of money in the process, what might convince them not to do so?

If fans know that match-fixing is taking place, but do not know which matches are fixed, the entire sport—a bastion of escapism, hope, and community—loses its value. Whatever the odds, spectators and bettors participate with the assumption that the game is subject to an open future. Think about the most extraordinary match you ever witnessed: How would you feel knowing the outcome was predetermined? Match-fixing turns fans away, and without fans there is no sport. Even athletes and coaches who cheat know their world depends on having fans; they just rely on not getting caught and on keeping those fans in the dark. But if the most powerful people in the sports universe can be bought, and sometimes caught in the act, who is safe?

13 Universities Gone Wild

Big Money, Big Sports, and Scandalous Abuse

at Penn State

■ HENRY A. GIROUX AND
SUSAN SEARLS GIROUX

Too many universities are now beholden to big business, big sports, and big military contracts. And it is within this new set of contexts that we must read the Penn State scandal. Much media attention has been drawn to the fact that Penn State pulls in tens of millions of dollars in football revenue, but nothing has been said of the fact that it also receives millions from Defense Department contracts and grants, ranking sixth among universities and colleges receiving funds for military research.[1] Or that as a result of considerable influence by corporate interests, the academic mission of the university is now less determined by internal criteria established by faculty researchers with the knowledge expertise and a commitment to the public good than by external market forces concerned with achieving fiscal stability and, if possible, increasing profit margins. The excesses to which such practices have given rise have proven obscene to the point of the pornographic. One has only to look closely at the unfolding tragedy at Penn State University to understand the potentially catastrophic consequences of this decades-long transformation in higher education for universities more generally.

The Penn State crisis may well prove one of the most serious scandals in the history of college athletics and university administration, while it also reinforces the claim, made by Paul Krugman, "that democratic values are under siege in America."[2] Jerry Sandusky, who coached the Nittany Lions for more than 30 years, allegedly used his position of authority at the university as well as at his Second Mile Foundation, a foster home, to lure vulnerable minors into situations in which he preyed on them sexually, having gained unfettered access to male youths through a range of voluntary roles.[3] Sandusky has been charged with sexually abusing at least a dozen boys, all of whom were 12 years old or younger when they were victimized. On at least three occasions, extending from 1998 to 2002, Sandusky was caught abusing young boys on the Penn State campus. These incidents have been the consistent focus of media attention. In 1998, a distraught mother of a boy who had showered with Sandusky reported the incident to the campus police. A janitor also observed Sandusky performing oral sex on a young boy in a Penn State gym in 2000. Finally, according to the grand jury report in the Sandusky case, Mike McQueary, a 28-year-old graduate assistant for the Penn State football team, alleged that in 2002 he saw Sandusky raping a young boy in the shower in the Lasch Football Building on the University Park campus. It has, therefore, taken 9 years for the police to investigate and finally arrest Sandusky, who has now been charged with over 50 counts of sexual abuse.

As tantalizingly sensational as the media have found these events, the scandal is about much more than a person of influence using his power to sexually assault innocent young boys. This tragic narrative is as much about the shocking lengths to which rich and powerful people and institutions will go in order to cover up their complicity in the most horrific crimes and to refuse responsibility for egregious violations that threaten their power, influence, and brand names.[4] The desecration of public trust is all the more vile when the persons and institution in question have been assigned the intellectual and moral stewardship of generations of youth.

The most recent cover-up appears to have begun in 1998 when Centre County District Attorney, Ray Cricar, did not file charges against Sandusky, in spite of obtaining credible evidence that Sandusky had molested two young boys in a shower at Penn State. Then, in 2000, the janitor who witnessed similar abuse and his immediate superior, whom he told about it, both failed to report the incident to the police for fear of losing their jobs, only to reveal the story years later. But the cover-up that has attracted the most attention took place in 2003 after Mike McQueary reported to celebrated coach Joe Paterno that he saw Sandusky having anal intercourse with a 10-year-old boy in one of the football facility's showers. Paterno reported the incident to his athletic director, Tim Curley, who then notified Gary Schultz, a senior vice president for finance and business. Both informed President Spanier about the incident. In light of the seriousness of a highly credible and detailed report alleging that a child had been raped, the Penn State administration simply responded by barring Sandusky from bringing young boys onto the university campus. At the end of the day, neither Paterno nor any of the highly positioned university administrators reported the alleged assault of a minor to the police and other proper authorities. Within a week after the story broke in the national media 8 years later, Paterno, Schultz, Curley, and Spanier had all been fired. Sandusky "now faces more than 50 charges stemming from accusations that he molested boys for years on Penn State property, in his home and elsewhere."[5] The charges include involuntary sexual intercourse, indecent assault, unlawful contact with a minor, corruption of minors, and endangering the welfare of a minor.

In the most shameful of ironies, the national response to the story has similarly engaged in a covering up of the violent victimization of children that lay at its core. The young boys who have been sexually abused have been relegated to a footnote in a larger and more glamorous story about the rise and sudden fall of the legendary Paterno, a larger-than-life athletic icon. Their erasure is also evident in the equally sensational narrative about how the university attempted to hide the horrific details of Sandusky's history of sexual abuse by perpetuating a culture of silence in order to protect the privilege and power of the football and academic elite at Penn State. If any attention was paid at all to distraught and disillusioned youth, it was to focus on the Penn State students who rallied around "JoePa," not on the youth who bore the weight into their adulthood of being victims of the egregious crimes of rape, molestation, and abuse. As many critics have pointed out, both dominant media narratives fail to register just how deeply this tragedy descends in terms of what it reveals about our nation's priorities about youth and our increasing unwillingness to shoulder the responsibility—as much moral and intellectual as financial—for their care and development as human beings.

Michael Bérubé rightly asserts that the scandal at Penn State and the ensuing "student riots on behalf of a disgraced football coach" should not be used to condemn the vast majority of teachers, researchers, and students at Penn State, "none of whom had anything to do with this mess."[6] Equally pertinent is his observation that Penn State has a long history of rejecting any viable notion of shared governance and that "decisions, even about academic programs, are made by the central administration and faculty members are 'consulted' afterward."[7] The American Association of University Professors extended Bérubé's argument, insisting that the lack of faculty governance has to be understood as a consequence of a university system that favors the needs of a sports empire over the educational needs of students, the working conditions of faculty, and health and safety of vulnerable children.[8]

The call for forms of shared governance in which faculty through their elected representatives are treated with respect and exercise power alongside administrators signals an important issue—namely, how many university administrations operate in nontransparent and unaccountable ways that prioritize financial matters over the well-being of students and faculty? At the same time, it is not uncommon for entrepreneurial faculty members to transgress established strategic priorities and circumvent layers of university oversight and adjudication altogether by bringing in earmarked funding for a pet project (through which she or he stands to gain), confident no administrator can refuse cash up front, whatever the Faustian bargain attached to it.

Big money derived from external sources has changed the culture of universities across the United States in still other ways. For example, in 2010, Penn State made $70,208,584 in total football revenue and $50,427,645 in profits; moreover, it was ranked third among American universities in bringing in football revenue. As part of the huge sports enterprise that is NCAA (National Collegiate Athletic Association) Division I Football, Penn State and other high-profile "Big Ten" universities not only make big money but also engage in a number of interlocking campus relationships with private-sector corporations. Lucrative deals that generate massive revenue are made through media contracts involving television broadcasts, video games, and Internet programming. Substantial profits flow in from merchandizing football goods, signing advertising contracts, and selling an endless number of commodities from toys to alcoholic beverages and fast food at the stadium, tailgating parties, and sports bars. Yet the flow of capital is not unidirectional.

Universities also pay out impressive amounts of money to support such enterprises and to attract star athletes; they hire support staffing from janitorial positions to top physicians in sports medicine to celebrity coaches; they pay to maintain equipment, grounds, stadia, and myriad other associated services. Consider Beaver Stadium—the outdoor college football monument to misplaced academic priorities—which has a capacity of 106,572 seats that require cleaning and maintenance. The stadium holds as many people as the entire population of State College, including Penn State students—all of whom require armies of staff to accommodate their needs. In this instance, the circulation of money and power on university campuses mimics its circulation in the corporate world, saturating public spaces and the forms of sociality they encourage with the imperatives of the market. Money from big sports programs also has an enormous influence on shaping agendas within the university that play to their advantage, from the neoliberalized, corporatized commitments of an increasingly ideologically incestuous central administration to the allocation of university funds to support the athletic complex and the transfer of scholarship money to athletes rather than academically qualified, but financially disadvantaged students. As *Slate* writer J. Bryan Lowder puts it, big sports

> wield too much influence over college life. In an institution that is meant to instill the liberal values of critical thinking and an egalitarian sense of equality in its students, having special dining rooms or living quarters for athletes . . . is a bad idea.[9]

What should be deeply unsettling and yet remains unspoken in mainstream media analyses is that the youth have also learned these lessons *at the university,* where they have been immersed in a culture that favors entertainment over education—the more physical and destructive, the better; competition over collaboration; a worshipful stance toward iconic sports heroes over thoughtful engagement with academic leaders, who should inspire by virtue of their intellectual prowess and moral courage; and herd-like adhesion to coach and team over and against one's own capacity for informed judgment and critical analysis. The consolidation of masculine privilege in such instances enshrines patriarchal values and exhibits an astonishing indifference to repeated cases of sexual assaults on college campuses.

Sexual assault is a problem on college campuses across the United States, as revealed in national statistics demonstrating that "one in five women [was] sexually assaulted while in college and approximately 81% of students experienced some form of sexual harassment during their school years."[10] However, in the years we taught at Penn State, it reached alarming proportions. According to the Center for Women Students on the university's main campus, "At Penn State approximately 100 students sought assistance for sexual assault during the 1996–97 academic year."[11] For those familiar with the behavior often exhibited by victims of sexual violence, the fact that 100 students came forward in a single year is simply shocking, given the overwhelming reticence most victims feel about reporting attacks. In addition to feeling fear and shame, the reluctance to report an assault is reinforced when the victim believes that it will seldom result in arrest or conviction. Put simply, this means that the extent of cases and many of the consequences of sexual assault, physical abuse, hazing, and violence on college campuses are probably much greater than what is actually known.

Claire Potter, writing in the *Chronicle of Higher Education,* argues that Penn State and universities in general have a vested interest in safeguarding their reputations by covering up acts of sexual violence. For Potter,

> Universities substitute private hearings, counseling and mediation for legal proceedings: while women often choose this route, rather than filing felony charges against their assailants, it doesn't always serve their interest to do so. But it always serves the interests of the institution not to have such cases go to court.[12]

Given how events have unfolded at the university, Potter's withering charge that Penn State has a greater interest in protecting its brand name than in protecting students—who are reduced to revenue-producing entities rather than seen as young people to whom it has the responsibility intellectually and ethically to shape and inspire—gains considerable force. For Potter, social power at universities dominated by a big sports culture often expresses itself not just in the glory of the game, the reputation of the coaches, or the herd-like devotion to a team, but also in forms of sexual power aimed at abusing female students. Potter wants to move these incidents away from the sports pages and popular media into classrooms where they can be understood within a larger set of economic, social, and political contexts and appropriately challenged.

The hardened culture of masculine privilege, big money, and sport at Penn State is reinforced as much through a corporate culture that makes a killing off the entire enterprise as it is through a retrograde culture of illiteracy—defined less in terms of an absence of knowledge about alternatives to normative gender behavior and more in terms of a willfully embraced ignorance—that is deeply woven into the fabric of campus life. Even and especially in higher education, one cannot escape the visual and visceral triumph of consumer culture, given how campuses have come to look like shopping malls, treat students as customers, confuse education with training, and hawk entertainment and commodification rather than higher learning as the organizing principles of student life. Across universities, the ascendancy of corporate values has resulted in a general decline in student investment in public service, a weakening of social bonds in favor of a survival-of-the-fittest atmosphere, and a pervasive undercutting of the traditional commitments of a liberal arts education: critical and autonomous thinking, a concern for social justice, and a robust sense of community and global citizenship.

As academic labor is linked increasingly to securing financial grants or down-sized altogether, students often have little option than to take courses that have a narrow instrumental purpose and those who hold powerful administrative positions increasingly spend much of their time raising money from private donors. All the while, students accrue more debt than ever before; student debt, in fact, has now surpassed the accumulated credit card debt in a nation of notoriously robust consumers. The notion that the purpose of higher education might be tied to the cultivation of an informed, critical citizenry capable of actively participating and governing in a democratic society has become cheap sloganeering on college advertising copy, losing all credibility in the age of big money, big sports, and corporate influence. Educating students to resist injustice, refuse antidemocratic pressures, or learn how to make authority and power accountable remains at best a receding horizon—in spite of the fact that such values are precisely why universities are pilloried by moneyed Republicans as hotbeds of Marxist radicals.

The displacement of academic mission by a host of external corporate and military forces surely helps explain the spontaneous outbreak of rioting by a segment of Penn State students once the university announced that Joe Paterno has been fired as the coach of the storied football team. Rather than holding a vigil for the minors who had been repeatedly sexually abused, students ran through State College, wrecking cars, flipping a news truck, throwing toilet paper into trees, and destroying public property. J. Bryan Lowder understands this type of behavior as part of a formative culture of social indifference and illiteracy reinforced by the kind of frat house insularity that is produced on college campuses where sports programs and iconic coaches wield too much influence. He writes,

> Building monuments to a man whose job is, at the end of the day, to teach guys how to move a ball from one place to another, is . . . inappropriate. And, worst of all, allowing the idea that anyone is infallible—be it coach, professor or cleric—to fester and infect a student body to the point that they'd sooner disrupt public order than face the truth is downright toxic to the goals of the university. . . . Blind, herd-like dedication to a coach or team or school is pernicious. Not only does it encourage the kind of wild, unthinking behavior displayed in the riot, but it also fertilizes the lurid collusion and willful ignorance that facilitated these sex crimes in the first place. But what to do? As David Haugh asked in *The Chicago Tribune*: "When will [the students] realize, after the buzz wears off and sobering reality sinks in, that they were defending the right to cover up pedophilia?"[13]

Phil Rockstroh extends Lowder's analysis, rightfully connecting the political illiteracy reflected in the student rampaging at Penn State to a wider set of forces characterizing the broader society to the obvious detriment of students. He writes,

> Penn State students rioted because life in the corporate state is so devoid of meaning . . . that identification with a sports team gives an empty existence said

meaning.... These are young people, coming of age in a time of debt-slavery and diminished job prospects, who were born and raised in and know of no existence other than life as lived in U.S. nothingvilles i.e., a public realm devoid of just that—a public realm—an atomizing center-bereft culture of strip malls, office parks, fast food eateries and the electronic ghosts wafting the air of social media. Contrived sport spectacles provisionally give an empty life meaning.... Take that away and a mindless rampage might ensue.... Anything but face the emptiness and acknowledge one's complicity therein and then direct one's fury at the creators of the stultified conditions of this culture.[14]

A number of critics have used the Penn State scandal to call attention to the crisis of moral leadership that characterizes the neoliberal managerial models that now exert a powerful influence over how university administrations function. As the investment in the public good collapses, leadership cedes to reductive forms of management, concerned less with big ideas than with appealing to the pragmatic demands of the market, such as raising capital, streamlining resources, and separating learning from any viable understanding of social change. Anything that impedes profit margins and the imperatives of instrumental rationality with its cult of measurements and efficiencies is seen as useless. Within the logic of the new corporate-driven managerialism, there is little concern for matters of justice, fairness, equity, and the general improvement of the human condition insofar as these relate to expanding and deepening the imperatives and ideals of a substantive democracy.[15] Discourses about austerity, budget shortfalls, managing deficits, restructuring, and accountability so popular among college administrators serve largely as a cover "for a recognisably ideological assault on all forms of public provision."[16]

If university administrators cannot defend the university as a public good, but instead, as in the case of Penn State, align themselves with big money, big sports, and the instrumental values of finance capital, they will not be able to mobilize the support of the broader public and will have no way to defend themselves against the neoliberal and conservative attempts by state governments to continually defund higher education. In recent years, universities have not thought twice about placing the burden of financial shortfalls on the backs of students— even as that burden grows apace, wrought by austerity measures, or by internal demands for new resources and space to keep up with record growth, or by new competition with international and online educational institutions. All this amounts to a poisonous student tax, one that has the consequence of creating an enormous debt for many students. Penn State has one of the highest tuition rates of any public college—amounting to $14,416 per year. But it is hardly alone in what has become a pitched competition to raise fees. Some public colleges such as Florida State College have increased tuition by 49% in 2 years! The lesson here is that abuse of young people comes in many forms, extending from egregious acts of child rape and sexual violence against women to the creation of a generation of students burdened by massive debt and a bleak, if not quite hopeless, jobless future.

The Penn State scandal is symptomatic of a much larger set of challenges—and the abuses they almost invariably invite—which are deeply interconnected and mutually informing. On the one hand, Penn State symbolizes the corruption of higher education by big sports, governmental agencies, and corporate power with vested interests and deep pockets. On the other hand, the tragedy can surely be seen as a part of what we have been calling the war on youth. The media emphasis on the fall of Paterno, the firing of high-ranking university administrators, and the alleged failure of a chain of command, although not incidental to the ongoing abuse of over a dozen boys, serves ironically to deflect attention from the egregious sexual assault of young boys, who have carried this grievous burden into their adulthood. Students, faculty, and administrators also pay a terrible price when a university loses its moral compass and refashions itself in the values, principles, and managerial dictates of a corporate culture.

Neither the media accounts of the rise and fall of a celebrity coach nor what many insiders would like to characterize as a woeful series of administrative miscommunications tells us much about how Penn State is symptomatic of what has happened to a number of universities since at least the mid-1940s and at a quickened pace since the 1980s. Penn State, like many of its institutional peers, has become a corporate university caught in the grip of the military-industrial complex rather than existing as a semiautonomous institution driven by an academic mission, public values, and ethical considerations.[17] It is a paradigmatic example of mission drift, one marked by a fundamental shift of the university away from its role as a vital democratic public sphere toward an institutional willingness to subordinate educational values to market values. As Peter Seybold has suggested, the Penn State scandal is indicative of the ongoing corruption of teaching, research, and pedagogy that has taken place in higher education.[18] Beyond the classroom and the lab, evidence of ongoing corporatization abounds: bookstores and food services are franchised; part-time labor replaces full-time faculty; classes are oversold; and online education replaces face-to-face teaching, less as a pedagogical innovation and more as a means to deal with the capacity issues now confronting those universities that pursued financial sustainability through aggressive growth.[19] It gets worse. The corporate university is descending more and more into what has been called "an output fundamentalism," prioritizing market mechanisms that emphasize productivity and performance measures that make a mockery of quality scholarship and diminish effective teaching—scholarly commitments are increasingly subordinated to bringing in bigger grants to supplement operational budgets negatively affected by the withdrawal of governmental funding.

In addition, the student experience has hardly been untouched by these shock waves, which have further undermined the genuinely intellectual, financial, social, and democratic needs of undergraduate and graduate students alike.

Young people are increasingly devalued as knowledgeable, competent, and so-cially responsible, in spite of the fact that their generation will inevitably be the leaders of tomorrow. Put bluntly, many university administrators demonstrate a notable lack of imagination, conceiving of students primarily in market terms and showing few qualms about subjecting young people to forms of education as outmoded as the factory assembly lines they emulate. Campus extracurricular activities unfold in student commons designed in the image of shopping cen-ters and high-end entertainment complexes. Clearly, students are not perceived as worthy of the kinds of financial, intellectual, and cultural investments nec-essary to enhance their capacities to be critical and informed individual and social agents. Nor are they provided with the knowledge and skills necessary to understand and negotiate the complex political, economic, and social worlds in which they live and the many challenges they face now and will face in the future. Instead of being institutions that foster democracy, public engagement, and civic literacy, universities and colleges now seduce and entertain students as prospective clients, or, worse yet, act as recruitment offices for the armed forces.[20] In other words, students are being sold on a certain type of collegial experience that often has very little to do with the quality of education they might receive, although university leaders appear content to have faculty provide entertainment and distraction for students in between football games.

Against the notion that the neoliberal market should organize and mediate every human activity, including how young people are educated, we need to develop a new understanding of democratic politics and the institutions that make it possible; we also need to organize individually and collectively to create the formative cultures that teach students and others that "they are not fated to accept the given regime of educational degradation" and the eclipse of civic and intellectual culture in and outside of the academy.[21] What is crucial to recognize is that higher education may be the most viable public sphere left in which demo-cratic principles and modes of knowledge and values can be taught, defended, and exercised. Surely, public higher education remains one of the most impor-tant institutions in which a country's commitment to young people can be made visible and concrete. The scandal at Penn State illuminates a profound crisis in American life, one that demands critical reflection—for those inside and outside the academy—on the urgent challenges facing higher education as part of the larger interconnecting crisis of youth and democracy. It demands that we con-nect the dots between the degradation of higher education and those larger eco-nomic, political, cultural, and social forces that benefit from such an unjust and unethical state of affairs—and which, in the end, young people will pay for with their sense of possibility and their hope for the future. Learning from the Penn State scandal requires that faculty, parents, artists, cultural workers, and others listen to students who are mobilizing all across the country and around the world as part of a broader effort to reclaim a democratic language and political vision. These insightful and motivated youth are rejecting the narrow prescriptions and heavy burdens that would be foist on them, and choosing instead to invent a new understanding of what it means to make substantive democracy possible.

■ AUTHORS' DECLARATION

The author(s) declared no potential conflicts of interest with respect to the research, authorship, and/or publication of this article. The author(s) received no financial support for the research, authorship, and/or publication of this article.

■ NOTES

1. For an excellent analysis of the weaponizing of higher education, see David H. Price, *Weaponizing Anthropology* (Oakland: AK Press, 2011). See also, Henry A. Giroux, *The University in Chains: Confronting the Military-Industrial-Academic Complex* (Boulder, CO: Paradigm, 2007).

2. Paul Krugman, "Depression and Democracy," *New York Times*, December 12, 2011, p. 23.

3. Center County Grand Jury Indictment against Gerald A. Sandusky. December 20, 2011, p. 3. http://www.freep.com/assets/freep/pdf/C4181508116.pdf

4. Ibid.

5. "Jerry Sandusky Arrested on New Charges of Child Sex Abuse: The Former Penn State Assistant Football Coach Faces More than 50 Child Sex Abuse Charges," *Los Angeles Times*, December 7, 2011. http://www.latimes.com/sports/la-sp-newswire-20111208,0, 265641. See also, "Penn State Charges: News on the Cases against Sandusky, Curley and Schultz," State College website, December 20, 2011. http://www.statecollege. com/news/penn-state-charges-sandusky-curley-schultz/

6. Michael Bérubé, "At Penn State, a Bitter Reckoning," *New York Times*, November 17, 2011, p. A33.

7. Ibid.

8. Cary Nelson and Donna Potts, "The Dangers of a Sports Empire," AAUP Newsroom, November 29, 2011. http://www.aaup.org/AAUP/newsroom/2011PRs/psu.htm

9. Bryan J. Lowder, "The Danger of Joe Paterno's 'Father-Figure' Mystique," *Slate*, November 2011. http://www.slate.com/blogs/xx_factor/2011/11/10/the_danger_of_joe_paterno_s_father_figure_mystique.html

10. Katherine Greenier, "From Fear to Safety: Confronting Sexual Assault and Harassment on Campuses," *RH Reality Check*, November 21, 2011. http://www.rhreality-check.org/article/2011/11/18/schools-must-protect-tudents-from-sexual-violence

11. Penn State Division of Student Affairs. "Know the Facts—Rape and Sexual Assault," Penn State Center for Women Students, December 20, 2011. http://studentaffairs.psu.edu/womenscenter/awareness/rapeandassault.shtml

12. Claire Potter, "The Penn State Scandal: Connect the Dots Between Child Abuse and the Sexual Assault of Women on Campus," *Chronicle of Higher Education*, November 10, 2011. http://chronicle.com/blognetwork/tenuredradical/2011/11/1401/

13. Bryan J. Lowder, "The Danger of Joe Paterno's 'Father-Figure' Mystique," *Slate*, November, 2011. http://www.slate.com/blogs/xx_factor/2011/11/10/the_danger_of_joe_paterno_s_father_figure_mystique.html

14. Phil Rockstroh, "The Police State Makes Its Move: Retaining One's Humanity in the Face of Tyranny," *Common Dreams*, November 15, 2011. http://www.commondreams.org/view/2011/11/15

15. Henry A. Giroux, *Against the Terror of Neoliberalism* (Boulder, CO: Paradigm, 2008).

16. Stefan Collini, "Browne's Gamble," *London Review of Books* 32.21 (November 4, 2010). http://www.lrb.co.uk/v32/n21/stefan-collini/brownes-gamble

17. Giroux, *University in Chains*.

18. Peter Seybold, "The Struggle against Corporate Takeover of the University," *Socialism and Democracy* 22.1 (March 2008): 1–11.

19. Seybold, quoted in Steven Higgs, "The Corporatization of the American University," *CounterPunch*, November 21, 2011. http://www.counterpunch.org/2011/11/21/the-corporatization-of-the-american-university/

20. See Price, *Weaponing Anthropology*; and also Nick Turse, *The Complex: How the Military Invades Our Everyday Lives* (New York: Metropolitan, 2008).

21. Stanley Aronowitz, *Against Schooling: Toward an Education That Matters* (Boulder, CO: Paradigm, 2008), p. 118.

14 Investigating Corruption in Corporate Sport

The IOC and FIFA

■ ANDREW JENNINGS

■ PROLOGUE

Investigative journalism? Here's how we do it. We find a gap between the polished public face and the sordid reality of a commercial enterprise, a government institution, a global sports body, whatever. We work assiduously acquiring confidential documents, legal affidavits from witnesses, the best of academic research, assembling a package of evidence that is scrutinized by media lawyers and reviewed by sceptical editors. All those tests passed, we publish our disclosures, are not sued and the cause of public knowledge is advanced.

My conference address on this theme at the University of Otago, New Zealand, was well received by the assembled scholars.[1] I duly sent footnotes and signed away copyright for my contribution to be included in a special issue of *Sport in Society*.[2] The guest Editor, Steven Jackson, a highly regarded scholar in this field, accepted my piece and prepared it for publication.

Some time later the Executive Editor, a Mr Majumdar, whose contribution to research in my area I remain unaware of, wrote rejecting my presentation, stating that he enjoyed reading my work 'in bits' but it needed rewriting to come up to his 'academic' standards. He also claimed there were legal reasons. Two FIFA officials were said to be 'well-known' litigants. I knew this to be factually incorrect. These men had never and would never risk being cross-examined on oath.

I wasn't surprised to discover later that Mr Majumdar and some of his Routledge/Taylor and Francis colleagues had made reverential presentations to FIFA's Blatter and the IOC's Samaranch, both of whose organizations in the past have been unable to resist torrents of corruption allegations in the media and in courtrooms. In April 2010 the *Financial Times* published my by-lined obituary of Samaranch in which I drew attention to his habit, when climbing the greasy pole of sports administration in Franco's Spain, of signing his letters to government officials: *'Siempre a tus ordenes te saluda brazo en alto'*—'I am always at your service with my arm raised.' I do not believe this fact was referenced in Mr Majumdar's presentation to Samaranch.

I circulated Steve Jackson and some of the Otago participants, making clear I wouldn't dream of rewriting my work to satisfy someone for whom I lacked any professional respect. This view was reinforced when I discovered that Mr Majumdar venerated sports officials who my research revealed were not worthy of such exaltation.

I went back to researching, filming, publishing and accepting worldwide invitations to lecture at universities and contribute to academic journals not associated with Mr Majumdar. Not all academics have the luxury of a freelance career to fall back on.

I have no idea if Mr Majumdar's approach to editing this special issue was influenced by his apparent admiration for Samaranch and Blatter, or that the publication suffered without my contribution. But other editors and academic publishers continue to request I write for them on the topics where I failed to meet his standards.

There's something I need to get off my chest. I should come clean with you. I'm delighted to be here, thanks for inviting me; you've kindly flown me all the way out here. You're entitled to know that I'm not all that I seem.

I'm a criminal. Yes, I'm a convicted criminal. And this is my crime. A court in Lausanne, in Switzerland, ruled in 1994 that I had shown 'a deep contempt towards the International Olympic Committee, its president and its members, criticizing their personalities, their behaviour and their management. I was guilty of telling lies for profit.' I got a five-day suspended jail sentence from that court.[3]

I'm a criminal because I wrote a book that told the truth. A book that revealed Juan Antonio Samaranch was a loyal Franco fascist for 37 years.

■ IN 1974

He was an IOC vice-president then. Six years later they made him President.

And I revealed that IOC members took bribes. And they did. It's all true.

But they're not the criminals. I am. And, what's more, the IOC banned me. I was banned from their press conferences, from covering their meetings, from doing my job as a reporter. And if you think they're beginning to sound a little heavy-handed, a little, shall we say, on the totalitarian side, then get this.

They illegally got hold of my phone records, identified some of my contacts. And *then* they used *their* police contacts to try to dig dirt on my friends. This is true! Samaranch personally called a Spanish police chief to get some dirt on my friend and fellow journalist Jaume Riexach. At least, that's what Samaranch *tried* to do. Instead he got a little muddled and by mistake called Jaume's number and started talking to Jaume as if he were the chief of police. Jaume had to tell him, Look, Mr President, you've made a mistake. . ..[4] I know it sounds like something the Marx Brothers dreamed up, but it's not. This is the real world of sport. These people have real power and the money to do as they want, and here's how they're using it.

Samaranch and his IOC were not the only ones. Now, it's happening with FIFA. I published a truth about FIFA. I said that President Sepp Blatter pays himself a secret bonus. They banned me. I carried on publishing. Their agents stole my phone records.[5] They identified people they thought might be my contacts and tried to intimidate them. I carried on. They used FIFA funds to attack me with their lawyers.[6] And on, and on. And don't forget, these people are supposed to be running *sports* events. That's their *job*, isn't it? Running sport for the benefit of humanity?

So what's all this got to do with foreign policy? Why am I here? I'll give you one small clue. I'm not the first person who suspects that, across the world, in countries rich and poor, policy, foreign and domestic, is, more than ever these days, run in the interests of the big corporations. Now, you'll know that I'm not an academic. I'm not an ideas man. You wouldn't put me in charge of a Think Tank.

I'm an investigator. I sniff something rotten and I go after it, like a detective, like a prosecuting magistrate. I go after the documents and the good people who might help me. They're the ones who've got the raw intelligence. They've got the documents, they know what's going on. I find them, persuade them, cajole them, find out what they know, digest it, go searching for more—more good people, more documents. I put the allegations to the bad guys. More sifting, more digesting.

Then, when I think I've got the material I need, I hang up my detective's mac, I go to my desk and become a storyteller. You know, someone once said that writing is easy. You just stare at a blank sheet of paper until your forehead bleeds. I turn storyteller and I try to tell my story in the most entertaining way I know. That's quite a job. And it's difficult to do all that while at the same time answering the big questions. What's their game? What's the big picture? Why are these people doing what they're doing? And lately I've been thinking hard about this. And the answers I've come up with are rather scary. But first I want to tell you a little about how I got here. How I came to sport. Why, of all the gin joints in all the towns, in all the world, I walked into this one.

Here's how I get started on a story. I spot a gap between the public face of an organization and its private reality. That piques my curiosity. I start digging. When I came across this line from the French sociologist and activist Pierre Bourdieu, I thought, Yes! He wrote: 'Among the tasks of a politics of morality [is] to work incessantly toward unveiling hidden differences between official theory and actual progress—between the limelight and the backrooms of political life.'[7] I learned my trade investigating crooked businessmen. During the Iran Contra affair I researched secret intelligence services.[8] Through the 1980s I explored corruption among top-level police officers in London and revealed their close relationships with the gangsters they were *supposed* to be catching. I investigated the mafia in Palermo and their heroin shipments to London.[9]

When I began investigating the IOC nearly 20 years ago some of my friends in journalism laughed: 'Sport? We investigate governments, big business, the police. Why poke around in sport?' I said, 'Sports organizations are in the public sphere. They're backed by public money. They wield power. Why should they escape scrutiny?' And the gap I'd spotted between the Olympic limelight and its backrooms had piqued my curiosity with such force I could barely sleep at night. I discovered that IOC President Juan Antonio Samaranch had been a loyal hard-working and successful fascist in Franco's murderous regime.[10] Here was the Olympics, an international organization pledged to sport and peace and youth and all things good. And here was its leader . . . I've got other pictures of Samaranch in his blueshirt and jackboots . . . a card-carrying fascist. Ludicrous? Unbelievable? True. I had to go digging.

Part of me wants you to believe that I suffered for this story that made my name around the world, I had to apply my brilliant brain, it was so tough outwitting the bad guys. Well, here's a secret. It *wasn't* that difficult. Samaranch's fascist past was a fact, just sitting there—if you'll excuse the expression—like a turd on a well-manicured lawn. All I had to do was pick it up. And there was no hurry, no competition. The beat reporters had their hands full already. Full of press releases, full of goody bags, full of hope—some of them—that one day they might land a job as a spokesman or a press officer for the people they report about to us. They were well-mannered guests at a party who weren't about to spoil the fun by asking embarrassing questions of the host, still less by digging up his lawn. Journalists aren't the only deferential guests.

For decades *some* academics have been turning education funding into unread volumes about 'Olympic Idealism', the 'Unifying power of the Games', perpetuating the myth that IOC members 'do it all for the athletes'. You know, these partygoers also got a little gift to take home: a preface of praise rounded off with a florid signature from Juan Antonio that they could paste in the front of their academic eulogies. What an endorsement! As for getting hold of original and confidential documents that might reveal what Bourdieu called 'hidden differences', dear me, no! That would definitely spoil the party. Reporters and academics should never be guests of the powerful. We shouldn't desire their invitations. We reporters must not forget who we are. We are honest brokers of information or we are worse than useless. We serve the people, not the power elites. Sure, power is seductive, that's one way it works. *We* don't succumb to that. We *resist*. We do our job. We investigate. And then we share our discoveries in the most entertaining way we know.

Back to Samaranch. I'd spotted my gap and soon I had the pictures that proved it. That wasn't difficult. I picked up my phone and called Barcelona. So, here, I thought, was the story: the fellow who ran the Olympics—peace, youth, goodness, all that jazz—had a history that conflicted with all of those values in every respect. I carried on digging and analysing, digging and analysing, learning more about Samaranch and how the Olympics worked.

I pondered that public–private gap. It wasn't as simple as I'd thought. I came to understand that this story went deeper and wider and it was dark. I studied Horst Dassler, once head of Adidas. I learned how Dassler, back in the 1960s, began investing his company's time, money and influence in putting useful men into positions of power in sport. He employed a secret team of fixers. Elections were manipulated and Dassler's placemen soared to the top of sports politics on thermals of Adidas money and influence.[11] And here's what Dassler wanted in return: Exclusive contracts for ISL, the sports marketing company he founded, and world domination for his sports kit company Adidas. Dassler was a visionary. He understood, years before the Harvard Business School started preaching it, the importance of strategic alliances. What's more, the true nature and value of Dassler's alliances was covert. Juan Antonio Samaranch was one of Dassler's placemen. Does that matter? I'd say so.

The Olympics is supposed to be a force for good in the world, something for all of us, not a front for boosting sales and making rich men even richer.

And there was more. Dassler's commercial imperative and Samaranch's fascist skills worked beautifully together. If you wanted to run the Olympics as a money machine, you had to keep things close, recruit loyalists and keep them loyal. Nothing buys loyalty like money. And, there's dirt; if you've got some on your subordinates, terrific. One way or another many Olympians went on the payroll. First-class air travel, the biggest limousines, five-star hotels, the full VIP-treatment. Fear and favour, absolute obedience to the leader, an appeal to youth and fitness. Sound familiar? The values that formed Juan Antonio Samaranch—totalitarianism, repression, respect for capitalism, all *that* jazz—were perfectly in tune with the way the Olympics really operated. This man's fascism *wasn't* an aberration. It was his supreme qualification for the job. Now and then bidding cities would complain about being asked to buy the Olympians' votes. The information was sitting there. Did the beat reporters pick it up? Not until Salt Lake, when the stink was so eye-watering that President Samaranch himself was forced to acknowledge it. Do you remember that? The things IOC members would trade for their votes? Cash. Sex. College places for the kids. Hip replacement operations. Cosmetic surgery. And—yes, really—one visiting party of IOC members demanded, and got, a violin, piles of Viagra and a vibrator![12]

I have to say I enjoyed those times. I took calls from journalists all around the world: 'Mr Jennings. You must feel very vindicated.' At last, the corruption of IOC members, an institutionalized corruption, created by Samaranch in exchange for total support at last, all that made global headlines. I was interviewed by around 150 TV networks, profiled all over the place. *The Wall Street Journal* sent a reporter to my front door! I was in *The New York Times*! The IOC lifted the ban! I did feel vindicated. Very vindicated.

Hurriedly, Samaranch announced a 'reform programme', a project built so heavily on lies that it could, alone, make a 300-page case study of Bourdieu's 'hidden differences'. That study is called *The Great Olympic Swindle,* my fourth book. This time, probing the gap, taught me more. Much more. I learned that sport was much bigger, far more important than I'd ever imagined. President Samaranch's reform programme was organized by Hill & Knowlton and one of its figureheads was Henry Kissinger.[13] I'll say that again: President Samaranch's reform programme was organized by Hill & Knowlton and one of its figureheads was Henry Kissinger. These are not the kind of people you employ to help launch a new brand of mascara. Hill & Knowlton are *the* spin-doctors of choice for global capitalism in trouble. When big tobacco wanted us to believe that smoking wasn't a health issue, Hill & Knowlton did the spinning. They've spun for McDonalds, Coca-Cola, Adidas. And now Hill & Knowlton were master-minding Samaranch's reform programme. Let's reflect on that for a moment. Feeling comfortable? And Henry Kissinger was there too. Henry Kissinger hasn't changed since he made his name carpet-bombing Cambodia, making the world safe for American capital. He hasn't retired. He's gone freelance! His international consulting firm, Kissinger Associates, has advised, among others, Coca-Cola, American Express, Freeport-McMoRan Minerals and J.P. Morgan-Chase. Hill & Knowlton based one team in New York, another in Washington and a third in Lausanne to keep a grip on the IOC members and massage the media. 'Safe' reporters were selectively leaked 'good news' documents.

Other American heavyweights drafted in to restore our confidence included former Republican Senator Howard Baker. His law firm ranked among the ten most powerful influence peddlers in Washington. Taking care of business for the US Olympic Committee was former Democratic Senator George Mitchell. George sits on the boards of many big companies including Walt Disney, Federal Express, Unilever and Olympic sponsor Xerox.

To head the new 'reform commission' Samaranch appointed ... himself. Among the honourable members was then FIFA President João Havelange, who, over a 20-year period, allegedly pocketed huge bribes from Horst Dassler's ISL marketing company in return for World Cup contracts. Watch my BBC *Panorama* documentary; read my book.[14] Many of the sponsors were drafted on to the commission—to keep control of the process. NBC's Dick Ebersol was there. Helping with the window-dressing was Olympic scholar Professor John MacAloon.

A question. When Hill & Knowlton and Henry Kissinger and Dick and João helped Samaranch with his reform programme, what values, whose interests do you suppose they had at heart?

A. Justice?
B. Fair Play?
C. Sports fans?
D. The youth of the world?
E. None of the above?

When the Salt Lake [City] scandal blew up, the interests most imperilled were those of the corporations who owned the brands. Coca-Cola, IBM, Kodak, McDonalds, Panasonic, Visa. . . . It wasn't just the hundreds of millions of dollars they'd invested in this particular event that were in jeopardy. The value of their *brands* was at risk. And these brands are worth billions. The Olympics was in trouble, so corporations were in trouble. So capital's master mercenaries of mind control, Henry Kissinger and Hill & Knowlton, rode to the rescue.

After months of phoney debate Hill & Knowlton presented the 'Fifty Reforms'.[15]

'A substantial travelling exhibition of the Olympic Movement and Olympic history to be installed in host cities', was one root and branch reform. Another was demanding 'Greater recognition of the educational importance of the flame relay'. The Fabulous Fifty continued with radical measures like, 'During the Closing Ceremony of the Olympic Games, the Elected Athletes [to the IOC Athletes Commission] should be recognized by their peers and by all the Olympic Family'. And, you know, journalists bought the Hill & Knowlton line. '50 Stunning Reforms'. That *many*? Hadn't they been thorough!

Reporters took the press-releases about Samaranch's new reformed IOC, keyed them in to their computers, and filed them to their news desks. We like to think we live in free societies. No-one shoots us for asking questions. I wonder, really it baffles me, this is not a rhetorical question: why, in a society like mine, is media—and academic—scepticism in decline? If you have answers I'd love to hear them. But back to sport.

Why is capital so keen on sport? I'm not a social anthropologist, I'm not a psychologist. I'm not an expert on Stone Age Man. But here's my theory: sport is as old as we are. It's how we trained ourselves for the hunt and for battle. It's one of the ways we have fun. For some it's part of the mating ritual. When we watch sport we're more than spectators. When Pelé scored a goal, I scored. When Ali knocked out Sonny Liston, young, black, disenfranchised people all over America threw that punch. In my kitchen at home is a leather recliner, broken (it doesn't recline anymore) since the late 1980s when my friend Dave leapt up and crashed down the moment Manchester United scored in the English Cup Final. He wasn't watching the match. He was living it. When we're enjoying sport we're all open, we're vulnerable, we're small children again, we're sucking it up, we are so open to suggestion. And that's how Big Capitalism likes us to be. I think it was Antonio Gramsci, who said that you can't have a revolution when the enemy has an outpost in your head. *Sport* gives the corporations that outpost in our heads.

Do you remember, decades ago we'd read reports of exploited peasants in the developing world who wanted to strike a blow against American imperialists? They were no match for the well-armed Marines guarding the American embassy in their capital cities—the symbol of their repression. So what did they do? They marched to their local Coca-Cola bottling plant and burned the place down. Why don't they do that anymore? Go to a football event in the developing world. Odds are that it will be draped in Coke emblems and slogans. The sports federation leaders who trouser the cash never miss a chance to talk up their generous 'partners'. Coke brings you sport. Development funding, the Olympic torch relay was sold to Coca-Cola long ago. Coke is no longer a symbol of capitalist exploitation. The message is soft, warm and persuasive. Coke brings you football, the Olympic Games, the world track and field championship. Coke is your friend and benefactor.

Sport these days is a tool of capitalism, part of the machine that persuades us to buy stuff we don't need, fuelling economic growth that may or may not be in our true interests—but most certainly serves the interests of a growing clique of corporate executives and shareholders whose individual wealth amounts to hundreds of millions of dollars. Do these people have common cause with the rest of us? Do corporations care? These people who flog obesity burgers to our children, rot their teeth with Coca-Cola, promote economic growth to the point where the very planet is in jeopardy? Do they care? Are they with us? The multi-millionaire executives who invest corporate money in sports advertising and sponsorship are doing what the law demands, looking after the interests of their shareholders. And they're doing what the law permits—helping themselves, big-time. Are these the kind of people who watch sport with enough joy and passion to break my leather chair when Manchester United scored? I don't think so. Here's one reason why.

The corporations need to reach millions of customers, they demand big television viewing figures; crowds require record-breaking heroes; the human race evolves too slowly to break records with sufficient frequency. . . .. Here are the dope doctors at hand—with a cure. Sportsmen don't need doping. Sponsors do. And so to football . . . the beautiful game. And it is, isn't it? When you watch world-class football, and you see the perfect header meet the perfect cross and the ball rockets into the goal. Isn't that beautiful? When you see your kids out there in the garden, sweaters for goal-posts, arguing over who's going to be Ronaldo today, tearing up the lawn—don't you see beauty there?

The corporations see it too. *They* see the beauty. And *they* know how to use it. To harness the beauty of the game, the beauty of our children's sweat and dreams, the beauty of an athlete's body . . . and don't forget, the passion of our tribal loyalties. They know how to harness all that, to whip it up—and get it pulling their brands. Gary Lineker, one of *our* footballing heroes, used to be in Britain a symbol of decency, fair play. Not any more. To our children in Britain Gary Lineker is Walkers Crisps. What's David Beckham? I'd say he's a brand. And Beckham's stupendous personal wealth? That reflects how his success on the pitch, his physical beauty and his 'private' life's news worthiness combine to produce a power strong enough to compel us to buy Vodafone or Gillette. David Beckham, the brand, is a tool of capitalism—capitalism, whose survival depends on growth, no matter what. And so, running world football, we've got an operation, very like Samaranch's, that's designed to serve the corporations.

Like Samaranch, FIFA President Sepp Blatter runs a tight ship; he recruits loyalists and keep them loyal. Nothing buys loyalty like money. And, there's dirt; if you've got some on your subordinates, terrific. And here we go again. First-class air travel, long limousines, five-star hotels, the full VIP-treatment. As for the critics: ban them, intimidate them, get their phone records, identify their contacts, threaten their publishers and try to destroy them.

FIFA is now a multi-billion dollar business operating under Swiss charitable association rules. That guarantees minimal disclosure about what they do with the money. But they make a lot of *noise* about their commitment to transparency. A couple of years ago I thought my newspaper readers might like to know how much money President Blatter pockets from FIFA. The obvious person to ask was FIFA General Secretary and Director of Finance, Mr Urs Linsi. You can trust Mr Linsi. In 2003 he told FIFA's website:

> We should always remember to let the media and the public know what we are doing. There is huge public interest in FIFA, therefore we have to be as transparent as possible. We will try to communicate in a more open way concerning football matters so the world can believe us and be proud of their federation.

I emailed the transparent Mr Linsi: 'Please tell me what President Blatter earns in salary, pension contributions, cars, bonuses and any other perks?' Mr Linsi didn't reply. So I emailed FIFA Director of Communications, Markus Siegler. You'll see his transparency in action, in the BBC film I've bought here with me.[16] Here is our exchange of emails!

JENNINGS: 'Please will you disclose how much Sepp Blatter is paid.'
SIEGLER: 'We can answer your question as follows: The matter of the compensation of the President was dealt with and decided unanimously at the Finance Committee at its meeting on 15 December 2002 in Madrid. The respective minutes have been ratified by the Executive Committee at its last meeting on 6 March 2003 here in Zurich.'
JENNINGS: 'Thanks for your understanding.'
Siegler hadn't begun to answer the question. So I tried again.
JENNINGS: 'I don't understand. Why won't you tell me what Blatter earns?'
SIEGLER: 'We must abide by internal rules and cultural traditions. In Switzerland, salaries or income are simply *not* published. Also, you must *not* question FIFA's dedication to transparency.'
I tried again:
JENNINGS: 'How much is Blatter paid?'
SIEGLER: 'We told you already.'
JENNINGS: 'No you didn't.'
SIEGLER: 'Yes we did.'
JENNINGS: 'So how much is he paid?'
SIEGLER: 'We told you already. And, anyway, who wants to know?'

I gave up and went digging again. I acquired a document proving that Blatter pays himself a huge, secret bonus. I wrote a story under the headline: 'Revealed: Blatter's Secret Bonus that FIFA Tried to Cover Up'. My story said that former FIFA president Havelange had arranged, in great secrecy, for Blatter to get this payment every year. I disclosed this in the London *Daily Mail* on 18 March 2003. Within hours FIFA's website announced, dramatically, at the top of the homepage: President Blatter has 'instructed their lawyers to file law suits against Andrew Jennings and the *Daily Mail*'. His press release said I published . . . 'fiction'. And they declared me *persona non grata* at all FIFA buildings, press conference and events. I still am. But they didn't sue.

They won't talk to me but they're having to talk to a determined Swiss Investigating Magistrate, Thomas Hildbrand. He's probing allegations that senior FIFA officials were systematically bribed for nearly two decades by the ISL Marketing company. Over that period ISL was given the exclusive marketing contracts to the football World Cup—and the Olympic Games and the world track and field championships. In November 2005 Hildbrand and a squad of detectives raided Blatter's office at FIFA HQ. It is quite possible that before long FIFA president Sepp Blatter and other officials will be indicted as part of the kickbacks scandal.

If the cops do their job, the head of the FIFA serpent will soon be cut off. Will they reform? Will anybody press them to? It doesn't look as if the International Olympic Committee is perturbed. Earlier this month IOC President Jacques Rogge was a welcome guest at FIFA's congress in Munich. He gushed to the delegates, 'FIFA has a wonderful role in the world of sport'. Rogge then praised FIFA for its *exemplary* efforts with regard to *ethics* and *transparency* . . . and in the *fight* against corruption, manipulation, racism and doping.[17] Perhaps Mr Rogge's aides neglected to tell him that one of FIFA's seven vice-presidents is a noisy anti-Semite and another, a foul-mouth racist.[18] Maybe, Mr Rogge doesn't care. The Congress also approved the FIFA financial report—currently under scrutiny by Magistrate Thomas Hildbrand. FIFA assures its members that every item has been checked by their Internal Audit Committee. Its chairman is Franco Carraro, recently forced to quit as president of deeply corrupt Italian football. He's a long-time member of the IOC, long-time ally of Samaranch. And the big picture. The big picture . . .

Some pictures that have stayed in my mind lately are the ones of two frail, old, decent, black men, two heroes of our time, two examples of humankind at our best, kowtowing to FIFA, begging FIFA to bring the World Cup to South Africa for 2010. Nelson Mandela and Archbishop Desmond Tutu both defied medical advice and travelled to Trinidad at FIFA's behest, to beg for one executive committee member's vote. And what do Mandela and Tutu represent? Surely, the people. If George W. Bush serves, as he puts it, 'the haves and the have mores', Mandela serves—and has truly suffered for . . . the have-nots. Well, Sepp Blatter's trusted vice-president, Jack Warner, had Mandela suffer a little more. I don't think I'm putting it too strongly when I say that if you disrespect Mandela, as FIFA's Jack Warner did, you disrespect not just South Africa, not just all Africa, but all of us.

Earlier this year, a comment in the *New Yorker* magazine caught my eye. Writer Nancy Franklin had been watching the Torino Games on NBC, the biggest single paymaster of the IOC. She said, 'The network made a nice profit from the Games, helped along with ads for health foods like Coke and McDonald's fried-chicken sandwiches and by dozens of ads for gas-guzzling Sports Utility Vehicles, the automotive shame of America, whose emissions do their part to melt the snow and ice that make the Winter Olympics possible.'[19] Allow me please, one last digression, would you? An awful lot of people, let's say 30 million of them, rely on the NBC television network for news. Can they trust NBC to tell them what's going on in the world? Is NBC an honest broker? Well, they're owned by General Electric, a gigantic global corporation that's into transportation, aircraft engines, lighting, nuclear reactors, medical equipment, plastics and money-lending. GE, along with McDonalds, Visa, Samsung and a few other global friends, is one of the leading Olympic sponsors. 'Partners', they call themselves. According to the Center for Public Integrity, in 2002 a study of misconduct by the leading 43 government contractors ranked GE top of the list of 'repeat offenders.'[20] GE had to pay $982 million in fines, judgments and out-of-court settlements for environmental violations, fraud in dealings with the government and consumers, workplace safety violations and employment discrimination. The Center tells us that in 2001 and 2002, General Electric spent more than $31 million lobbying Congress and other government agencies. So that's General Electric, the parent. Is NBC an honest broker?

When, a couple of years ago, Thomas Hoog, chairman of Hill & Knowlton's Washington office, picked up the public relations industry's highest award—they call it the Gold Anvil—at a glitzy banquet in New York, the master of ceremonies was one Al Roker, a host of NBC's *Today Show*. Al needs to earn a crust, but still . . .

As we hurtle towards environmental catastrophe, Big Capitalism wants us to carry on consuming regardless of the consequences. Sport, opening us up, exposing our childlike, suggestible selves, is a powerful force. And it's controlled by some frightening fellows. So, let's investigate our governments, corrupt police officers, environmental polluters. And let's take a closer look at sport. As I said at the beginning, I'm not a great thinker. I'm not an academic. Please, explore this area. Open it up. Please, shine some light on what seems to me a dark and dangerous place where international sport and governments and big business intersect. And, if they invite you to their party, may I make a suggestion? Leave your manners at home. Take your spade. You see that manicured lawn? Come on. Let's dig.

▪ NOTES

1. 41st University Otago Foreign Policy School, "Sport and Foreign Policy in a Globalising World", 23–26 June 2006.

2. Sport and foreign policy in a globalising world, *Sport in Society* 11.4 (2008).

3. Reuters, 8 December 1994.

4. *El Triangle,* 18 December 1992.

5. *Daily Mail*, 18 March 2003.

6. Evidence of attempts to access my phone records, in Jennings, *Foul,* 300.

7. Bourdieu, *Practical Reason.*

8. Granada TV, *Very British Mercenary.*

9. Granada TV, *Mafia in Palermo.*

10. Jennings and Simson, *Lords of The Rings.*

11. Jennings, *Foul;* Jennings and Simson, *Lords of The Rings.*

12. *Salt Lake Tribune*, 30 September 2000.

13. BBC, *Panorama;* Jennings, *Foul.*

14. IOC report, 1999.

15. Canton of Zug, press release, 2005.

16. BBC, *Panorama.*

17. Rogge speaking at FIFA Congress, Munich, June 2006.

18. On allegations that Julio Grondona is an anti-Semite, see Jennings, *Foul,* 245–248; on allegations that Jack Warner is a racist, see *Trinidad Express*, 10 May 2006.

19. Franklin, *New Yorker,* 3 March 2006, 89.

20. Center for Public Integrity.

▪ REFERENCES

BBC. (2006). *Panorama: The Beautiful Bung.*

Bourdieu, P. (1998). *Practical Reason.* Stanford, CA: Stanford University Press.

Canton of Zug. (2005). Judicial Department of Economic Crime. Press release.

Center for Public Integrity. (n.d.). Available at http://www.publicintegrity.org/default. aspx.

Daily Mail. (2003). Blatter's secret bonus. 18 March.

El Triangle. (1992). Samaranch plays at spies. 18 December.

Franklin, N. (2006). New Yorker. 6 March.

Granada TV. (1997). *World In Action: With the Mafia in Palermo.*

Granada TV. (1998). *World In Action: A Very British Mercenary.*

IOC. (1999). Report by the IOC 2000 Commission to the 110th IOC session, Lausanne, December.

Jennings, A. (2006) *FOUL! The Secret World of FIFA: Bribes, Vote Rigging and Ticket Scandals.* London: Harper Collins.

Jennings, A., and Simson, V. (1992). *The Lords of The Rings.* London: Simon & Schuster.

Salt Lake Tribune. (2000). Viagra. *Salt Lake Tribune.* 30 September.

Trinidad Express. (2006). 10 May.

15   ¿Plata o plomo?

Why Do Footballers Fix Matches?

■ DECLAN HILL

> Because then you're fucking him around, and he won't like it, and
> he'll tell his Short Man ... and then you get the chop and then you
> better watch it. You better get a bullet proof fucking vest, then....
> That's how fucking big it is.... This is how fucking dangerous it
> is.... When you're playing with fucking dangerous men, its fucking
> dangerous.
>
> —BRUCE GROBBELAAR, *cited in* Foul Play *by David Thomas*

Mexican drug dealers ask a simple question to potential collaborators in corrupt
deals—"¿*Plata o plomo?*"—Money or lead? That's accept a bribe or take a bullet in
the head.

It is a good model to examine the question: "Why do players participate in
fixed matches?" Do match-fixers (corruptors) make players "offers they cannot
refuse" or are players willing participants in the corruption?

In the popular literature on gambling match-fixing there is a theory that corruption is generated by violence. However, the evidence presented in the first
section of this paper shows that although violent recruitment may occasionally
occur, these stories are often media creations or an alibi created by the players to
cover their willing involvement.[1]

The second section of the paper is an examination of *why* the players choose to
accept bribes and *which* players are most likely to do so.

■ METHODS

This paper is based on a mixture of quantitative and qualitative research techniques. The author conducted over four hundred interviews with players, referees, coaches, team managers, league officials, policemen, prosecutors, bookmakers, gamblers and match-fixers who have direct experience in match-fixing. The
interviews are numbered and identified using the following codes: Corruptors
(COR1), Sports Officials (SO1), Players (P1), Law Enforcement (LE1).

Along with the interviews, there was also a text analysis of a "confession databank" consisting of documents—over 450,000 words—gathered from thirty-
one jurisdictions. One of the important sources in the databank was a collection
of previously unexamined witness statements collected by the Royal Malaysian
Police when they investigated match-fixing in their football league in 1995.

The research was also shaped by behavioural observation when the author directly witnessed match-fixers attempting to corrupt matches at major international football tournaments.

There is also a quantitative analysis from the construction of several databases. The two key databases used are Fixed/Non-fixed Games and Fixing/Non-fixing Players, referred to here as the FPD database.[2]

■ **MATCH-FIXING DEFINED**

An accurate definition of "match-fixing" is:

> When a player or referee deliberately underperforms during a sporting contest to ensure that one team loses or draws the match.

Given this definition, there are two different types of match-fixing in football. These types are:

> *Arranged match-fixing*: when corruptors manipulate a football match to ensure that one team wins or draws the match.

> *Gambling match-fixing*: when corruptors manipulate a football match to profit-maximise on the gambling market.[3]

In corrupted football matches, an arrangement fix will directly benefit one particular team—in the same way corporate executives can deliberately ignore environmental regulations to boost the value of their company.

While in gambling fixes, a team can be effectively sabotaged by its own players acting for their own profit—in the same way corporate fraud can devalue a company.

Match-Fixing Is Not Cheating

Match-fixing is *not* cheating. Match-fixing is where one person agrees to help one side lose. Cheating is using unscrupulous means to win.

In many cultures, cheating in sport is encouraged. What differs between sporting cultures is *how* someone cheats. For example, in some countries, to fake an injury to get an opponent unfairly sanctioned is accepted.

An example—Mauricio Taricco, was an Argentine defender playing in England:

> I had a problem with an opposing player and he pushed me . . . he raised his hand to me and I threw myself to the ground. . . . The ref saw me and sent him off. So everyone told me, "You're a cheat" (including his own team-mates and coach). The mentality of the people is different. Here they don't accept that. . . . I can't completely agree with

it. . . . In Argentina, if you get someone sent off . . . the coach will see it as a good move. (Taylor 1998, 58–59)

The implication is that only Argentinean players cheat to win. However, that argument ignores the English game's reputation for violent play. In English football kicking and elbowing opponents is considered a masculine, "fair" form of cheating. One symbolic example of this cheating is the widely-purchased photo of an English player—Vinnie Jones (later an actor known for tough-guy roles)—grabbing the testicles of a better player.

The point then is not that the Argentine game is fairer than the English game. It is that both sporting cultures condone cheating, just *different* kinds of cheating. Yet neither culture regards match-fixing as anything but deviant.

■ COERCION

In the media, there are a wide range of anecdotes that seems to support the idea that gambling corruptors coerce players into fixing matches—snakes in a player's car, a goalkeeper dying in a "mysterious" car accident. Some of the Malaysian players' confessions also seem to support the idea that violence is used for recruitment:

September 1993—it was during training time. Two Chinese men, maybe 5 feet 6 inches (167.6 centimetres), thirty years old, came up to me and congratulated me. They said they knew Mike and Frankie [Two Singapore corruptors]. They were Frankie's men. They had just met some of the other players. They asked me to cooperate with a fix against Singapore. I refused. I left. The two Chinese [men] followed me and forced me to stop. One of them took out a Rambo-style knife and threatened to kill me and my wife, if I did not agree to help them. (Royal Malaysian Police 1995, confession no. 5)

Stories of players being coerced by gambling corruptors also exist among different sports in different eras. For example, during the *President's Commission on Organised Crime* that followed the U. S. college basketball fixing scandals of the 1970s, a player who helped fix games testified that one of the organised crime operatives connected to the corruptors had said, "You can't play basketball with a broken arm. . .".

These excerpts and others seem to indicate that gambling corruptors frequently use coercion to persuade players to take part in gambling match-fixing. However, when the interviews were analysed by "role," none of the players who were directly involved in fixing matches, regarded coercion as a motivation. This excerpt from an interview with one player is typical, when asked if players were threatened by corruptors, he replied:

P6: Oh no. It is like a business to them.

QUESTION: So they don't threaten a player right away?
P6: Oh no . . .

The two other groups of interviewees who claimed there was little coercion during recruitment were law enforcement officers and the corruptors themselves—the two groups who were closest to the corrupt deals.[4] It could be argued that it is in a corruptor's best interests to claim not to use violence. Or those corruptors who did use violence to recruit players were less likely to be caught. However, even in the covertly taped confessions, where the corruptor does not know they are being recorded, violence is not explained as a recruitment tool.

A senior Singaporean policeman, who led many match-fixing investigations, also claimed that violence was not used in the recruitment of players:

> I don't think many players were forced into the fixing. [In the] Initial stages anyone could have acted with impunity. After we started enforcement, then there was a lot more apprehension. And then they started to enforce cooperation, but before we began operations there was no fear. It was only then that the players became fearful of the muscle behind the bookies. (LE5)

In the confession databank there are similar examples. Frequently, the police officers who interrogated the players wrote in that they felt the stories of violent coercion were an attempt to excuse the players' actions. For example, in the Royal Malaysian Police (1995) confession no. 5, the player was the head of the corruption network on his team, so he needed a strong exculpatory reason to explain why he had become involved. According to the police, the player's claim that he was the victim of extortion was an attempt to excuse his involvement.

There are cases of coercion in the confession databank, and there are mentions in some interviews in each group of interview subjects. However, a closer analysis of the American basketball case is typical: the gangster threatened the player with a broken arm after a "trial game" had not succeeded. In other words, it was coercion used to enforce the player's "continued involvement" rather than an initial recruitment ploy.

The confession databank was analysed using the following distinction: 'coercion used for recruitment' versus 'coercion used to enforce agreements.'

There are thirty-nine different incidents of coercion mentioned in the gambling section of the confession databank. Only five of these examples report incidents of coercion being used as an initial recruitment tactic.

However, of these five cases, three are where the police felt they were dealing with a "cover" story. A fourth was explicitly denied by an organised crime confederate in an interview with the author (although, of course, this is what they would say). The fifth incident is a report of an anonymous player in the British leagues of the 1960s being forced to fix matches by a betting syndicate to pay for his extensive gambling debts.

TABLE 15.1. *Coercion for Recruitment vs. Coercion for Ongoing Agreement (N = 39)*

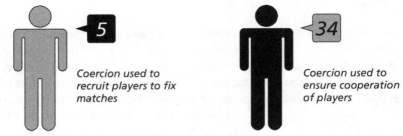

Coercion used to
recruit players to fix
matches

Coercion used to
ensure cooperation
of players

Source: Confession Databank.

The other thirty-four incidents of coercion follow the pattern where an arrangement did not work out and only then were the players threatened or felt that the possibility of extreme danger existed. See Table 15.1 for a breakdown of the recruitment versus enforcement results.

But what about the players who said no to corrupt deals? Was coercion used against them?

Among the interview subjects and confession databank, there are twenty-five cases of players who refused to fix matches when approached by gambling corruptors. Only one of them was exposed to coercive methods after he had turned down the first offer of fixing. Ironically, this came from his corrupt team-mates, rather than a gambling corruptor. They said in the 1915 fix between players of Manchester United and Liverpool, "If you score a goal you are—well—finished with Liverpool."

The experience of Laurent Wuillot, a midfielder for the Belgian team Brussels FC, who was approached in 2005 by alleged organized crime corruptors, is more typical:

> Two days before the match, I received a telephone call from an old acquaintance. He asked me if I would accept to not play the game to my fullest. . . . I refused immediately. I did not want to fall that low. But it was clear. The person and his commander respected my decision. I had known them for a long time and I was never threatened, *contrary to what people would have you believe.* (Delepierre 2006; emphasis added)

The data does indicate that *internal corruptors* (team management) use coercion to recruit players to fix matches. This finding was substantiated by the 2012 FIFPro report on fixing in Eastern European football leagues in a survey of over 3,000 of their members on match-fixing.[5] To those authors' surprise, not only did 11% of the survey group report being approached to fix matches, they also a reported a consistent pattern of harassment of the players by club owners. The authors stated,

> Even the most battle hardened of us, who had worked in player unions for many years, were astonished at the scale of the problems the players face. Non payment of salaries,

match fixing, violence, discrimination were all too common. . . . Many players were too scared to respond and many of the players' unions face hostile reactions from the clubs who would not allow their players to participate. FIFPro would also like to comment [on?] the players who have agreed to be interviewed. . . . [M]any of these players have been threatened and bullied. (FIFPro 2012, 4)

■ WHY WOULD A PLAYER PARTICIPATE IN A GAMBLING FIX?

If players are not forced into fixing, why would they fix?

It is not an easy question if one uses theories from classic criminology. Robert Merton, who was influential in shaping the field, argued that criminal deviant acts are, largely, committed by working-class males who lack status in society. The perpetrator has little legitimate means of acquiring status and thus turns to a criminal pathway.

It seems that Merton and his disciples would say that professional athletes are exactly the *last* people to commit an act of corruption. Professional sportsmen command enormous amount of status in their societies. Their place of work is watched by tens of thousands of fans. They are, purportedly, well-rewarded. Yet across a range of different leagues, countries and cultures, athletes at the very height of their careers have decided to fix matches. We saw in the last section that most of the time players are not coerced into corruption, so why would so many players decide to fix a match?

The data shows that the best way to understand why some footballers agree to fix matches for gambling corruptors is to see them as economically-motivated criminals who choose to participate in fixing matches for a set of financial reasons. The best comparison of footballers is not disadvantaged working-class males, but a mixture of business executives and professional ballet dancers.

Financial Motivation

The data indicates that in general, footballers take part in corrupt deals not because they are coerced but also for financial gain. The desire for money is shown throughout an analysis of the Fixing/Non-fixing Player Database (the FPD database mentioned earlier). The database has 117 players who responded either "yes" or "no" to a specific invitation to fix a football match: twenty-five who declined, and ninety-two who accepted. In the database there are 24 variables. One of these variables is "decision points," or a specific answer to a directly asked question related to gambling fixes "Why did you fix, or not fix, a match?"—for seventy-six of the players. These decision points come from varying sources in the database: some come from interviews; some are found in the equivalent of "life-histories"; in twenty-three of the cases, the players are answering this question in a court of law or a police confession.

The cases do show that the consistent, almost universal motivation for match-fixing is money.

The precise motivation for acquiring that money varies in each case, from conditions of relative deprivation to simple greed. There are various reasons, like private schools or clothes for children, investment in another business or inability to sell a house, given by the players to justify their decisions. The phrases that are repeated throughout the confession databank, in leagues of both high and low corruption, are variations of this theme:

> You have to understand these types. They can make more money on one fixed game than in an entire season, they are so badly paid at these clubs they are desperate to survive. (Delepierre 2006)

> It took a lot of heart-searching before I finally made up my mind to go through with the deal. I love football. It is my whole life. But I was in debt, and finding it difficult to manage. I thought of our money troubles. (Gabbert 1963)

> He had a fucking Rolex on his arm. I said, "Give it to me, I want to weigh it." It was the fucking business—three grands' worth of watch. He said, "This is yours, the next time you do the business [fix a match]." (Bruce Grobbelaar, quoted in Thomas 2003, 93)

This finding leads to two specific questions: If the players are mostly bribed into match-fixing, *why* do players accept bribes? *Which* players will accept bribes?

Is It All Just Anomie?

There are a range of theories that attempt to describe why some players chose to participate in gambling match-fixing. For example, the one most widely cited by Malaysian and Singaporean football officials is the "good-young-boys-entering-into-bad-circumstances."

This is a version of the "sex, drugs and rock n' roll ruining the lives of young men" argument that has assumed various guises since the Biblical prophets mentioned it to the young Israelites. It is, essentially, Emile Durkheim's theory of anomie.[6] The idea goes as follows: The players are young men who suddenly receive attention and financial rewards beyond their wildest dreams. They hang out with bad company. They drive fast cars. They are tempted by faster women. It all goes to their heads. Suddenly, they are fixing football matches and ruining the integrity of the sport that has given them so much. A senior Malaysian football official, outlines the structure of this argument:

> Most players are dropouts. Country boys. They would probably be working in the fields or rubber estates, if it were not for football. They are completely lost when they

become big football players. They visit discos. It is all new surroundings. Lots of girls. There is a lot of naiveté. They are not hard criminals. (SO1)

This lack of economic opportunity certainly describes the background of many professional football players in Malaysia. They tend to be disproportionately from both poor backgrounds and socially marginalized groups like the Tamil community in Malaysia or the Malaysian community in Singapore. The argument of the sports officials is strengthened by the strong sense of hierarchy in professional football in Malaysia and Singapore.

The players, from their mostly disadvantaged backgrounds, are given little status within the football community. At times, they have to kiss the hands, literally, of some league officials. These officials often do not hide their class-conscious contempt of the players. Another football official when interviewed said, "Most of the players are sharecroppers who without football would be cutting rubber trees in the jungle."

To summarize this argument: a group of young working-class men, who normally would be unable to enjoy a middle-class lifestyle, are suddenly catapulted into a profession that gives them relatively large financial rewards, but uncertain status. The players have no set of firm rules that can guide them in this new situation. Their state of moral confusion is so overwhelming that they commit acts of deviancy and match-fixing.

If the theory of individual anomie leading to match-fixing were correct, match-fixing would be negatively correlated with age. Because players generally enter the league between the ages of 19 and 22, then the younger a player is, the more likely he would be to fix matches. Does the quantitative data support this hypothesis?

The text of Percy Seneviratne's (2000) history of the Malaysian football league, (published with the financial backing of the Football Association of Malaysia,

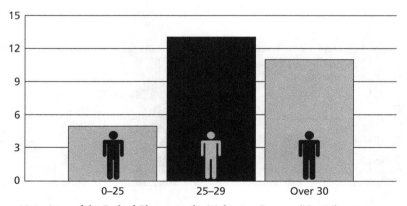

Figure 15.1. Ages of the Bribed Players in the Malaysian League (N = 29). *Source:* Seneviratne, *History of Football in Malaysia.*

or FAM) generally supports the idea of young players losing their heads and fixing matches. However, as shown below in Figure 15.1, it also reveals that of the twenty-nine players suspended by the FAM in 1994, only five of them were 24 or under. The other twenty-four players were senior professionals with years of experience both as players and in enjoying "the high life."

This finding is supported by the Fixing/Non-fixing Player Database for different leagues and playing eras. In the database there are sixty-six players who committed acts of gambling-related match-fixing whose ages we know. When broken down, the figures of the Malaysian-Singaporean league are, roughly, replicated. They show that match-fixing is largely the purview of older players: of the players who fixed matches, twelve (18.2%) were under the age of 25; twenty-one (31.8%) were between 25 and 28; and a further thirty-three (50%) players were 29 years old and over.

In Figure 15.2, these numbers are also contrasted with the age breakdown of players in a typical league of relatively high corruption—the Football League Fourth Division, operating in England & Wales in 1961—as a control group. In that league, 23.8% of the players were under 24, 56.7% were between 24 and 29, and only 19.5% of players were 30 and over. Yet this last group—players 30 and over—accounts for almost 45% of the match-fixing players in the database. In other words, a player 30 and over is more than twice as likely to be engaged in match-fixing as a player under the age of 25. These results are shown in Figure 15.2.

These findings do not, of course, mean that we can completely dismiss the theory of individual anomie. Figures 15.1 and 15.2 indicate only when the players were either caught or confessed to match-fixing, not when they started match-fixing. Players may have begun match-fixing at an earlier age because of individual anomie, but carried on fixing for other reasons. To further test the hypothesis that match-fixing is caused by youthful anomie, there was data for

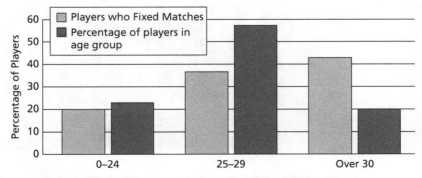

Figure 15.2. Ages of Bribed Players vs. Average Age of Players (N = 66).
Source: Fixing/Non-fixing Players Database.

TABLE 15.2. *Age Started Fixing and Years of Career Before Fixing (N = 41).*

	Average age of player in League	Age when started fixing	Age when caught fixing	Years of fixing	Years Playing before fixing
Average age	26.3	26.8	28.1	2.5	**7.3**

Source: **Fixing/Non-fixing Players Database (N = 41).**

forty-one of the players that give both their ages when they were caught match-fixing and when they started fixing. The results of this analysis are shown below in Table 15.2:

If a match is to be fixed, it is easier for a player with the most "playing capital" (the ability to most influence the game) to fix the match. It is the younger, less experienced players who, generally, lack playing capital since their place in the team is uncertain, their talent is undeveloped, and their ability is unknown.

The confessions and interview subjects also confirm that it was the senior players on the team who were generally the most prominent in fixing matches. These senior players were the players who had the longest amount of time to become used to the "high lifestyle."

Sexual Anomie

There is one qualification concerning these results. The statistics are accurate. However, they have an underlying sample bias. The data is, perforce, mostly from leagues of high corruption. The more corruption there is, the more players there will be who are fixing; the more fixing players there are from one league, the more the database will reflect situations of high corruption. However, there are four examples in the interviews and database of anomie leading to match-fixing. The examples are not related to age; rather, they are linked to leagues or circumstances of low corruption. An example, from one of the corruptors who was, allegedly, able to corrupt matches at the Olympic Games:

> There are some players who won't do it for money, but they will do it for women. I fixed the XXX team in 1996 against YYY at the Olympics in Atlanta. They wouldn't do it, when I offered lots of money. They said, "No, no, no . . . I am praying to God . . .". Finally, I got this beautiful Mexican girl. I paid her 50,000 dollars for the whole tournament. She would hang out in the lobby. She met him (the player from the XXX team) and then went up to his room, did it [had sex] and then she proposed to him. Then I went in. . . . "Will you do one game for me?" He said, "Yes." And they lose to YYY. (COR1)

The significance of this example is that sexual anomie was successfully created, not against a younger player in a league of high corruption, but against an older religious player in a competition where corruption was relatively difficult. In other words, in leagues/competitions where corruption is widely practiced, the decision to fix games comes mostly from the older players for financial reasons. However, in leagues/competitions with little corruption, anomie can be used as a motivation to get players to fix matches.

The general, correlated relation between age and match-fixing echoes other studies in the literature on economic crime and corruption ("white collar crime"). For example, in their study at Yale University, David Weisburd and colleagues examined the criminal conviction records of several hundred business executives. They looked at variables such as house ownership, marital status and societal position—which produced no significant difference. However, the one variable that did show a positive correlation was age: the older a person was, the more likely they were to commit economic crimes. As Weisburd et al. wrote:

> as offenders move into middle age they gain a growing awareness of time as a "diminishing, exhaustible resource" (Shover 1985, 211). Goals and aspirations change for these offenders as for other people as they get older. We suspect that such changes influence the willingness of offenders to be involved in criminality, irrespective of opportunity structures and other prerequisites for offending. (Weisburd et al. 2001, 41)

Advancing age makes economic crime unique. It is in direct opposition to most "street" crimes—burglary, murder, rape—where youth is directly related to the criminal's propensity to commit them. As business executives' propensity to commit economic crime is linked to their age, so footballers' success is directly linked to their physical ability, and professional footballers effectively become "middle aged" by their late twenties.

It is because of this physical factor that there is a link between match-fixing footballers and professional dancers. The British academics Steve Wainwright and Bryan Turner (2006) discovered in their study of professional ballet dancers, "Just Crumbling to Bits?", that many dancers have an acute sense of "physical capital." In a typical excerpt a dancer says:

> I retired at 38. I would say the last three years [I was] increasingly aware of aches that hadn't been there in the past, and also the fact that you take a little bit longer to get over from a particular exertion. . . .. [A]s I got older my wife would always notice when I got out of bed and creaked! (Wainwright and Turner 2006, 244)

Linked to this idea is the sense that physical ability is not only of relatively short duration but also vulnerable. Harry Gregg, a successful goalkeeper of the era when match-fixing was relatively common in the British game (including on Gregg's own team), revealed in an interview the attitude to injured players in the Manchester United squad: "when you get injured nobody will talk to you . . . you shouldn't get injured. That was just the unspoken thing. . . ."

It is this sense of the vulnerability and risk of imminent injury that is seen in the "fear of falling" that Stanton Wheeler et al. write of in their 1988 study of the motivation of economic criminals. Wheeler et al. claim that it is not only money that motivates economic criminals but also a sense of imminent failure. The FIFPro study also mentions this sense of failing. Older footballers have a strong sense that their careers may be over in the next game or practice. They need to make as much money as possible now. This is the key to why they fix matches.

Public Expression of Morality

One final question: Are players who publicly express religious or moral views less likely to fix a game?

The popular myth that surrounds match-fixing is that players who take part must be "lowlifes", while those who decline to take part have a far better moral code. As the Norwegian academic Jon Elster observes, morality is very difficult to measure accurately. It is, for example, quite possible for people to be guided by two or more moral codes simultaneously. However, what is clear in the specific case of match-fixing is that publicly professed personal morality is not a primary indicator of whether a player will fix a match; in fact, the exact opposite may be true.

As with coercion, morality does at first seem to play a part in the decision to fix a match. In the database, there are twenty-five instances where a player chose not to fix a match. In all of them some form of publicly professed morality is mentioned as a reason for turning down the fix. A few examples:

> Money would have been given to me if I had been willing to secure the loss of my team. The negotiations ended quickly. "I answered right away—no thank you. I can't hear you." *This kind of idea is so strongly against my morals that it wasn't a temptation..* (Staff writer, Ilta-Sansomet 2005; emphasis added)

> In the dressing room before the start of the game, he [the goalkeeper] was cornered, told what was about to happen and asked quite bluntly. "Do you want in?" Hastie Weir [the goalkeeper] went berserk [saying no]. . . *Weir was raging and ranting like some fire-and-brimstone preacher.* (St. John and Lawton 2006, 64; emphasis added)

> Two days before the match, I received a telephone call from an old acquaintance. He asked me if I would accept to not play the game to my fullest. . .. I refused immediately. *I did not want to fall that low.* (Delepierre 2006; emphasis added)

However, a closer examination of this evidence suggests that morality is not the only factor that prevents these players from corrupting matches. In all of these examples, as in most of the cases in the database, the "confessor" goes on to describe that in their own case they had enough money not to be tempted. The first example is a Finnish goalkeeper who reveals later in his confession that he had just signed a contract for several years with a professional team. In the second example, the financial position of Hastie Weir, the goalkeeper who turned down the fix, like "some fire-and-brimstone preacher", was compared to the other, poorer, fixing players:

> He [Hastie] had a good job as a works manager and when he joined us from the amateur club Queen's Park, he reputedly signed for £10,000, which was rather more generous than the bonus received by the rest of the dressing room. . . . The pros [who were organizing the fix] joined for a mere £20. (St. John and Lawton 2006, 63)

The Belgian player, whose confession was the final one listed, said, "Me, I had a chance. I made a career that took me to foreign places [i.e., he was well-paid]. It made it easy for me to refuse." A good summation of this mixture of morality and finance was given by Maurice Cook, a player for the English team Fulham, who was approached by representatives of Everton to fix a match in 1961. Cook claimed in his affidavit that, "Because of the smallness of the sum and my reputation for being a completely 'straight' player I could hardly believe that [the offer] was serious" (Gabart and Campling 1964). In other words, it was both the lack of money and Cook's own internal morals that did not allow him to take the corrupt offer seriously.

This is not to say that all morality has a price or that any player who refuses to take part in fixed matches is practicing a morality that is only achieved with financial security. But it is to say that the data from the confession databank is inconsistent on whether it is only morality or a combination of other intertwined factors that make players refuse to fix matches.

There is a similar comparison in the wider literature on corruption where Johann Lambsdorff points out that "corrupt people tend to be involved in a variety of charitable institutions." Thus publicly professed morality might on occasion be an indicator of corruption. However, the specific data on match-fixing at this moment is simply not clear enough.

▪ CONCLUSION

In this paper, we have seen that, in general, players are not forced into gambling match-fixing. Rather, the players decide to accept bribes as a rational choice. The key to understanding *which* players are more likely to accept bribes lies with Robert Merton (2005) and his academic followers. They are partly correct in describing why a player might consider accepting a bribe. The footballers are not under strain or anomie in their *current* circumstances. Nor are they thinking about trying to gain status; however, they are thinking about the *near* future, where they may be in a situation of anomie—no career, relatively uneducated and little opportunity for both the status and pay that they enjoyed as players. Given these circumstances, it then becomes a rational choice for the players to accept corrupt deals.

▪ NOTES

1. Peter Reuter did similar work in his study *Disorganized Crime* on the illegal gambling industry of New York, finding that many of the tales of violence were media creations.

2. For a more detailed examination of the research methods, please see pp. 14–27 in Hill, *The Fix*.

3. There is also a sub-group of gambling match-fixing called spot-fixing. This is when a player or referee deliberately underperforms specific events during a sporting contest to profit-maximise on the gambling market. However, the overall result of the contest may not be affected by spot-fixing.

4. The groups of interview subjects who claimed that players had been forced into match-fixing were people all removed from the corrupt deals: journalists, commentators or sports officials.

5. FIFPro is the International Federation of Professional Footballers, comprising 58 national players' associations.

6. Merton would later adapt Durkheim's theories to produce the Strain Theory of criminal behaviour.

▪ **REFERENCES**

Adler, F., and Laufer, W. S., eds. (1999). *The Legacy of Anomie Theory: Advances in Criminological Theory.* Vol. 6 of *Advances in Criminological Theory,* edited by F. Adler and W. S. Laufer. New Brunswick, NJ: Transaction Publishers.

Atkinson, Robert. (1998). *The Life Story Interview. Qualitative Research Methods.* Edited by John Van Maanen. London: Sage.

Biggs, Michael. (2005). "Dying Without Killing: Self-immolation 1963–2002." In *Making Sense of Suicide Missions,* ed. Diego Gambetta, 173–208; 320–324. Oxford: Oxford University Press.

Cole, Stephen. (1975). "The Growth of Scientific Knowledge." In the *Idea of Social Structure,* ed. Lewis A. Coser, 175. New York: Harcourt Brace Jovanovich.

Cressey, Donald. (1960). "Epidemiology and Individual Conduct: A Case from Criminology." *Pacific Sociological Review* 3(2): 47–58.

Cressey, Donald. (1967). "Methodological Problems in the Study of Organized Crime." *Annals of the American Academy of Political Science* 374: 101–112.

Delepierre, Frederic. (2006). "'On M'a Proposée 200,000 Euros': C'est Une Première. Un Joueur Approche Par La Mafia Des Paris Truques Ose Parler. Il a Refusé Le Jackpot." *Le Soir,* February 7, p. 36.

Denzin, Norman. (1989). *Interpretive Biography.* Newbury Park, CA: Sage.

Durkheim, Emile. (1952/1897). *Suicide: A Study in Sociology.* Translated by George Simpson and John A. Spaulding. London: Routledge & Kegan Paul.

Europol. (2013). European Police Press Conference, The Hague, Netherlands, February 6.

FIFPro. (2012). *Black Book: Eastern Europe—The Problems Professional Footballers Encounter: Research.* Hooffddorp, The Netherlands. January.

Ford, Trevor. (1957). *I Lead the Attack.* London: Stanley Paul.

Gabbert, Michael, and Peter Campling. (1963). Series of articles in *The People,* May 8, August 4, and August 11.

Gabbert, Michael, and Peter Campling. (1964). Offer That Was a Joke in *The People* 1: 8–9, October 10.

Gabbert, Michael, and Peter Campling. (1964). Series of articles in *The People,* August 4, August 11, May 3, and October 10.

Hill, Declan. (2010). *The Fix: Soccer and Organized Crime.* Toronto: Mclleland and Stewart.

Hill, Declan. (2013). *The Insider's Guide to Match-Fixing in Football.* Toronto: Anne McDermid & Associates.

Hobbs, Dick. (2003). *Bad Business: Professional Crime in Modern Britain.* Oxford: Oxford University Press

Hoffman, John. (2002, March). "A Contextual Analysis of Differential Association, Social Control, and Strain Theories of Delinquency." *Social Forces* 81(3): 753–785.

Katz, Jack. (1988). *Seductions of Crime: Moral and Sensual Attractions in Doing Evil.* New York: Basic Books.

Kuper, Simon. (2002, October 28). "Corruption? You Bet." *The Times,* p. 20.

Kuper, Simon (2005, July 23). "Pain, Humiliation and Fear—For a Few Moments of Glory." *Financial Times: London.*

Lambsdorff, Johann Graf. (2001). "Exporters' Ethics: Some Diverging Evidence." *International Journal of Comparative Criminology* 1(2): 27–44.

Lambsdorff, Johann Graf. (2007). *The Institutional Economics of Corruption and Reform: Theory, Evidence and Policy.* Cambridge: Cambridge University Press.

Maguire, Mike. (2000). "Researching "Street Criminals": A Neglected Art." In *Doing Research on Crime and Justice,* ed. Emma Wincup and Roy D. King. Oxford: Oxford University Press.

Merton, Robert K. (1967). *Social Theory and Social Structure.* New York: Free Press.

Merton, Robert. (2005). "Social Structure and Anomie." In *Social Deviance: Readings in Theory and Research,* ed. Henry Pontell, 37–44. Upper Saddle River, NJ: Pearson-Prentice-Hall.

Platini, Michel. (2011). Testimony before the Council of Europe, Strasbourg.

Reuter, Peter. (1985). *Disorganized Crime: Illegal Markets and the Mafia.* Cambridge: The MIT Press.

Ruggiero, Vincenze, South, Nigel, and Taylor, Ian. (1998). *The New European Criminology: Crime and Social Order in Europe.* London: Routledge.

Sanders, Teela. (2005). *Sex Work: A Risky Business.* Portland, OR: Willan Publishing.

Seneviratne, Percy. (2000). *History of Football in Malaysia.* Kuala Lumpur: PNS Publishing Sdn Bhd.

Shover, Neal. (1985). *Aging Criminals* (Sociological Observations). Beverley Hills: Sage.

St. John, Ian, and Lawton, James. (2006). *The Saint: My Autobiography.* London: Hodder & Stoughton.

Staff Writer. (2005). "Kaksi maalivahtia kertoo IS Urheilulle, että lahjuksia on tarjottu' and 'Maalivahti Sami Sinkkonen: Kieltäydyin kolmest lahjukssta." *Ilta-Samsonet,* December 2–3: 1–3.

Taylor, Chris. (1998). *The Beautiful Game: A Journey through Latin American Football.* London: Weidenfeld & Nicolson.

Taylor, Ian. (1970). "Football Mad." In *The Sociology of Sport,* ed. E. Dunning. London: Frank Cass.

Thomas, David. (2003). *Foul Play: The Inside Story of the Biggest Corruption Trial in British Sporting History.* London: Bantam.

Thomas, William Issac, and Znaniecki, Florian. (1918). *The Polish Peasant.*

Varese, Federico. (2001). *The Russian Mafia: Private Protection in a New Market Economy.* Oxford: Oxford University Press.

Wainwright, Steve P., and Turner, Bryan S. (2006). "'Just Crumbling to Bits?' An Exploration of the Body, Ageing, Injury and Career in Classical Ballet Dancers." *Sociology: Journal of the British Sociological Association* 40(2): 237–256.

Walton, Paul, Taylor, Ian, and Young, Jock. (1994). *The New Criminology: For a Social Theory of Deviancy.* London: Routledge and Paul Kegan.

Weisburd, David, Waring, Elin, and Chayet, Elin. (2001). *White-Collar Crime and Criminal Careers.* Cambridge Studies in Criminology. Cambridge: Cambridge University Press.

Wheeler, Stanton, Mann, Kenneth, and Sarat, Austin. (1988). *Sitting in Judgement: The Sentencing of White-Collar Criminals.* New Haven: Yale University Press.

Zainal, Mohamed, Ali, Mohamed, and Lomri, Ali. (2003). Disciplinary Hearing No.1-3/ 2003, 6. Disciplinary Committee, Football Association of Singapore.

PART V

Risk, Choice, and Coercion

All sports involve some risk. At minimum, there is the risk of losing or under-performing. Without it, there is nothing to gain. Many sports include additional risks to health and safety. As a society, the United States is relatively lenient in letting individuals accept risks. Despite high statistics of injury and fatality, we are allowed to hang glide, ride motorcycles, and compete in rodeos. However, they are limited allowances. We cannot hang glide anywhere we want, motorcyclists must be licensed (and helmeted in some states), and rodeos must be certified by organizing bodies. While ethics and the law are not mirror images, they are both concerned with consent and with knowing the consequences of risks. Society wants risk-takers to understand what they are giving up, and to isolate potential harm to the risk-taker.

Consent sounds good, but can a motorcyclist or hang glider, especially one who is young and feeling indestructible, actually understand his or her probabilities of serious injury or what life would be like as a quadriplegic? Are risks ever completely isolated when most citizens pay into a health-care system that is at least somewhat strained by reckless adventurers? Sports like American football, boxing, mixed martial arts, and even cheerleading lead to injuries that pose similar questions.

Some sports in history do not exist in modern civilized society because the risks are deemed too great. Gladiators are no longer allowed to fight to the death. Jousting at renaissance fairs bears minimal resemblance to the severe maiming that took place between actual knights. For much of human history, the length of a human life was largely unpredictable. Conditions like tuberculosis and pneumonia, or events like famine and earthquakes, brought swift ends to life and paid little attention to age. The relatively recent arrival of effective medical treatments, rapid transportation, and reliable physical and social infrastructure has also brought expectations for longer and fuller lives. It is possible that earlier societies were willing to tolerate more dangerous sports because sudden death was a more regular and accepted part of life. Modern society accepts sports with less, but still significant, risk. Do these risks correspond with our social expectations for informed consent and limited consequences? Are we tough enough on risk when it comes to sports like soccer, football, hockey, and wrestling—sports in which head trauma is common?

What must an athlete know about risk to give true informed consent? Recent revelations about concussions are putting the severity and permanence of head injuries in a different category from fractured ribs, torn tendons, and persistent aches. Starting as youth, athletes in American football become well acquainted with the latter risks. Several of them also receive concussions. They may think that a brief stint out of the game or a few days rest means full recovery. These players accept the possibility of temporary wooziness, as well as longer-term back stiffness, knee cracking, and limited range of arm and leg motion. If someone told them early on that playing high-level football would increase their chances of head-splitting migraines, extreme insomnia, violent mood swings, and/or suicidal depression, how many of them would continue with the sport? Many retired professionals, including present and future hall-of-famers like Harry Carson and Brett Favre, have become advocates for concussion awareness, and have indicated they do not want their children and grandchildren to play football.

Youth sports further complicate questions of both consent and consequences. As bad as many adults are at evaluating risk, children are worse. Adults are responsible for protecting children from each other and from themselves. This requires tailoring rules of play to age, such as we are seeing in some youth American football programs that limit full-pad tackle practice or in a few youth soccer programs that are requiring head protection. As Douglas Abrams explains in chapter 18, expectations for sportsmanship and respect can improve young athletes' communication and in-game choices, which can reduce aggressive contact and improve safety. Protecting children also requires appropriate role modeling. If adults and professional athletes exhibit disrespectful and dangerous behavior, or indulge fan expectations for hyper-aggressive contact, the rules governing youth sports will have limited effect. Youth athletes emulate their collegiate and professional counterparts, then those youth become their adult counterparts. It is clear that cultivating standards for respect and sportsmanship at all levels is beneficial for enhancing the value of sports and improving safety. Perhaps new medical science discoveries indicate that certain modern sports, regardless of their rules, are too dangerous in their present forms for kids and adults.

A. Dangerous Sports

16 The Organization and Regulation of Full-Contact Martial Arts

A Case Study of Flanders

■ JIKKEMIEN VERTONGHEN,
MARC THEEBOOM, ELS DOM,
VEERLE DE BOSSCHER,
AND REINHARD HAUDENHUYSE

■ 1. INTRODUCTION

Several studies have indicated that there is a high participation rate in martial arts (e.g., judo, karate, taekwondo, kickboxing) in a variety of countries (e.g., Australia [1]; Canada [2]; Europe [3]).* A participation study including all countries in the European Union revealed that martial arts are often situated in the top 10 of most practiced sports in a club-related context (e.g., France, Spain, Italy, Slovenia, Poland [3]). It is interesting to note that, throughout the years, the practice of harder variations (or types) of martial arts in particular (e.g., boxing, kickboxing, Thai boxing), referred to later in the paper as full contact martial arts,[1] has become increasingly popular [5, 6]. And while in many countries most of these full contact martial arts are not recognized or supported by the government, nor are they on the list of Olympic disciplines, these sports receive a lot of attention internationally. Illustrative here is the organization of the World Combat Games, including not only more "traditional" martial arts (e.g., judo, karate, taekwondo, aikido, wrestling), but also harder martial disciplines, such as boxing, kickboxing, Muay Thai, savate. The first edition of this high-level international multi-sport event was organized in 2010 in Beijing and included 13 Olympic and non-Olympic martial arts. The second edition, which was held in Saint Petersburg (2013), featured 15 different sports. The World Combat Games are organized by SportAccord, the umbrella organization for international sports federations, which works in close collaboration with the International Olympic Committee (IOC). This clearly shows the increased international recognition of martial arts in general, and harder types in particular.

In light of this trend, it is worthwhile noting that some controversy exists with regard to the organization and practice of these martial arts. On the one hand, there is a belief that involvement in these types of martial arts can lead to positive socio-psychological outcomes (e.g., development of social capital, improved personal well-being) [7, 8], and as such belief in their educational value. From this perspective, among other things, full contact martial arts are regarded as a developmental tool in working with youth at risk [9]. On the other hand, the practice of these types of martial arts raises distinct ethical and medical concerns for many. Most of the ethical concerns have been based on the assumed detrimental effects of full contact martial arts practice to the personal and social well-being of participants, in terms of aggressive and violent behavior [10]. This has often been linked specifically to youth involvement, which has resulted in an ambiguous public view as to their value as a youth activity. It has been indicated that these views are often largely based on perceptions created by the media and entertainment industry [11, 12]. According to some, popular media have created a distorted image of martial arts for mere (commercial) entertainment purposes [13–15].

With regard to medical concerns, which have been raised concerning the practice of full contact martial arts, reference has often been made to the prevalence of injuries in these types of martial arts. Although it is often assumed that full contact martial arts participants are more susceptible to injury [16, 17], to date sound empirical proof is still lacking. For example, it remains unclear whether or not there is a higher occurrence of injuries in full contact martial arts compared to other sports. While some studies reported higher injury rates in full contact martial arts [17], other research did not [18, 19]. Injury rates of full contact martial artists and other martial arts have also been compared. Findings have not always pointed in the same direction, however. While some studies reported a higher injury incidence among full contact martial arts compared to other martial arts (e.g., karate, taekwondo) [20], other research indicated that there were no differences [21].

Next to the ethical and medical concerns, full contact martial arts are confronted with some complex organizational issues. First, a wide variety of martial arts styles and disciplines exist, making it difficult to organize and regulate full contact martial arts. Several authors have attempted to develop a classification system, using a number of criteria (e.g., physical, functional, cultural, historical, philosophical). Some have made a distinction between martial arts and so-called "combat sports," with the former being described as "systems that blend the physical components of combat with strategy, philosophy, tradition, or other features, thereby distinguishing them from pure physical reaction" [22]. On the other hand, for the definition of combat sports reference could be made to "human target" [23]. This means that the objective of most combat sports is to show one's superiority over the rivals directly on the rivals' bodies (by employing different sets of techniques, such as throws, strangles, joint-locks, holds, punches, kicks, *etc.*) However, by far the most popular classification system divides martial arts according to cultural differences, such as "Eastern" *versus* "Western"

[24]. In this context, as also indicated by Theeboom [4], a dichotomization often exists between the "good" and the "bad." The Eastern martial arts (e.g., karate, taekwondo, aikido), which are often more associated with positive and educational outcomes, are mostly considered as "good." The Western martial arts (e.g., boxing, kickboxing), which are characterized by a strong emphasis on physical power and are more linked to aggression, violence, and health-compromising behavior, are regarded as "bad." For these reasons, the latter are often viewed from a negative perspective [10, 25]. In this context it is interesting to refer to a number of authors who have described an evolution towards increasingly harder variants or types of martial arts. This trend, also described as "brutalization" [26] or "desportization" [27] of martial arts, not only entailed more medical concerns [28] but it also led to a moral debate about the social acceptability of such types of martial arts [29–32]. In light of this, several authors have called for youngsters to be banned from participating in full contact martial arts, because of their assumed negative influences, based on medical, ethical, legal, and moral arguments [25, 33, 34]. However, as several authors have indicated, it is not clear that a ban would produce a better state of affairs. A ban may force the sport underground, where medical controls would be non-existent [35, 36].

Furthermore, the wide variety of martial arts styles and disciplines is one of the reasons why many different associations and federations are involved in the organization of full contact martial arts. As a result, a fragmentation of the full contact martial arts structures exists [37, 38]. For example many international boxing federations exist for boxing (e.g., World Boxing Council, WBC; World Boxing Association, WBA; World Boxing Organization, WBO; World Boxing Federation, WBF; International Boxing Federation, IBF; Women's International Boxing Federation, WIBF; Women's International Boxing Association, WIBA; International Boxing Union, IBU), while only one federation is recognized by SportAccord (*i.e.,* International Boxing Association or Association Internationale de Boxe, AIBA). As a result, the federations without a controlling organization above them can escape certain regulations and are less controllable regarding, among other things, the ethical and medical concerns previously indicated. This situation occurs not only at an international level, but also at a national level (e.g., France [37], The Netherlands [38]). The fragmentation of the full contact martial arts sector creates a lack of clarity in their organization making it difficult for administrators and policy makers to support and regulate martial arts, especially full contact martial arts, in a clear-cut manner.

As a result, it is not surprising that policy makers struggle with the governance of full contact martial arts. According to Kikulis [39], "sports governance" is the responsibility for the functioning and overall direction of the organization, and is a necessary and institutionalized component of all sports codes from club level to national bodies, government agencies, sports service organizations, and professional teams around the world. Despite the lack of clarity in a number of issues related to full contact martial arts, it is interesting to note that in several countries, policy makers endeavor to develop (or rethink) their strategy towards the regulation and support of full contact martial arts (The Netherlands [38], US [40, 41], France [37]). However, governments sometimes do not know which stance to take regarding the legitimacy of full contact martial arts (e.g., in terms of recognition or banning), which often results in an ambiguous position. In The Netherlands, for example, on the one hand the government supports martial arts by subsidizing and licensing, yet on the other hand they have attempted to limit and even to ban full contact martial arts events [38].

Furthermore, in this context it is also interesting to consider the changing point of view of policy makers with regard to the legitimacy of, for example, Mixed Martial Arts (MMA) in the United States (US). Hess [42] indicated that MMA began in the nineties more as a spectacle than a legitimate sport, and the shocking nature of the practice led initially to statewide bans on MMA competition in the US. According to Varney [41], the introduction of more rules, weight classes, and eventual state regulation, also described as re-sportization [27], ensured that MMA became more popular and visible, and as a result many states lifted their ban on MMA. Although much has been accomplished in making the sport a mainstream success, there are still areas that need to be/could be improved upon (e.g., public image, the boundary between "real" and "mock" fighting, influence on spectators, point of view of politicians [27, 41, 43]).

In conclusion, the full contact martial arts sector deals with some critical issues on a medical, ethical, and organizational level. These concerns are often the main reason why governments do not know which stance to take regarding the legitimacy of full contact martial arts (e.g., in terms of recognition/subsidizing or banning).

2. PURPOSE OF THE STUDY

In order to obtain a better understanding of the ethical, medical, and organizational concerns with which the full contact martial arts sector is confronted, scientific research into the governance of full contact martial arts is required. Although scientists from a wide range of disciplines (e.g., biomechanics, psychology, history, physiology, sociology, pedagogy, epidemiology of injuries) [44] have been paying increased attention to martial arts, until now only a limited number of studies have been conducted with regard to governance in martial arts [38, 40, 41].

By means of a case-study approach, the present paper will discuss some of the key issues regarding the regulation of a number of full contact martial arts which are considered to be problematic for (sports) authorities, and which confront sports policy makers in Flanders.[2] We decided to focus specifically on the situation in Flanders as the Flemish government has undertaken several steps in an attempt to tackle some of these concerns. In describing the Flemish case, this paper aims to highlight the need to develop a sound martial arts policy that can provide a legitimation base for the provision and organization of these full contact martial arts.

3. METHOD

In the period from October 2012 to February 2014 data were collected to obtain a better understanding of the specific situation with regard to the governance and organization of full contact martial arts in Flanders. More specifically, we attempted to list the problems, which confront the full contact martial arts sector, and to identify how policy makers have responded to this.

After conducting a literature review with regard to the organization and regulation of full contact martial arts, and analyzing sports participation data for these sports in Flanders, a document analysis regarding legislative and governance initiatives regarding full contact martial arts in Flanders as well as in other countries (particularly The Netherlands, US, England) was performed.

In addition, 58 interviews were conducted in order to obtain more insight into the experiences, problems, needs, expectations, and opinions of different relevant stakeholders (in)directly involved in the regulation or organization of full contact martial arts in Flanders. More precisely, these stakeholders were representatives of all known full contact martial arts federations ($n = 10$), experts[3] ($n = 5$) and referees ($n = 2$), representatives of the Flemish ($n = 4$) and local governments ($n = 13$), physicians who have experience with full contact martial arts ($n = 12$), experts with regard to full contact martial arts in The Netherlands ($n = 6$), and representatives of other organizations indirectly involved in the organization of full contact martial arts (e.g., insurance companies, coordinating organizations responsible for medical examinations of sports participants, organization involved in the domain of ethics in sports) ($n = 6$). Full contact martial arts participants or athletes are not included in this research as a separate group because a sufficient number of the interviewees are (were) active as participants.

In order to gain an overview of how full contact martial arts are regulated and organized in other countries beyond Flanders, an international survey was sent to (1) researchers involved in martial arts research and (2) national and international full contact martial arts federations which are linked to Flemish sports federations. In total, 12 researchers and 24 representatives of federations were asked to respond to the questionnaire. The response rate was, however, quite low, namely 31%. This can be attributed to the fact that none of the full contact martial arts federations responded. In contrast to the federations, 11 out of the 12 researchers that we contacted filled in the questionnaire. These researchers were from different countries all over the world (*i.e.*, Spain, Italy, Great Britain, Poland, Japan, USA, Russia, and The Netherlands).

In addition, four focus group discussions were organized, three regarding medical aspects related to full contact martial arts in which several physicians with experience of this group of sports participated ($n = 4$, $n = 4$, $n = 19$). Another focus group was held regarding the guidance and education of those involved in the organization of full contact martial arts (*i.e.,* teachers, referees, physicians) ($n = 5$). Present at the latter were representatives of different organizations: 2 full contact martial arts teachers, 1 member of the Flemish sport administration and 2 representatives of the department of the Flemish government that is responsible for the organization of courses for trainers.

Finally, 14 martial arts training sessions (3 for boxing and 11 for kick-/Thaiboxing), and 13 competitions of different full contact martial arts were attended, as well as 1 meeting of the executive board and 2 annual general assemblies of full contact martial arts federations.

Many different methods were used to gather the data of the present study. As indicated by Zohrabi [45], it is believed that using different types of procedures for collecting data and obtaining information through different sources augment the validity and reliability of the data and their interpretation. All interviews and focus groups were tape-recorded and most relevant aspects were transcribed verbatim. Afterwards the information was organized, processed, and discussed with the different authors of the present study. The results of this study are often based on the discrepancies between (a) different interviewees and (b) what was told and what was seen during competitions and trainings.

■ 4. RESULTS

Before starting to describe the Flemish case, it is interesting to first take a look at the lessons that could be learned from other countries outside Flanders with regard to the regulation and organization of full contact martial arts.

4.1. An International Survey Regarding the Organization and Regulation of Full Contact Martial Arts

The international questionnaire revealed a number of general findings relating to organization, competition, and coaches' education in full contact martial arts.

A first finding was that full contact martial arts are organized by recognized (by the government) or unrecognized (national) federations or organizations. Furthermore, it is reported that in most cases, full contact martial arts are organized within more than one sport federation, often with no collaboration. This results in a fragmented organizational setting per country and type of full contact martial art. Only in the United States does a particular structure exist today at governmental level, more specifically the State Athletic Commissions. Such a commission has a regulatory (umbrella) role with regard to full contact martial arts in particular states, regardless of the federations that are active in those states. As also indicated by Maher [40] and Berg and Chalip [46], the various state legislatures pass laws regulating full contact martial arts and commonly delegate authority to an administrative body, often a state athletic commission, to perform rule-making, licensing, operational, and enforcement functions.

Secondly, there appear to be a variety of providers of full contact martial arts competitions, such as federations and private organizations. If organized by the latter, a majority reported that little to no control exists with regard to the regulation of such events by local and national administrators.

Thirdly, in all the participating countries a coaches education program for full contact martial arts teachers exists, which is mostly coordinated by a (governmental) coordinating organization responsible for the organization of trainer courses.

There may be several explanations for the fact that only limited information could be collected. First, as indicated in the introduction, researchers investigating the regulation and organization of full contact martial arts are scarce and, as a result, a limited number of researchers have knowledge regarding this topic in their country (The Netherlands [38]; US [40, 41], France [37]). Secondly, most of those who do possess such knowledge are focused on only one full contact martial arts style and cannot provide a general view of how these sports are organized and regulated in their country. The latter limitation might also be applicable for the different full contact martial arts federations. Representatives of these federations can describe their particular situation, but they might not be able to give (objective) information on other federations. And thirdly, a language barrier exists, as most of the representatives of the federations do not speak English.

In conclusion, in most countries no coordinating federation or organization exists, which makes it difficult to obtain a general overview of the governance of full contact martial arts in other countries. Consequently, it seems even more relevant to obtain greater insight into how full contact martial arts are organized and regulated in one particular country.

4.2. The Flemish Case

Over a period of 17 months, we attempted to obtain a deeper insight into the organization and regulation of full contact martial arts in Flanders, using a number of means (*i.e.*, document analysis, interviews with key witnesses, focus group discussions, and observations of training sessions, competitions, and events). In the following paragraphs we will first provide a list of the key issues that are considered to be problematic for (sports) authorities, and which confront the full contact martial arts sector as well as sports policy makers in Flanders. These key issues will be discussed from an organizational, pedagogical, ethical and medical, and governmental perspective. Secondly we will describe the different initiatives that Flemish policy makers have undertaken in response to the difficult issues related to full contact martial arts.

4.2.1. Concerns Regarding Full Contact Martial Arts in Flanders

4.2.1.1. Organizational Perspective

The full contact martial arts sector is confronted with some complex organizational issues, which make it difficult to regulate and organize full contact martial arts in a clear-cut way. Some examples:

- As a consequence of the wide variety of federations involved in the organization of full contact martial arts in Flanders, the full contact martial arts sector is fragmented. Despite the fact it is difficult to gain insight into which federations are involved with the organization of full contact martial arts, we made an attempt to provide a brief overview of the Flemish federations which have been identified until now (see Table 16.1):
  - Four martial arts federations are recognized but not subsidized in Flanders. One of them offers only full contact martial arts (*i.e.,* Flemish Boxing League). Two federations offer next to full contact martial arts, also other (styles of) martial arts (*i.e.,* Flemish wushu federation and ABC Flanders). Finally, one of the four recognized federations is a multi-martial arts federation, which offers different martial arts, of which full contact martial arts are one.
  - Three multi-sports federations offer, among other sports, full contact martial arts. Those sports federations are recognized and subsidized by the Flemish government. In Flanders, however, the regulations which multi-sports federations are required to meet in order to be recognized and subsidized are less comprehensive than those imposed on uni-sports federations, because they are not involved in multiple tasks, such as the organization of competition on a local, national, and international level, talent development, and elite sport development, *etc.* The focus of those multi-sports federations is particularly on the organization of recreational sports participation.
  - Four martial arts federations, offering full contact martial arts are not directly recognized, but are affiliated with a recognized multi-sports or multi-martial arts federation.
  - Finally also not recognized full contact martial arts federations exist in Flanders. Today, we could only identify one federation. Probably more full contact martial arts federations exist, but because they do not wish to be known, it is hard to obtain an overview of them.
- Some sports clubs do not have any affiliation with a sports federation. Even more so than full contact martial arts clubs that are a member of a sports

TABLE 16.1. Overview of Flemish Federations Offering Full Contact Martial Arts (Boxing, Kick-/Thaiboxing, Mixed Martial Arts (Mma), Cage Fighting, K1, Full Contact Karate and Sanda). *

Recognized Martial Arts Federations (Offering Full Contact Martial Arts)	Flemish Multi-Sports Federations (Recognized and Subsidized) (Offering among Other Sports, Full Contact Martial Arts)	Martial Arts Federations Not Directly Recognized, but Affiliated with a Recognized Multi-Sports or Multi-Martial Arts Federation	Not Recognized Martial Arts Federations
1. ABC Flanders** (Kickboxing...)	1. Federation for Recreational and Omnisports (FROS)** (Kick-/Thai boxing, MMA, shoot boxing, K1, Full contact American Kickboxing ...)	1. Flemish Kickboxing, Muaythai & MMA Organization (Kick-/Thai boxing, MMA, shoot boxing, K1, Full contact American Kickboxing ...)	1. International Martial Arts Federation Belgium
			2. ...
2. Flemish Boxing league (Boxing)	2. SPORTA** (Muaythai, Boxing...)	2. Belgian Karate Organisation Shinkyokushin (full contact karate)	
3. Flemish wushu federation** (Sanda)	3. Federation Dance and Sport** (Kyokushinkai karate)	3. Belgian Kyokushin Organisation (full contact karate)	
	4. ...	4. Belgian Mixed Martial Arts Federation (Kick-/Thai boxing, MMA, full contact karate...)	
4. Flemish martial arts federation** (Kick-/Thai boxing, MMA, full contact karate ...)		5. ...	

* Only those federations known by the Flemish government are included in this table; ** Offers, next to full contact martial arts, also other (styles of) martial arts; *** Affiliated with . . .

federation, clubs without any affiliation are hard to control and regulate, because they are difficult to reach and less information is available about them. Particularly, in such clubs the ethically and medically sound sports participation is highly questionable.

- A profound distrust exists between the different full contact martial arts federations, which makes it difficult to set up any form of collaboration. This distrust has been historically grown. Often it is a slight disagreement (such as conflicts regarding competition results, financial disputes, *etc.*) which results in the impossibility of any kind of collaboration.

He is a renowned person in our martial arts style. But we, as a federation, could not continue to pay his personal expenses such as the wheels of his car. That is why he is split off from our federation. (a representative of a martial arts federation)

- Full contact martial arts participants and clubs can be a member of different federations. Because the federations do not have any information about each other, this leads to some critical issues. For instance, when a participant of a full contact martial art is suspended in one federation, he or she can participate at competitions organized by other federations. If the participant was suspended because of medical reasons (e.g., after a knock-out) this can have consequences for the health of the participant. Moreover, each federation has its own competition rules and system to classify competitors according to their level of experience (e.g., elite-amateur, A-B-C-D). The phenomenon of "federation shopping" can raise several questions: How can the level of experience of a competitor be determined when each federation uses its own classification system? How can a competitor prepare him/herself thoroughly if he/she has to adapt him/herself to the rules that are applied?

4.2.1.2. Pedagogical Perspective: Full Contact Martial Arts Coaches' Education

In Flanders, a department of the administration of the Flemish government leads the organization of a trainer course with regard to full contact martial arts. In order to guarantee the quality, the organization of trainer courses is based on a collaboration between the sports administration of the Flemish government, the recognized Flemish sports federations, three Flemish universities, and 14 colleges offering an education in Physical education and Movement Sciences. The trainer course with regard to full contact martial arts focuses on historical, medical, ethical, didactical, safety, juridical, mental, and deontological aspects of full contact martial arts, as well as on how to train youth practicing a full contact martial art. However, some concerns exist with regard to this course. Some examples:

- Because of the fragmentation as well as the wide variety of full contact martial arts, the trainer course is a general course for different full contact martial arts. This implies that no sports specific training course exists for boxing, kick-/Thaiboxing, MMA, *etc.*
- Only a limited number of full contact martial arts trainers have followed the trainer course organized by the department of the administration of the Flemish government. This is an issue concerning demand for—as well as supply of—the trainer course. With regard to the former, there is only limited interest and motivation to follow the training course, because the content of the existing course is not sufficiently well-known in the federations, or supported by specific federations. Regarding the supply chain, the training course is not accessible enough for full contact martial arts teachers, because many of them are low-skilled and/or immigrants. With regard to the latter also a language barrier exists.
- Very few full contact martial arts federations require recognized certification for a trainer to start a sports club. This carries the risk that participants of full contact martial arts are trained by insufficiently qualified trainers, meaning the safety of the participant cannot be ensured.

4.2.1.3. Ethical and Medical Perspective

In Flanders, a number of aspects suggest that the safety of participants is insufficiently guaranteed today. Some examples:

- In some full contact martial arts clubs and federations in Flanders, members are not obligated to have insurance. Some clubs and federations require this only of their competitors.
- Furthermore, a lack of clarity exists regarding compulsory protection (e.g., is it compulsory to wear a helmet?). Furthermore, differences exist in the protection material (e.g., leg protection: thick *versus* thin).

The shin protection is sometimes treated in a stepmotherly way. Some have really very thin, other very thick protection. There is a big difference between the impact of a blow to the head with such a light protection, that has mostly moved to the wrong side during the fight, as compared with a thick shin protection. (a physician)

- No clear agreement exists with regard to the medical examination of a participant of a full contact martial art (*e.g.*, before a competition, after a medical suspension period, *etc.*)
- Because of the fragmentation of the full contact martial arts sector and the problem of "federation shopping," discussed previously, no general system exists, with regard to checking the medical status of participants. Each federation has its own system, and as a result there is no general registration of the total number of competitions with an indication of wins/losses,

injuries sustained, knock-outs, - A lack of clarity exists with regard to the authority of a physician during competition.

- In most federations, the specific regulations with regard to youth are vague. For example, in some federations punching to the head is allowed, but participants are not allowed to hit "hard."

It is written in the rules that youth cannot make hard contact, but in fact this is bullshit, because what is "hard"? "Hard" for the one is different for another. (expert in full contact martial arts)

Some additional ethical issues related to full contact martial arts are interesting to note:

- The commercialization of full contact martial arts events can be considered as an ethical issue. The commercial gain of such events is often considered more important than the safety of the participants.
- In Flanders, popular media have created a distorted image of full contact martial arts, by focusing on a one-sided, negative account, primarily with regard to the negative medical impact of practicing full contact martial arts [47–49].

4.2.1.4. Governmental Perspective

Finally, also from a governmental perspective some issues which confront the full contact martial arts sector, as well as sports policy makers, in Flanders could be raised. Some examples:

- There is lack of clarity in the vision of the Flemish government. For more than a decade, one of the pillars of the Flemish sports subsidization policy relies on the existence of a selected list of 54 sports that are eligible for official recognition and financial support by the Flemish government. The list includes 10 different martial arts (aikido, amateur boxing, fencing, jiu-jitsu, judo, karate, kendo, taekwondo, wrestling, and wushu). Apart from amateur boxing (because of its Olympic status), no other full contact martial arts are included. This is mainly because of distinct medical and moral concerns that were raised. The lack of clarity in the vision of the Flemish government relates to the fact that on the one hand, limited recognition and no support is allowed for participants of full combat martial arts, such as Thai and kickboxing (because they are not on the official sports list), while on the other hand, the same government supports a number of sports-based developmental initiatives that make use of these sports.
- The Flemish government uses a specific term to refer to full contact martial arts, namely "risk" martial arts. This term refers to those martial arts that have specific techniques which permit punching or kicking an opponent with the intention of reducing his/her physical or psychological integrity

(Decree of 13 July 2007 on medically and ethically sound sports participation, Art. 2, §13). Based on the interviews with expert witnesses, as well as on what was heard during attendance of different competitions, trainings, and meetings, we can indicate that the introduction and the use of this term has caused consternation among different individuals involved with martial arts practice. According to many of those involved in full contact martial arts the use of this term promotes negative stereotyping, and is not positive for the image of this kind of martial arts.

In order to improve the image of our martial arts, we have to take our own responsibility and emphasize the positive aspects. . . . This is however very difficult when you are called "risk martial arts." (a representative of a martial arts federation)

Besides the Flemish government, the local authorities are also confronted with some difficulties regarding the regulation of full contact martial arts.

- Municipalities and cities are unaware of the problems and the possible abuses that occur in full contact martial arts (*e.g.*, rental of locations to organizations which are not practicing/organizing martial arts in a medically sound way).
- Municipalities and cities can determine the criteria that sports clubs have to fulfill in order to obtain financial support. Often a sports club is not required to be a member of a recognized sports federation. Because of this, it is possible for a local sports club to receive the financial support of the local authorities without being a member of a sports federation. As they receive the financial support of the local authorities, they do not feel the need to be affiliated with a sports federation. As indicated earlier, such clubs are less controllable and often, even more than those that are a member of a sports federation, the ethically and medically sound sports participation is highly questionable in these clubs.

4.2.2. Initiatives of the Flemish Government Regarding Full Contact Martial Arts

Despite the complex and numerous difficulties with regard to full contact martial arts in Flanders, the practice of these sports has become increasingly popular. Flemish participation data show that the number of participants practicing full contact martial arts (e.g., kick-/Thaiboxing, boxing, and MMA) has increased from 783 in 2002 to 5,718 participants in 2011. Since 2007, the Flemish government has undertaken different steps with regard to the governance of full contact martial arts. These different steps will be described more in detail below.

In 2007, the Flemish government passed a decree regarding medically and ethically sound sports participation in which the term "risk" martial arts was introduced. Two years later, as a consequence of this decree, Flanders set up an expert committee including policy officers, martial arts representatives, and physicians. Its task is to advise the Minister of Sports regarding the conditions for a medically sound practice and delivery of full contact martial arts instruction in Flanders. Among other things, the committee has proposed a set of generic guidelines with a dual purpose. On the one hand it should give the Flemish government standards that allow her to test the obligations that sports federations have, in order to guarantee medically and ethically sound sports participation. On the other hand, those guidelines have to give more clarity to sports federations who organize full contact martial arts on how they can comply with the decree regarding medically and ethically sound sports participation. To date, however, there is no formal obligation that requires sports federations to act according to these guidelines. If it were a formal obligation, the Flemish government would control the fulfillment of these guidelines, with financial implications.

Additionally, in 2011 a round table conference was organized on behalf of the Minister of Sports. In total, 94 participants attended the conference. The aim of this conference was to create more public support for the generic guidelines, and to offer the possibility to representatives of different sectors (*i.e.,* government, martial arts, health, welfare, education, youth, *etc.*) to exchange relevant information regarding the practice and the organization of martial arts. Furthermore, by listing the experiences, problems, needs, expectations, and opinions of relevant stakeholders it was aimed to obtain a better understanding of the specific issues with which the martial arts sector is confronted.

Finally, based on the results of this conference, at the beginning of 2013 the Flemish government decided to set up a Flemish Platform on full contact martial arts. This platform was formed in the context of an experimental project in which two full-time employees were appointed for a duration of two years. In general, the platform aims to provide more professional and qualitative support to those involved in the organization of full contact martial arts in Flanders, and to encourage collaboration between the various actors involved. More specifically, this is reflected in three major assignments:

- The platform is a knowledge center to extend knowledge with regard to the different aspects of full contact martial arts;
- The platform is a communication center and contact point: a center which will inform and communicate regarding full contact martial arts with all sorts of stakeholders (e.g., federations, government, *etc.*) on a regular basis;
- The platform is a service and support center for stakeholders involved in the organization or the practice of full contact martial arts.

Finally, it should be noted that the Flemish government should pay attention that, besides the fragmentation of the full contact martial arts sector itself, no fragmentation occurs at policy level, as the role of the different initiatives (e.g., expert committee, Flemish Platform on full contact martial arts) is not always very clear.

■ 5. CONCLUSIONS

Despite the increasing popularity of full contact martial arts, today the full contact martial arts sector is confronted with some ethical, medical, and organizational concerns which make it difficult for administrators and policy makers to support and regulate these sports in a clear-cut manner. The aim of the present paper was to highlight the need to develop a sound full contact martial arts policy. This was achieved by describing the Flemish situation, more specifically by describing (1) the key issues considered to be problematic for the full contact martial arts sector as well as sports policy makers in Flanders and (2) how the Flemish government has responded to these problems since 2007. It can be concluded that a number of concerns exist in Flanders with regard to the organization and regulation of full contact martial arts. However, a positive evolution is noticeable, as the Flemish government has undertaken different steps in order to outline a policy with regard to the regulation of full contact martial arts. One of the policy tools used by the Flemish government in their attempt to regulate the full contact martial arts sector was the formation of the Flemish Platform on full contact martial arts. However, it should be noted that several difficulties still need to be overcome in Flanders, at the level of the government (*e.g.*, how to pursue a full contact martial arts policy and obligate sports federations to act according to this policy?), of the martial arts sector (*e.g.*, how to increase the limited number of well-educated full contact martial arts teachers?), as well as at the level of the martial arts clubs (*e.g.*, how to deal with safety matters in the sports club?). Furthermore, it will be necessary to refine the data used in the present study because the underlying reasons behind certain aspects need further clarification. For example, (a) the influence of international federations at the national level and (b) which responsibilities should be taken by the government and which by the martial arts sector?

The Flemish case is not a single one, however. In other words, the difficulties with regard to governance in full contact martial arts are not bound to geographical places or limited to specific countries [50]. It will not be enough to tackle these difficulties at the local and national levels, because it leaves the possibility for full contact martial arts organizations to escape from more regulated countries to less strict regulated countries. Therefore the governance of full contact martial arts should be regarded as a transnational issue. Consequently, the question can be raised as to which role the European Union (EU) can fulfill. In this context, it is interesting to note that one of the programs of the European Commission aims to tackle cross-border threats to the integrity of sport and to promote and support good governance in sport [51]. Within this scope, it might be relevant to think in terms of the development of an international coherent policy with regard to full contact martial arts. However, it will be difficult to achieve the right balance between the rules enforced by the EU and the freedom of local and national self-regulation.

Furthermore, the deterritorialization and globalization of full contact martial arts requires research at a supranational level. This kind of research could be helpful to gain more of an insight into solving the problems related to governance, regulation, and management of martial arts, especially within an international context. The increased need to exchange knowledge and experience concerning the regulation and support of full contact martial arts can be illustrated by the organization of a workshop on the organization and regulation of martial arts during the 21st annual conference of the European Association of Sport Management (EASM) in 2013. At the end of this workshop, it was concluded that more initiatives are needed to initiate and stimulate research cooperation, to exchange relevant information, and to consider the option of developing an international network of researchers and policy makers involved in organizing, managing and regulating martial arts [50]. Consequently, more research is necessary with regard to the regulation of full contact martial arts from an organizational and governance policy perspective. In this kind of research, several issues could be raised, such as should full contact martial arts be banned by law or not? If so, what would be the consequences? If not, which rules and conditions are necessary in order to guarantee medically and ethically sound sport participation? In addition, it would be relevant to examine whether the regulation and the organization of full contact martial arts is the responsibility of the government or the martial arts sector itself. Alternatively, as suggested by Berg and Chalip [46] and Koppenjan and Klijn [52], it might be preferable for the full contact martial arts sector to work together with governments to tackle the difficulties with regard to these sports. In this case it would be necessary to examine how the government and the sector relate to each other.

Finally, we would like to focus on the increasing interest in the use of full contact martial arts as a developmental tool [53]. Despite the fact this is a positive evolution with regard to full contact martial arts, this should be viewed from a critical point of view. The simple fact that people engage in a sport setting does not automatically imply that improvements in personal or social outcomes can be expected. It therefore becomes clear that more attention must be paid to the structural components and processes of management and guidance within the sports context in general, in our case within full contact martial arts, in order to provide greater insight into the complexity of the underlying processes that are presumed to generate social benefits [54–56]. A more modest perspective and more research that tries to obtain insight into the underlying conditions and processes producing developmental outcomes would contribute to a deeper understanding of any effects.

In conclusion, the complex issues that confront full contact martial arts need a local and international approach, as well as further investigation. By stimulating research cooperation and exchanging knowledge and experience, more insight could be obtained into the governance, provision, and organization of full contact martial arts, which in turn can provide a legitimation base for the development of a sound martial arts policy. Better organization and regulation of the full contact martial arts sector might be helpful in developing towards a more accepted, respected, and recognized group of sports.

The authors declare no conflict of interest.

▓ NOTES

1. Many different terms and definitions are used to refer to martial arts [4]. For the remainder of the present paper, we will use "martial arts" as a generic term, and use the term "full contact martial arts" to refer to sports such as boxing, kick-/Thaiboxing, mixed martial arts (MMA), cage fighting, K1, full contact karate, and sanda.

2. Flanders is the Dutch-speaking northern part of Belgium.

3. Someone was considered an expert when he or she had more than 20 years of experience with full contact martial arts as an athlete and more than 10 years of experience as a teacher. Moreover, most had experience with the practice of more than one full contact martial art.

▓ REFERENCES

1. Australian Bureau of Statistics. *Children's Participation in Cultural and Leisure Activities, Australia, April 2009.* Available online: http://www.abs.gov.au/AUSSTATS/abs@.nsf/DetailsPage/4901.0Apr%202009?OpenDocument (accessed on 21 January 2010).

2. Ifedi, F. *Sport Participation in Canada 2005.* Culture, Tourism and the Centre for Education Statistics: Ottawa, ON, Canada, 2008.

3. Van Bottenburg, M.; Rijnen, B.; van Sterkenburg, J. *Sports Participation in the European Union. Trends and Differences.* Mulier Institute: Amsterdam, The Netherlands, 2005.

4. Theeboom, M. A closer look at effects of martial arts involvement among youth. *Int. J. Sport Manag. Mark.* **2012,** *11,* 193–205.

5. Brent, J.; Kraska, P. Fighting is the most real and honest thing: Violence and the Civilization/Barbarism Dialectic. *Br. J. Criminol.* **2013,** *53,* 357–377.

6. Theeboom, M.; Vertonghen, J.; Dom, E. The regulation of "risk" martial arts: The case of Flanders. In *Book of Abstracts*, Proceeding of the 21th Conference of the European Association for Sport Management (EASM), Istanbul, Turkey, 11–15 September 2013, pp. 79–80.

7. Fulton, J. "What's your worth?"—The development of capital in British boxing. *Eur. J. Sport Soc.* **2011,** *8,* 192–218.

8. Haudenhuyse, R.; Theeboom, M.; Coalter, F. The potential of sports-based social interventions for vulnerable youth: Implications for sport coaches and youth workers. *J. Youth Stud.* **2012,** *15,* 437–454.

326   ▪   Risk, Choice, and Coercion

9. Theeboom, M.; Wylleman, P.; de Knop, P. Martial arts and socially vulnerable youth: An analysis of Flemish initiatives. *Sport Educ. Soc.* **2008**, *13*, 301–318.
10. Endresen, I. M.; Olweus, D. Participation in power sports and antisocial involvement in preadolescent and adolescent boys. *J. Child Psychol. Psychiatry* **2005**, *46*, 468–478.
11. Grady, J. Celluloid katas: Martial arts in the movies—A practitioner's prejudices. *J. Asian Martial Arts* **1998**, *7*, 86–101.
12. Smith, R. *Martial Musings: A Portrayal of Martial Arts in the 20th Century.* Via Media Publishing: Erie, PA, USA, 1999.
13. Fu, P.; Desser, D. *The Cinema of Hong Kong: History, Arts, Identity.* Cambridge University Press: Cambridge, UK, 2000.
14. Taylor, K. Martial media. In *Martial Arts of the World: An Encyclopedia of History and Innovation*; Green, T. A., Svinth, J. R., Eds. ABC-CLIO: Santa Barbara, CA, USA, 2010; pp. 527–554.
15. Hunt, L. *Kung Fu Cult Masters: From Bruce Lee to Crouching Tiger.* Wallflower Press: London, UK, 2003.
16. Ngai, K. M.; Levy, F.; Hsu, E. B. Injury trends in sanctioned mixed martial arts competition: A 5-year review from 2002 to 2007. *Br. J. Sports Med.* **2008**, *42*, 686–689.
17. Junge, A.; Engebretsen, L.; Mountjoy, M. L.; Alonso, J. M.; Renstrom, P.; Aubry, M. J.; Dvorak, J. Sports injuries during the Summer Olympic Games 2008. *Am. J. Sports Med.* **2009**, *37*, 2165–2172.
18. Pappas, E. Boxing, wrestling, and martial arts related injuries treated in emergency departments in the United States, 2002–2005. *J. Sports Sci. Med.* **2007**, *6*, 58–61.
19. Porter, M.; O'Brien, M. Incidence and severity of injuries resulting from amateur boxing in Ireland. *Clin. J. Sport Med.* **1996**, *6*, 97–101.
20. Gartland, S.; Malik, M. H. A.; Lovel, M. E. A prospective study of injuries sustained during competitive Muay Thai kickboxing. *Clin. J. Sport Med.* **2005**, *15*, 34–36.
21. Gartland, S.; Malik, M. H. A.; Lovel, M. E. Injury and injury rates in Muay Thai kick boxing. *Br. J. Sports Med.* **2001**, *35*, 308–313.
22. Green, T. A.; Svinth J. R. Introduction. In *Martial Arts of the World: An Encyclopedia of History and Innovation*; Green, T. A., Svinth, J. R., Eds. ABC-CLIO: Santa Barbara, CA, USA, 2010; p. xix.
23. Parlebas, P. *Jeux, Sports et Sociétés, Lexique de Praxeologie Motrice [Game, Sports and Society, Lexicon of Motor Praxeology].* Institut National du Sport, de L'expertise et de la Performance (INSEP): Paris, France, 1999.
24. Donohue, J.; Taylor, K. The classification of the fighting arts. *J. Asian Martial Arts* **1994**, *3*, 10–37.
25. Pearn, J. Boxing, youth and children. *J. Paediatr. Child Health* **1998**, *34*, 311–313.
26. Förster, A. The nature of martial arts and their change in the West. In *Mind and Body: East Meets West*; Kleinman, S., Ed. Human Kinetics: Champaign, IL, USA, 1986; pp. 83–88.
27. Van Bottenburg, M.; Heilbron, J. De-sportization of fighting contests: The origins and dynamics of no holds barred events and the theory of sportization. *Int. Rev. Sociol. Sport* **2006**, *41*, 259–282.
28. Buse, G. J. No holds barred sport fighting: A 10 year review of mixed martial arts competition. *Br. J. Sport Med.* **2006**, *40*, 169–172.
29. Sheard, K. G. Aspects of boxing in the Western "Civilizing Process." *Int. Rev. Sociol. Sport* **1997**, *32*, 31–57.

30. Carr, D. What moral significance has physical education? A question in need of disambiguation. In *Ethics and Sport*; McNamee, M. J., Ed. E. & F.N. Spon: London, UK, 1998; pp. 119–133.
31. Parry, J. Violence and aggression in contemporary sport. In *Ethics and Sport*; McNamee, M. J., Ed. E. & F.N. Spon: London, UK, 1998; pp. 205–224.
32. Steenbergen, J. *Grenzen aan de Sport: Een Theoretische Analyse van het Sportbegrip* [*Frontiers to Sport: A Theoretical Analysis of the Sport Concept*]. Elsevier: Maarssen, The Netherlands, 2004.
33. American Academy of Pediatrics. Boxing participation by children and adolescents. *Pediatrics* **2011**, *128*, 617–623.
34. World Medical Association. WMA statement on boxing. Available online: http://www.wma.net/en/30publications/10policies/b6/index.html (accessed on 1 September 2010).
35. Gauthier, J. Ethical and social issues in combat sports: Should combat sports be banned? In *Combat Sports Medicine*; Kordi, R., Maffulli, N., Wroble, R., Wallace, A., Eds. Springer: London, UK, 2009; pp. 151–172.
36. Jones, K. A key moral issue: Should boxing be banned? *Sport Soc.* **2001**, *4*, 63–72.
37. Collinet, C.; Delalandre, M.; Schut, P.; Lessard, C. Physical practices and sportification: Between institutionalisation and standardisation. The example of three activities in France. *Int. J. Hist. Sport* **2013**, *30*, 989–1007.
38. Dortants, M.; van Bottenburg, M. Aanzien en overleven in een sport vol passie [Respect and survive in a sport full of passion]. In *Over Regulering van Full Contact-Vechtsporten* [*Regulation of Full Contact Martial Arts*]. Arko Sports Media: Nieuwegein, The Netherlands, 2013.
39. Kikulis, L. Continuity and change in governance and decision making in national sport organizations: Institutional explanations. *J. Sport Manag.* **2000**, *14*, 293–320.
40. Maher, B. *Understanding and Regulating the Sport of Mixed Martial Arts*. University School of Law: Oklahoma City, OK, USA, 2010.
41. Varney, G. Fighting for respect: MMA's struggle for acceptance and how the Muhammad Ali act would give it a sporting chance. *West Va. Law Rev.* **2010**, *112*, 269–305.
42. Hess, P. The development of mixed martial arts: From fighting spectacles to state-sanctioned sporting events. *Willamette Sports Law J.* **2007**, *4*, 1–23.
43. Sanchez Garcia, R.; Malcolm, D. Decivilizing, civilizing or informalizing? The international development of mixed martial arts. *Int. Rev. Sociol. Sport* **2010**, *45*, 39–58.
44. Distaso, M.; Maietta, A.; Giangrande, M.; Villani, R. The state of the art of scientific research in combat sports. In *Book of Abstracts*, Proceedings of the 14th annual Congress of the European College of Sport Science, Oslo, Norway, 24–27 June 2009; p. 599.
45. Zohrabi, M. Mixed method research: Instruments, validity, reliability and reporting findings. *Theory Pract. Lang. Stud.* **2013**, *3*, 254–262.
46. Berg, B. K.; Chalip, L. Regulating the emerging: A policy discourse analysis of mixed martial arts legislation. *Int. J. Sport Policy Polit.* **2013**, *5*, 21–38.
47. De Smedt, L. *Wij Krijgen Onterecht Stempel Crimineel* [*We Obtain Unfairly the Stamp of a Criminal*]. Available online: http://www.nieuwsblad.be/article/detail.aspx?articleid=DMF20131009_00782826 (accessed on 11 October 2013).

48. Op de Beek, H. 20 *Redenen Waarom deze Gevechtsport zo Gevaarlijk is [20 reasons Why Martial Arts Are Dangerous]*. Available online: www.hln.be/hln/nl/956/Meer-Sport/article/detail/1777518/2014/01/20/20-redenen-waarom-deze-gevechtssport-zo-gevaarlijk-is.dhtml (accessed on 3 February 2014).
49. Vermeiren, M. *Sugar Jackson werd Jarenlang Slecht Begeleid [Sugar Jackson Was Poorly Guided for Many Years]*. Available online: http://www.vandaag.be/sport/137822_sugar-jackson-werd-jarenlang-slecht-begeleid.html (accessed on 3 February 2014).
50. Vertonghen, J.; Dortants, M. Report on the workshop "Organising, Managing and Regulating Martial Arts" during the 21st EASM Conference. *Rev. Artes Marciales Asiáticas* **2014**, *8*, 480–483.
51. European Commission. *Erasmus + Programme Guide*, 2014. Available online: http://ec.europa.eu/programmes/erasmus-plus/documents/erasmus-plus-programme-guide_nl.pdf (accessed on 19 February 2014).
52. Koppenjan, J.; Klijn, E. *Managing Uncertainties in Networks. A Network Approach to Problem Solving and Decision Making*. Routledge: London, UK, 2004.
53. Theeboom, M.; Verheyden, E. *Vechtsporten met een Plus: Extra Kansen voor Kwetsbare Jongeren [Martial Arts with a Plus: Additional Opportunities for Socially Deprived Youth]*. Vubpress: Brussels, Belgium, 2011.
54. Chalip, L. Toward a distinctive sport management discipline. *J. Sport Manag.* **2006**, *20*, 1–21.
55. Theeboom, M.; Schaillée, H.; Nols, Z. Social capital development among ethnic minorities in mixed and separate sport clubs. *Int. J. Sport Policy Polit.* **2011**, *4*, 1–21.
56. Vertonghen, J.; Theeboom, M. How to obtain more insight into the true nature of outcomes of youth martial arts practice? *J. Child. Serv.* **2013**, *8*, 244–253.

B. Football and Concussions

17 Concussion and Football

Failures to Respond by the NFL and

the Medical Profession

■ DAVID ORENTLICHER
AND WILLIAM S. DAVID

■ INTRODUCTION

While medical experts have come to a better understanding of concussion in recent years, there still is much more to learn. We know that some football players develop a form of dementia (chronic traumatic encephalopathy) that appears to result from the repeated and mild head injuries that are a routine part of the sport.[1] However, we do not know the likelihood that a player will suffer from football-related dementia, nor do we know the extent to which genetic or other factors place some players at a greater risk than other players of developing dementia.

In reviewing the response of the National Football League (NFL) to concussion, one can easily think that the league was too slow to worry about the medical consequences of head trauma. Despite concerns being raised for many years about the risk to player health, it took until December 2009 for the NFL to advise its teams that players should not return to play or practice on the same day that they suffer a concussion.[2]

But the NFL was not alone in viewing concussion as a relatively mild problem; physicians also did not worry very much about the medical consequences of concussions. For some time, neurologic experts disagreed as to whether concussions could cause permanent injury, with many attributing patient symptoms to psychological issues or to the incentives created by compensation programs for people with disabling conditions. Team owners and league officials could have found articles or books that would have put them on notice about the effects of concussion, but they also could have found articles or books that would have given them a false sense of security.

Indeed for decades, concussion was viewed as a benign phenomenon without any structural damage to the brain and whose symptoms resolved fully within a short period of time.[3] Moreover, people typically assumed that concussions required some kind of collision between the head and another object and that a loss of consciousness was always part of a concussion. Over time, however, it has become clear that concussions result in damage to the brain, that the damage may be permanent, and that concussions can occur without any impact to the head or without any loss of consciousness.

Accordingly, the NFL now recognizes that concussions entail some degree of brain injury and that players should not be placed at risk of further trauma to the brain until all evidence of the injury has disappeared. As long as the player experiences any signs or symptoms of the concussion, additional brain trauma may place the player at risk for even greater injury.[4]

To be sure, there are experts who believe that the brain never fully heals from a concussion, that there is always some permanent loss of brain capacity. In this view, repeated head injury increases the extent to which brain capacity is diminished with players suffering greater problems in neurologic functioning as the diminution increases.[5] Thus, some neurologists believe that players should no longer play football (or other sports) once they have had three concussions. But there is currently not a consensus on this question.[6]

While the NFL may have responded slowly to problems from concussions, the extent to which its response was unreasonable is unclear. If many medical experts did not worry about concussions, it is difficult to fault the NFL for not worrying either. Moreover, the NFL did not ignore concerns about head injuries. It imposed helmet requirements and banned types of blocking and tackling that were particularly dangerous.[7] The NFL also convened an expert committee to study the issue.[8] Still, one can question the NFL's failure to adopt concussion guidelines in the late 1990s, when guidelines were issued by medical experts.

■ CONCUSSION

Although concussions need not involve any impact to the head, they do involve a collision between the brain and the inside of the skull. When a person's head or body is jolted suddenly and forcefully, the brain can crash against the skull causing small tears and other damage to the brain tissue and disrupting the balance among chemicals in the brain.[9] Both kinds of injury can cause neurological dysfunction.

The neurological dysfunction from a concussion can cause a variety of symptoms. People may temporarily lose consciousness, have headaches, feel dizzy or disoriented, and experience sensitivity to noise or light.[10] Individuals may also experience nausea and vomiting, have difficulties concentrating, or fail to remember what happened just before and after the concussion.[11] The symptoms may resolve within minutes, hours, or days; they may also persist for months or longer.[12]

Researchers believe that the disrupted chemical balance (metabolic dysfunction) leaves brain cells vulnerable to further injury. As a result, a second concussion in the next days or weeks can cause much more damage than a single concussion alone. In some cases, the second concussion can be lethal ("second impact" injury).[13] In addition, the repetitive brain trauma associated with football and other sports can lead to severe and permanent neurological impairment (chronic traumatic encephalopathy).[14]

Concussions are considered to be a relatively mild type of traumatic brain injury, with more severe types, including subdural hematoma, having the potential to cause devastating brain injury immediately. At one time, concussions were viewed as the mildest form of traumatic brain injury, but harm can also occur from blows to the brain that are not severe enough to cause a concussion ("subconcussive" trauma).[15]

■ MEDICAL UNDERSTANDING OF CONCUSSION

As mentioned, the medical profession was slow to recognize the significance of concussions. Consider, for example, what people would have learned about concussion in 1975 by consulting the fourth edition of Walton's *Essentials of Neurology*: concussion is "a temporary and largely reversible disorder of brain function which is not apparently associated with any striking pathological change in the brain."[16] Or consider what was written in 1981 by Cartlidge and Shaw in *Head Injury*:

> There are also those who believe that the postconcussional syndrome not only lacks an organic basis but is due to frank malingering. Miller . . . advanced in forthright terms the view that patients with postconcussional syndromes were simulating or at least consciously exaggerating their symptoms. In his own case studies he established a relationship between the occurrence of the syndrome and the incidence of claims for compensation . . . and he was struck by the absence of the syndrome as a sequel to sporting injuries.[17]

Some discussions of concussion reflected greater concern but also did not suggest that the problems were serious. In the chapter on concussion in Cooper's 1982 *Head Injury*, the text distinguished between mild cerebral concussion, for which consciousness was maintained, and classical cerebral concussion, which involved a "transient and reversible" loss of consciousness. After a mild cerebral concussion, the athlete would recover completely except for amnesia for the time periods just before and after the concussion. After a classical cerebral concussion, the great majority of athletes would have no long-term effects other than the brief amnesia, but "some patients may have more long-lasting though, subtle neurological deficiencies. Further investigation of these sequelae must be done."[18]

Even experts who counseled caution sent mixed messages. In a leading text on head injuries in football that was published in 1973, the authors observed that some players should stop playing football entirely after a single severe concussion (e.g., one that involved a loss of consciousness for more than five minutes) but also described concussion as a "reversible physiologic condition" that reflected "brief neurologic dysfunction."[19] And the authors advised that for mild or moderate concussions, it would be permissible for the player to return to the game once symptoms resolved.[20]

Interestingly, the authors acknowledged that players could return to action after concussions that would trigger a twenty-four-hour hospitalization for the average citizen.[21] As one reads the literature on concussion, one cannot help notice that experts are reluctant to prevent players from participating in athletic competition.[22] Of course, individuals assume risks in many occupations, and it may be the case that the risks from concussion are worth bearing in view of the potential benefits from playing football. But it also may be the case that the risks from concussion were discounted in a society that has glorified the hard hits of football.[23]

Skepticism about the harms from concussion reflected a number of factors. There did not appear to be a good correlation between the apparent severity of head trauma and the extent of symptoms. Some individuals did not develop persistent symptoms, despite the loss of consciousness and other neurological abnormalities that can accompany mild head trauma, while other people developed persistent symptoms without any loss of consciousness or other evidence of significant injury.[24] In addition, the medical profession had not developed a good definition for post-concussion syndrome. In a 1994 article, the author reported that only twenty-four percent of neurologists agreed that the post-concussion syndrome was "a clearly defined syndrome with a solid basis for determining prognosis."[25]

To be sure, there were experts who sounded the alarms. In 1962, for example, *The Lancet* published "Concussion and Its Sequelae." That article described the commonly held view that patients recover from concussion with no lasting deficits but then went on to observe that "[t]he concept of concussion as a transient and benign affair" is "no longer tenable." Rather, it was actually the case that the effects of concussion "may be severe and long-continued and are not always completely reversible."[26] Similarly, while the previously mentioned chapter on concussion in Cooper's 1982 *Head Injury* seemed reassuring, a later chapter in the same book, *Behavioral Sequelae of Head Injury*, raised greater concerns. It discussed evidence of significant and permanent neurologic damage from concussion, especially for athletes who sustained multiple concussions.[27] And by 1986, a leading expert on concussion in sports, Robert Cantu, had issued guidelines on the management of concussion that generally advised minimum waiting periods before resuming play after a concussion (e.g., one week), with longer waiting periods for more severe concussions (e.g., one month), and even longer waiting periods after multiple concussions (e.g., two weeks instead of one week or terminating the season instead of one month).[28] Still, it would have been easy for league officials and team owners to find comfort from the medical profession, particularly if they were looking for reassurance.

By the mid- to late-1990's, public and professional understandings had shifted, and concussion injuries were taken more seriously. Consider, for example, the approach of the American Academy of Neurology ("Academy"), which took a harder line than other groups. The Academy published guidelines in March 1997 for the management of concussion sustained during athletic competition. While the Academy concluded that an athlete could resume play after a concussion when symptoms lasted no more than fifteen minutes and there was no loss of consciousness, it also said that a second such concussion in the same contest should result in the athlete abstaining from play until a week passed with no symptoms at rest or with exercise. Moreover, if symptoms of concussion lasted more than fifteen minutes, the athlete should abstain from play until two weeks passed with no symptoms at rest or with exercise.[29]

If a player lost consciousness, then greater precautions should be taken. For a loss of consciousness that lasted a matter of seconds, the Academy wrote that athletes should abstain from play until a week passed without symptoms at rest or with exercise. If athletes lost consciousness for a matter of minutes, they should abstain from play until two weeks passed without symptoms at rest or with exercise. Finally, if an athlete sustained a second concussion with loss of consciousness, the athlete should abstain from play until at least one month passed without symptoms at rest or with exercise.[30]

While the Academy's guidelines represented important progress, they reflected some failures in the response to the problem of concussion by medical experts. For example, the Academy recommended weaker precautions for concussions without loss of consciousness than for concussions with loss of consciousness. Also, the focus was much more on management of concussion than on its prevention. Finally, there was not much consideration of the possibility that playing football might pose risks to brain functioning that were too high. Rather, the main concern was how long an athlete should be kept out of competition after a concussion before returning to play—for fifteen minutes, the rest of the game, a week, or longer? In short, the Academy's primary concern was to ensure that athletes avoided contact that might aggravate their concussions by having the athletes refrain from play until it appeared that they had fully healed.

Indeed, when it came to recommendations for future research, the Academy said nothing about concussion prevention. Rather, it called only for the development of better ways to assess concussions in athletes on the sideline of the field immediately after the concussions occurred and for studies that would document the health consequences of concussion.[31]

Of course, concussions are an inherent risk to playing football,[32] so attention must be paid to their management. Still, the Academy might have recommended that regulations be adopted to reduce the risks of concussion, as it did in a later position statement on sports such as boxing that involve intentional trauma to the brain.[33] And indeed, the NFL has taken or is considering measures to reduce the number of concussions. For example, full-contact practices may be held only about once a week during the season, and the league is con-templating the elimination of kickoffs, which have an especially high rate of concussion injuries.[34]

Nine months after the Academy's report, in December 1997, the American Orthopaedic Society for Sports Medicine (AOSSM) convened a "Concussion Workshop Group," with representatives from major sports organizations and leading physician associations. Neurologists, neurosurgeons, orthopedic sur-geons, pediatricians, and emergency physicians were represented, as were the NCAA, NFL, and NHL.[35] Like the Academy, the workshop group focused its attention on treatment of athletes after they sustained a concussion. The group published the results of its deliberations in 1999, and it identified some key areas of concern:

- Athletes should not be allowed to resume competition after a concussion while the brain was still recovering from the injury. In rare cases, a second concussion shortly after the first concussion could cause death.[36] In addi-tion, repeated concussions could have a cumulative effect over time that was disabling.[37]
- There were no objective measures that could identify whether a player ac-tually suffered a concussion or how much harm was caused by the head trauma.[38]
- Most athletes recovered completely after a concussion, but an "unknown number" would experience chronic symptoms, which for some players would be permanent and disabling.[39]

After discussing the medical profession's understanding of concussion and the ways that doctors should evaluate an athlete who may have suffered a concussion, the workshop group provided guidelines for when teams should allow players to resume competition after a suspected concussion. Surprisingly, the guidelines were not as strict as those issued by the American Academy of Neurology two years earlier:

- Athletes could return to play immediately if any symptoms resolved within fifteen minutes, they had a normal neurologic examination, and there was no loss of consciousness.[40]
- For athletes with loss of consciousness or more than fifteen minutes of symptoms, the working group urged caution but did not provide clear guidance. For example, the group observed that:

Current medical knowledge does not adequately address this situation. While some athletes may benefit from 5 to 7 days of rest after experiencing initial symptoms in excess of 15 minutes, others may be able to safely return to play much sooner.[41]

- In short, "[c]urrent neuroscience knowledge in humans does not give a safe, firm timetable for return to play after concussion in most circumstances."[42]

Hence, the working group called for more research and an individualized assessment of each athlete. Individualized assessments were to include repeated neurological assessments during gradual increases in physical exertion to see if the exertion triggered symptoms.[43]

Once again, the main issue was not whether athletes were placed at too great a risk of brain injury from playing football but how long they should rest after a concussion before returning to play. Notably, the working group did not suggest a different approach to the athlete who had suffered multiple concussions. Nor did it offer any suggestions by way of preventing concussions.

Indeed, the lack of recommendations for measures to reduce the frequency of concussion injuries is striking. In a 2004 article, "Unreported Concussion in High School Football Players: Implications for Prevention," the authors concluded that prevention initiatives "should focus on education to increase athlete awareness of concussion and its risks and promotion of open lines of injury report."[44] Robert Cantu had sounded a similar theme seven years earlier. After discussing the need to educate parents and athletes about the symptoms of concussion, he wrote that "education remains the most important preventive tool we have."[45] In other words, prevention was viewed as a form of concussion management.

The emphasis on management rather than prevention of concussion likely reflected the fact that concussion generally did not appear to result in lasting harm. Thus, according to Goetz and Pappert's *Textbook of Clinical Neurology* in 1999, concussions "are infrequently associated with structural brain injury and rarely lead to significant long-term sequelae."[46] The text also advised that when "patients have unusual or persistent complaints, the possible contributions of personality disorder, psychosocial problems, or secondary gain should be considered."[47]

To be sure, the text identified two exceptions to the typical outcome. When athletes experienced a concussion in competition, they faced two significant risks: (1) the possibility of death from a second concussion shortly after the first one and (2) cognitive disability from multiple concussions.[48] But even then, the risks were not taken seriously enough. With respect to the effects of multiple concussions, the Goetz and Pappert text observed that:

> The cumulative effects of multiple minor [head injuries] is recognized in boxing as the *punch drunk syndrome* . . . ; however, the occurrence of this syndrome in association with other sports is controversial.[49]

Just as in earlier periods, there were experts in the late 1990's who expressed greater concern about the harms from concussion. As Cantu observed, some neurologists believed "that there is no such thing as a minor head injury," that intellectual functioning "may be reduced after a minor head injury," and that repeated head injuries cause more severe and more persistent impairment.[50] Hence, he republished his 1986 guidelines with its recommended waiting periods before resuming play after a concussion.[51]

While medical understanding of concussion had not fully caught up with reality even by the late 1990's, medical experts by then had put the NFL on notice that players needed to be assessed carefully once they had suffered a concussion and that play or practice should not be resumed as long as symptoms or signs of the concussion persisted either at rest or upon exertion. As discussed, the American Academy of Neurology and the Concussion Working Group had issued their guidelines in 1997 and 1999, respectively.[52] An important question is why the NFL did not respond by adopting return-to-play guidelines for its players.

To be sure, the NFL did take some action. It formed its Committee on Mild Traumatic Brain Injuries in 1994, and the committee undertook a detailed study of concussion over a six-year period. But a second important question is whether the committee was correct when it concluded in 2005 that concussion management guidelines issued by other groups "may be too conservative for the NFL."[53] The committee reported that players did not appear to be at an increased risk of injury when they returned to a game after concussion even if it took more than fifteen minutes for their symptoms to resolve or even if they had lost consciousness with their concussions.[54] As mentioned earlier, the American Academy of Neurology's guidelines precluded a return to the same game when symptoms lasted more than fifteen minutes or there was a loss of consciousness.[55]

In the past decade, concern about concussion has generated more research studies and more consensus statements. To some extent, the guidelines have become tougher; in other ways, they have become weaker. For example, the National Athletic Trainers' Association (NATA) suggested in 2004 that players should be disqualified for the remainder of the season once they sustained three concussions during the season. NATA also observed that three concussions in a career might be grounds for permanent disqualification of the athlete.[56] On the other hand, the NATA consensus statement equivocated on the question whether athletes should refrain from play for a minimum amount of time after their first concussions. While NATA acknowledged data indicating that repeat concussions tend to occur within seven to ten days after an initial concussion, the report suggested that an earlier return to play might be appropriate if the athlete was symptom free on exertion, and activities were restricted for the first few days to avoid a repeat head injury.[57] As with other guidelines, the NATA statement focused on management rather than prevention of concussion, though it did call for the use of properly fitting helmets and mouth guards.[58]

Where does medical understanding stand today? Any concussion should be taken seriously, and players should cease play or practice immediately. Moreover, play or practice should not be resumed until the brain has had a chance to heal. For some experts, that means a minimum period of rest (e.g., one week for a first concussion) plus the absence of any symptoms of head injury, either while resting or with exertion, and no evidence of injury during neurologic testing. For other experts, a minimum period of rest is not required, as long as there are no symptoms of head injury, either while resting or with exertion, and sophisticated neurologic testing is normal.[59]

There still is considerable uncertainty as to the long-term consequences of concussion. It appears that multiple concussions can cause permanent and severe neurologic dysfunction, but it is unclear why only a small number of players appear to be at risk for that level of injury.[60] Perhaps there are genetic or environmental factors that work in combination with concussion to cause dementia or other problems. Indeed, genetic factors affect the likelihood that a boxer will develop the punch drunk syndrome.[61] Or perhaps the likelihood of severe dysfunction has been underestimated. It also may be the case that just one concussion can result in permanent and severe neurologic dysfunction, but medical understanding cannot answer that question yet either.[62]

Part of the reason for the uncertainty is the medical profession's incomplete understanding of brain functioning and the imperfection of tests that are used to measure brain functioning. Researchers have developed more sophisticated ways to measure neurologic function, but they cannot be certain that they are measuring it fully. The other important cause of uncertainty reflects the fact that it can be difficult to distinguish between correlation and cause and effect. We know that many former athletes suffer from early dementia (a correlation), but it is impossible to conduct the kind of studies that prove cause and effect—one cannot randomize people in a study in which half of the subjects are spared concussion and half of the subjects are given one or more concussions.

■ CONCLUSION

Medical understanding of concussion has evolved considerably over the past few decades. While neurologists once viewed mild traumatic brain injury as a largely benign event with symptoms that were temporary, a growing body of evidence indicates that concussions can have serious consequences, especially when a person sustains multiple concussions over time. At one time, boxers were thought to be the only athletes at risk for sport-related dementia; now, medical experts understand that dementia may be a consequence of competition in football, hockey, soccer or many other sports.[63]

Even with the greater understanding that has developed, there is much more to be learned about concussion. What is the actual risk to a football player of permanent brain damage from concussion? To what extent does the risk depend on the number of concussions or the severity of the concussions? Do genetic factors make some players highly susceptible to injury while leaving other players very resilient after head trauma?

As we wait for more data, the NFL and the public must grapple with other important questions. Has football become too dangerous?[64] What changes should be implemented to reduce the risk of concussion?[65] How conservative should the NFL and other football associations be in dealing with an uncertain risk? Should they err on the side of caution and take very strong precautionary measures? The answers to these questions are difficult, but they must be sorted through.

■ NOTES

1. Steven T. DeKosky, Milos D. Ikonomovic, & Sam Gandy, *Traumatic Brain Injury—Football, Warfare, and Long-Term Effects*, 363 NEW ENG. J. MED. 1293, 1295 (2010).

2. The guideline also states that players should not return to play or practice on a later date until cleared by the team physician and an independent neurologist. In a 2007 guideline, the NFL advised teams that players should not return to play or practice the same day as a concussion when the concussion was accompanied by a loss of consciousness. *See* Todd Neale, *NFL Institutes New Concussion Policy*, MED PAGE TODAY (Dec. 3, 2009), http://www.medpage today.com/Neurology/HeadTrauma/17302.

3. ROLLAND S. PARKER, CONCUSSIVE BRAIN TRAUMA: NEUROBEHAVIORAL IMPAIRMENT AND MALADAPTATION 50–51 (2001).

4. It is important to note that while the data on the effects of repetitive concussion are not definitive, there is growing evidence indicating that players need to fully heal after concussions to protect themselves against permanent neurologic injury.

5. Ultimately, repeated concussions can lead to severe neurological dysfunction and chronic traumatic encephalopathy. *See* Ann C. McKee, et al., *The Spectrum of Disease in Chronic Traumatic Encephalopathy*, BRAIN: A JOURNAL OF NEUROLOGY (Dec. 2, 2012), http://brain.oxfordjournals.org/content/early/2012/12/02/brain.aws307.full.

6. P. McCrory, et al., *Consensus Statement on Concussion in Sport—The 3rd Int'l Conference on Concussion in Sport, Held in Zurich, November 2008*, 16 J. CLINICAL NEUROSCIENCE 755, 760 (2009).

7. Richard S. Polin & Nidhi Gupta, *Athletic Head Injury, in* NEUROLOGY AND TRAUMA 506, 513 (Randolph W. Evans ed., 2nd ed. 2006).

8. Ira A. Casson, et al., *Concussion in the Nat'l Football League: An Overview for Neurologists*, 26 NEUROLOGIC CLINICS 217, 217–218 (2008).

9. ROBERT C. CANTU & MARK HYMAN, CONCUSSION AND OUR KIDS: AMERICA'S LEADING EXPERT ON HOW TO PROTECT YOUNG ATHLETES AND KEEP SPORTS SAFE 2–8 (2012).

10. Most concussions do not result in a loss of consciousness.

11. CANTU & HYMAN, *supra* note 9, at 8–9.

12. *Id.* at 71.

13. Edward M. Wojtys, et al., *Concussion in Sports*, 27 AM. J. SPORTS MED. 676, 677–78 (1999). There has never been a second impact death in the NFL. *See* Casson, et al., *supra* note 8, at 227.

14. Paul McCrory, *Sports Concussion and the Risk of Chronic Neurological Impairment*, 21 CLIN. J. SPORT MED. 6, 6 (2011).

15. CANTU & HYMAN, *supra* note 9, at 111.

16. JOHN N. WALTON, ESSENTIALS OF NEUROLOGY 242 (4th ed. 1975). Seven years, later, Walton's fifth edition included the same assessment of concussion. *See* SIR JOHN WALTON, ESSENTIALS OF NEUROLOGY 258 (5th ed. 1982).

17. N. E. F. CARTLIDGE & D. A. SHAW, HEAD INJURY 148 (1981). Cartlidge and Shaw did not themselves subscribe to this view. Rather, they believed that individuals vary in their

responses to concussion, with some suffering real physical injury and others having symptoms of psychological origin. *Id.* at 153.

18. Thomas A. Gennarelli, *Cerebral Concussion and Diffuse Brain Injuries, in* HEAD INJURY 83, 85–87 (Paul R. Cooper ed. 1982). While Gennarelli did not say anything about athletes suspending their play after a concussion in his HEAD INJURY chapter, he wrote a similar chapter for another book in which he advised that after a mild cerebral concussion, players "should not be permitted to participate in the remainder of the contest" and that after a classic cerebral concussion, players should abstain from play for one to two weeks. *See* Thomas A. Gennarelli, *Cerebral Concussion and Diffuse Brain Injuries, in* ATHLETIC INJURIES TO THE HEAD, NECK, AND FACE 93, 96–97 (Joseph S. Torg ed. 1982). However, nine years later, Gennarelli removed his recommendations about players temporarily suspending play after a concussion and said nothing on that question. *See* Thomas A. Gennarelli, *Cerebral Concussion and Diffuse Brain Injuries, in* ATHLETIC INJURIES TO THE HEAD, NECK, AND FACE 270, 272–74 (Joseph S. Torg ed., 2nd ed. 1991).

19. Richard C. Schneider & Frederick C. Kriss, *First Aid and Diagnosis—The Treatment of Head Injuries, in* HEAD AND NECK INJURIES IN FOOTBALL: MECHANISMS, TREATMENT, AND PREVENTION 163, 164–165 (Richard C. Schneider ed. 1973).

20. *Id.* at 164–165.

21. *Id.* at 165.

22. LINDA CARROLL & DAVID ROSNER, THE CONCUSSION CRISIS: ANATOMY OF A SILENT EPIDEMIC 127 (2011).

23. *Id.* at 40–41 (describing the NFL's "Greatest Hits" videos and a "Headcracker Suite" video).

24. PARKER, *supra* note 3, at 50. In fact, concussions that do not cause a loss of consciousness are just as serious as concussions that do cause a loss of consciousness; *see also* CANTU & HYMAN, *supra* note 9, at 106–107.

25. Randolph W. Evans, *The Postconcussion Syndrome: 130 Years of Controversy*, 14 SEMINARS NEUROLOGY 32, 32 (1994).

26. Sir Charles Symonds, *Concussion and Its Sequelae*, 279 LANCET 1, 1 (1962).

27. Thomas J. Boll, *Behavioral Sequelae of Head Injury, in* HEAD INJURY 363, 368–369 (Paul R. Cooper ed. 1982).

28. Robert C. Cantu, *Guidelines for Return to Contact Sports after a Cerebral Concussion*, 14 PHYSICIAN & SPORTSMED. 75, 79, 82 (1986).

29. American Academy of Neurology, *Practice Parameter: The Management of Concussion in Sports (Summary Statement)*, 48 NEUROLOGY 581, 583 (1997).

30. *Id.* at 583–584.

31. *Id.* at 584.

32. According to Pittsburgh Steeler Troy Polamalu, "When people say they feel a little buzzed or dazed, it's considered a concussion. I wouldn't [think that]. But if that is a concussion, any football player has 50–100 concussions a year." Dan Patrick, *Just My Type*, SI VAULT (Dec. 31, 2012), http://sportsillustrated.cnn.com/vault/article/magazine/MAG1206651/index.htm.

33. *Position Statement on Sports that Include Intentional Trauma to the Brain*, AMERICAN ACADEMY OF NEUROLOGY (June 21, 2008), http://www.aan.com/globals/axon/assets/7466.pdf.

34. Judy Battista, *'Train Wreck of a Play' Collides with Consciences*, N.Y. TIMES (Dec. 15 2012), http://www.nytimes.com/2012/12/16/sports/football/tradition-vs-player-safety-

in-nfl-kickoff-debate.html?_r=0; Casson, et al., *supra* note 8, at 224; Collective Bargaining Agreement 143, NFL PLAYERS ASSOCIATION (Aug. 4, 2011), http://images.nflplayers.com/mediaResources/files/PDFs/General/2011_Final_CBA_Searchable_Bookmarked.pdf.

35. Wojtys, et al., *supra* note 13, at 676.

36. This is the "second impact" phenomenon. Richard L. Saunders & Robert E. Harbaugh, *The Second Impact in Catastrophic Contact-Sports Head Trauma*, 252 JAMA 538–539 (1984).

37. Wojtys, et al., *supra* note 13, at 676–677, 681.

38. *Id.* at 677.

39. *Id.* at 681.

40. *Id.* at 684.

41. *Id.*

42. *Id.* at 685.

43. *Id.* at 684–685.

44. Michael McCrea, et al., *Unreported Concussion in High School Football Players: Implications for Prevention*, 14 CLIN. J. SPORT MED. 13, 16 (2004).

45. Robert C. Cantu, *Reflections on Head Injury in Sport and the Concussion Controversy*, 7 CLIN. J. SPORT MED. 83, 83–84 (1997). Some experts did call for measures to prevent concussion. For example, there were recommendations for better helmet design. Jennifer M. Hootman, Randall Dick & Julie Agel, *Epidemiology of Collegiate Injuries for 15 Sports: Summary and Recommendations for Injury Prevention Initiatives*, 42 J. ATHL. TRAIN. 311, 316 (2007).

46. Randolph W. Evans & Jack E. Wilberger, *Traumatic Disorders*, in TEXTBOOK OF CLINICAL NEUROLOGY 1035, 1036 (Christopher G. Goetz & Eric J. Pappert eds. 1999).

47. *Id.* at 1041.

48. *Id.* at 1039.

49. *Id.* Evans & Wilberger use minor head injury as an alternative term for concussion. *Id.* at 1036. The punch drunk syndrome also is known as "dementia pugilistica." DeKosky, et al., *supra* note 1, at 1295.

50. Robert C. Cantu, *Return to Play Guidelines After a Head Injury*, 17 CLIN. SPORTS MED. 45, 51 (1998).

51. *Id.* at 53–57.

52. *See supra* pages 7–11.

53. Elliott J. Pellman, et al., *Concussion in Professional Football: Players Returning to the Same Game—Part 7*, 56 NEUROSURGERY 79, 88 (2005).

54. *Id.*

55. Although the NFL did not implement guidelines for the management of concussion, it had made some rule changes to reduce the risk of concussions or more severe brain injuries. As mentioned earlier, *supra* page 3, the league banned "spearing," or the use of the head to block or tackle another player. *See* Polin & Gupta, *supra* note 7, at 513, 516.

56. Kevin M. Guskiewicz, et al., *Nat'l Athletic Trainers' Ass'n Position Statement: Mgmt. of Sport-Related Concussion*, 39 J. ATHLETIC TRAINING 280, 282, 291 (2004). While the guidelines were issued by an association of athletic trainers, leading medical experts participated in the development of the guidelines.

57. *Id.* at 286. The report did recommend a 7-day minimum waiting period after a repeat concussion, especially if the second one occurred in the same season. *Id.*

58. *See id.* at 292–293.

59. *Id.* at 281–282.

60. McCrory, *supra* note 14, at 10.

61. DeKosky, et al., *supra* note 1, at 1295.

62. Brandon E. Gavett, et al., *Mild Traumatic Brain Injury: A Risk Factor for Neurodegeneration*, 2:18 ALZHEIMER'S RESEARCH & THERAPY 1, 1 (2010).

63. CANTU & HYMAN, *supra* note 9, at 19–52.

64. A number of NFL players think so. For example, Green Bay Packer and former Indianapolis Colt Jeff Saturday won't let his son play youth football. *Id.* at 144–145. Robert Cantu believes that no child should play tackle football before age fourteen. *Id.*

65. And for those head injuries that cannot be prevented, what steps can be taken to make athletes more comfortable reporting their symptoms? Unfortunately, there are strong pressures to remain silent in a culture in which injuries are downplayed so players can remain in the game. DeKosky, et al., *supra* note 1, at 1295.

C . Managing Risk

18 Player Safety in Youth Sports

Sportsmanship and Respect as

an Injury-Prevention Strategy

■ DOUGLAS E. ABRAMS

■ INTRODUCTION

The night was November 3, 1999, and only seconds remained in a junior varsity hockey game between two bitter local rivals, New Trier High School and Glenbrook North High School, at the Rinkside Sports Ice Arena in Gurnee, a suburb of Chicago.[1] New Trier was comfortably ahead, 7–4, in the teams' first encounter since Glenbrook North had edged New Trier 3–2 for the Illinois State Junior Varsity Title a season earlier.[2]

Junior varsity contests do not normally provide lasting memories in any sport, but this early-November game would be different. Beginning shortly after the opening faceoff, "violence flared repeatedly" and "the mood grew ugly."[3] Eyewitnesses would later describe the game as "an intense battle,"[4] with each team's parents and students heckling rival fans and players.[5] The teams themselves traded taunts and squared off in altercations, unrestrained by their respective coaches[6]—leaders that pediatric professionals recognize as "the most important individuals for maintaining safety" in youth leagues.[7]

One coach reportedly left the bench and strode onto the ice in the middle of the game to confront a referee,[8] and the Glenbrook North coach allegedly "incited his players to "take special action'" against New Trier's fifteen-year-old sophomore, cocaptain Neal Goss, whose three goals helped seal his team's ultimate victory.[9] In total, the referees called sixteen penalties,[10] a particularly high number for a junior varsity hockey game.[11]

When the final buzzer sounded to end the contest, or within a second or two thereafter, a fifteen-year-old Glenbrook North player skated full speed across the ice, blindsided Neal Goss, and cross-checked [12] him headfirst into the rink's sideboards.[13] "This is what you get for messing,"[14] the player allegedly said as Goss laid on the ice, permanently paralyzed from the neck down.[15]

Neal Goss' catastrophic spinal cord injury introduces this article's two conclusions, drawn from my experiences and concerns about player safety, both as a lawyer for the last thirty-five years and as a volunteer coach of youth league and high school hockey teams for more than forty years. Both conclusions concern injury prevention, the first obligation of parents and coaches who conduct and supervise games for the estimated twenty-five to thirty million boys and girls who participate in organized sports leagues in the United States each year.[16]

First, society should not exaggerate the law's role in preventing avoidable injury to "youth leaguers"—players in sports events conducted by public and private schools, private organizations, and public agencies such as parks and recreation departments.[17] Americans often look to the law for enforceable standards to help govern personal behavior, but, as Part I of this article discusses, the law provides youth leaguers only limited protection.[18] A civil action for damages and a criminal prosecution were filed shortly after Goss' injury, but neither proceeding did anything to prevent the student's lifelong paralysis.

Second, the protections afforded to players through the national safety standards established by safety experts—such as equipment designers, physician groups, and national youth sports governing bodies—are similarly limited.[19] As Part II of this article discusses, parents and coaches who behave irresponsibly can neutralize safety standards and put players in harm's way in a matter of moments.[20] Protective equipment is designed and playing rules are conceived with sound medical advice at the national level,[21] but young athletes wear equipment and compete at the local level.

For years, schools and national youth sports governing bodies (USA Hockey, US Youth Soccer, the American Youth Soccer Organization, and others) have influenced local behavior through adult-education programs that emphasize sportsmanship and mutual respect among competitors and their families.[22] Posters, videos, DVDs, brochures, website entries, and similar materials provide the framework for mandatory parent meetings that local leagues and teams often conduct, usually during the preseason period.[23] These materials typically cast parents and coaches as role models for the players they raise and supervise.[24]

The "role model" approach[25] makes sense because youth leaguers are not born with preconceived attitudes about sportsmanship and respect, but instead, like all other children, learn from what they see and experience.[26] These athletes react not only to media reports of foul play in professional sports but also to the verbal and nonverbal cues passed on to them by their parents and coaches—the most influential adults in their athletic lives.[27] While adults carefully watch their children as they play organized sports, the children also watch the adults.

Sportsmanship and mutual respect indeed teach children citizenship, but they do much more than that. Adherence to sportsmanship and mutual respect can also help prevent many avoidable injuries that may disrupt and even devastate the lives of young athletes and their families.[28] If New Trier and Glenbrook North had played hard but clean, Neal Goss would likely have walked out of the rink that night because sportsmanlike, respectful teens trained by responsible adults do not blindside opponents or drive the opponents' heads into the ground at the end of a game.

My years of coaching experience support the conclusion that adult-education materials created and distributed by schools and national youth sports governing bodies do, in fact, successfully influence many adults to embrace sportsmanship and respect. More work, however, still needs to be done. According to a 2010 poll that Reuters and Ipsos, a market research company, conducted in twenty-two nations, parents in the United States still rank as the world's "worst behaved" parents at children's sports events.[29]

As they seek new ways to influence adult attitudes, schools and national youth sports governing bodies should combine the time-tested and assuredly valuable citizenship-based "role model" message with new safety-based messages that prominently and directly link sportsmanship and respect to injury prevention. When sportsmanship and respect prevail, children striving to win are less likely to get hurt.[30]

New safety-based messages may strike a receptive chord in parents and coaches, reminding them that maintaining sportsmanship and respect during games and practice sessions remains every family's concern, even families whose children play clean.[31] Avoidable injury arising from local abandonment of these values frequently strikes youth leaguers at random.[32] Neal Goss was simply in the wrong place at the wrong time, a victim of an opponent's impetuous violence. The victim lying paralyzed on the ice at the end of the New Trier–Glenbrook North hockey game could have been any parent's child because the volatility that the adults encouraged and tolerated throughout the contest deprived every player of the safety provided by protective equipment and carefully crafted national safety standards.[33]

Finally, this article's conclusion discusses why adult-education materials, which now stress citizenship but draw a link to safety only in passing, if at all, should be recast to sensitize parents and coaches to a straightforward formula:Sportsmanship + Respect = Safety.[34]

■ I. THE LAW'S LIMITED ROLE
    IN INJURY PREVENTION

"If your only tool is a hammer," the old saying goes, "all your problems will look like nails."[35] Because the litigation model[36] dominates law school curricula, lawyers sometimes spend their entire careers reflexively viewing accidents and other significant problems as potential lawsuits destined for the courtroom.[37] Nonlawyers also tend to visualize civil or criminal trials as the tools of choice because most Americans develop their impressions of the legal system from either watching television law dramas or serving on jury duty.[38]

The law's role in promoting youth leaguers' safety, however, can be overstated. Lawyers, economists, and other commentators participating in the national "tort reform" debate disagree about the capacity and propriety of negligence law to influence corporate and individual conduct before injury occurs and to compensate victims afterwards.[39] Without entering that debate, it seems clear that civil actions for damages can only compensate youth leaguers, such as Neal Goss, for injuries that have already occurred. Moreover, a third or more of a victim's recovery after settlement or trial often goes not to the injured, but to the plaintiff's lawyer, under the contingent fee retainer agreements common in personal injury suits.[40] For their part, criminal prosecutions can only punish wrongdoers for inflicting prior injuries.[41]

Prevention thus remains the most child-protective strategy because litigation cannot necessarily make an injured youth leaguer's life good; the most it can often do is make that life less bad.

A. Premises Liability

The law's impact on youth leaguers' safety begins with an analysis of premises liability, the obligation of both owners and managers to assure that safe conditions mark fields, gymnasiums, and other similar venues.[42] The prospect of premises liability may help prevent some injuries by encouraging school districts, parks and recreation departments, and other public agencies and private businesses to impose greater safety measures on the venues that they manage.[43] The professionals in charge of these entities are more likely than laypersons to be familiar with legal proceedings and to retain lawyers and insurance risk managers who understand that potholes, poor lighting, rotted benches, and similar hazards invite litigation, much of it avoidable or made less costly by exercising reasonable care and foresight.[44]

Settlements or judgments after trial in premises liability suits following youth sports injuries are certainly not unknown, and it may be difficult or impossible to deter a plaintiff's lawyer from filing suit against owners or managers even with weak evidence.[45] In more than forty years, however, I cannot recall ever having coached a youth hockey game in an ice rink that appeared unsafe or genuinely contributed to an injury. No media report, and no later allegation in the civil or criminal filings, suggested that conditions at the Rinkside Sports Ice Arena had anything to do with the injury that confined Neal Goss to a wheelchair, unable ever again to walk or care for his daily needs.

B. National Safety Standards

What about potential negligence liability based on either the quality of protective equipment or the sufficiency of playing rules established by schools or national youth sports governing bodies? These national safety standards remain central in contact sports such as hockey or football, but these sports do not hold a mo-nopoly on injuries—or lawsuits.[46]

Concern about negligence liability doubtlessly influences engineers who design protective equipment, and schools and national youth sports governing bodies that establish and periodically refine playing rules.[47] Decision makers act not only from a genuine desire to prevent injury but also because they know that their organizations typically have "deep pockets" that attract plaintiffs' lawyers seeking damages.[48]

For example, USA Hockey's steady march toward more protective safety stan-dards,[49] since I first laced on skates nearly fifty years ago, has undoubtedly spared many youngsters avoidable injury. Neal Goss was injured while he wore a helmet, face cage, and other protective equipment that met USA Hockey safety specifica-tions, whose sufficiency was not questioned.[50] Further, regardless of whether the performance of the coaches or referees during the New Trier–Glenbrook North game met the minimum expectations for responsible adult leadership, no report indicated that any coach or referee had evaded or failed USA Hockey's nationally-mandated criminal or child abuse background checks,[51] or lacked the classroom training certification required of coaches and officials.[52]

Nor was negligence evident in USA Hockey's national playing rules,[53] which provide penalties for both "checking from behind"[54] and "cross-checking,"[55] the particular violations committed by Neal Goss' opponent when he delivered his blow at the end of the game.[56] The Glenbrook North player who injured Neal Goss received a penalty for "checking from behind" and a thirty-day suspension pend-ing a hearing before state amateur hockey officials.[57]

C. The Legal Process

With the sufficiency of USA Hockey national safety standards not in issue,[58] the law reacted to Neal Goss' life-changing injuries as best it could. Concluding that the blindside hit occurred seconds after the game ended while Goss was skating to his team's bench, the state prosecutor charged the opponent with two felony counts of aggravated battery.[59] One count alleged great bodily harm, and the other alleged use of the hockey stick as a deadly weapon.[60] The opponent (who re-mained unnamed by the media because he was a minor) entered an Alford plea[61] to one count of simple misdemeanor battery.[62] The juvenile court judge sentenced him to 120 hours of community service at a facility for paralyzed patients and placed him on probation for a period of two years, during which he could not play contact sports.[63]

Facing lifetime costs for medical and around-the-clock personal care, Neal Goss and his family filed a multimillion dollar civil action for dam-ages. The suit alleged that five defendants—the Glenbrook North opponent; the Glenbrook North coach; the Illinois Hockey Officials Association; the Northbrook Hockey League, which sponsored the Glenbrook North team; and the Amateur Hockey Association of Illinois—negligently failed to maintain adequate control over the game.[64] The parties reached private settlements in some of the civil suits, and USA Hockey's insurance also helped meet Gross' ongoing expenses.[65]

■ II. THE CENTRAL ROLES OF SPORTSMANSHIP AND RESPECT IN INJURY PREVENTION

The national safety standards fashioned by equipment designers and USA Hockey did not fail Neal Goss, nor did the legal process that played catch-up after his injury.[66] Instead, players on both teams were left vulnerable by rabid local adults who let the game get out of hand and abandoned effective control, neutralizing the national standards that were designed to prevent injury.[67]

In their adult-education materials produced for local parents and coaches, national youth sports governing bodies should explicitly link sportsmanship and respect with player safety. A simple analogy demonstrates the need for this link.

In purpose and form, a sport's rulebook resembles the statutes and laws that influence other aspects of our daily lives. "The life of the law," said former Harvard Law School Dean Roscoe Pound, "is in its enforcement."[68] Pound meant that achieving a statute's protective purpose depends on responsible public and private enforcement because words protect no one and statutes do not apply themselves.[69] Similarly, a youth sport's playing rules are merely words on paper, and achieving their protective purpose depends on parents, coaches, officials, and league administrators—all of whom, by responsibly enforcing standards of sportsmanship and respect, remain committed to injury prevention.

A. Prevention Strategies in the Upbringing of Children

1. Existing Prevention Strategies in American Life

If adult-education materials stressed sportsmanship and respect as an injury-prevention strategy in youth sports, these materials would follow a path already familiar in American life. A wide range of public and private prevention strategies already seek to protect children from conduct dangerous to themselves or others.[70]

For example, organized after-school activities and other prevention programs enable adults to reduce rates of juvenile delinquency, eliminating much conduct by minors that would be a crime if committed by an adult.[71] Researchers have also demonstrated the effectiveness of classroom curricula that enable teachers to help prevent violence and bullying in the nation's elementary and secondary schools.[72]

Like these and other juvenile prevention programs, new initiatives that link sportsmanship and respect to player safety will not prevent all unfortunate incidents.[73] Juvenile prevention programs achieve success through reduction, not perfection.[74] Reduction—motivating much of the targeted audience to modify their behavior[75]—remains a realistic and worthwhile goal when the unpalatable alternative would be toleration of unacceptably high rates of incidents.[76]

2. A New Injury Prevention Strategy for Youth Sports

a. The Existing Framework

Parents and coaches might feel tempted to dismiss Neal Goss' paralysis as extraordinary, and not as a meaningful predicate for sustained safety-based prevention initiatives in youth sports generally. The disregard for sportsmanship, respect, and safety that marked the New Trier–Glenwood North hockey game, however, helped produce consequences that remain extraordinary only in their severity.[77]

Sports medicine specialists and other pediatric professionals understand how runaway emotions during a game can endanger player safety.[78] The "Safety Checklist" provided by the National Athletic Trainers' Association, for example, includes these measures: "Coaches should strictly enforce the sports rules,"[79] and leagues should "develop a sports/parent "code of conduct,'" that encourages the adults to "always show good sportsmanship."[80]

A provocative 2008 study conducted by the Center for Injury Research and Policy at Nationwide Children's Hospital underscores how local adherence to a youth sport's national playing rules enhances player safety.[81] The study focused on nine high school sports: boys' football, soccer, basketball, wrestling, and baseball; and girls' soccer, volleyball, basketball, and softball.[82] Researchers estimated that between 2005 and 2007, more than 98,000 injuries in these sports were directly related to an act that a referee, official, or disciplinary committee ruled illegal.[83] Thirty-two percent of these injuries were to the head or face, and twenty-five percent were concussions.[84]

"Each sport has ... rules developed to promote fair competition and protect participants from injury," the Children's Hospital researchers concluded.[85] "Enforcing rules and punishing illegal activity is a risk control measure that may reduce injury rates by modifying players' behavior."[86]

The overheated New Trier–Glenbrook North hockey game demonstrates, as the Children's Hospital researchers suggest, that adherence to sportsmanship and respect helps assure youth leaguers' safety by promoting competition within the letter and spirit of playing rules developed over time.[87] Paralysis and other catastrophic injuries are indeed rare, but observers continue to report "innumerable cases ... throughout the country every month ... of games turning tragic at the hands of enraged parents"[88] during brawls and other similar encounters. "Waves of head-butting, elbowing and fighting have been reported at youth sporting events across the country."[89] With improper adult conduct disturbingly common in youth sports, it is not unreasonable to think that for every reported incident other such incidents never reach the media.

As this article's Introduction noted, the 2010 poll that Reuters and Ipsos jointly conducted underscores the prevalence of adult misbehavior at youth sporting events.[90] Out of the twenty-two nations polled, parents in the United States ranked as the world's "worst behaved" parents at these events.[91] Sixty percent of American adults who attended youth sports contests reported that they saw parents become either verbally or physically abusive toward coaches or officials.[92] Runner-ups were parents in India (59%), Italy (55%), Argentina (54%), Canada (53%), and Australia (50%).[93]

"It's ironic that the United States, which prides itself in being the most civilized country in the world, has the largest group of adults having witnessed abusive behavior at children's sporting events," said an Ipsos senior vice president.[94]

The Reuters-Ipsos' poll confirmed earlier estimates of adult misbehavior. For example, in a Survey USA poll conducted in Indianapolis, Indiana, 55% of parents reported that they observed other parents engaging in verbal abuse at youth sporting events and 21% witnessed a physical altercation between other parents.[95] Likewise, in a Minnesota Amateur Sports Commission survey, 45.3% of youth leaguers said that adults called them names, yelled at them, or insulted them while they played in a game; 21% said that they played with an injury because they were pressured to do so; 17.5% said that an adult had hit, kicked, or slapped them during a game; and 8.2% said that they were pressured to harm others intentionally.[96]

The National Alliance for Youth Sports has estimated that about fifteen percent of youth league games involve at least one confrontation between a parent and a coach or official.[97] The National Summit on Raising Community Standards in Children's Sports concluded that youth sports are a "hotbed of chaos, violence and mean-spiritedness."[98] In a survey conducted by *Sports Illustrated For Kids* magazine, 74% of youth athletes reported watching out-of-control adults at their games; 37% of the athletes witnessed parents yelling at children; 27% saw parents yelling at coaches or officials; 25% observed coaches yelling at officials or children; and 4% saw violence by adults.[99]

Linking cause and effect in sports can be imprecise, but precision is not necessarily a prerequisite for initiatives designed to improve the circumstances of youth athletes. These consistent poll and survey numbers give ample justification to infer the existence of a relationship between adult behavior and player safety, even where the avoidable injuries would not approach the severity of Neal Goss' injury.

On the first anniversary of the fateful New Trier–Glenbrook North rematch, a veteran hockey referee said that "nothing" had changed in Chicago-area high school hockey.[100] "It's just as bad as it ever was," the referee concluded.[101] "There's kids being carried off the ice every night. You have parents acting like animals in the stands, coaches acting like animals on the bench . . . but when their kid gets hurt, they can't figure out why.'"[102]

b. The Outlook for the Future

As a longtime youth-league coach, I remain confident that thoughtful adult-education materials can lead many—though certainly not all—parents and coaches to link sportsmanship and respect to player safety. At one end of the spectrum, some adults will likely continue to resist messages urging sportsmanship and respect, including safety-based messages.[103] At the other end, some adults need no reminders about sportsmanship and respect because the two virtues already define their lives.[104] In the vast middle, however, parents and coaches remain unsure about how to behave, perhaps from their own inexperience in youth sports, or perhaps because their own children only recently began playing.[105]

Before and during the New Trier–Glenbrook North hockey game, responsible adult enforcement of national safety standards could have scripted a happier ending. Media reports did not indicate that, as game day approached, any adult sought to cool tempers and prepare for a spirited yet sportsmanlike contest. The adults needed only to listen to what their children said at home because taunting, trash talking, and threats of violence do not arise for the first time by spontaneous combustion when players arrive at the game. As the game itself spiraled out of control for an hour or more, the press did not report that any adult in the rink—any parent, coach, referee, or league administrator—possessed the ethical compass, emotional strength, or common sense to stop the game, deliver a public announcement requesting calm, instruct the players to regain their composure, or take any other steps to move the teams back from the brink before it was too late.

The enduring lesson of the New Trier–Glenbrook North donnybrook is that when local adults compromise sportsmanship and mutual respect and let the "hot blood of emotions" get the better of them,[106] these adults undermine the capacity and efficacy of national safety standards that are designed to protect the safety of youth athletes. When safety-based adult education induces parents and coaches to do better, every injury prevented will spare some youth leaguer short-term disability, long-term distress, or both. Players and families spared this damage will be much better off, even though they may never know of their good fortune. "An ounce of prevention," taught Benjamin Franklin, "is worth a pound of cure."[107]

B. Crafting Safety-Based Prevention Messages Grounded in Sportsmanship and Respect

Where do we go from here? As they design and disseminate adult-education materials, schools and national youth sports governing bodies often produce effective messages in hard copy brochures, on DVDs, on league websites, or on posters displayed at the fields and other venues where children play organized sports.[108] Creating messages that link sportsmanship and respect to player safety presents a convenient opportunity because it requires only that the creators recast the materials that these governing bodies already use.[109]

1. Sportsmanship

Effective parent-education materials stressing safety would recognize that embracing sportsmanship from the relative security of a keyboard, speaker's podium, or preseason parents' meeting takes only words, which can come easily because they carry no consequences. Maintaining sportsmanship while watching games from the stands, directing the team from the bench, or playing on the field can be much tougher because impulses toward self-restraint clash with equally strong—and sometimes stronger—passions to win.

The clash is real because maintaining sportsmanship with a lit up scoreboard depends on willpower—as President Abraham Lincoln put it on the eve of the Civil War—to overcome passion and heed "the better angels of our nature."[110] In a national sports culture that values winning, rewards winners, and sometimes views winners as "good people" and losers as "bad people,"[111] living up to Lincoln's admonition can be a tall order.

Effective safety-based adult-education materials would also acknowledge what every athlete and youth leaguer's parent and coach already knows—that winning is preferable to losing.[112] Wanting to win is a perfectly natural impulse, and indeed defines the essence of sportsmanship at any age and at any level of amateur or professional play.[113] The integrity of sport depends on competitors who each care about the scoreboard. Athletes unconcerned about the score should not play because they deny their opponents the spice that comes from physically and emotionally invigorating competition.

Effective safety-based appeals for sportsmanship would also recognize, however, that the integrity of sports depends on each player's resolve to pursue victory within the rules, and then to shake hands with the opponent and accept the outcome gracefully—win, lose or draw. The British National Association of Coaches has it right: "Sport without fairplay is not sport and honours won without fairplay can have no real value."[114]

2. Respect

Even if Neal Goss had emerged unscathed that cold November night, the suburban Chicago hockey game brought no honor to anyone in the ice rink because the game proceeded without mutual respect, the cornerstone of sportsmanship.

By tolerating and indeed encouraging trash talking and physical confrontations, the hockey players and their families did not live up to the aspiration to "respect the game" by playing or rooting vigorously while trying their best to win within the rules.[115] "Respect the game" has almost become a term of art and, indeed, was the title of Ryne Sandberg's acceptance speech when the Chicago Cubs second baseman was inducted into the Baseball Hall of Fame in 2005.[116]

The New Trier and Glenbrook North hockey players did not respect their opponents as fellow competitors entitled to a hard, spirited contest. The players did not respect their families or themselves by playing clean. Parents, coaches, and league administrators did not respect one another or the players by maintaining decorum in the stands and on the benches.

Collective disrespect endangered every New Trier and Glenbrook North player, even ones who played within the rules that night. Local breakdowns in sportsmanship and respect bring a shared risk on the field. As catcher Crash Davis, played by Kevin Costner in the award-winning movie *Bull Durham*,[117] said: "You don't respect the game, and that's my problem."[118]

3. Building on Existing Citizenship-Based Messages

National youth sports governing bodies, schools, national youth sports reform organizations, and local leagues already advance sportsmanship and respect as the lodestars for athletic competition.[119] Some of these organizations have also explicitly linked sportsmanship and respect to safety.[120] With some tailoring, existing adult-education materials can combine citizenship-based and safety-based messages for the first time or can stress the combination more prominently.

For example, one national governing body, USA Hockey, already instructs that "fair play and respect are the backbone of any successful amateur sports program."[121] The ultimate goal is a compact among "all participants and spectators [to] have respect for all players, coaches, officials, administrators, spectators and the sport of hockey."[122] Specifically, USA Hockey emphasizes that: (1) "players are encouraged to develop a deep sense of respect for all (opponents and officials),"[123] (2) "coaches are responsible for instructing their players to play the sport in a safe and sportsmanlike manner,"[124] (3) "each official should enforce all playing rules fairly and respectfully,"[125] and (4) "spectators are encouraged to support their teams while showing respect for all players, coaches, officials and other spectators."[126]

Turning to youth sports reform organizations, the nationally recognized Positive Coaching Alliance (PCA) advances "Honoring the Game" as "the governing precept in youth sports."[127] The precept is grounded in "respect for Rules, Opponents, Officials, Teammates and one's Self."[128] Several national sports governing bodies, including Little League Baseball,[129] USA Water Polo,[130] and USA Rugby have embraced PCA's call for honor and respect.[131] The American Youth Soccer Organization (AYSO) similarly strives to "create a positive environment based on mutual respect rather than a win-at-all-costs attitude, and ... to instill good sportsmanship."[132] "A key component of ethical behavior," adds U.S. Lacrosse, "is respect."[133]

Local leagues and concerned parents and coaches have created citizenship programs bearing such names as "Respect Sports,"[134] "Respect the Game,"[135] and "Respect My Game."[136] As it receives players from youth sports programs, the National Collegiate Athletic Association (NCAA) introduced its RESPECT Sportsmanship Initiative in 2009.[137] Through its credo—"RESPECT. It's the Name of the Game"[138]—the NCAA Initiative aims to "address sportsmanship head-on" by reinforcing the importance of a respectful competitive environment.[139]

With sportsmanship and respect already prominent in youth sports, recasting existing citizenship-based messages to stress player safety seems to be a natural step in the effort to serve the best interests of youth leaguers.

■ CONCLUSION

A. "One Word—Respect"

In the wake of Neal Gross' injury, *Chicago Tribune* writer Bob Verdi challenged his readers with a direct question: "Where did our children learn disrespect for the games and opponents they play?"[140] Paraphrasing cartoonist Walt Kelly, Verdi blamed the adults: "We have met the enemy and it is us."[141]

New safety-based adult-education materials should squarely confront "the enemy," the attitudes of many parents and coaches in youth sports. The first step for these adults is to recognize that fidelity to sportsmanship and respect does not indicate softness toward opponents, or lack of passion to win. Ryne Sandberg took the lead during his induction to the National Baseball Hall of Fame in Cooperstown in 2005. "If there was there was a single reason I am here today," the Chicago Cubs star told the audience in his acceptance speech, "it is because of one word—respect."[142]

> I was in awe every time I walked on to the field. That's respect. I was taught you never, ever disrespect your opponent or your teammates or your organization or your manager and never ever your uniform. . . . I played [the game] right because that's what you're supposed to do—play it right and with respect.[143]

Sandberg's abiding respect guided his will to win throughout his sixteen-year major league career, though he too recognized that respect has taken a hit in recent years. "When we all played," said the new Hall of Famer at the Cooperstown ceremony, respect for the game "was mandatory. It's something I hope we will one day see again."[144]

B. "Torment . . . for the Rest of Their Sad Lives"

The second step in confronting "the enemy" within us is to recognize that the ultimate goal of youth sports is to leave the players with memories to savor during a lifetime of good health. The final score of the New Trier–Glenbrook North game has long since faded from memory, a meaningless statistic when compared with the catastrophic injury suffered by fifteen-year-old Neal Goss. Every person in the Rinkside Sports Ice Arena that night—including many adults whose passion to win overwhelmed concern for sportsmanship, respect, and safety—learned a bitter lesson.

The lesson, articulated by President George Washington in his Farewell Address in 1796, is that self-discipline means tempering passion with reason.[145] Glenbrook North parents came to their senses once they saw the human costs of a breakdown in sportsmanship and mutual respect. When their team faced off against Evanston a few days after Neal Goss lay facedown on the ice, the chastened Glenbrook North parents cheered as their rivals scored the first goal, a generous gesture grounded in reason but delivered too late.[146]

The New Trier–Glenbrook North junior varsity hockey game had no winners, only losers. Neal Goss and his opponent were both reportedly clean players not known for skating at the edge of the rules.[147] The opponent received only one penalty during the prior season.[148] According to Nancy McMahon, whose son played on the Glenbrook North team, and whose husband Jim was a former Chicago Bears quarterback, the opponent was "just the sweetest thing."[149]

"Both of these children," said one writer about Neal Goss and the opponent who blindsided him, "will be tormented by this for the rest of their sad lives."[150] "I can never say 'sorry' enough," read the opponent from a prepared statement at the juvenile court dispositional hearing.[151] "I pray every day for Neal and a medical miracle that could end this suffering."[152] "Part of me has survived," Neal Goss responded in the prepared statement he read in court, "and part of me has been lost forever."[153] Each young man likely spoke from the heart after learning the grim consequences of casting aside sportsmanship and respect.

Neal Goss remains confined to a wheelchair, dependent on around-the-clock caregivers to bathe and dress him and help with other daily activities because he has no use of his legs, no movement in his fingers, and only limited movement in his arms and wrists.[154] Despite these obstacles, he achieved a perfect score on the mathematics part of the Scholastic Aptitude Test (SAT), earned a business degree at the University of Pennsylvania's Wharton School of Business, and secured a position as a financial analyst at a Chicago investment firm.[155] "When you look at what he has had to overcome," says the firm's general manager, "it's inspirational."[156]

Neal Goss' story thus proceeds more heroically than many of the attendees at that early-November junior varsity game might initially have expected. The story demonstrates that the indomitable human spirit has an uncanny capacity to overcome adversity, and that athletes fortified by years of physical and emotional discipline sometimes demonstrate the greatest resilience of all.

C. Teachable Moments

Wise parents and coaches of youth leaguers seek out "teachable moments," opportunities to educate their children with positive lessons drawn from bad events. Sometimes, however, the adults can learn as well as teach.

Neal Goss' injury holds two important lessons for the parents and coaches who guide young players. First, the law usually cannot make an injured youth leaguer whole because the civil or criminal proceeding happens only after the injury.[157] Second, and perhaps more important, parents and coaches who behave irresponsibly can put the players in harm's way when passion unrestrained by reason neutralizes the safety measures built into national equipment standards and a sport's rulebook.[158]

With these lessons in mind, schools and youth sports governing bodies would serve the teaching process best by coupling existing citizenship-based messages in their print and electronic adult-education materials with a strong, clear, and prominent new message that also stresses injury prevention:

"Sportsmanship + Respect = Safety."

People who cringed as Neal Goss left the ice rink on a stretcher that cold November night undoubtedly wished that they could turn back the clock and script a different ending to the game. Goss' story might have had a much happier ending if the players on the ice that night had been protected not only by national equipment safety standards, but also by local adherence to principles of sportsmanship and respect that help ensure a safe, spirited athletic competition.

▪ **LEGAL TOPICS**

For related research and practice materials, see the following legal topics:

Criminal Law & Procedure
Guilty Pleas
Alford Pleas
Education Law
Athletics
Recruitment
Torts
Public Entity
Liability
Liability General Overview

▪ **NOTES**

1. Susan Dodge & Robert C. Herguth, *N. Trier Hockey Player Paralyzed*, Chi. Sun-Times, Nov. 5, 1999, at 151, available at Factiva, Doc. No. chi0000020010826dvb500ycd.

2. Megan O'Matz, *Teen Charged with Battery in Hockey Hit: Intent to Injure Is Cited; Foe Paralyzed from Check*, Chi. Trib., Dec. 8, 1999, at 1, available at Factiva, Doc. No. trib000020010830dvc802bdw; Bryan Smith et al., *Emotions High Before Hockey Tragedy*, Chi. Sun-Times, Dec. 9, 1999, at 1, available at Factiva, Doc. No. chi0000020010826dvc90128n.

3. Mike Robinson, *Hockey Player Enters Plea Agreement in Case of Paralyzed Rival*, Associated Press, Aug. 7, 2000, available at Factiva, Doc. No. aprs000020010803dw870g7a7.

4. Debbie Howlett, *Teen May Face Trial in Sports Injury: Body Check in Hockey Game Left Boy Paralyzed*, USA Today, May 5, 2000, at 3A, available at Factiva, Doc. No. usat000020010813dw55009je.

5. *Id.*; Robinson, *supra* note 3; *see also* Smith et al., *supra* note 2.

6. Richard Roeper, *Decatur Fight Child's Play Next to Hockey Violence*, Chi. Sun-Times, Dec. 13, 1999, at 11, available at Factiva, Doc. No. chi0000020010826dvcd012rg; Smith et al., *supra* note 2.

7. Charles H. Tator et al., *Spinal Injuries in Canadian Ice Hockey: An Update to 2005*, 19 Clinical J. Sport Med. 451, 455 (2009).

8. Doug Abrams, *A Winning Equation*, USA Hockey Mag., Aug. 2011, at 20.

9. Megan O'Matz, *Hockey Suit Detailed: Family Seeks Damages*, Chi. Trib., Dec. 9, 1999, at 1, available at Factiva, Doc. No. trib000020010830dvc902ce7.

10. Rummana Hussain, *Probation for Teen Who Delivered Hockey Hit*, Chi. Trib., Oct. 27, 2000, at 1, available at Factiva, Doc. No. trib000020010813dwar029p1.

11. Based on the author's own experiences as a coach.

12. A "cross-check" occurs whenever a player "delivers a check to an opponent using the stick with both hands on the stick and no portion of the stick on the ice." USA Hockey, *2011–13 Official Rules of Ice Hockey* r. 609(a), at 60 (2011), available at http://usahockey. com/uploadedfiles/usahockey/southeast48/docume nt_library/2011—13 rulebook.pdf.

13. Tony Gordon, *Plea Deal Ends "Emotional" Hockey Case: Boy Pleads Guilty to Misdemeanor Battery Charge*, Daily Herald (Arlington Heights, Ill.), Aug. 8, 2000, at 1, available at Factiva, Doc. No. dhld000020010805dw8801084; Howlett, *supra* note 4.

14. Dirk Johnson, *Hockey Player, 15, Is Charged After Seriously Injuring a Rival*, N.Y. Times, Dec. 9, 1999, at A21, available at Factiva, Doc. No. nytf000020010828dvc901vih.

15. *Id.*; O'Matz, *supra* note 9.

16. *See* Tom Farrey, *Game On: The All-American Race to Make Champions of Our Children* 16 (2008); Glyn Roberts, *Motivation in Sport: Understanding and Enhancing the Motivation of Children*, in *Handbook of Research on Sport Psychology* 405, 411 (Robert N. Singer et al. eds., 1993).

17. Douglas E. Abrams, *Achieving Equal Opportunity in Youth Sports: Roles for the "Power of the Permit" and the "Child Impact Statement*," in *Learning Culture Through Sports: Perspectives on Society and Organized Sports* 32, 32 (Sandra Spickard Prettyman & Brian Lampman eds., 2d ed. 2011).

18. *See* discussion *infra* Part I.C.

19. *See* discussion *infra* Part I.B.

20. *See* discussion *infra* Part II.

21. *See, e.g., Sports Medicine*, U.S. Soccer, http://ussoccer.com/about/federation-services/sports-medicine.aspx (last visited Nov. 30, 2011) (discussing the role of medical professionals in adopting youth sports safety regulations); *Sports Standards and Recreation Standards*, ASTM Int'l, http://astm.org/Standards/sports-and-recreation-standards.html (last visited Nov. 30, 2011) (same).

22. *See, e.g.,* Greg Bach, *The Parents Association for Youth Sports: A Proactive Method of Spectator Behavior Management*, J. Physical Educ., Recreation & Dance, Aug. 2006, at 16, 16; *Parent Education Information*, USA Hockey, http://usahockey.com/template_

usahockey.aspx?nav=pl_ 06&id=19212 (last visited Nov. 30, 2011); *Parents*, US Youth Soccer, http://usyouthsoccer.org/parents (last visited Nov. 30, 2011).

23. *See, e.g.*, Bach, *supra* note 22, at 16; Parent Education Information, *supra* note 22; Parents, *supra* note 22.

24. *See, e.g.*, USA Hockey, *Sportsmanship: Why It Matters* (8/11 rev. 2011), http://usa-hockey.com/uploadedfiles/usahockey/menu_membership/sportsmanship2011.pdf (presenting "Parent's Code of Conduct"); *Referees, Coaches and Parents: Role Models for Life*, US Youth Soccer, http://usyouthsoccer.org/downloads/national_office/rolemodelsforlife.pdf (last visited Nov. 30, 2011) ("referees, coaches and parents form a trio of role models from which many of our young men and women learn behaviors that they will carry into adulthood").

25. The "role model" approach is premised on the social theory of learning, which theorizes that individuals process information "through the observation of others' actions" and that as individuals "observe other actors, they often imitate their behavior." Sarah A. Soule, *The Diffusion of an Unsuccessful Innovation*, Annals Am. Acad. Pol. & Soc. Sci., Nov. 1999, at 120, 124.

26. Michael A. Messner & Donald F. *Sabo, Sex, Violence & Power in Sports: Rethinking Masculinity* 91 (1994) (recognizing that "violent adult athletic role models and rewards from coaches, peers, and the community for the willingness to successfully use violence creates a context in which violence becomes normative behavior").

27. *See* Tator et al., *supra* note 7, at 451, 455.

28. *See* C. L. Collins et al., *When the Rules of the Game Are Broken: What Proportion of High School Sports-Related Injuries Are Related to Illegal Activity?*, 14 Injury Prevention 34, 34 (2008).

29. *US, India Parents Seen as Worst Behaved at Kids' Sports*, Reuters, Apr. 7, 2010, available at Factiva, Doc. No. LBA0000020100407e6470007u [hereinafter *Parents Worst Behaved*].

30. *See* discussion *infra* Part II.B.

31. *See* discussion *infra* Part II.A. 1–2.

32. Jason R. Schuette, *Adolescent Sports Violence—when Prosecutors Play Referee. Making Criminals out of Child Athletes, but Are They the Real Culprits?*, 21 N. Ill. U. L. Rev. 515, 533 (2001) (recognizing that "what happened in Gurnee could happen anywhere in America").

33. *Id.* (noting that society must be able to admit the pervasiveness of violence in youth sports before it "can begin to reassert a sense of ethical order" to the problem").

34. *See* discussion *infra* Conclusion.

35. Charles Pollard, *If Your Only Tool Is a Hammer, All Your Problems Will Look Like Nails*, in *Restorative Justice and Civil Society* 165 (Heather Strang & John Braithwaite eds., 2001).

36. The litigation model focuses on the outcomes of a court case, "usually expressed in terms of winners and losers." Susan Jacobs Jablow, *Newly Formed Collaborative Law Committee to Educate Attorneys*, 13 Law. J. 3 (2011). This model "works well in many areas of law, where there are clear-cut disputes about money or property. However, in legal matters involving personal relationships, the litigation model may intensify painful emotions and fail to address the issues that are most important to the parties involved." *Id.*

37. *See* Jean R. Sternlight, *Separate and Not Equal: Integrating Civil Procedure and ADR in Legal Academia*, 80 Notre Dame L. Rev. 681, 688–689 (2005).

38. *See* Douglas E. Abrams, *Picket Fences, in Prime Time Law: Fictional Television as Legal Narrative* 129, 141 (Robert M. Jarvis & Paul R. Joseph eds., 1998).

39. *See* generally Kenneth S. Abraham, *The Forms and Functions of Tort Law* (3d ed. 2007) (discussing various provisions taken by participants in the "tort reform" debate).

40. *See* Model Rules of Prof'l Conduct R. 1.5(c) (2010) (contingent fees).

41. *See, e.g.*, Kenneth C. Sears & Henry Weihofen, *May's Law of Crimes* 3 (4th ed. 1938).

42. For a discussion on premises liability, *see* generally Walter T. Champion, Jr., *Fundamentals of Sports Law*§§2:6, 7:1–7:5 (2d ed. 2004); Glenn M. Wong, *Essentials of Sports Law* 122–126 (4th ed. 2010).

43. John R. Braley III & John R. Braley IV, *It's All Fun and Games Until Someone Gets Hurt: Tort Liability and Managing Recreational Activity Risk in Virginia*, 10 Appalachian J. L. 1, 1, 25 (2010).

44. *See* generally *id.*

45. See Richard B. Schmitt, *Truth Is First Casualty of Tort-Reform Debate*, Wall St. J., Mar. 7, 1995, at B1, available at Factiva Doc. No. j000000020011028dr37000cm.

46. *See, e.g.*, Consumer Prods. Safety Comm'n, *2009 NEISS Data Highlights* (2009), http://cpsc.gov/neiss/2009highlights.pdf (discussing injury rates for various sports, including ones not considered to be contact sports).

47. *See, e.g.*, James H. Andrews, *Injury Lawsuits Said To Cause Financial Crisis for Many US Companies*, Christian Sci. Monitor, Jan. 25, 1994, at 11, available at Factiva Doc. No. chsm000020011028dq1p001k1.

48. *See* Linda S. Calvert Hanson & Charles W. Thomas, *Third Party Tort Remedies for Crime Victims—Searching for the "Deep Pocket" and a Risk Free Society*, 18 Stetson L. Rev. 1, 33 (1988) (arguing that "in an era during which the search for "deep pockets' and a society free of risk is accepted by many as a worthy goal . . . it appears to advance a definition of foreseeability" in premises liability "that is so tortured that it often has the effect of blurring the edges between negligence and strict liability").

49. See, e.g., Glen Colbourn & Lois Kalchman, Pashby Changed the Face of the Game: Hockey Pioneer Saved Many Players, Toronto Star, Aug. 25, 2005, at A1, available at Factiva, Doc. No. TOR0000020050825e18p0004v.

50. O'Matz, *supra* note 9 (discussing the Goss family's lawsuit, which named only participants responsible for the Nov. 3 game, without naming USA Hockey).

51. *See, e.g.*, Rachel Snyder, *More Than a Whistle: Law Regarding Certification for Coaches May Raise the Bar for Youth Activities*, Chi. Trib., Jan. 4, 1998, http://articles.chicagotribune.com/1998-01-04/features/9801040126.

52. *See id.*

53. *See* generally USA Hockey, *supra* note 12.

54. *See id.* r. 608, at 60 (prohibiting "checking from behind").

55. *See id.* r. 609, at 60 (prohibiting "cross checking").

56. *See* Schuette, *supra* note 32, at 529.

57. Cornelia Grumman, *Gurnee Cops Investigating Hockey Hit Against Teen: New Trier Player to Undergo Surgery*, Chi. Trib., Nov. 9, 1999, at 1, available at Factiva, Doc. No. trib000020010830dvb90247e.

58. *See* discussion *supra* Part I.B.

59. Robert C. Herguth, *Hockey Player, 15, Charged: Opponent Partially Paralyzed*, Chi. Sun-Times, Dec. 8, 1999, at 3, available at Factiva, Doc. No. chi0000020010826dvc801241; Schuette, *supra* note 32, at 529.

60. Herguth, *supra* note 59; Hussain, *supra* note 10; O'Matz, *supra* note 9.

61. North Carolina v. Alford, 400 U.S. 25 (1970) (affirming the constitutionality of an Alford plea in which a defendant pleads guilty while maintaining his or her innocence, conceding that prosecutors had enough evidence to convict).

62. Rummana Hussain, *Plea Agreement For Hockey Player In Cross-Checking*, Chi. Trib., Aug. 8, 2000, http://articles.chicagotribune.com/2000-08-08/news/0008080240.

63. Hussain, *supra* note 10.

64. O'Matz, *supra* note 9.

65. Lisa Black & Susan Berger, *Turning Tragedy Into Victory*, Chi. Trib., Jan. 4, 2007, http://articles.chicagotribune.com/2007-01-04/news/0701040288.

66. *See* discussion *supra* Part I.B-C.

67. "Children's sports are in many respects becoming less of a game and more an extension of their parents' lives." Schuette, *supra* note 32, at 523. "When parents focus on sport and winning in these terms (that being as a means of realizing external goals), they are . . . consequently increaseing the probability or tendency that children will employ unfair, unethical, and unsportsmanlike behavior in the quest to seize the glory and prestige that is at the end of the winning rainbow." *Id.*

68. Roscoe Pound, *Mechanical Jurisprudence, 8 Colum. L. Rev. 605, 619 (1908)*.

69. *Id.* at 605 (noting that the law "must be valued by the extent to which it meets its end, not by the beauty of its logical processes or the strictness with which its rules proceed from the dogmas it takes for its foundation").

70. *See, e.g.,* James Alan Fox et al., *Bullying Prevention Is Crime Prevention* (2003), http://pluk.org/Pubs/Bullying2.pdf (discussing bullying prevention in the public schools); Christopher Slobogin & Mark C. Fondacaro, *Juvenile Justice: The Fourth Option*, 95 Iowa L. Rev. 1 (2009) (discussing juvenile delinquency prevention); *Note,* Jessica P. Meredith, *Combating Cyberbullying: Emphasizing Education Over Criminalization*, 63 Fed. Comm. L.J. 311, 334 (2010) (discussing cyberbullying prevention in the public schools).

71. *See, e.g.,* Peter W. Greenwood, *Changing Lives: Delinquency Prevention as Crime-Control Policy* 49–83 (2006).

72. *See, e.g.,* Douglas E. Abrams, *A Coordinated Public Response to School Bullying, in Our Promise: Achieving Educational Equality for America's Children* 399, 414–419 (Maurice R. Dyson & Daniel B. Weddle eds., 2009) (discussing the success of the Olweus Bullying Prevention Program in public elementary and secondary schools).

73. *See* O'Matz, *supra* note 2 (quoting Alan Kray, president of the Northbrook Hockey League, as acknowledging that "there are penalties every game," including "checking-from-behind (penalties)," and that "it happens in hockey . . . in football," and "in lots of [other] contact sports").

74. "Reduction, the most realistic outcome of prevention efforts, remains a worthwhile goal when the alternative is tolerating unacceptably high rates of injury to person or property." Abrams, *supra* note 72, at 411.

75. Deborah Prothrow-Stith, *Strengthening the Collaboration Between Public Health and Criminal Justice to Prevent Violence*, 32 J. L. Med. & Ethics 82, 84 (2004).

76. Abrams, *supra* note 72, at 411.

77. Schuette, *supra* note 32, at 533 (acknowledging that absent the severity of Gross' injuries "it is unlikely that [his] case would have ever made headlines").

78. *See infra* notes 79–86.

79. *See, e.g.,* Nat'l Athletic Trainers Ass'n & N. Am. Boosters Club Ass'n, *Sports Safety Checklist to Help Prevent Common Athletic Injuries* 2 (n.d.), http://boosterclubs.org/PDF/NATA-NABCA Checklist.pdf.

80. *Id.* at 5.

81. *See* Collins et al., *supra* note 28, at 34.

82. *Id.*

83. *Id.*

84. *Id.* at 36.

85. *Id.* at 34.

86. *Id.*

87. *See* Collins et al., *supra* note 28, at 34.

88. Gwen Morrison, *Parent Rage in Youth Sports: Giving the Game Back to Our Children*, Psychol. Sports (July 13, 2002), http://psychologyofsports.com/2002/07/13/parent-rage-in-youth-sports-giving-the-game-back-to-our-children-2.

89. Michael S. James & Tracy Ziemer, *Are Youth Athletes Becoming Bad Sports?*, ABC News (Aug. 8, 2000), http://abcnews.com/sports/story?id=99665.

90. *Parents Worst Behaved, supra* note 29.

91. *Id.*

92. *Id.*

93. Press Release, Ipsos, Four in 10 (37%) Global Citizens Have Been to Children's Sports Events (Apr. 7, 2010), http://marketwire.com/press-release/four-in-10-37-global-citizens-have-been-to-childrens-sports-even-1143748.htm.

94. *See Parents Worst Behaved, supra* note 29.

95. Morrison, *supra* note 88.

96. Fred Engh, *Why Johnny Hates Sports: Why Organized Youth Sports Are Failing Our Children and What We Can Do About It* 140 (2002).

97. *See, e.g.*, Jeanie Tavitas-Williams, *Play Ball (Not Brawl): Adults Often Forget To Be Good Sports*, San Antonio Express-News, Apr. 27, 2004, at 1C, available at Factiva, Doc. No. SAEN000020040428e04r00007.

98. Jim Thompson, *The Double-Goal Coach* 5 (2003).

99. Buzz Bissinger, *Bench the Parents*, N.Y. Times, Aug. 23, 2008, http://nytimes.com/2008/08/23/opinion/23bissinger.html; Doug Wrenn, *Violent Parents—the New Contact Sport*, Magic City Morning Star (Feb. 5, 2007, 8:16 AM), http://magic-city-news.com/Doug_Wrenn_44/Violent_Parents_-_The_New_Contact_Sport7433.shtml; *see also* Press Release, Sporting Kid, Survey: Parents Believe Rash of Adult Violence at Youth Sporting Events Requires Nationwide Solution (Mar. 19, 2003), http://www.prnewswire.com/cgi-bin/stories.pl?acct=104&story=/www/story/03-19-2003/0001910938 (discussing survey of adults and players conducted by SportingKid magazine reporting "more than 84% of respondents [reported that they] have personally witnessed parents acting violently (shouting, berating, using abusive language) toward children, coaches and/or officials during youth sporting events").

100. Barry Rozner, *One Year After a Hockey Tragedy, What Has Changed?*, Daily Herald (Arlington Heights, Ill.), Nov, 3, 2000, at 1, available at Factiva, Doc. No. dhld000020010805dwb301ekb.

101. *Id.*

102. *Id.*

103. *See, e.g.*, Bill Wells, *Zealous Parents Troubling*, The Republican (Springfield, Mass.), Mar. 7, 2010, at B8, available at Factiva, Doc. No. SUNW000020100309e6370001v ("75% of all people involved in youth sports are quality, first-rate people . . . . 5% are just nuts . . . . 20% consists of good people . . . but when it comes to youth sports, something happens. Something gets triggered."). Fred Engh, president of the National Alliance for Youth Sports, has estimated that the number of problem youth sports parents has increased

from about 5% to about 15%. Chat Transcript: Fred Engh on Sports Rage, ABC News (Sept. 11, 2000), http://abcnews.com/US/story?id=94468&singlePage=true.

104. Douglas E. Abrams, *Lessons from the "Hockey Dad" Trial*, San Diego Union-Trib., Jan. 16, 2002, at B11, available at Factiva, Doc. No. sdu0000020020118dy1g0000w.

105. *Id.*

106. Bob Bigelow et al., *Just Let the Kids Play* xii (2001).

107. *See* [Benjamin Franklin], *On Protection of Towns from Fire*, Pa. Gazette, Jan. 28–Feb. 4, 1735, at 1.

108. *See supra* notes 23–24.

109. *See supra* text accompanying notes 22–24.

110. Abraham Lincoln, First Inaugural Address (Mar. 4, 1861), in *Lincoln: Speeches and Writings 1859–1865*, at 215, 224 (1989).

111. Bernie Schock, *Parents, Kids and Sports* 31–32 (1987); see also Thomas Tutko & William Bruns, *Winning Is Everything and Other American Myths* 8 (1976) (describing positive characteristics attributed to winners and negative characteristics attributed to losers).

112. Schuette, *supra* note 32, at 515 (noting that in the American society "winning is rewarded and athletes revered").

113. *Id.* at 519 (noting that a "moral and physical ethos" were cornerstones to "the initial rise of organized youth sports").

114. *The Growing Child in Competitive Sport* 8 (Geof Gleeson ed., 1986) (quoting the British National Association of Coaches).

115. *See, e.g.*, Rosie DiManno, *DiManno: Wells' Bat Quiets the Boobirds*, Toronto Star, Apr. 13, 2010, http://thestar.com/sports/baseball/mlb/bluejays/article/794376 (quoting Toronto Blue Jays outfielder Vernon Wells: "All we ask of everyone is to respect the game . . . As long as you have this uniform on, go out there and play as hard as you can . . ."); Jim Massie, *Women's Basketball: Buckeyes Are Bruised, not Beaten in Big Ten*, Columbus Dispatch, Jan. 17, 2010, http://dispatch.com/content/stories/sports/2010/01/17/osu_wbk_1-17.ART_ART_01-17-10_C3_QIGAMDF.html (quoting Ohio State University women's basketball coach Jim Foster: "When you respect the game, that stuff [starters' failure to shake hands before the game] doesn't come into play"); Scott Akanewich, *Montgomery Creates a Band of "Brothers"*, San Diego Union-Trib., Apr. 8, 2010, http://signonsandiego.com/news/2010/apr/08/montgomery-creates-a-band-of-brothers/(quoting San Diego high school baseball coach Manny Hermosillo: "We respect the game here"); Lois Kalchman, *Pilot Project Shows Way to Clean Up Kids' Hockey*, Toronto Star, Apr. 24, 2010, at S6, available at Factiva, Doc. No. TOR0000020100424e64o00068 (quoting Scott Oakman, executive director of the Greater Toronto Hockey League: "We want a safer, more respectful hockey").

116. Ryne Sandberg, *Respect the Game*, Yahoo! Sports (Aug. 1, 2005), http://yahoo.com/mlb/news?slug=rs-speech080105.

117. Bill Durham (The Mount Company 1988).

118. Memorable Quotes for Bull Durham (1988), IMDb, http://imdb.com/title/tt0094812/quotes (last visited Nov. 30, 2011); *see also* Awards for Bull Durham (1988), IMDb, http://imdb.com/title/tt0094812/awards (last visited Nov. 30, 2011).

119. *See* sources cited *infra* notes 121–139.

120. *See, e.g.*, Little League Baseball, *Play It Safe: A Practical Approach to Leadership Responsibility in an Effective Little League Safety Program* 4:11 (1998), http://littleleague.org/Assets/forms_pubs/asap/Section4 _PlayItSafe_2010.pdf ("Good sportsmanship and

courtesy, which are necessary for a harmonious and safe environment, can be taught best through the good example set by all adults on and off the field."); Respect Sports, http:// respectsports.com (last visited Nov. 30, 2011) ("respectful behavior in youth athletics will result in the establishment of standards that foster a healthy and safe environment").

121. *See* USA Hockey, *supra* note 12, at vii.

122. *Id.*

123. *Id.* at viii.

124. *Id.*

125. *Id.*

126. *Id.*

127. Thompson, *supra* note 98, at 110.

128. *Id.*

129. *See* Principle #3: *Honoring the Game*, Little League Online, http://littleleague. org/managersandcoaches/double_goal_coaching/pcahonoringthegame.htm (last visited Nov. 30, 2011).

130. *See Positive Coaching Alliance*, USA Water Polo, http://usawaterpolo.org/pro-gramshome/positivecoachingalliance.a spx (last visited Nov. 30, 2011).

131. *See Coach the Game*, USA Rugby, http://usarugby.org/#goto/coaches (follow "Coach the Game" hyperlink; then follow "Certification" hyperlink) (last visited Nov. 30, 2011).

132. *See AYSO's Six Philosophies*, Am. Youth Soccer Org., http://ayso.com/aboutayso/ ayso_philosophies.aspx (last visited Nov. 30, 2011).

133. *See Code of Ethics*, US Lacrosse, http://uslacrosse.org/utilitynav/aboutusla-crosse/codeofethics.aspx (last visited Nov. 30, 2011); see also St. Louis Sports Comm'n Sportsmanship Initiative, http://sportsmanship.org (last visited Nov. 30, 2011) (discuss-ing a focus on respect); *History*, Athletes for Better World, http://abw.org/about-us/his-tory (last visited Nov. 30, 2011) (discussing "commitment to the positive values of disci-pline, integrity, respect, cooperation, and compassion").

134. *See, e.g.*, Judy Pfitzinger, *Disrespect a Continuing Problem: Trash Talking in Athletics Is a Byproduct of an Increasingly Crass Culture, Those Involved in Youth Sports Say*, Star Trib. (Minneapolis, Minn.), Feb. 13, 2007, at 1E, available at Factiva, Doc. No. MSP0000020070213e32d000dz; Respect Sports, *supra* note 120.

135. *See, e.g., Respect the Game*, Md. Pub. Secondary Schs. Athletic Ass'n, http:// mpssaa.org/respectthegame (last visited Nov. 30, 2011) ("The ultimate indicator of the value of school athletic programs must be the level of citizenship displayed by those who participate."); *Respect the Game*, Ohio High Sch. Athletic Ass'n, http://ohsaa.org/RTG/ default.asp (last visited Nov. 30, 2011) ("When people involved in high school sports treat each other badly, disrupt games, or generally behave in a manner unworthy of the game itself, they are devaluing what you, and all of us, care so much about.").

136. *See, e.g., Softball Ontario's Respect My Game Is Launched!*, Lifestyle Info. Network, http://lin.ca/resource-details/14297 (last visited Nov. 30, 2011) ("An innovative program geared to create and build mutual respect between all participants in the great game of Softball.").

137. *See* generally *Respect: It's the Name of the Game* (n.d.), NCAA, http://fs.ncaa.org/ docs/di_champs_sports_m_gmt_cab/2010/june 2010/supp_1_respect pamplet.pdf.

138. *See* generally *id.*

139. *Id.* at 2.

140. Bob Verdi, *Adults Guilty of Cross-Checking Morality*, Chi. Trib., Dec. 12, 1999, http://articles.chicagotribune.com/1999-12-12/sports/9912120271.

141. *Id.* (paraphrasing cartoonist Walt Kelly, creator of "Pogo").

142. Sandberg, *supra* note 116.

143. *Id.*

144. *Id.*

145. See George Washington, *Farewell Address* (Sept. 17, 1796), in 1 *A Compilation of the Messages and Papers of the Presidents* 205, 213 (James D. Richardson ed., 1897) ("The Government sometimes . . . adopts through passion what reason would reject.").

146. Smith et al., *supra* note 2.

147. *Id.*

148. Grumman, *supra* note 57.

149. Verdi, *supra* note 140.

150. Barry Rozner, *What Can Be Learned from Ill-Fated Hit?*, Daily Herald (Arlington Heights, Ill.), Dec. 16, 1999, at 1, available at Factiva, Doc. No. dhld000020010826dvcg01mlw.

151. Hussain, *supra* note 10.

152. *Students' Statements*, Chi. Sun-Times, Oct. 27, 2000, at 3, available at http://highbeam.com/doc/1P2-4571538.html.

153. Hussain, *supra* note 10.

154. Black & Berger, *supra* note 65.

155. *Id.*

156. *Id.*

157. See discussion *supra* Parts I, II.A. 1–2.

158. See discussion supra Part II.B.

19 Health and Sports Law Collide

Do Professional Athletes Have an Unfettered Choice

to Accept Risk of Harm?

■ KEN J. BERGER

▦ 1.1 APPLICATION OF PRINCIPLES IN FORM OF HYPOTHETICAL EXAMPLE

The main issue is whether the Detroit Red Wings Hockey Club or their physicians ("Red Wings") had a positive duty at law to prevent a player with a serious medical disability from returning to play despite the player agreeing to accept the risk.

▦ 1.2 THE FACTS OF HYPOTHETICAL CASE

1. The respondent, the Detroit Red Wings Hockey Club ("Red Wings") are a professional hockey team in the National Hockey League ("NHL"). JF was at all material times a six-foot-five, twenty-five-year-old defenseman on the Detroit Red Wings.

2. JF died from a cardiac arrest during a National Hockey League game. This was not his first cardiac arrest. He survived the first cardiac arrest, after immediate CPR and defibrillation from an Automatic External Defibrillator device (AED) were applied to his chest by his team physicians.

3. JF was found to have a pre-existing (congenital) heart abnormality during a pre-season physical in September 2002. After its discovery JF told the media, "I wasn't scared about the abnormality. But I was scared about not playing hockey again." Further testing, back in 2002, revealed that he was fit to play, but he was asked to sign a waiver.

▦ 1.3 THE ISSUES

4. The broad issue in this appeal is when the risk of serious injury or even death is too high despite the signing of a waiver to be considered unacceptable. Further, can a professional athlete accept a high risk such as serious injury or death? Waivers are contracts and present a conflict between a person's rights to have

freedom to contract as they so desire and negligence, that one should be responsible for negligent acts which cause injury to another.

5. Soldiers go to war and the family is barred from suing because death is an accepted risk. Evil Knievel did his dangerous stunts despite high risk of serious injury or death. Why should professional athletes not make their own choices? Why should disabled athletes like JF not have an equal opportunity to practice their profession and have a "right to risk"? Why should he be prevented from playing with a congenital heart disability especially if there are methods of treatment to reduce risk? How does advanced medical technology or treatment affect a player's rights to accept risk?

6. For policy reasons, at the far end of the spectrum, society may not want to go as far with the exercise of individual autonomy as euthanasia in the Netherlands. Euthanasia is the deliberate putting to death of a person after voluntary consent. The goal is to terminate the suffering of a person from an incurable disease. How far can individuals go in the athletic context before society will intervene? Is high risk of serious injury or death in the athletic context equivalent to voluntary euthanasia or are there differences? Euthanized death is a predictable consequence of deliberate action. Therefore, it is easily distinguishable from the sports context where athletes accept high or uncertain risk of serious injury or death but it is not deliberate action with certain death. Athletes are often more likely able to make voluntary decisions without the burdens of incurable pain and clouding medications that can affect the voluntariness of a terminally ill patient's consent. Should policy reasons, nonetheless, preclude professional athletes from accepting high or uncertain risks of serious injury or death?

7. Advanced medical technologies are allowing athletes back more quickly from injury or illness, in a greater number of circumstances. From NBA basketball players like Alonzo Mourning's return to the National Basketball League after a kidney transplant to JF return to the NHL. What standard of medical certainty or legal certainty is appropriate regarding the "right to risk" and what principles of law should win: *contract* principles or *tort* law?

8. The higher the risk of serious injury or death and the greater the medical uncertainty, the more tort law might trump contract principles. In contrast, less risky and medically certain outcomes would be easier to knowingly and voluntarily assume by way of a contract that waives liability for negligence. That does not mean that tort law should trump contract principles whenever there is either a high risk of harm or death or when it is not medically clear that there is no high risk of harm or death. The absence of any foreseeable harm is complete safety. But all of us would be in straitjackets. Cigarettes are harmful, but they remain on the shelves. Athletes knowingly engage in sports that may have a reduced life expectancy and quality of their lives on a daily basis; weightlifting, boxing, and race car driving are typical examples.

9. Society wants individual autonomy and less paternalism, but it also wants individual protection from foreseeable harm using adequate means. How can

courts resolve this inherent conflict among different philosophies? Tort law is a means of preventing harm through deterrence and victim compensation, but contract law does not eliminate all means of protecting an individual from harm. The benefit of contracts and waivers is that it respects an individual's inherent autonomy, provided they are truly voluntary. Contracts just shift the risk. A player can still purchase disability and life insurance or obtain assistance through the NHL collective bargaining agreement.

10. The narrow issue in this appeal is the liability of the Red Wings for JF death and whether the waiver signed by JF exempts them from liability. It depends on the context, the circumstances, and the balancing and addressing of a number of sub issues:

> Did the Red Wings team physicians owe a duty of care to JF?
> If a duty existed, what standard of care is required in the circumstances?
> Was the standard of care breached? If there was a breach of the standard, did it cause JF death?
> Was the death too remote to extend liability?
> Did JF voluntarily assume the risk?
> Was JF contributory negligent?
> If the Red Wings were liable, can they rely on the waiver as a contractual defense to the tort claim?

11. In terms of analysis, the legal issues apply to all different legal systems. The arguments on the issues will use Canadian common law principles to try to resolve the dilemma that this legal problem creates. Equally well, civil law in non-common law jurisdiction would likely use its civil codes to resolve the very same issue, however, the same general principles and policies likely apply.

■ 1.4 DUTY OF CARE

12. A duty of care arises when there is a relationship of sufficient proximity. The Supreme Court of Canada has adopted the two-part Anns[1] test to establish when the law will recognize that parties are of sufficient proximity, to find that there is a duty of care.

13. The main issue as far as the duty of care is concerned is whether the Red Wings had a duty to control the conduct of JF by preventing him from returning to the ice. This action, as alleged by JF, is not based on negligent conduct (*misfeasance*), but a failure of the Red Wings to take affirmative action, or take positive steps, (*nonfeasance*) to prevent harm to JF.

14. In fact, the action is not based on risk created by the Red Wings (either negligent conduct or a failure to warn), but rather is based on protecting JF from something intrinsic to him: A pre-existing congenital heart disability, that he knew and appreciated the consequences of, that increased his own risk of serious injury or death.

15. The common law was reluctant to extend the reach of legal obligations to affirmative action and protection because of a philosophy of individualism. Negligent conduct creates risks and makes the defendant's position worse. In the case of inaction or a failure of affirmative action, a person has merely failed to possibly benefit a person by not interfering in his affairs. In *Osterlind*[2], the defendant rented a canoe to drunken people and had no duty to refuse because they were drunk or rescue them when they were in danger.

16. However, due to an increased sense of social obligations, there has been a growing group of special relationships, which import an obligation to engage in positive action for the benefit of another. Today, there is a duty to rescue when one innocently or negligently created a perilous situation, physically worsened a person's position, denied the person other rescue opportunities, or induced the person to rely to their detriment. Normally, there is some element of control or economic benefit to the person as a result of the relation, which justifies the creation of a duty of care. In *Bain*[3], the court found the teachers liable in *nonfeasance* for failing to take positive steps to protect students under their control when a 19-year-old learning disabled child fell, on a forestry tour, on a mountain. However, in another case the court found no affirmative duty for the parents to control a 16-year-old's snowmobile driving. The 16-year-old drove 40 miles per/hour and one person died, another was seriously injured. A duty to take affirmative action has been found in the social host's liability, because of an inviter-invitee relationship. In *Crocker*[4], a duty of care was established to control the conduct of a drunken competitor and remove him from a downhill skiing competition.

17. Do physicians have an affirmative duty to protect patients from their own foolishness or bad decisions? If physicians do not have a general affirmative duty of protection, then should team physicians or professional sports teams have an affirmative duty to protect their players from their own risks?

■ **1.5 STANDARD OF CARE**

18. What standard of care should be applied in the circumstances of professional hockey players when they assume the risk of harm? Should the standard of care be lowered because of the assumption of risk?

19. Negligence assesses liability on the basis of a breach of a duty of care arising from a foreseeable and unreasonable risk of harm to one person created by the act or omission of another. Negligence arises when a person fails to safeguard others against an unreasonable risk. In *Paris*[5], the court looked at standard of care of an employer with regards to a particularly vulnerable employee. The employee had only one functioning eye. The employer had knowledge of the employee's medical disability. The frequency of injury was very low, but the seriousness of the consequences of failing to provide protective safety goggles was catastrophic. The standard of negligence does vary depending on the circumstances.

20. The main issue is what standard of care to apply in professional sports when athletes accept risk of harm? Does modifying the standard from a subjective player to an objective one, assist the court in applying the standard of care to sports or should negligence law even be applied? If negligence law is applied, is the 'reasonable person standard', whether subjective or even objective, too easily breached?

21. In *Zapf*[6], the defendant appealed the verdict of the trial court regarding the standard of care to apply to ice hockey, arguing that the court applied the wrong standard. The plaintiff broke his neck while playing in a Junior A hockey game and is quadriplegic. The court tried to resolve this issue by explaining that it is not every careless act causing injury that will give rise to liability, it is acts outside the risks assumed, but the courts have difficulty consistently applying a consistent standard. In *Wilson*[7], the court held that the standard of care was higher than just negligence when a collision during recreational baseball caused a compound fracture. The judge found that persons participating in sporting events accept risk of injury. The defendant's conduct must amount to a reckless disregard for the others safety or was deliberately intended to cause injury. Similarly, in *Hackbart*[8], a Colorado state court agreed that negligence, inadvertence, or a failure to take precautions does not belong in the sports world. "Professional sport is a species of warfare not actionable in court". However, the appeal court reversed Hackbart, holding that tort-law principles were not inapplicable merely because the injury took place during a professional football game. Overall, the case law is not particularly consistent. It does not unanimously point to a narrower, lower standard of care. Therefore, the appropriate standard is negligence. The "mythical" *reasonable person* test is supposed to be applicable to all different contexts and circumstances.

▧ 1.6 BREACH OF STANDARD OF CARE

22. The breach of a standard of care is a question of fact determined by the trier of fact on the balance of probabilities.

23. In *Pichardo*[9], in a wrongful death action, parties running a summer league baseball game were not responsible for a baseball player being struck and killed by lightning. Lightning while rarely striking, posed an unreasonable risk, but the assumption of risk denied the defendant's liability. In *Parmentier*[10], the promoter of a boxing match between minors, a fight in which each contestant sought to gain an advantage over the other by injuring him by means of blows, was not liable for the death of one of the minors between the fifth and sixth rounds. While the minor may not have fully and knowingly understood and appreciated his own risk, the court felt that when entering a boxing match, both the participants and their parents accepted serious risk, so the court denied liability.

24. The history of the role of the team physician is relevant to this inquiry. In the past, the return to the sport arena was more vital than complete recovery of the patient. Athletes would not seek any treatment at all. Doctors were seen as

evil. If an athlete saw the team physician, the first recommendation was, "Well, give up football" so that doctors and athletes were seen as incompatible. Also, coaches, management and sometimes players resisted a doctor's involvement. In *Robitaille*[11], the court awarded $435,000 in damages for a neck injury that did not have an adequate chance to heal. The physician was pressured from the team and management, and insisted that Robitaille return to the ice. In the newspaper the coach stated ". . . Of course, we were short a defensemen with Robitaille out (sore shoulder). I don't know exactly how bad it is but I tell you he'd better start playing. If he doesn't, I'm going to have to consider suspending him . . .". Today, a more contemporary approach is used.

25. The majority of sudden cardiac deaths in young athletes are cause by either inherited or congenital cardiac disorders. This is a common problem among young professional athletes. The implantable defibrillator, a device that provides excellent protection from sudden death, has revolutionized the treatment of athletes with life-threatening ventricular arrhythmias but defining the athletes who would benefit is not always clear.

26. The cost of avoiding the risk would not be a barrier for the Red Wings. The Red Wings could have offered JF a job in administration, as a non-player. However, the cost to JF was not insignificant. As he had mentioned to the media previously, he would have been psychologically devastated if he did not return to the game, a game he had devoted his life to.

27. There is social utility in allowing JF to make his own choice. The NHL is a form of public entertainment and performs a social good. It gives young players hope that one day their dreams of becoming an elite athlete will be realized rather than turning to drugs or alcohol. This would be based on their own choices without undue interference from others. Provided it does not affect the safety of others, players feel that they should be entitled to assume their own risk and achieve their goals and dreams.

▪ 1.7 CAUSATION

28. Before liability can be proven, the negligent conduct by the Red Wings must have caused JF death. Causation can be proven in two ways. First, was the Red Wings' conduct the causal factor, or proximate cause, of JF death? *But for* the Red Wings' allowing F back on the ice, JF would not have died. The Supreme Court of Canada, in *Snell v. Farrel*[12], found that medical causation does not have to reach scientific precision, but is a question of fact to be determined on the balance of probabilities. But here the trial court was not permitted to infer causation from little affirmative evidence as in *Snell*, because knowledge in this case was not one sided, within the knowledge of the Red Wings alone. JF was knowledgeable and had independent legal and medical experts who advised him. Second, even if the Red Wings' conduct of not preventing JF from returning to the ice did not alone

cause JF death, causation could be established if the negligent conduct of failing to protect JF materially contributed to his death. It is enough that the negligent conduct amounted to one of the material contributing causes. The *thin skull rule* applies, whereby the Red Wings are still fully liable even if the death is more serious than their conduct alone as compared to the seriousness of JF preexisting congenital heart condition. The Red Wings must take JF as they found him, and as they diagnosed him. The Red Wings were aware of the risks that his heart condition posed, as they consulted with independent lawyers and medical experts.

■ 1.8 VOLUNTARY ASSUMPTION OF RISK

29. The courts are reluctant to find, in tort, that the plaintiff voluntarily assumed the risk because it is a complete bar to recovery. Voluntary assumption of risk may also operate unfairly when, in one situation, the plaintiff is contributory negligent and in another the plaintiff is not, because it is a complete bar to recovery. The courts prefer apportionment under the *Negligence Act*. In *Dube*[13] and in *Seymour,* the plaintiff agreed to accept the risk when he accepted a ride from a drunk driver, but the court found that the plaintiff did not waive his legal rights. In *Crocker,* the burden is on the defendant to show that the plaintiff not only was aware of the physical risk, but also accepted all of the physical risk without compensation and knowingly waived his rights to have any legal recourse.

■ 1.9 CONTRIBUTORY NEGLIGENCE

30. The burden is on the Red Wings to prove that on the balance of probabilities the plaintiff was negligent himself for returning to the ice. One expects a reasonable person to take reasonable precautions for their own safety. JF did just that. He sought medical treatment, the implantable defibrillator, and medical advice before returning to the ice. JF was not contributory negligent.

■ 2.0 WAIVER AS CONTRACTUAL DEFENSE

31. Waivers are contracts, so contract principles apply. Waivers are offered and accepted. Waivers need to have consideration and the intention that they will be legally binding to be enforceable. Consideration is usually the right of the athlete to participate after he/she contractually waives the risk. In exchange for participating, the athlete as part of the bargain knowingly waives his right to sue. Especially if an athlete relinquishes a lot, there should be some evidence that there was a bargain. Similar to contracts, waivers are struck down if there is fraud, duress, undue influence, or unconscionability. The party bound by the waiver must be given adequate notice or the party seeking to rely on the waiver must take reasonable measures to draw the waiver to the bound party's attention

and take reasonable steps in the circumstances to ensure the bound party understands the waiver. The bound party must have clear knowledge and appreciation of the nature and character of the risk to be assumed and voluntarily accept the risk. The waiver should express what the parties intended or contemplated regarding the scope of the conduct of the potential defendant and the severity and type of injuries or damages that were to be accepted. Unless it is plain and obvious that the conduct and injuries are clearly within the ambit of the waiver, a motion's court may refuse to dismiss the claim on summary judgment, as there may be a genuine issue for trial. For negligent conduct, a court will generally look at the drafting of the waiver to ensure that a participant has willingly given up his or her rights to be legally protected from personal injury caused by negligence. Courts have upheld waivers that cover negligent acts and this is not unique to the sport's context. However, courts have not always been consistent on deciding on the validity of waivers.

32. In the absence of a signed waiver, participants assume only the ordinary risks of doing the activity from the perspective of the average reasonable participant. For instance, a golfer who gets hit by a stray ball will likely lose his/her negligence claim even without having signed a waiver because it is an ordinary risk of the average golf enthusiast. In *Everett*[14], an ice hockey player who sustained a serious head injury sued in both negligence and strict liability for a defective hockey helmet design. While the jury ruled in the plaintiff's favor for negligence, the judge immediately disagreed as a matter of law that the plaintiff voluntarily assumed the risk of injury. Defendants are not required to be shielded by waivers if a sport or activity has been deemed inherently dangerous by the courts, such as skydiving, white water rafting or bungee jumping, since a participant should know the serious dangers. However, if an unusual danger causes injury, the defendant is liable, without a waiver. In *Haley*[15], a tobogganer riding a crazy carpet was injured when she fell into a hole just off of the groomed portion of the slope. A hole is not a risk inherent in the sport of tobogganing. She sustained a broken leg. The resort knew about the hole and should have foreseen a risk to the tobogganers. They marked the hole with a danger warning, but this was insufficient to discharge their duty of care. The defendant should have drawn the hazard to the attention of the tobogganers before permitting them to proceed down the slope. The plaintiff was found to be 50% contributory negligent, as she did not look to see if hazards existed on the slope. In *MacCabe*[16], a 16-year-old girl was rendered quadriplegic by trying a back flip in gymnastics class. She was 25% contributorily negligent as she was aware of the dangers. In *Rudd*[17], the plaintiff sustained a serious acquired brain injury after falling off a horse missing a shoe. She was 33.3% contributorily negligent. But in *Msuya*[18], no contributory negligence was granted because it was unreasonable to expect a 12-year-old, who was a newcomer to a group, to assert herself, not to take part in a cross-country bike trip.

33. In *Ivo*[19], the court analyzed the issues differently. The defendant had a duty to completely and accurately inform the plaintiff of the condition of a racetrack.

Here, there was a depression in the racetrack. The defendant, who had special knowledge, made an incomplete representation of the safety of the racetrack, inducing him to enter into a contract to the defendant's detriment. Ivo suffered injuries, and the defendant was liable. Assumption of risk did not apply, because he was not fully informed of the danger and therefore could not fully appreciate the risk that he was accepting.

34. In *Murray*[20], the plaintiff was rendered paraplegic when a cattle-roping chute fell on her. The agreement only provided for the assumption of risk of using the arena, not the acceptance of both the physical and legal risk of injury from the defendant's negligence. Similarly in *Llewellyn*[21], a trail riding accident waiver did not cover negligence and thus was irrelevant and the defendant was liable. In *Hutchison*, the park was negligent in failing to instruct the plaintiff how to enter the waterslide. He fractured his ankle. While he paid a fee to enjoy the slide and accepted the risk of injury, he did not abandon his legal rights.

35. If the risks, injuries or conduct are beyond the ordinary risk of the activity, and includes negligence, a waiver is usually required to exempt the defendant from liability. In *Dyck*[22], the court found negligence because the conduct and injuries were beyond the usual ordinary risk, but the court exonerated the claim due to the waiver clause in a snowmobile race entry form. In *Dyck*, the plaintiff signed the waiver with full knowledge of its intention, to exempt the defendant from liability; including negligence. The waiver was found not to be against public policy, a fundamental breach, nor was there an unconscionable transaction.

36. Waivers are generally disfavored by the courts, unless they are unambiguous (*contra proferentem*—construing an ambiguous provision most strongly against the drafter), not against public policy and entered into knowingly and voluntarily. In *Crocker,* the waiver was not drawn to the plaintiff's attention, he had not read it thinking it was an entry form. The court in *Crocker* invalidated the waiver because it was entered into unknowingly and involuntarily.

37. Even if a waiver is valid on its face, the court will generally not release the defendants from intentional, willful, reckless or wanton acts for want of public policy. Courts do not want to allow reckless potential defendants from getting a free way out by using waivers of liability. There are concerns that an injured party cannot be made whole just because he signed a piece of paper or it was on the back of an admission ticket. There is a concern that waivers may lower the standard of care. As far as public policy is concerned, a counter-argument is that the courts have to be mindful that sports are not peripheral to society; they are central to life and have become an important unique institution for the transmission of social and political concerns. Civil liability should not, therefore, pose an undue burden on the development of sport at both an amateur and professional level just because of unproven fears.

38. Waivers have been upheld in ultra hazardous activities, such as racecar driving, otherwise it would increase the liability of the sporting event to such a

degree that all the similar events would be cancelled. This would not be in the public interest. In the United States, some sports have been shut down or made more expensive as a result of the high cost of defending lawsuits. Also, it is inappropriate for today's court to re-watch a video frame by frame and then decide whether liability should, in retrospect, be pinned on a defendant.

39. Dale Earnhardt died at the Daytona 500 car race, but his death was not unpredictable. He risked his life and limb every time he entered into a race. In *Williams*, a law student signed a waiver voluntarily with knowledge and appreciation of the risk before entering a 10,000-meter road race in the heat. He argued that there was no choice but to sign the waiver, otherwise he could not enter the race. He sustained permanent impairment of motor functions from heat exhaustion. The waiver was valid. The waiver was particular enough of the risks, not against public policy and there was no unequal bargaining power. Courts have generally held that entering a race or participating in sports at the amateur level is discretionary. Professional or elite athletes do have an argument that it is of financial necessity shifting the risk back to the defendants on the ground that the waiver is unconscionable. However, independent legal advice may save an otherwise unconscionable waiver or a waiver entered into under duress or undue influence.

40. In *Blomberg*[23], a skier signed a contractual waiver of all claims including negligence. The skier claimed that he did not read it before signing. The court held that the waiver was valid and enforceable. The waiver was a bar to the action. The defendant took reasonable steps to bring notice of the waiver to the skier by having it witnessed by an employee who went over the reasons for having it signed. The skier knew that he was signing a waiver, but chose not to read it. This is not a case of *non est factum*. The plaintiff was well educated and a sophisticated businessman. There was no misrepresentation or fraud. The plaintiff knew the risk inherent in skiing. The court held that the waiver was not unconscionable or divergent from community standards of commercial morality and not against public policy. In *Ocsko*[24], a British Columbia appeal court drew a similar conclusion with a skier that signed a waiver. Some courts have found in recent cases that the use of exempting conditions on the back of ski lift tickets suffice to avoid liability.

41. In *Cowes*[25], a student and exotic dancer visited the African Lion & Safari and were attacked by Siberian tigers. The park was strictly liable for severe physical and psychological injuries of the plaintiff because the Siberian tigers were wild and dangerous animals. Since the park kept the Siberian Tigers free, rather than in cages, the park was held to strict liability and the court was more reluctant to apply contributory negligence. There were signs outside the park and brochures stating: "All visitors enter the park at their own risk. No responsibility for damage to vehicle or person however caused". Like *Crocker*, the plaintiff neither recalled seeing the signs or reading the brochures, nor did anyone working at the park draw the sign or the brochure to their attention. Because there were issues

with consent, voluntariness and notice, the courts in *Cowes* and *Crocker* did not uphold the waiver or the assumption of risk.

42. Under public policy, waivers may not be upheld if there is an industry practice that is unconscionable. While individuals who elect to participate in ultra-hazardous activities like bungee-jumping are exempted from suing under a waiver, cheerleading groups who are forced to participate in dangerous stunts are not, mainly because the waivers are unconscionable.

43. Moving to the use of waiver in the sports medicine context. In *Lewis*[26], the estate of former Boston Celtic NBA player Reggie Lewis lost a wrongful death suit against several physicians. Reggie Lewis saw several specialists about his heart condition and was aware of his risk. The physicians after treatment recommended a monitored game plan which never occurred. Instead, Lewis, against medical advice, died while playing unmonitored basketball with friends on July 27, 1993.

44. In *Thomas*[27], a student was rendered quadriplegic after sustaining a broken neck after making a football tackle. The risk was within the ambit of the "Interscholastic Athletic Permission Form". The injury was within the limits of risk inherent in tackle football. It is of interest that the plaintiff may have had a pre-existing "lean swan neck", which increased his risk especially if he played defensive-back. The court found that this "lean swan neck" theory was not common knowledge among coaches and, therefore, the court did not find the coaches negligent. The plaintiff participated in tackle football under his own free will with knowledge of the risk. Thomas did not sign a waiver, which would overcome negligent conduct by his coaches, but the coaches were not found to be negligent and his lawsuit was unsuccessful.

45. In the health law setting, waivers have been upheld. In *Hobbs*[28], despite malpractice and a negligently performed surgery that resulted in bleeding during a laparoscopically assisted vaginal hysterectomy, the patient preoperatively signed a refusal to permit blood transfusion and she was aware of the dangers of surgery without available blood transfusion. She died. The estate argued that the waiver of blood transfusion did not intend to excuse the physician's negligence. The transfusion would have saved the patient's life. The court could not accept that a person should be able to deny a doctor's use of every tool to overcome the effects of negligence.

46. In the medical treatment context, informed consent is the standard expected of a reasonable physician in discussing and implementing treatment decisions. In *Hopp*[29], the nature of the proposed treatment, its gravity, any material risks and any special or unusual risk should be disclosed. In *Reibl*[30], the court changed the standard from what a reasonable medical doctor would disclose to what a reasonable patient should receive. Certain cosmetic procedures require a higher standard the Reibl.

47. In the treatment of sports athletes, some would argue a higher standard than *Reibl*, but if one appreciates the complexity of the dynamics in the sports

world, between team physician, the team and the athlete, *Reibl* is a more reasonable and sufficient standard that properly balances all the interests. For instance, an athlete wanting to return to the ice after treatment should be expected to receive all the risks that a reasonable player in the circumstances should receive before deciding whether or not to accept the risk.

48. The team physician generally has the primary responsibility for medically clearing athletes to play. Athletes have either threatened to sue or sued their physician for negligent advice. The estate of a H. Gathers, a college basketball player, alleged that the physicians improperly cleared him to resume playing college basketball with a serious heart condition. Since there is no currently well-defined judicial precedent establishing specific parameters of a physician's legal duty of care in clearing athletes to participate in competitive athletics, a case-by case assessment is recommended. In *Classen*[31], the ringside physician's failure to stop a boxing match when the participant received several blows to the head resulting in death may have constituted malpractice. In *Mikkelsen*[32], the physician was negligent for allowing an athlete to return to ski jumping after hip replacement surgery.

49. The courts have determined the standard to be within the bounds of acceptable or reasonable sports medicine practice governed by the obligation to protect the athlete from medically unreasonable risks of harm. Appropriate considerations include: the intensity and physical demands of a sport; the athlete's physiology; the available clinical evidence, conference or customary guidelines; the probability and severity of harm; and whether medication, monitoring or protective equipment will minimize the potential health risks of the participant and enable safe athletic participation.

50. In terms of a waiver, physicians cannot insist on a waiver in the regular routine treatment of their patients for public policy reasons. But the team physician-adult athlete relationship is different and the parties should be able to establish their relationship by a waiver. If an athlete is fully informed of all the risks of playing with an illness or injury, or the player desires a physician to utilize innovative treatment, an athlete should be able, if willing, to release a physician from potential negligence and be cleared to play. Doing so may contravene a team physician's fiduciary obligation to protect an athlete's health by not discouraging participation that exposes them to risk of serious harm. But if a team or a physician denied treatment or denied allowing the player to compete, a player should have the option of challenging the exclusion by requesting that the sport or physician provide accommodation to allow participation in the sport. Teams are generally able to defend these challenges or claims if the athlete's participation in the sport creates a significant increased risk of substantial harm to the athlete or other players. In *Knapp*[33], a basketball player suffered a cardiac arrest while playing basketball. He survived after defibrillation. He had an implantable defibrillator and he

played successful recreational basketball. The doctors refused to let him play intercollegiate basketball. Even with the defibrillator he was at significant risk of ventricular fibrillation or cardiac arrest during competitive sports. The implantable defibrillator had not been tested in intercollegiate basketball. The court found that the University could establish legitimate physical qualifications that an individual must satisfy before competing. It held that an athlete could be disqualified if necessary to avoid a significant risk of injury to himself that cannot be eliminated through reasonable medical accommodations. The court in closing stated that its decision may not be the right one, only that it is not an illegal one under the Rehabilitation Act. The problem is that physicians tend be conservative and if the decision is left solely in the hands of the physician, without any input from informed athletes, many otherwise disabled players would be refused participation when realistically they could participate safely, albeit with a high risk.

2.1 CONCLUSION

51. There is a positive duty at law to prevent a player with a serious medical disability from returning to play. The Red Wings had a duty of care to JF and failed to discharge that duty. However, if a player is able to seek medical treatment that reduces the risk and does so, a player's will to return cannot be ignored. The team must substantiate the restriction by justifying the risk as a relatively certain and substantial risk. A player may agree to accept high risk of serious injury or death through a contractual waiver to insulate others from liability in negligence. JF signed a valid contractual waiver that exempts the Red Wings and their physicians from liability in negligence. Independent legal advice and advice from medical experts ensured that the waiver was voluntary, understood and appreciated and that both the team and player bargained on a relatively equal platform. While the principles and arguments apply to Canadian common law, the principles and policies are applicable to all other common-law countries and civil law countries throughout the world, as the problems and issues addressed in this paper are not local. Each legal and medical system should try to resolve the issues using the framework of its own rules of law, but the principles and policies should be broadly accepted.

APPENDIX I

Table of Legislation

Negligence Act R.S.O. 1990, N.1.
Occupiers' Liability Act, R.S.O. 1990, c. 0.2.

Table of Cases

Arland v. Taylor, [1955] 3 D.L.R. 358 (Ont. C.A.).

Assiniboine South School Division, No. 3 v. Greater Winnipeg Gas Co., [1971] 4 W.W.R. 746 (Man. C.A.).

Athey v. Leonati (1996), 140 D.L.R. (4th) 235 (S.C.C.).

Bain v. Calgary Board of Education, [1994] 2 W.W.R. 468.

Blomberg v. Blackcomb Skiing Enterprises Ltd., [1992] B.C.J. No. 196.

Buchan v. Ortho Pharmaceutical (Canada) Ltd., [1986] 25 D.L.R. (4th) 658 (Ont. C.A.).

Car and General Insurance Corp. Ltd. v. Seymour, [1956] S.C.R. 322.

Classen v. Izquierdo, 520 N.Y.S. 2d 999 (Sup. Ct. N.Y. County 1987).

Cowles v. Balac, [2005] O.J. No.229.

Crocker v. Sundance Northwest Resorts Ltd, [1988]1 S.C.R. 1186, [1988] S.CJ. No. 60.

Donoghue v. Stevenson, [1932] A.C. 562 (H.L.).

Dube v. Labar, [1986] 27 D.L.R. (4th) 653 (S.C.C.).

Dyck v. Manitoba Snowmobile Association Inc., [1985] 1 S.C.R. 589.

Everett v. Bucky Warren, Inc., [1978] 380 N.E. (2nd) 653.

Gagnon v. Beaulieu, [1977] 1 W.W.R. 702 (B.C.S.C.).

Hackbart v. Cincinnati Bengals, Inc., [1979] 601 F2nd 516.

Haley v. London Electricity Bd., [1965] A.C. 778 (H.L)

Haley v. White Hills Resort Ltd, [1999] N.J. No. 157.

Hobbs v. Robertson, [2004] B.C.J. No. 1689.

Hopp v. Lepp, [1980] 2 S.C.R. 192.

Hutchison v. Daredevil Park Inc., [2003] O.J. No. 1570.

Ivo v. Halabura, [1990] S.J. No. 384.

Jane Doe v. Metro Toronto Comm. Of Police, [1998] O.J. No. 2681 (Gen. Div.).

J.G. v. Stathcona, [2004] A.J. No. 664.

Kauffman v. T.T.C., [1959] 18 D.L.R. (2d) 204 (Ont. C.A.).

Knapp v. Northwestern University, 010 F. 3d 473 (7th Cir. 1996).

Knockwood v. Cormier, [1995] 167 N.B.R. (2d) 147, 427 A.P.R. 147.

Law Estate v. Simice, [1994], 21 C.C.L.T. (2d) 228 (B.C.S.C.).

Lewis v. Mudge, [2003] 60 Mass. App. Ct. 480, 803 N.E. 2d 735.

Llewellyn v. MacSwain, [1993] P.E.I.J. No. 38.

MacCabe v. Westlock Roman Catholic Separate School District No. 110, [2001] A.J. No. 1278.

Menow v. Jordan House Ltd., [1974] S.C.R. 239.

Mikkelsen v. Haslam, 764 2 d 1384 (Utah CT. Aoo. 1988).

Msuya (Litigation guardian of) v. Fraser, [2000] O.J. No.3304.

Murray v. Bitango, [1996] A.J. No. 418.

Nairne v. Wagon Wheel Ranch Ltd., [1995] O.J. No. 1234.

Norberg v. Wynrib (1992), 12 C.C.L.T. (2d) 1 (S.C.C.).

Ocsko v. Cypress Bowl Recreations Ltd., [1992] B.C.J. No. 1992.

Osterlind v. Hill, (1928) 160 N.E. 301 (Mass.S.C.).

Paris v. Stepney Borough Council, [1951] A.C. 367 (H.L).

Parmentier v. McGinnis [1914] 157 Wis 596.

Pascoe v. Ball Hockey Ontario Inc., [2005] O.J. No. 1253.

Pichardo v North Patchogue Medford Youth Athletic Assoc., Inc. [1991, 2d
    Dept] 172 App Div 2d 814.

Reibl v. Hughes, [1980] 2 S.C.R. 88.

Robitaille v. Vancouver Hockey Club Ltd., [1981] B.C.J. No. 555.

Rudd v. Hamiota FeedLot Ltd., [2006] M.J. No. 36.

Snell v. Farrell, [1990] 72 D.L.R. (4th) 289 (S.C.C.).

Tarasoff v. Regents of University of California, [1976] 17 Cal. 3d 425, 551 P.2d
    334, 131 Cal. Rptr. 14.

Thomas v. Hamilton (City) Board of Education, [1994] O.J. No. 2444.

U.S. v. Carroll Towing Co., [1947] 159 F-2d 169 (2d Cir).

Waldick v. Malcolm, [1991] 83 D.L.R. (4th) 114 (S.C.C.).

Wilson v. Haddock, [1998] B.C.J. No. 1036.

Zapf v. Muckalt, [1996] B.C.J. No. 2402.

◼ **APPENDIX III**

Secondary Authorities

Barnes, J. *Recent developments in Canadian sports law*. 23 Ottawa L. Rev. 623
    (1991).

Champion, W. *Car race waivers' checkered flag on third party loss of
    consortium claims*. 14 Seton Hall J. Sports & Ent. L. 109 (2004).

Cheerleading group wants stunt restrictions. Associated Press report, MSNBC
    broadcast, Mar. 8, 2006. http://cheerwiz.com/ap4.htm

Dent, J. *Congenital heart disease and exercise*. 22 Clin. Sports Med. 81–99
    (Jan. 2003).

Elvin, C. *United Kingdom: A question of sports law—what happens next?*
    Monday Business Briefing, Sept. 6, 1999.

Firoozi, S., et al. *Risk of competitive sport in young athletes with heart disease*.
    89 Heart 710–714 (July 2003).

Garson, A. *Arrhythmias and sudden cardiac death in elite athletes*. American
    College of Cardiology, 16th Bethesda Conference, 20 Pediatr. Med Chir.
    101–103 (Mar.-Apr. 1998).

Grazis, S. *Liability of participant in team athletic competition for injury to or death of another participant.* 55 A.L.R. 5th 529. (1998).

Jaffey, J. *Minor league plaintiff sues hockey league for injury after signing waiver.* 25 The Lawyers Weekly 4.

Iacono P. *The municipality as occupier of recreational property.* 6 Advocates' Soc. J. 27–34.

Liberthson, R. *Arrhythmias in the athlete with congenital heart disease: Guidelines for participation.* 50 Ann. Rev. Med. 441–452 (1999).

Ling, M. et al. *Ventricular arrhythmias in the athlete.* 16 Curr. Opin. Cardiol. 30–39 (Jan. 2001).

Lorvidhaya, P. *Sudden cardiac death in athletes.* 100 Cardiology 186–195 (2003).

Mitten, M. *Emerging legal issues in sports medicine: A synthesis, summary, and analysis.* 76 St. John's L. Rev. 5 (2002).

Neumann, J. *Disclaimer clauses and personal injury.* 55 Sask. L. Rev. 312 (1991).

Piantanida, N., et al. *Sudden cardiac death: Ethical considerations in the return to play.* 3 Current Sports Med. Rep. 89–92 (Apr. 2004).

O'Donoghue, D. *Treatment of injuries to athletes.* Toronto: W.B. Saunders, 1976.

Rovell, D. *Doctor will recommend more detailed hear tests.* ESPN broadcast. ESPN.com. (2006). Retrieved from http://espn.go.com/nba/news/story?id=2333051.

Sethi, D. *Please release me: Prospective exculpatory covenants in Arizona.* American Bar Association website, (Aug. 2005). www.abanet.org.

Tomlinson J., and Machum, G. *Participants, organizers must consider potential exposure: Door open to high damages in sports activities.* 14 The Lawyers Weekly 44.

University of California, Berkeley. "Waiver of liability, assumption of risk and indemnity agreement." Online example from University of California, Cal Sport Club.

■ NOTES

1. *Arland v. Taylor*, [1955] 3 D.L.R. 358 (Ont. C.A.).
2. *Osterlind v. Hill*, [1928] 160 N.E. 301 (Mass.S.C.).
3. *Bain v. Calgary Board of Education*, [1994] 2 W.W.R. 468.
4. *Crocker v. Sundance Northwest Resorts Ltd*, [1988] 1 S.C.R. 1186, [1988] S.CJ. No. 60.
5. *Paris v. Stepney Borough Council*, [1951] A.C. 367 (H.L).
6. *Zapf v. Muckalt*, [1996] B.C.J. No. 2402.
7. *Wilson v. Haddock*, [1998] B.C.J. No. 1036.
8. *Hackbart v. Cincinnati Bengals*, Inc. 601 F2nd 516.
9. *Pichardo v North Patchogue Medford Youth Athletic Assoc.*, Inc. (1991, 2d Dept) 172.

10. *Parmentier v. McGinnis* [1914] 157 Wis 596.
11. *Robitaille v. Vancouver Hockey Club Ltd.,* [1981] B.C.J. No. 555.
12. *Snell v. Farrell,* [1990] 72 D.L.R. (4th) 289 (S.C.C.).
13. *Dube v. Labar,* [1986] 27 D.L.R. (4th) 653 (S.C.C.).
14. *Everett v. Bucky Warren, Inc.,* 380 N.E. (2nd) 653.
15. *Haley v. White Hills Resort Ltd,* [1999] N.J. No. 157.
16. *MacCabe v. Westlock Roman Catholic Separate School District No. 110.* [2001] A.J. No. 1278.
17. *Rudd v. Hamiota FeedLot Ltd.,* [2006] M.J. No. 36.
18. *Msuya (Litigation guardian of) v. Fraser,* [2000] O.J. No.3304.
19. *Ivo v. Halabura.* [1990] S.J. No.384.
20. *Murray v. Bitango,* [1996] A.J. No. 418.
21. *Llewellyn v. MacSwain.* [1993] P.E.I.J. No. 38.
22. *Dyck v. Manitoba Snowmobile Association Inc.,* [1985] 1 S.C.R. 589.
23. *Blomberg v. Blackcomb Skiing Enterprises Ltd.,* [1992] B.C.J. No. 196.
24. *Ocsko v. Cypress Bowl Recreations Ltd.,* [1992] B.C.J. No. 1992.
25. *Cowles v. Balac,* [2005] O.J. No.229.
26. *Lewis v. Mudge,* 60 Mass. App. Ct. 480. 803 N.E. 2d 735.
27. *Thomas v. Hamilton (City) Board of Education.* [1994] O.J. No. 2444.
28. *Hobbs v. Robertson,* [2004] B.C.J. No. 1689.
29. *Hopp v. Lepp,* [1980] 2 S.C.R. 192.
30. *Reibl v. Hughes.* [1980] 2 S.C.R. 88.
31. *Classen v. Izquierdo,* 520 N.Y.S. 2d 999 (Sup. Ct. N.Y. County 1987).
32. *Mikkelsen v. Haslam,* 764 2 d 1384 (Utah CT. Aoo. 1988).
33. *Knapp v. Northwestern University,* 010 F. 3d 473 (7th Cir. 1996).

PART VI

Medicine and Sports

Sports can promote health, but athletes at the elite level are often required to push themselves to unhealthy extremes. Injuries are a routine part of sports as well. College and professional athletes experience intense physical strain, often for several hours a day, and like all machines, the human body is subject to breaking down. Good maintenance practices like proper workout techniques and biomechanics, high-quality protective equipment, proper warm-up and stretching, and diet help prevent deterioration, but they cannot prevent blunt-force compound fractures or concussions. Sports physicians regularly mitigate permanent impairment and even save lives through accurate diagnosis and treatment of high-impact injuries. However, sports physicians sometimes send players who are not incapacitated, but in bad shape, back into the game. Why would a respected health-care professional, whose duty (fixed by the Hippocratic Oath) it is to prioritize his or her patient's well-being, intentionally put broken athletes in harm's way by returning them to play?

Just as a professional athlete is a replaceable employee, a sports physician is also a team employee and may incur pressure to clear athletes to play. Nothing can guarantee an athlete's complete safety during games, but modern medicine can prevent athletes who are injured from feeling the full extent of their pain. If that athlete can make one more key play despite the risk of exacerbating an injury, it might clinch a victory that would ensure the coach or other players keep their jobs for another year. Athletes might also lose their starting positions if they let injuries keep them off the field, so there is a huge incentive to ignore health risks and play through an injury.

This means sports physicians are pressured by their employers and their patients. If the physician stands by principles of protecting the athlete's health, little prevents the team from finding a more compliant physician. Knowing that, is it the physician's ethical responsibility to protect the athlete and lose his or her job? Perhaps a longer-term solution is requiring that all physicians be employed by leagues and report to and get assessed by an independent medical committee, thus preventing team leadership from exercising undue influence. But this does not solve the problem of how to reconcile the athlete-patient's conflicting wishes.

As Bruce Greenfield and Charles West point out in chapter 20, coaches and athletes might reframe what it means to sacrifice for the team. Some athletes *want* to return too early. If the athlete acknowledges and accepts the possible consequences of playing injured, should a physician indulge them?

Modern medicine prioritizes patient autonomy on par with beneficence, largely because the meaning of the concept "patient's best interest" has been evolving. For example, two patients with significant pain might have drastically different treatment desires. One prefers medication that eases the pain while clouding thought, and the other does not want to sacrifice presence of mind for comfort. Both are legitimate forms of well-being informed by patient values, which treating physicians should respect. Similarly, professional athletes who have built their lives around their sports might consciously choose to risk their long-term health to play injured for a critical moment in an important game. This creates an argument for ensuring that athletes are fully informed about the possible consequences of short-term treatments so they can make their own treatment decisions. But, with the expectations of the manager and fans bearing down, and a second-string replacement champing at the bit, as well as the possibility of glory for years to come only one analgesic injection away, can an athlete be expected to make rational decisions on the sideline as the time-out clock runs down? Physician paternalism may have a bigger role in sports than in other areas of life.

20 Ethical Issues in Sports Medicine

A Review and Justification for Ethical Decision Making and Reasoning

■ BRUCE H. GREENFIELD
AND CHARLES ROBERT WEST

In the United States, college coaches and athletic administrators are under significant pressure from students, fans, boosters, and politicians to succeed and are paid exorbitant salaries, often exceeding those of their respective college presidents [13]. Similarly, professional sports offer municipalities, team owners, stockholders, coaches, and athletes the prospects of huge financial gains [8]. And while the professional athlete is the direct economic beneficiary of his or her athletic ability, agents and family members serve to benefit as well from an athlete's success. Successful sports teams can arrange lucrative television contracts and attract and expend large sums of money to highly visible and successful coaches and athletes. In turn, the pressure to perform is exceedingly strong. Given the economic climate surrounding professional athletics, we should not be surprised that athletes are often viewed as commodities that are bought, sold, and traded. Not least, organizations that invest large sums of money on athletes expect returns on their performance, which include proper maintenance of their physical and mental status for ongoing competition.

Pressures for athletes to perform in high-impact sports such as football, where injuries are ubiquitous, have contributed to the rapid evolution of medicine in sports [7]. Health care professions have developed societies and interest groups within their mainframe organizations specifically for health care professionals focusing on care for athletes. These societies have developed journals in sports medicine, have been instrumental in developing formal residencies and fellowships, and, in many cases, have developed a cottage industry of continuing education courses in sports medicine. What has emerged is the concept of the team physician and the health care team [4]. College and professional sports teams routinely hire a professional health care staff that includes physicians, psychologists, physical therapists, and athletic trainers to attend to the ongoing physical, emotional, and mental needs of their athletes. In some cases, large health care entities and private practitioners pay for the privilege of being the team physician, often as part of a marketing agreement between a health care center and a sports team franchise. The unique structural relationship of sports franchises has challenged the traditional fiduciary role of health care professional and their patients and has given rise to potential ethical conflicts. At the core of these conflicts are the competing obligations faced by a health care professional deciding when an athlete is ready to return to full competition. A team physician must decide: What are the rights of the athlete, family, agent, or coach to be involved in that decision? Where does the locus of control ultimately lie? Dunn et al. [7, p. 840] capture potential conflict of interest in writing that the "ethics of the classic doctor-patient dyad" and, by extension, the physical therapist–athletic trainer dyad, "in which the physician has the primary obligation to the patient's well-being, is challenged by the emergence of the doctor-patient-team triad."

Notwithstanding the fact that health care professionals face conflicting obligations from stakeholders, we argue that team physicians and other health care professionals involved in college or professional sports are under unique pressures to navigate the multiple layers of team management to return an athlete to sport, particularly when he or she might not be ready. The dynamic and unique relationships of sports organization members result in potential conflicts of interest between the obligations of team physicians to their patient/athletes and those to the team organization. Because of this unique organizational structure, the ethical principles of autonomy and confidentiality do not easily translate into sports medicine because of competing obligations and lack of clarity of ethical guidelines.

To address the issues raised above, the purpose of this article is to explore ethical issues faced by health care professionals who work with professional athletes. To begin, we present an overview of current research describing ethical issues in sports medicine. We then offer some suggestions to help health care professionals improve their ethical decision-making abilities. Brief examples illustrate and provide practical decision-making strategies.

▣ ETHICAL PROBLEMS IN SPORTS MEDICINE

Many of the ethical issues in the care of athletes often result from the unique and dynamic interrelationship of multiple stakeholders associated with sports franchises. These include the health care professionals (team physician, athletic trainer, and physical therapists); the athletes themselves; and management, including coaches, general manager, and, in professional sports, the team owner. Additional stakeholders include agents, families, the media, and fans. Because these various stakeholders often have different interests and goals, health care professionals are often conflicted about the proper course of treatment for an injured athlete. Conflicts of interest are common in these situations. Swisher et al. [14] sequentially surveyed a group of athletic trainers with experience working with sports teams to identify the types of ethical issues that these trainers commonly faced in working with athletes. Qualitative examination of 154 ethical issues yielded 7 themes. Among top-rated themes were interdisciplinary conflicts, including miscommunication about roles, conflicts of interest due to divided loyalties, conflicts in acting in the athlete's best interest, and pressure to return to play from the coach, parent, supervisor, administration, or athlete.

Anderson and Gerrard [3] surveyed a sample of 18 sports team physicians in New Zealand to identify and map ethical issues. The physicians identified ethical issues related to confidentiality and privacy concerns manifested by tension between medical requirements to the patients and demands to play from the patients and other stakeholders associated with the team. The physicians reported conflicts about their responsibilities as doctors and about the precise nature of their relationship between the physician and the patient/athlete. Confidentiality was the most common issue related to the health information of players from the organization and from media. Privacy was also an issue in trying to provide care in a shared facility such as a training room. The next issue was the fiduciary responsibility to care for the patient and the pressure from the organization to return the athlete to the sport as soon as possible. Many reported that the source of pressure to return athletes to sports too soon came from the athlete, coaches, and other players. Responsibility to athletes, coaches, and even player unions can create conflicts. Problems related to this pressure included the use of analgesics to allow injured players to continue, the problem of inadequate assessment on the field due to time pressure, and the high expectations of national and regional teams when stakes are high.

In a conversation with Dr. John Xerogeanes, chief of sports medicine at Emory University, Atlanta, Georgia (January 22, 2012), he identified conflict of interest as the most significant issue faced by the team physician in both the college and professional levels. He spoke about the pressure that many coaches and owners can place on a team physician to return an athlete to sport with minimal recovery time. Although some athletes desire a quick return to sport regardless of the severity of injury or the need for surgery, he said that it is not uncommon for the physician to be pressured from team management for an early return to sport. In such cases, the athlete develops mistrust in the judgment of the team physician to properly care for his best interests. As a result and at times unfairly, an athlete will choose not to see his team physician but choose instead to see a physician who is not associated with his team.

In reviewing the relationship of management to team physicians, Polsky [11, pp. 4–6] reported that, not surprisingly, management often places pressure on team physicians to return an athlete quickly to competition. Although most sports organizations have the best interest of their athletes in mind, Polsky reported some instances when an organization pressures its medical team to choose a less-than-ideal procedure to treat an athlete to promote shortened recovery time and faster return to play. Polsky reported cases of pressure from team management containing the implicit threat that the physician will be replaced if he or she does not support management policies. Likewise, management would exert significant pressure on the athletes themselves for a speedy recovery. Athletes may also have the specter of terminated employment or loss of salary due to loss of playing time. In this way, they also may place pressure on the medical team for a faster recovery via a less intense procedure. These short-term gains pose long-term risks, however.

Pressure to play early comes not only from management (and even ownership) but also, as mentioned above, from the athlete and his or her peers. McKenna et al. [9] interviewed practicing physiotherapists in the United Kingdom to explore their experiences of rehabilitating elite athletes. In response to in-depth interviews, the therapists reported that many of the athletes during rehabilitation were somewhat fragile emotionally, with their entire focus being on their ability to return to their sport. The therapists all perceived that the athletes were impatient with rehabilitation and favored a rapid return to sport, often at the detriment of ideal rehabilitation. Significant injury often had large effects on their mental states, with effects sometimes being similar to those of individuals who had experienced a natural disaster. On the other hand, responses varied widely, with some athletes viewing injury as merely a slight setback. Rehabilitation for these individuals was viewed as a return, rather than as a gain or improvement. Additionally, their time spent while injured was viewed as "missing out" on all the positive aspects of professional athletics. Athletes were described as often being very talented and somewhat arrogant, to a fault, in that they sometimes believed that they had some knowledge of what would improve them that the physical therapist did not. The physical therapist, in contrast and as a result, typically exhibited concern about projecting one's confidence in regard to the treatment to the athletes, Polsky [11] provides several examples of quotes from team physicians and athletic trainers about the tremendous pressure that athletes feel to play with pain. Those athletes who did return early were more respected and admired, and those who did not were often stigmatized and ridiculed by teammates. Because there is no real job security in the National Football League, the greatest threat that players feel if they do not play with pain is replacement.

An interesting source of pressure is the pressure that team physicians often place on themselves. There are 2 reasons, according to Polsky [11]. First, team physicians routinely believe that they are part of the team and therefore sacrifice a player's health for the sake of the team. Second, a team physician may put undue pressure on himself to please management so he or she can keep one's position because of the many benefits received from the status as a professional sports team doctor. The strong pressure creating conflicts of interest for the team physician may cause one to compromise one's medical judgment. But as Polsky correctly reminds us, although conflicts of interest may increase risks of unethical conduct, they are not inherently unethical but rather a fact of practice reality. Physicians and other health care professionals must always act in the best interest of the patient whether she or he is an athlete or not, regardless of setting, and irrespective of incentives.

Because of conflict of interests, the team physician faces a unique situation related to the ethical principles of autonomy and to confidentiality and informed consent. To what extent do team management and related stakeholders have a right to medical information about the athlete? Without doubt, the team has a stake in the medical decisions affecting the care of the athlete. As Dunn et al. [7] described, an athlete with a torn meniscus will often best be treated with a meniscal repair than with a meniscectomy based on long-term outcomes. After explaining the procedure, the risks and benefits, and alternatives, the athlete may opt for a meniscal repair, ready to sacrifice short-term playing time for longer rehabilitation and better long-term outcomes. Yet, when advised of the athlete's decision, the coach, agent, and owner may disagree, hoping for a quicker return. Ultimately, the loyalty of the physician must be toward the wishes of the athlete, despite pressures exerted on the physician to change the athlete's mind. In such a case, the physician must advocate for the most appropriate course of medical treatment given the evidence. If when given full disclosure and informed consent, the athlete decides for a meniscectomy, the physician must weigh the benefits and risks of doing an alternate procedure based on his or her best judgment. As mentioned above, in the final analysis the physician has the right to refuse a medical treatment that one judges to be inappropriate. We must remember that physicians should never agree to a medical procedure that is not considered standard and appropriate care. It is always the ethical obligation for health care professionals to justify their medical decisions based on sound professional judgment.

What is particularly unsettling is that sports physicians are often bombarded from the press and public with suggestions to use the latest fads in medical technology, some valid and some not. The field of sports medicine is evolving constantly due to innovative research, emerging technology, and financial investments from commercial enterprises. Certain emerging medical interventions and technologies are in the experimental stages or have little clinical evidence supporting their efficacy in long-term outcomes. Not too long ago, thermal capsular shrinking techniques developed a vocal following in orthopaedics and media hype, in lieu of the more invasive but successful surgically tightened stabilization procedures for athletes with recurrent shoulder dislocations [7]. Orthopaedic team physicians can be placed under extreme pressure from coaches, owners, agents, media, and athletes to use current "sexy" procedures with very little evidence to support their use. With emerging technology, the physician must obtain full consent of the patient, which requires full knowledge of all aspects of the procedure, including its less proven nature. The physicians themselves must conduct a careful review of the new technology before administration to a patient.

In traditional medical settings, confidentiality about medical conditions is a general obligation that physicians and other health care professionals owe to their patients [4]. Most health care codes of ethics support the inviolability of confidentiality except under conditions in which the health care professional judges that the withheld information may result in harm to the patient or someone else [12]. In addition to being ethically obligated to maintain patient confidentiality, health care professionals are legally bound by state laws, as well as federal law (Health Insurance Portability and Accountability Act, or HIPAA) to maintain patient medical confidentiality [6, 7].

In sports medicine, numerous occasions arise to challenge the patient/athlete's rights to confidentiality. Bernstein et al. [6] raised an interesting hypothetical scenario and subsequent question: Say that during an on-campus medical evaluation at a major college, a recruited athlete discloses to a team physician that he experienced 3 concussions while playing high school football, each of which required hospitalization. In spite of the athlete's urgent request that the physician keep the information confidential—to avoid jeopardizing his college football career and potential scholarship—does the physician have an obligation to tell the team coaches and athletic director?

Certainly, coaches for a college team recruiting an athlete for a scholarship have a legitimate right to know about the potential athlete's fitness to compete. It is morally permissible and in fact morally required that the team physician tell the coaches about the significant past medical history of this student athlete to avoid future harm. The operative phrase in this case and in many cases of confidentiality is "significant past [or current] medical history" that is relevant to provide. Certainly, the physician should never tell a coach about a potential student athlete's personal history that has no bearing on his or her ability to perform athletically, if in fact that information was given in confidence. But a physician is under no such obligation of strict confidentiality if, for example, an athlete discloses that he is illegally taking performance-enhancing drugs. This action is directly in violation of rules controlling the use of banned substances, and it moves toward a legal issue taking precedence over any ethical concern about confidentiality. Bernstein et al. [6] suggested that prior to any examination or care of an athlete, the team physician or any health care professional has a duty to clarify the nature of the relationship with the athlete before the examination, indicating that he or she is not the patient's private health care professional and confidentiality is not guaranteed. The same should be done with team management, who should be apprised of the nature and limits of confidentiality requirements. If an athlete is seeing a private health care professional not employed directly by the team, then the limits of confidentiality are based on the type of information judged by the health care professional that affects the athlete's overall health and welfare to compete.

■ SUGGESTIONS FOR ETHICAL CONDUCT

Having brought forward the issues of ethics in sports medicine, we turn now to suggestions to improve the ethical decision-making abilities of health care professionals working with sports teams. First, we advocate that sports medicine fellowship programs include an ethics component dealing with the conflict-of-interest issues presented by high-level athletics. We examined the webpage offerings of several high-profile sports medicine fellowships in the United States. While we were unable to view their curriculum in any sort of depth, none made any mention of ethics in any part of the publicly available information about their fellowships. One did indicate that among its core values were patient care and professionalism, but it did not go into detail about whether there was an ethical component or not.

We suggest that the fellowship train physicians in ethical reasoning and present cases that involve ethical content. Current research in expert practice, a goal of fellowship training, clearly indicates that expert practitioners use multiple sources of reasoning, including technical, narrative, and ethical reasoning as part of patient care.

Second, there should be clear rules governing relationships between medical practitioners/facilities and athletic teams/organizations. There is evidence that in cases where physicians are employed directly by the sports team or where a physician or facility pays a premium to treat a team's athletes, a conflict of interest may arise in which the ultimate well-being of the patient athlete may be compromised in favor of short-term gains for the sporting organization. The problem herein lies when physicians are beholden to the interests of someone other than the patient. These physician-team relationships should function under clear rules to prevent the alteration of medical treatment based on nonmedical concerns. This should tie in with the American Medical Association's oversight committee.

We also suggest that health care professionals entertaining thoughts of working with sports teams be trained in basic principles and concepts of applied ethics [5]. Codes of ethics provide a moral template for professional conduct [1, 2, 10]. The principles and rules contained in professional codes can help health care professionals clarify their obligations toward the patient and to other stakeholders. The American Medical Association's code of ethics [1] contains a subsection on sports medicine. For example, opinion 3.06 (sports medicine) states,

> The professional responsibility of the physician who serves in a medical capacity at an athletic contest or sporting event is to protect the health and safety of the contestants. The desire of spectators, promoters of the event, or even the injured athlete that he or she not be removed from the contest should not be controlling. The physician's judgment should be governed only by medical considerations.

Similarly, the National Athletic Trainers' Association's code of ethics states the principles of ethical behaviors that should be followed in the practice of athletic training [10]. Physical therapists working with athletes in sports teams should be guided by the principles and rules in the American Physical Therapy Association's code of ethics [2]. In addition, state practice acts can further clarify legal commitments.

Yet, it should be remembered that codes of ethics have limits applied to ethical decision making to solve ethical dilemmas because they do not provide any particular hierarchy of principles that govern in all situations. Simply put, codes of ethics are not designed as a framework of ethical decision making. Most health care professionals balance ethical principles of the patient's right to autonomy, with fairness, and their obligations to avoid doing harm (non-maleficence) and doing good (beneficence) [5]. To balance these principles for a favorable outcome, health care professionals turn to utilitarianism, balancing potential benefits versus risks and judging a decision based on maximizing positive outcomes. Before acting on a decision, the health care professional should confer with trusted colleagues, preferably those who are not directly associated with the case. A helpful approach is to present the case to a colleague and brainstorm possible alternatives. It is helpful to compare alternative suggestions to what is decided to do. Make certain that the actions are ethically justifiable (based on ethical and legal principles and rules and consistent with the threshold of using sound professional judgment), while at the same time addressing the needs of the major stakeholders in the best way possible. Once an action is taken, it is important that the health care professional judge the consequences of the action and reflect on the results. The health care professional should ask herself if the best action was taken; given the results, might a different action be called for in the future? Self-reflection is important in ethical decision making and an excellent way to learn how to navigate similar problems in the future.

A basic framework of ethical decision making should be integrated into continuing education certification courses in sports medicine. At the very least, sports medicine practices should be encouraged to integrate in-services that provide opportunities for health care professionals to discuss and reflect on ethical issues they encounter in practice. The use of narrative is particularly effective. Health care professionals can be encouraged to write stories about difficult ethical situations. These stories can be shared with colleagues as points of discussion to help clarify the issues and to work through solutions for the future. As pointed out, experienced clinicians are well versed in practice skills and knowledge, as well as technical reasoning and ethical reasoning. Part of best practice is being able to not only navigate ethical issues but effectively address ethical concerns of the athlete and other stakeholders in sports.

▨ CONCLUSIONS

It is clear that sports medicine presents unique challenges for health care professionals because of the organizational pressures involved in returning an athlete to competitions as quickly and as safely as possible. Physicians, like all health professionals who work with sports teams (particularly at a high level), need to be prepared to deal with ethical issues as they arise. The successful practice of sports medicine depends not only on the knowledge and skills in differential diagnoses of medical conditions and the assessment of impairments and functional losses but also on skills in ethical decision making. Given that ethical issues are ubiquitous in sports medicine, health care professionals must be properly trained and adequately well versed in the ethical issues they will face.

▨ NOTE

For reprints and permission queries regarding this article, please visit SAGE's Web site at http://www.sagepub.com/journalsPermissions.nav.

▨ REFERENCES

1. American Medical Association. Opinion 3.06: sports medicine. http://www.ama-assn.org/ama/pub/physician-resources/medical-ethics/code-medical-ethics/opinion306.page. Published June 1983. Updated June 1994. Accessed March 1, 2012.
2. American Physical Therapy Association. Code of ethics. http://www.apta.org/ethics. Published 2011. Accessed March 6, 2012.
3. Anderson LC, Gerrard DF. Ethical issues concerning New Zealand sports doctors. *J Med Ethics*. 2005;31(2):88–92.
4. Attarian DE. The team physician: ethics and enterprise. *J Bone Joint Surg Am*. 2001;83(2):293.
5. Beauchamp T, Childress JF. *Principles of Biomedical Ethics*. 6th ed. New York, NY: Oxford University Press; 2005.
6. Bernstein J, Perlis C, Bartollozi AH. Normative ethics in sports medicine. *Clin Orthop Rel Res*. 2004;420:309–318.
7. Dunn WR, George MS, Churchill L, Spindler KP. Ethics in sports medicine. *Am J Sports Med*. 2007;35:840–844.
8. Leeds M, Allmen PV. *The Economics of Sports*. 2nd ed. Boston, MA: Pearson Addison Wesley; 2005.
9. McKenna J, Delaney H, Hillips S. Physiotherapists' lived experience of rehabilitating elite athletes. *Phys Ther Sports*. 2002;3:66–78.
10. National Athletic Trainers' Association. Code of ethics. http://www.nata.org/codeofethics/code-of-ethics.pdf. Published 2005. Accessed March 1, 2012.
11. Polsky S. Winning medicine: professional sports team doctors' conflict of interest. *J Contemp Health Law Policy*. 1998;14:503–529.

12. Purtilo RB, Doherty RF. *Ethical Dimensions in Health Professions.* 5th ed. St Louis, MO: Elsevier; 2011.
13. Ramares K. Big-time college sport is big business: a university makes money and gains prestige by having a big time sports program. http://globalresearch.ca/index.php?context=va&aid=22442. Published December 17, 2010. Accessed January 28, 2012.
14. Swisher LL, Nyland J, Klossner D, Beckstead J. Ethical issues in athletic training: a foundational descriptive investigation. *Athletic Ther Today.* 2009;14(2):3–9.

PART VII
What About Animals?

As if trying to figure out the definition of sport were not difficult enough, the use of animals makes it harder. In some animal-related sports like sled racing, horse racing, fence jumping, and herding trials, animals are used as tools for comparing human performances. In other animal-related sports, like racing camels and greyhounds, and fighting dogs or roosters, the animals are pitted against each other as competitors. Another category that includes bullfighting and bull and bronco riding pits humans against other animals as competitors. Hunting employs animals as tools, like dogs to sniff out game, and pits the hunted animals against humans. Of these activities, which demonstrate the necessary qualities of sport? All were designed for human entertainment, but as discussed in chapter 1, this quality is not sufficient to define a sport. They all involve competition, but many of the "competitors" are not willingly engaged. To be a sport, must the competitors be consenting?

As described in the context of hunting, John Cohan (chapter 22) might say yes. If any participants are forced to compete, then they are not agreeing to engage according to the rules of the game. Hunters designate rules of engagement, like limiting the kinds of allowable weapons. In this hunt, we can only use short-range shotguns, or bows and arrows, and we cannot use machine guns or grenades. We will not hunt maimed, sick, or baby animals. Bullfighters get only a cape and javelins. These limitations exist to ensure challenge, uncertainty of outcome, and a certain degree of fairness, some of which seem essential to the definition of sport. Whatever the limitations that hunters or bullfighters self-impose, the animals never agree to the definition of fair, in the same way that human slaves did not agree to fight animals or each other in competitions of the past. Deadly gladiatorial combat by slaves, and lions chasing and killing human prey—both seem to cross over from "sport" to "repugnant exhibition."

If we believe, as Cohan does, that consent is necessary for sport, which animals in which sports have the capacity to consent? Perhaps hounds "agree" to participate in a hunt by virtue of their apparent enjoyment: wagging tails, eagerness to begin the search, proud gait after retrieving a kill. Some dogs engage in herding behavior even when there is nothing meaningful to herd, like encircling and barking at playing children. Perhaps this could be understood as a form of consent to entering the dog into a herding competition. As questionable as these consent processes are, it is far more difficult to devise a consent method for animals who might be captured or killed in the activity.

The question remains: If the sport demonstrates fair competition and risk, and is challenging, physical, and entertaining, is it a sport despite lack of consent? It is easier to allow that sports can exist even without all participants' consent, as Kutte Jönsson might (chapter 21), claiming that consent only bears on whether a sport is ethical (not whether it is actually a sport). Sport activities involving animals can employ standards or expectations for how the animals should be treated. We can (although often do not) require that race animals be given a certain number of days rest and a high-quality diet, and that animals injured in the hunt be killed as swiftly and humanely as possible. Regardless of what animal-care standards are established, sport animals are unanimously used as means for human enjoyment in ways that humans should not be ethically used. This means that, for animal sports to be ethical, animals must be different from humans in crucial ways. What are these ways?

Scientists and philosophers point to sentience, or self-awareness, as a distinguishing factor. It is true that animals experience negative emotion—it can be seen in a dog's eyes as its family leaves for work in the morning, and in the moans of both a mother cow and her baby as the latter is taken away to slaughter. To what extent is suffering implied by these negative emotions? If you were to stalk a hare, its heart would race as you drew near and it would dash to avoid you, which might indicate shock and fear; its siblings might cry out after it was shot, indicating sadness; and it would certainly feel pain. If you were to stalk and shoot me, my family and I would likely feel more complicated emotions, including betrayal, contempt, and rage. Do the hare's less complicated emotions reach a threshold for moral consideration? Do those of sled dogs, greyhounds, racehorses, or fighting roosters? Does the threshold impose a strict bar on animal use, or one that gives sport animals limited rights? It is hard to know whether we will ever have the tools to accurately gauge nonhuman animal experience. The tools we have indicate surprising similarity of experience, despite differences in expression. That fact ought to undergird our thinking about the ethics of sports involving animals.

21 Humans, Horses, and Hybrids

On Rights, Welfare, and Masculinity in

Equestrian Sports

■ KUTTE JÖNSSON

▨ INTRODUCTION

Animals are "entertaining". This is a well-founded truth in our culture, and the "theatres" in which we—as humans—can *look* at animals for our amusement are many.

We go to zoos to look at them; we enter the circus to watch them make astonishing tricks; some of them even become movie stars.

If we do not watch animals entertaining us at zoos and circuses, we may visit more "authentic" environments, such as national parks and safari routes to watch and even hunt so-called wild animals, sometimes described as "untamed" and "dangerous" animals. And if we do not want to "risk our lives", we can watch them on TV.

All of these examples contain a continuing separation from the animals. The message is that animals are essentially different from us. They are *the Others*.

Needless to say, the separation of humans and non-humans can be manifested in many ways—for example, through sports. And one of the prevailing sports we find in equestrian sports.

Without doubt, equestrian sports play a significant role in the big and growing sports industry, not least for commercial reasons. Successful horses may bring in great amounts of prize money, and after their careers they very often become valuable subjects in the breeding industry. This particular commerce is fuelled by another industry: the betting industry. Big money runs through the economic system, money that can be seen as serving everyone in society, simply based on the fact that tax money from the betting industry lands in the state's pocket. In other words, many people and entire states have strong interests to feed the equestrian sports industry.

But there are other values to consider as well; for example, the value of gender equality. Equestrian sports are one of few sports where men and women compete against each other on equal terms. But not only that: Equestrian sports also hold a potentiality for equality between humans and non-humans, based on the fact that there is a co-operative dimension imbedded in many equestrian sports disciplines.

But—can we be certain that this means that the rights and welfare of the horses are sufficiently met?

In this article, I will argue from a radical egalitarian point of view that it is possible to defend the existence of equestrian sports, but not without dismantling the masculinity norms that to this day govern modern sports culture. The premise of this article is based on the understanding of sport as a phenomenon founded in masculinity. I will suggest that it is masculinity norms that compromise the already complicated relationship between humans and animals, and therefore become an obstacle for a utopian idea of equality between humans and non-humans. This utopian suggestion can be described in several ways. One way of describing it is to use a mythological figure from Greek mythology.

According to Greek mythology there once was a group of creatures called the Centaurs, described as half-human, half-animal. A Centaur had a torso of a human joined at the waist to the horse's withers. This mythological creature does not just give us a symbolic hint of the leaky distinction between humans and animals; it also holds a moral message: there is no essential distinction between humans and animals.

Here I will argue in favour of what I will call the hybrid view. This particular view derives from an interspecies (or non-species, to be more accurate) radical egalitarian point of view. This view, I will suggest, implies a necessary breakdown of the masculinity ideology that today governs competitive sport, including equestrian sports. As part of the argumentation I will presuppose that masculinity and sport are intertwined concepts and therefore cannot be separated from each other, and that the masculinity ideology often enforces the rather harsh view on animals in sport in general.

I will begin the discussion from a much more general point of view, though; more exactly, with the question of animals' status as rights holders in the world of sport.

▪ ARGUMENTS FOR AND AGAINST THE USE OF ANIMALS IN SPORT

Animal sports can mean different things. In fact, there are three categories of animal sports:

1. Sports in which humans use animals in pursuit of athletic excellence (equestrian events, horse racing, polo, certain rodeo events)
2. Sports in which humans pit themselves against animals in tests of athletic skill (hunting, fishing, bullfighting)
3. Sports in which animals are pitted against other animals in contests of deadly combat or in contests to assess superior animal athletic prowess (cock fighting, dog racing) (Morgan and Meier 1995, p. 373).

It seems obvious that the examples above contain different moral standings dependent on which sport we are focusing on. Most of us would consider, for example, bullfighting as deeply immoral, whereas most consider equestrian sports as morally acceptable. The reason behind the differences is self-evident: bulls in bullfighting are being deliberately killed; in fact, it is the *goal* of the sport to kill the bull at the end of the show. In equestrian sports, it is not the goal of the sport to kill or in other ways harm the animals. Quite the contrary, to some extent humans and animals have to cooperate in order to be successful in equestrian sports. Therefore, it is easy to argue that there is a great moral difference between these two categories of animal sports.

Nonetheless, comparatively uncontroversial sports such as equestrian sports may still encourage certain behaviours that put animals at risk. Almost every week one can read about horses being harmed in the name of sport. It can be horses that have been harmed by doping or by illegal training methods; it can be horses that have been whipped during training or competition, and so on; or horses that simply die at the race track.

Of course, most participants in these sports would claim that such examples are exceptions. They would say that the majority of trainers, owners, coachmen, show-jumpers and jockeys take good care of their horses. Besides, every competition is supposed to be supervised by veterinaries. But should we be satisfied with that? Perhaps it all depends on how we understand the concept of caretaking. On what level can we say that horses are cared for? Or, what is the minimum level for morally accepting events where non-consenting animals are an essential part "of the game"? Where to draw the line? Is it sufficient to ban certain training methods, or to lean on anti-doping regulations? If we think that is sufficient, we still have to ask if we really can trust the supervising veterinaries at the racetracks. They may have other interests than the welfare of the horses at heart. In other words, it is not obvious that we should trust the persons involved in equestrian sports when we analyse the ethics of these sports.

Horses can be harmed in many ways; these can be narrowed down to two general groups of harm: (i) horses can be *literally* harmed, and by that I mean physically and mentally harmed; and (ii) they can be *symbolically* harmed, in that they are being subjected as a species for humans to use and perhaps even exploit for the benefit of human interests.

But what if we consider animals in sport as athletes among other athletes? Would that change anything? Probably not, for the simple reason that "animal athletes" differ from most other athletes in at least one respect: They have not chosen to become athletes; they are being forced by humans to become athletes.

In fact, animals are much in the same relatively powerless position in relation to humans as children are in relation to adults. And hardly anyone would seriously argue that we ought to force children to become athletes. At the same time, when it comes to relations between adult humans and subjected categories—such as *children* and *animals*—unequal power distributions may sometimes serve the interest of the subjected groups, and sometimes not. It is as simple as that.

However, there are also important differences between adult humans' relationship to children, on the one hand, and humans' relationship to animals, on the other. For example, children need adult humans in order to survive; animals generally do not. But as soon as humans have elected to care for animals' welfare, they have a moral responsibility towards animals to consider. Ideally, this means that adult humans should take the *animals' best interests* into consideration when decisions are made that concern the animals, in the same way as adult humans ideally take *children's best interest* into consideration when adults make decisions that concern children.

We may find the arbitrariness in the mentioned relationships unsatisfying, solely based on the fact that children as well as animals are in vulnerable positions. This stresses the question whether it is in the animals' interest to be a part of the sports world. Evidently, also "animal athletes" are in a vulnerable position towards humans. Many humans have strong interests in keeping this situation intact—not only owners, trainers and (human) athletes, but also punters and governments (who gain tax incomes from the betting industry). And, as claimed, the animals do not have the possibility to give their consent to be part of this industry.

At this point, I have established that (1) animals in sports are by definition coerced to be part of sports, and (2) they are subjected to arbitrary decisions made by humans. That is, animals in sports are subordinated to humans. Mostly, though, this is not a deep moral problem *per se*, given that the animals are well treated and are met with respect.

Nonetheless, it is still a possibility that animals in sport have rights that are being violated solely by making them parts of a competitive sports environment. However, if we claim that, we also have to accept that animal rights exist in the first place. But do they?

The Value of Animal Rights

Do animals, horses included, have rights? The question is crucial. According to the American philosopher Tom Regan they do. In his famous book *The Case for Animal Rights* (2004), he argues in favour of a strong rights-based principle.

But what does it mean to have rights? The classical liberal understanding of the concept of rights is that only humans have rights. Advocates of animal rights, such as Tom Regan, want to widen the circle so that also non-human species can be included in the faculty of moral rights holders.

Having moral standing, Regan argues, does not depend on the ability to make moral decisions or having the capacity to reason in rational terms about oneself and others. Based on this, Regan suggests that not only humans but also non-humans should be considered to possess what he calls *inherent value.*

This does not mean that he cannot see any difference between humans and non-humans when it comes to moral rights. But he distinguishes between two kinds of moral rights holders: one regarding *moral agents* and one regarding what he calls *moral patients.*

In line with this distinction, humans are moral agents, whereas non-humans, and especially mammals, are moral patients.

Moral agents, Regan argues, have moral responsibilities for which they can be accountable, while moral patients are (or, should be) protected by rights, but without being held responsible or accountable for how they act. In other words, you do not have to be a moral agent in order to have moral standing. According to Regan it is sufficient that you have passed what he calls *the subject-of-a-life criterion,* a concept he describes in the following way:

> To be the subject-of-a-life, in the sense in which this expression will be used, involves more than merely being alive and more than merely being conscious. (Regan 2004, p. 243)

And he continues:

> [I]ndividuals are subjects-of-a-life if they have beliefs and desires; perception, memory, and a sense of the future, including their own future; an emotional life together with feelings of pleasure and pain; preference- and welfare interests; the ability to initiate action in pursuit of their desires and goals; a psychophysical identity over time; and an individual welfare in the sense that their experiential life fares well or ill for them, logically independently of their utility for others and logically independent of their being the object of anyone else's interests. (Regan 2004, p. 243)

To some extent, Regan's statement may seem rather radical—perhaps too radical. Some have also questioned the empirical ground for some of the factors that need to be satisfied in order to fulfil the subject-of-a-life criterion. The Swedish philosopher Torbjörn Tännsjö is one of these critics. He wonders if it is really true that all mammals pass the test, and he argues: "It strikes me as very implausible that most mammals have 'a sense of the future, including their own future.'" (Tännsjö 2010, p. 40). Of course, one can claim that Tännsjö makes a good point. On the other hand, it does not seem clear whether every single one of the factors has to be satisfied. Moreover, one can argue that the strength of these factors varies. Perhaps certain animals have stronger preferences for living well than many humans, even if the given individual animal has not been "thinking" about it in the way that individual humans might have. We cannot know that. It is not even obvious that it is relevant to talk about the concept of future in this way, but focusing on what the moral obligations might be for humans to have towards animals.

According to Regan, humans—as moral agents—have moral obligations to prevent violations of the rights of animals. Animals do not have the same obligations. This means, for instance, that if animals harm each other—for example, when a wolf attacks a sheep—we do not have a moral obligation to rescue the sheep, because when this scenario occurs, no violation of rights has been taking place. But what does the rights view mean with respect to equestrian sports? Perhaps we should consider equestrian sports as a violation of animal rights. As a matter of fact, it is not an unreasonable thought.

First of all, there is no such thing as voluntariness for horses in sport. The horse's possibility to resist being a part of sport is strongly limited, if at all existing. If humans believe that a certain horse would be a perfect competitor, humans will force him or her to the race track. On the other hand, this argument falls back on a rather narrow interpretation of the concept of voluntariness. Some may say that trained people can "read" horses simply by looking at how the horses behave. Some may even say that horses are, in fact, able to resist. In some respect it is an understandable argument. Consider, for example, a horse in show-jumping who refuses to jump an obstacle. Or, consider a horse who bluntly refuses to take part in the sport altogether, that is a horse who is "difficult" to work with. These examples can very well be interpreted as examples of animal resistance, but it is not a resistance against being forced to take part of the sport as much as a resistance against being forced to act in a certain way. No matter what, one *could* understand the animal's behaviour in this respect as a form of (unintentional) act of resistance, and therefore as "evidence" for the argument that animals *do* have a choice within the individual animal's cognitive and perceptual limits. On the other hand, this argument can be an example of wishful thinking. By that I mean that humans may have an interest to rationalise the oppression of animals by arguing that animals—simply based on how they respond to force or to other oppressive actions—can "talk back" and refuse to take part in the human spectacle. I believe this is a critical way to argue, though. I do not think we should underestimate the strong interests of rationalising human behaviour for the sake of fulfilling human preferences on behalf of the interests of other species. But what if the very existence of horses depends on the existence of sports? Would that change the rights view in any relevant way?

The Value of Existence and Economy

The fact that horses are forced can be seen as a major moral problem for equestrian sports in general. But let us not jump to conclusions. Perhaps there are other values that may overrule the rights aspect of the issue. Consider, for example, the fact that most successful racehorses (measured by the amount of money they bring to owners and punters) have been *bred* in order to become racehorses. Here, one can consider the arguments the American philosopher Donald Scherer has articulated in defence of using animals in sport:

(1) the present uses of the animals are justified because they are better for the animals than the alternative, namely non-existence, or that
(2) breeding an animal for a purpose gives the breeders (transferable) rights over what they have bred. (Scherer 1995, p. 351)

Let us now confront these two arguments. Are they valid? Are they sustainable and strong?

The first argument, to begin with, says that existence is a better alternative than non-existence. Whether this is true or not can (of course) be difficult to say anything certain about. It all depends on how the grounds for existence occur. So, what does it mean to say that existence is better than non-existence?

Is it ever possible to proclaim a fixed welfare level and say that above this level, we have reason to choose existence over non-existence? Probably not. Humans, as well as non-humans, are not static entities in this respect. Our preferences can evidently change over time. Or, to use an example from Scherer, most humans who live what one could call miserable lives (that is, lives with a very low welfare level) do not commit suicide, but some do. An objectively low welfare level does not have to be the cause of the suicide, though. Otherwise, humans who "have it all" would not been committing suicide, but some of them do. Of course, this does not mean that objective welfare levels (based on things such as income, social services, and social security systems, et cetera) are irrelevant for individual welfare levels; it only means that it is not obvious that there is a causal connection between objective welfare and subjective welfare. The point here, though, is that it should not be considered as a general truth that non-existence is always better than living what many would consider lives of misery.

If we now return to the animal sports issue, Scherer argues:

> [S]ince the lives of these animals [that is, animals in sport] are (arguably) worth living despite what misery human beings inflict, human beings are entitled to treat these animals, within that limit, as they please, since they would not exist at all save for human beings bringing about their existence. (Scherer 1995, p. 352)

Now, the obvious objection to this is to say that it opens a gate towards legitimizing immoral behaviours. For instance, if the owner of a horse harms, abuses or neglects his or her horse, he or she could always say that it is better to exist than not to exist, even if it means a life in misery for the horse. This is not the case, though, Scherer argues. In fact, his response to that objection is clear: "One's behaviour is not acceptable merely because it leaves others with a life better than death" (p. 352). That is a fairly good response. But as a general principle it does not say much about the acceptable *welfare level* of the particular existence of the horse.

Even regarding horses that would not have existed without being bred into the sports industry, and even if these horses are not neglected by their owners in any meaningful sense of the word, it does not mean that the humans have maximized the welfare of the particular animals. But perhaps they should, for the simple reason that they have a moral responsibility to the animals, simply based on the fact that they are the owners of them. This is one objection to Scherer's argument. On the other hand, I must confess that my objection begs the question regarding the issue of *moral responsibility*.

So, what exactly is the moral responsibility of the humans in this case? Do the breeders have an owner's right to the animal they have brought into existence? Scherer claims that they do. And he uses an analogy with the creation of artefacts.

For example, consider an artist who paints a picture. In doing that, she has to use certain materials. She works the material into a picture, and she mixes her labour with the painting material. When she has finished painting the picture, she has the right to do whatever she wants with it (as long as she does not harm others with it; she is not allowed to use the painting as a weapon, for example). She can try to sell it, she can put it on her own wall, and she can destroy it, if she wants to do that. This is rather uncontroversial. But a painted picture is a "dead" object; horses (and other animals) are not. But does it mean that animals are self-owned?

Even if the creative process behind a painting and a racehorse differ from each other, we cannot escape the fact that both of these examples can be put in the context of ownership rights. According to the very same philosophy of ownership, human beings—so we have been taught—are self-owned and cannot be owned by others without violating human rights. But when it comes to ownership regarding animals, there are other rules in motion. When it comes to animals and the animal reproduction industry, we have no problem saying that they—that is, the animals—are properties, and that the only thing that matters is *how* the property is treated. But what if there is a connection between the view that animals can be owned (much as human slaves once upon a time) and the interest of animal welfare? What if violation of animal rights has an impact on how we value animal welfare?

The Value of Animal Welfare

As shown, the issue of animal rights raises many intriguing questions. Many of them are related to the issue of animal welfare. It is one thing that animals are bred for the sake of being athletes, another thing how their welfare needs are being met in that particular role.

If Tom Regan, as claimed earlier, focuses on the rights issue, other advocates of animal rights focus on other aspects. The Australian philosopher Peter Singer, for example, supports animal rights by using utilitarian arguments.

According to the classical understanding of utilitarianism, we should maximize happiness. In its most simple meaning this could mean that it would be morally permissible to breed racehorses *en masse,* and perhaps even treat them with cruelty, if it would serve the total amount of happiness in the world. I guess most would consider this to be too demanding and morally counter-intuitive in reality. Therefore, many modern utilitarians favour so-called *preference utilitarianism,* which simply suggests that we ought to weigh preferences against each other, and favour the strongest preferences, including the preferences of animals.

The idea of including the preferences of animals in the weighing process can be traced back to the "founding father" of modern utilitarianism, Jeremy Bentham (1748–1832). In a famous passage, Bentham writes:

> It may come one day to be recognized, that the number of the legs, the velocity of the skin, or the termination of the *os sacrum,* are reasons equally insufficient for abandoning a sensitive being to the same fate. What else is it that should trace the insuperable line? Is it the faculty of reason, or, perhaps the faculty of discourse? But a full-grown horse or a dog is beyond comparison a more rational, as well as a more conversable animal, than an infant of a day, or a week, or even a month, old. But suppose the case were otherwise, what would it avail? The question is not, Can they *reason?* Nor, Can they *talk?* But, Can they *suffer?* (Bentham 2002, ch. 17)

Along with Bentham, I think most of us would say that animals can suffer and feel pleasure. Why would we believe differently? Do we have any good reason for doing that? Animals in pain behave in much the same way as humans in pain, and we also know that especially mammals and birds have nervous systems very much like humans; so for good reasons we can assume that animals can suffer from pain, as Peter Singer claims in his famous book *Animal Liberation* (2002, p. 11).

However, even if it is a scientific fact that animals can suffer from pain, it does not imply that we should treat them in the same way as we treat humans. From an interspecies egalitarian point of view, it means that we should act in such a way that we do not inflict pain on non-humans. But perhaps not only that; we may also have a moral obligation to actively *promote* animal welfare. If we follow what Singer calls *the principle of equal consideration,* we may have to act in different ways in order to secure and promote animal welfare. He writes:

> It is an implication of this principle of equality that our concern for others and our readiness to consider their interests ought not to depend on what they are like or on what abilities they may possess. Precisely what our concern or consideration requires us to do may vary according to the characteristics of those affected by what we do: concern for the well-being of children growing up in America would require that we teach them to read; concern for the well-being of pigs may require no more than we leave them with other pigs in a place where there is adequate food and room to run freely. But the basic

element—the taking into account of the interests of the being, whatever those interests may be—must, according to the principle of equality, be extended to all beings, black or white, masculine or feminine, human or non-human. (Singer 2002, p. 5)

What can be made from this when we consider equestrian sports? Can anyone guarantee that the principle of animal welfare is met in equestrian sports? I believe it depends on how we choose to understand the human role in the making of animal welfare.

The problem is that it is humans who define the concept of animal welfare. Animals are subordinated to humans in that sense, and even if we think that we can guarantee the welfare of the animals, this may also be an interpretation derived from a self-given power position. Thereby, we can always claim that animals are subordinated to humans and can never be equals in a relevant meaning of the word. In fact, from the welfare argument, it does not seem evident that horses should never be a part of sports. Suppose we say (for good or bad reasons) that a given horse would be better off if she becomes an "animal athlete". Consider, for example, the following example:

Horse H is owned by owner O, who treats H with cruelty. Trainer T knows that he can buy H and later turn H into a racehorse that may win races. According to T's economical calculation, T will benefit from the transaction. So will H. Everyone benefits from this transaction. H will be better off being a racehorse than not being a racehorse, according to the premises of this example.

Of course, one can object to this argument by saying that this is not a typical case. But not only that, one can argue that it is still a form of animal exploitation. In other words, H becomes exploited by T for the simple reason that H doesn't have the cognitive possibility to give consent to the situation. And this exploitation may continue after the career as an athlete is over. Because if H become successful, she will most likely be used for breeding, which usually means being *forced to artificial insemination* (so-called "rape rack"), which in turn may be seen as a form of sexual exploitation of animals and therefore morally wrong.

In short, even if individual horses can benefit from being racehorses, it does not imply that we should support horseracing as such. In fact, even if the individual horse may benefit from being a racehorse on welfare grounds, there may be other aspects to consider that may compromise the issue. The aspects I am thinking of are related to another important element of all these—that is, the issue regarding sport masculinity.

■ SPORT MASCULINITY, GENDER EQUALITY, AND SYMBOLIC VALUES

Equestrian sports do not exist in an ideological vacuum. Equestrian sports are a product of a culture defined by masculinity norms, a gender ideology where animals easily become victims.

I will now continue the discussion by linking the rights view and welfare view to the masculinity ideology. First a few words on *sport masculinity* in general.

I believe we have no reasons not to think that sport plays a significant role in everyday constructions of gender stereotypes. Or, as the gender theorist R. W. Connell describes it:

> In historically recent times, sport has come to be the leading definer of masculinity in mass culture. Sport provides a continuous display of men's bodies in motion. Elaborate and carefully monitored rules bring these bodies into stylized contests with each other. In these contests a combination of superior force (provided by size, fitness, teamwork) and superior skill (provided by planning, practice and intuition) will enable one side to win. (Connell 1995, p. 54)

The kind of masculinity Connell describes gives us a picture of the gender hierarchy that every man and woman has to relate to, and that also excludes women from sport. Connell says:

> The institutional organization of sport embeds definite social relations: competition and hierarchy among men, exclusion or domination of women. These social relations of gender are both realized and symbolized in the bodily performances. Thus men's greater sporting prowess has become a theme of backlash against feminism. It serves as symbolic proof of men's superiority and right to rule. (p. 54)

I believe Connell's statement is relevant also for equestrian sports, simply in that the argument aims at, and concerns, general gender norms regarding *sport culture*. At the same time, when it comes to equestrian sports, we also have to consider not only relations between men and women but also relations between humans and non-humans, where the non-humans are used as tools in the construction of the masculinity norms of sport.

As I have stated above, animals do not have much of a chance in their contact with humans. And even *if* horses are better off being a part of sports than not being part of it, they may be symbolically harmed, at least if we de-individualize the horses and only see them as "anonymous" members of a certain species. Symbolically, equestrian sports may be considered as an example of humans' self-righteous dominion over other species. That should be seen as a moral problem in itself, I think, not least because it holds a threat. The actual symbolic subordination of the horses can easily be put into actual practice. In other words, the symbolic value is not harmless; it says something about the unequal relationship between humans and non-humans.

At the same time, equestrian sports can be said to represent one of the most egalitarian sports when it comes to gender, at least superficially.

As one of few sports where gender is not supposed to be relevant for the outcome of the competitions, equestrian sports plays an important, and to some extent radical, role in a gender-conservative sports world. In other words, *there are good and strong arguments for suggesting that gender equality can be enforced* thanks to equestrian sports. But in a broader meaning, the gender equality argument is rather weak, and for two reasons:

   i. Gender equality does not undermine the masculinity ideology upon which all sports are built; and
   ii. Gender equality should not automatically overrule the preferences of animals, not least considering the fact that animals are being forced to be part of sport; it simply does not seem fair that animals should pay the price for human (in) equality.

One should not underestimate the value of gender equality. The fact that the status of women's sports has increased over the last decade is of great importance for how we understand gender constructions overall. In this respect, I truly believe that sport has played an important role for women's liberation, as an arena for feminist struggle. This can be described in many ways. For example, for women who are "masculine" or have interests that are not traditionally feminine, sports can be a place for (personal) liberation and self-realization, which in turn may change how we understand gender constructions overall. Still, this does not mean that the gender-constructed *sports ideology* changes in its core. Sport still is a masculine arena.

The (sport) masculinity ideology has great impact also when it comes to the animal issue. When animals (by force) enter the sports world they are forced into a humanly defined masculinity. They are being controlled and dominated, and therefore they become mere means in the masculine construction of symbolic power. In fact, this is what competitive elite sports is all about: symbolic wars between individuals, nations and/or teams. Moreover, sports have always been educational as well. Many sports, and especially team sports (such as football, rugby and ice hockey), have been used as means to mould boys into men, and this in turn can be seen as a sign of how sports culture is very much like military culture. In this particular context, harming and abusing animals have often been considered as fruitful methods in the making of "real men", especially through so-called blood sports, such as hunting and fishing (Ryder 2000, p. 235).

This kind of gender construction contains an internal purpose, and that is to distance men from women as well as from non-humans. The most extreme form of this is of course, as mentioned, blood sports (such as hunting and other sports where killing plays an essential part of the sport). But the masculine ideology behind blood sports can be traced to "milder" forms of sports as well, such as equestrian sports.

To dominate and control *animals* (or to hunt and kill animals, or to breed what may become "winning" animals) can, in fact, be seen as a hyper-masculine form of modern sport. Perhaps it is all about a desire to control what is usually defined as "nature", whether it is the nature in humans or the nature placed outside the human body. And sports are much about taming and thereby taking control over the nature in humans. Idealists may even say that controlling is a way of celebrating humanity.

Because of the unfortunate constructional link between the concepts of "nature" and "animal", animals become tools for controlling nature, and by controlling nature humans can see themselves as much more important and valuable forms of living beings than members of other species.

In short, using living, and non-consenting, individuals for sport spectacles can be seen as an example of human arrogance, fuelled by the masculine ideology within modern sports culture. In this respect, gender equality seems to be a rather weak weapon. Fortunately, there are other, and more radical, views to consider.

■ THE HYBRID ARGUMENT

In her famous essay "A Cyborg Manifesto", the American philosopher and feminist writer Donna Haraway argues that humans and animals not only live in a symbiotic relationship; the boundaries between these two entities are in fact dissolved. In using the concept of cyborg, traditionally defined as a hybrid of organic life and technological systems, Haraway constructs an image in which humans and animals can be joined together as companions. She argues:

> By the late twentieth century [. . .], the boundary between human and animal is thoroughly breached. The last beachheads of uniqueness have been polluted if not turned into amusement parks—language, tool use, social behavior, mental events, nothing really convincingly settles the separation of human and animal. And many people no longer feel the need for such separation; indeed, many branches of feminist culture affirm the pleasure of connection of human and other living creatures. Movements for animal rights are not irrational denials of human uniqueness; they are a clear-sighted recognition of connection across the discredited breach of nature and culture. Biology and evolutionary theory over the last two centuries have simultaneously produced modern organisms as objects of knowledge and reduced the line between humans and animals to a faint trace re-etched in ideological struggle or professional disputes between life and social science. [. . .] The cyborg appears in myth precisely where the boundary between human and animal is transgressed. Far from signalling a walling off of people from other living beings, cyborgs signal disturbingly and pleasurably tight coupling. (Haraway, 1991, p. 152)

Haraway's theory is thought-provoking. By using the concept of the cyborg, she aims at very specific distinctions in human thought, represented in popular Cartesian dualisms. She challenges common distinctions such as the male/female distinction, the nature/culture distinction and the human/animal distinction. In challenging the Cartesian dualisms, she also indirectly challenges the work of many animal rights theorists as well, simply because many of the most popular animal rights theories are based on anthropocentric views, and therefore logically reflect the ideas and ideologies that lie behind animal exploitation. So, why not change views altogether, and approach animals as social constructions? This may also mean that animals can take pleasure in the relationships with human beings. In fact, one can argue that many animals are better off held in captivity than they would have been living in the free, not least already domesticated animals such as dogs and cats.

What we're faced with here is an ideological "conflict" between the animals' rights to be "free" and the animals' rights to high welfare levels. Sometimes these two aspects go hand in hand, but sometimes they do not.

However, irrespective of how we choose between these two (broadly formulated) aspects, they both rely on the presumption that animals are not more "natural" than humans. Animals too are social constructions. This line of argument is not the only one when it comes to the issue of the social making of animals. In a more abstract sense humans *construct* animals based on *conceptions* of how we *want* to understand animals (and nature) and thereby make quite loose distinctions between "wild" animals and "domesticated" animals, or between "dangerous" animals and "harmless" animals, and so on. "Wild" animals are often considered to be a (latent) threat to humans and their "domesticated" animals, and "domesticated" are often seen as more human-like than other animals.

A hybrid theory suggests something else. A hybrid theory suggests a dismantling of these common distinctions and conceptions—in short, a dismantling of the constructed boundaries of species, and logically a critique of perceiving "humans" and "animals" as belonging to completely different categories.

As I mentioned in the introduction, it can be useful to utilize Greek mythology as a metaphor for this philosophy. In the Greek mythology we find the Centaurs. This image may very well play a role in terms of ethics in equestrian sports.

To begin with, a Centaur is a figure described as half-human, half-animal. The torso of the human part is joined at the waist to the horse's withers. In other words, there is no relevant distinction between the human and the horse; they are the same body (and mind), and they cannot exist without one another. What we have here is a new species, albeit a mythological one.

Now, suppose we leave the anthropocentric view behind, and accept the existence of such a figure. What would it mean in terms of ethics? For one thing, one can argue that animals would not be subjected to the arbitrariness of human action, for the simple reason that there would not be any distinction between humans and animals. Also, it would mean that humans look at themselves as a part of the kingdom of animals, deeply connected to animals, and also interrelated to the welfare of animals. All of a sudden, it would not be possible to harm animals without harming oneself. Thereby, it would not be morally possible neither to objectify animals for sports nor other events where we today exploit what is supposed to be inferior creatures. Looking at animals in this way would also lead us away from the disturbing consequences of romanticizing animals. In this light, to speak about and actively support *animal rights* and *animal welfare* is not *that* radical, even if it serves an important political purpose.

■ ETHICAL CONCLUSIONS, PRACTICAL IMPLICATIONS, AND A UTOPIAN PROPOSAL

For all we know, we have reasons to be rather critical of the existence of equestrian sports (as well as other sports were animals are involved). But how to challenge the anthropocentric view that today forms our understanding of equestrian sports?

What we may need is a whole new set of analytical tools, tools that we can use in order to dismantle what I am inclined to call the fictional distinction between humans and non-humans. Perhaps it is a question of semantics. Do we really need to distinguish between the concepts of "humans" and "animals"? Is not the distinction in itself simply an illustration of a rather narrow-minded way of thinking?

What ethical conclusions are to be made from the argumentation in this article? Is it possible to say something concrete and action guiding on the basis of what's been discussed here? I like to believe it is.

A crucial point concerns the human/animal relationship. Whether we choose to take a rights view or a welfare view, or a combination of the two, we may have to draw the conclusion that it is morally difficult, if not impossible, to defend equestrian sports, based on the fact that we are dealing with a sports industry where horses always are inferior. But from a hybrid-theoretical point of view we may come to a different conclusion.

If we would consider that particular view seriously, it would most certainly mean that some of the disciplines of today would have to cease to exist—for example, cross-jumping (because of the risk of serious physical harm), harness racing and horseracing (because of the accepted use of whipping) and dressage (because of the degradation of animals in making them aesthetic artefacts).

Show jumping, on the other hand, seems to be more in a grey zone in this sense (based on the fact that the rider and the horse have to engage in more intimate teamwork). However, this does not mean that we escape the ideological problem imbedded in show jumping (and all the other disciplines): that equestrian sports are based on a masculine ideology, where it has become normalized to dominate and control animals in order to gain benefits on exploitative, and therefore unfair, grounds.

As I stated earlier, gender equality seems to be an all too blunt weapon for making sports culture de-masculinized. But that does not mean that nothing can be changed in this matter. Historically, we have seen a change of masculinity norms (both within and outside sports culture). Based on that, one can argue that something has changed also when it comes to equestrian sports. Consider, for example, the impact that popular "horse psychologists", such as Monty Roberts, the real-life "horse whisperer", have had on how to "break" (a word Roberts himself never would use) so-called wild horses to become "tamed" enough to be racehorses (see, for example, Roberts 2009). In contrast to the "traditional" ways of training racehorses, Roberts argues for softer methods. No beating or whipping is "allowed". Instead, he argues, the trainer should communicate by *listening* to the horse.

It is not difficult to sympathize with Monty Roberts' view on this. But how should we understand it from an ideological point of view? Evidently, Roberts represents a different kind of masculinity than the traditional form, where brute violence is an accepted method to elicit compliance. But does that mean that he's an example of a new trend where "feminine" qualities challenge the traditional masculine values? I am not convinced of that. What we *can* say, I guess, is that he represents a "new" form of masculinity within sports culture, a form with roots in the ethics of care, which traditionally is connected to feminist philosophy (see, for example, Rachels 2007; Tong 1993). The connection between feminism and ethics of care contain certain internal pitfalls. The most obvious of these is that not only is ethics of care connected to women as a social group in general, but it is also supposed to be a "soft" theory relative to other theories of ethics. But I think one can say that the example of Monty Roberts' "whispering" in the ears of the horses shows that it can mean something else. Because, even if he, and others like him, uses a "softer touch" when he works with the horses, the goal is still to make racehorses of them. He "works" a certain "material" in order to force the horses into a rather harsh sports culture. Is that really something we should applaud? I am not sure of that, even if it is arguably better than beating the horses to success.

In this respect one can claim that the hybrid view on equestrian sports offers another view on the human/animal relationship, with or without sports—a view that may be essentially and fundamentally truer than what the anthropocentric view offer us.

The hybrid view suggests a totally different approach: An elimination of gender (that is, distinctions between men and women, and masculinity and femininity). But not only that, this particular view also offers an elimination of the distinction between humans and non-humans. This view can, of course, easily be linked to a radical egalitarian ideology which may seem utopian—but nonetheless worth striving for, not least for moral reasons.

■ REFERENCES

Bentham, J. (2002 [1789]): *An Introduction to the Principles of Morals and Legislation.* London: Library of Economics and Liberty.

Connell, R. W (1995): *Masculinities.* Berkeley/Los Angeles: University of California Press.

Haraway, D. (1991): "A Cyborg Manifesto: Science, Technology, and Socialist-Feminism in the Late Twentieth Century". In *Simians, Cyborgs, and Women. The Reinvention of Nature*. New York: Routledge.

Morgan, W. J., and Meier, K. V., eds. (1995): "Part VII Summary". In *Philosophic Inquiry in Sport*. Champaign, IL: Human Kinetics.

Rachels, J. (2007): *The Elements of Moral Philosophy*. Boston: McGraw-Hill.

Regan, T. (2004 [1983]): *The Case for Animal Rights*. Berkeley/Los Angeles: University of California Press.

Roberts, M. (2009 [1996]): *The Man Who Listens to Horses. The Story of a Real-Life Horse Whisperer*. New York: Ballantine Books.

Ryder, R. (2000): *Animal Revolution. Changing Attitudes towards Speciesism*. Oxford/New York: Berg.

Scherer, D. (1995): "Existence, Breeding, and Rights: The Use of Animals in Sports". In *Philosophic Inquiry in Sport*, ed. Morgan, W. J., and Meier, K. V. Champaign, IL: Human Kinetics.

Singer, P. (2002 [1975]): *Animal Liberation*. New York: HarperCollins.

Tong, R. (1993): *Feminine and Feminist Ethics*. Belmont, CA: Wadsworth.

Tännsjö, T. (2010): *Animal Ethics. A Crash Course*. Stockholm: Thales.

22   Is Hunting a "Sport"?

■ JOHN ALAN COHAN

> When a man shoots a tiger to murder him, he calls it sport, but when
> a tiger attacks a man, he calls it a savage beast.
> —GEORGE BERNARD SHAW[1]

■ I. INTRODUCTION

Hunting has always been a source of social tension—tension concerning human power over nature, and tension over whether there is an intrinsic brutality of the hunt. In this essay I will show that it is incorrect to categorize hunting as a competitive sport.[2] I use competitive, or *agonistic,* sport as the focus of this topic because, if hunting is a sport, it would necessarily be a competitive sport because the hunter engages in the activity with an adversarial subject; that is, the hunter is pitted against the hunted animal, and one or the other ends up "winning" the "game."

I hope to accomplish a transformative shift in the way we *characterize* hunting, so that people will stop referring to hunting as a sport or as a form of amusement. I hope to show why hunting as a form of amusement is susceptible to moral criticism (except for indigenous populations that rely upon hunting for sustenance), and why it is a categorical error to refer to hunting as a "sport." It is my ultimate hope that hunting will cease to be a socially normative form of amusement, regardless of how it is characterized.

Many animal welfare issues are beyond the scope of this essay. I am not addressing whether eating animals is right or wrong, however humanely the animals might be killed. I am not addressing or propounding the view that animals should be granted a certain measure of legal rights pertaining to liberty and autonomy,[3] although animal welfare laws have increasingly expanded legal protections of animals against human incursions. Nor am I arguing that certain animal species such as chimpanzees or other animals with similar levels of consciousness should be considered "persons," and thus afforded a basic set of individual rights comparable to that of persons. Nor am I addressing other animal welfare issues, such as animal farming, however cruel some of its practices may be.[4] These issues are simply beyond the scope of my topic. Pain in creatures is something that humans should seek to end in the wild as well as in domestic contexts. There is a need, in my opinion, for greater protection of animals in the wild because anticruelty laws are largely confined to domesticated animals and farm animals.

I am not taking issue with the fact that hunters generally obey local regulations that effectively, for the most part, assure surpluses of harvestable animals for the future. I am not taking issue with the notion that hunters, perhaps more than most citizens, care deeply about ecosystem integrity, or that hunters have a deep reverence for nature and for all life, including the lives of the animals they seek to kill.[5] I *do* take issue, however, with the view that hunting is an "engagement" with nature, because to my mind the killing of wild animals is an "engagement" with nature only in the sense of constituting an attack, scuffle, fracas, skirmish, melee, or other hostile, rather than pacific, "engagement."

Apart from moral considerations, the entire business of killing animals has a strong connection to the global economy. The global economy is hugely dependent on food and clothing industries, which involve killing of animals in farm factories, as well as stalking and trapping of animals. Vast segments of society earn their livelihood in the breeding, feeding, raising, caring for, transporting, slaughtering, packaging, marketing, preparation, and advertising of animals in one form or another in the economic chain. The ranching, farming, fur, leather, and wool industries would change enormously if the exploitation of animals were completely forbidden. Even in the sparce population of the Northwest Territory, the economy of the Innuits is closely linked to the hunters who come from afar to hunt polar bears. It is hard to imagine how any thoroughgoing scheme of prohibiting the exploitation of animals could overcome these economic realities.

I will first discuss what I regard as an anthropocentric fallacy that human beings often make in justifying human domination over animals. I will then analyze the historical development of hunting, and show that for a long period of time hunting has ceased to be a mode of sustenance, but rather has been an activity of amusement, however cruel it may be. I will then show that over a period of time there has been moral progress in what people regard as acceptable forms of amusement. I will then discuss the modes and methods of hunting, with a view towards bringing into sharper focus the elements of deception and cruelty involved. I will then show that the techniques of hunting, widely practiced, constitute animal cruelty, and that animal cruelty is subject to moral criticism, so that it would be inappropriate to characterize hunting as "amusement."

Next, I will discuss the nature of sports, defining what constitutes traditional competitive sports, and in doing so I will show how hunting fails to come close to meeting the criteria that constitute competitive sports. I will then discuss wildlife management as a separate case, showing how hunting in that context is never referred to as "sport." I will then make some concluding remarks.

■ II.   THE ANTHROPOMORPHIC FALLACY THAT THE "SUPERIORITY" OF HUMAN BEINGS JUSTIFIES THE "RIGHT" TO EXPLOIT ANIMALS

A common idea of hunters is that animals in the wild are "fair game," that they have no autonomy rights, that wild animals become the property of those who capture (kill) them, that they can be freely killed at will, and that to do so is not susceptible to moral criticism. The justification for this view is that human beings constitute the "dominant" species in the world, and that dominion over all other creatures is simply a "right" based on this superior ranking of human beings. I refer to this as the anthropomorphic fallacy.

For many years the appropriateness of human domination over nature (kindly or not) has been the subject of scrutiny. Darwin removed humans from a privileged position in the world and designated humans as just another step in the evolutionary ladder, suggesting that we all participate in a common nature, and that there is a unity of human beings with all other creatures. He said: "There is no fundamental difference between man and the higher mammals in their mental faculties. In other words, the difference in mind between man and the higher animals, great as it is, certainly is one of degree and not of kind."[6] Rather than a hierarchy of being in the world, the theory of evolution shows that there is a seamless web of relations between animals and humans. Evolution teaches that the differences between species are incremental; there are no huge gulfs between species that are cousins or located on the same branch of the evolutionary tree. Moreover, the theory of evolution does not assert any value ascription as to the superiority of the human species to other species. The notion of survival of the fittest simply has to do with the ongoing process of the survival of individual species within their particular populations. As early as 1837 Darwin referred to animals as "our fellow brethren" and remarked that "we may be all melted together."[7] Ultimately, Darwin thought that, as ethics evolved, all sentient beings would come to be included in the moral community.[8] The ideas of Darwin were echoed by John Muir, who intuited that human beings are members of the natural community: "Why should man value himself as more than a small part of the one great unit of creation?"[9] The Russian philosopher P. D. Ouspensky (1878–1947) was convinced that "there can be nothing dead or mechanical in Nature. . . . [L]ife and feeling . . . must exist in everything." Furthermore, *a mountain, a tree, a river, the fish in the river, drops of water, rain, a plant, fire*—each separately must possess a mind of its own."[10] Henry David Thoreau's moral environmentalism embraced nature and its creatures as a *society*. In 1857 he wrote: "I do not consider the other animals brutes in the common sense."[11] He said, "What we call wildness is a civilization other than our own."[12]

There is controversy as to what criteria go into the scientific differentiation of species in the first instance. Clearly, there is an anthropomorphic bias in zoological classification. Chimpanzees, for example, are more closely related to humans than they are to gorillas, but chimpanzees and gorillas are placed into one family (Pongidae), while human beings are given their own (Hominidae).

Often enough, we see that other animals have superior skills and faculties, and are better adapted to living in the world than are humans, suggesting that our species is not necessarily the "fittest" for survival. For example, we are frail, we can live only within a narrow range of temperature, we cannot keep warm without clothing and fire, we have limited and clumsy mobility, we cannot survive under water, we need consistent hydration and nutrition in order to survive, we certainly cannot fly from branch to branch, or perch upon the water, we cannot carry much weight on our backs, and if we are attacked by a wild animal we have little means of escape. The camel can survive with much less water than humans; the giraffe can get food from foliage at greater heights; elephants can call warnings to one another at great distances; birds can take flight to avoid conflict with predators; fish can survive underwater, at great depths, and at cold temperatures; beetles can carry ten or twenty times their weight, bury themselves under the earth and survive, and not get crushed by objects many times their size and weight.

With anthropomorphic projection we may run the risk of getting things wrong. Aristotle and other philosophers have claimed that human beings are distinguished from all other creatures by the faculty of rational thinking, practical reason, and the ability to choose. But it is not entirely clear in what way rational thinking or other forms of "higher" cognition such as self-reflection operate to make human beings more advanced than other species, except from an anthropocentric perspective. In fact we do not know whether our cognitive abilities are "superior" to those of other species. Tom Regan, a popular animal rights theorist, has already thoughtfully laid out the idea that rationality, in and of itself, does not make humans morally superior to animals.[13] Moreover, the reasoning capabilities of some animals may be underrated because human researchers have not found appropriate ways to test such capabilities and then to accurately compare them to human skills.

Often enough, the quantum of rational thinking and practical reason in human beings is deficient. Humans frequently make mistakes in fulfilling their ends due to weakness of will (*akrasia*) and the failure to follow what reason dictates, while lower animals cannot make such mistakes; they instinctively know and automatically execute what they intuit to be for their own good. Moreover, human beings are prone to follow a teleology of irrationality, of bias, of cognitive dissonance, of "groupthink," and so on that fails to produce sound results.[14] Thus, the high stakes predicated of human rational thinking fails to show how rationality is a characteristic sufficient to justify a claim of superiority by humans against other animals.

Moreover, it is not at all clear that language as a tool, as a method of communication, is unique to humans. The evidence seems overwhelmingly to support the linguistic ability of many animals. How is it, for example, that schools of fish swim in extraordinary unison, or that flocks of birds fly in extraordinary synchronization, unless there is some sort of communication going on? What are we to make of the vocal sounds, such as squawks, shrills, calls, chirps, roars, howls, barks, buzzes, and so on of innumerable animal species, or the "bee dances" that have been commonly noted, or of the sharp bellows of dolphins? If these are not linguistic abilities, then what exactly counts as such? Is it conceivable that nature has endowed them with these vocal abilities without there being something functional posited with it? The fact that we may not understand the squawks or chirps of birds does not rule out the possibility that they are engaged in some form of linguistic practice. Perhaps the burden of proof is on us to show in what way their interpersonal squawks and verbal interactions do *not* constitute a language.

The trend towards a kinder treatment of animals, of greater respect toward animals, whether domesticated or in the wild, and the increasing outrage expressed towards hunting, seems to have followed from the Enlightenment itself. Animals are different from other kinds of property. We no longer accept Descartes's mechanized view of animals being soulless machines with no feelings of pain or emotions. Urbanization and the concomitant domestication of animals have enabled human beings to regard animals more as objects worthy of our love and respect. Animals are clearly more than just objects. We feel differently about animals than we do about inanimate things. Animals have a place in our emotional lives that is unique. People seem to attribute to animals "feelings such as love and affection, obedience and loyalty, trustworthiness and valor."[15] Mammals share with us many emotive and cognitive characteristics, and the higher primates are very similar to humans both neurologically and genetically. We observe that animals display playfulness, trust, courage, love, and other humanlike traits. Still, hunting, which very often involves practices that are inhumane, cruel, and unfair, prevails as a form of amusement for many who insist that it is a "sport."

■ III. HISTORICAL EMERGENCE OF HUNTING AS A "SPORT"

To early human beings, hunting was a necessity, and in many parts of the world that remains true today.[16] It was not only a means of obtaining food, but also provided many of the other necessities of life such as clothing, tools, and other artifacts made from animal bones. As civilization advanced, certain animals were domesticated, and livestock were bred and raised to provide ongoing sources of animal food, and hunting for sustenance subsided.

As new areas were opened up in America and Africa, hunting again became a principal means of survival. But again, as the colonies of America and the wilderness regions of the West began to flourish, organized cultivation of livestock soon made it unnecessary to hunt in order to acquire game to eat. And today there is an entire international industry devoted to raising livestock and poultry for human consumption (agrifarming), thus obviating the need to hunt except for certain remote regions of the world where indigenous peoples rely upon hunting and fishing for their sustenance.[17]

It is far from clear when hunting as a means of sustenance changed into hunting as "sport." The "sport" of stag hunting, formerly called "hunting at force," dates back 800 years in England. This "sport" entailed chasing of deer by horsemen with a pack of hounds. Stag hunting became the most fashionable of noble "sports." Edward II, while engaged in a war with France, maintained sixty pair of staghounds, which he took with him to the battlefields. Chasing the stag continued as an aristocratic "sport" up to and including the period of World War II in England, and was also pursued in France.

The hunt, for nearly the entire time of the second millennium, was a ritual celebration of the power of the monarch. The hunt was used to celebrate royal power and, more specifically, royal power over wild nature. Its dominant social justification was as preparation for war, and as a means of perpetuating the power of the landed elite. In Elizabethan England many viewed hunting as an arduous sport that subjected men to extreme physical hardship that thus served as a training ground in the arts of war.[18] From the Middle Ages to the end of the seventeenth century in England, hunting was one of the most significant royal activities and manifestations of royal power. "To read the history of kings," observed Tom Paine in the eighteenth century, "a man would be almost inclined to suppose that government consisted of stag hunting."[19]

Social tensions concerning the hunt were evident during the Elizabethan period, when hunting was a highly visible sign of privilege, and the vast parks and forests set aside for the pursuit of that privilege acted as an irritant, both literally and symbolically, to the less privileged. The law of the forests, which originated with the Norman kings and was separate from the common law, gave the monarch sole authority over every forest in the kingdom and all of the animals in the forest. Forests were essentially wildlife preserves for the royal hunt. The right to hunt in a forest could only be conferred by the monarch, and even the right to hunt in the boundaries of the forest, the so-called purlieus, was restricted to those of superior wealth and rank. Even the establishment of a private game park required a warrant by the monarch.[20] During the Civil Wars of England, one of the main causes of the wholesale destruction of hunting parks was the popular rage against a repressive social custom.[21] In his *Description of England* (1587), William Harrison referred to the general resentment of the hunt by commoners, and noted that the keeping of parks was dangerously destructive. The reduction of arable land necessary to the support of parks led owners to enclose common lands, which contributed to the impoverishment, dislocation, and depopulation of the common people. He criticized hunting of deer and stag as "pastimes more meet for ladies and gentlewomen to exercise . . . than for men of courage to follow, whose hunting should practice their arms in tasting of their manhood and dealing with such beasts as efstoons will turn again and offer them the hardest [danger] rather than their horses' feet, which many times may carry them with dishonor from the field."[22]

Fox hunting in England actually got going in earnest in the seventeenth century, and in the nineteenth century fox hunting became a national pastime that surpassed stag hunting in popularity. While fox hunting started as an upper-class pastime, it eventually became a national "sport." In England, the "sport" involves hunting of fox, either free or pre-released, by having packs of hounds and costumed hunters on horseback pursue the fox across the marshes until it collapses from exhaustion, at which point the dogs usually tear it to pieces.

Fox hunting has in recent years become a divisive, controversial, and emotional issue in England, facing substantial public outcry. Many are opposed to fox hunting as cruel and barbaric. Recently, the House of Commons voted overwhelmingly to outlaw fox hunting with dogs, although the ultimate fate of the measure is subject to further parliamentary hurdles in the House of Lords.[23]

In America, fox hunting was for many years considered a privileged "sport." Fox hunting became a favorite pastime of several presidents of the United States, cabinet members, justices of the Supreme Court, senators, congressmen, and high-ranking army and navy officers. George Washington devoted practically all of his spare time to the chase, having learned the "sport" from his friend Lord Thomas Fairfax, who came to Virginia in 1746. Washington often managed to enjoy a few hours of hunting between battles during the Revolution, according to his diary. Martha Washington also hunted occasionally. Thomas Jefferson was a keen hunter of foxes, as was Alexander Hamilton. In New York City, fox hunting was extremely popular before and after the Revolution. Many early newspapers carried accounts of hunting on Manhattan Island as well as Long Island, North Riding, and Westchester counties. Fox hunting was a social event for the landed gentry of Virginia, Maryland, and Pennsylvania. Hounds and hunt servants were imported from England, and a good deal of attention was paid to the formality of hunt protocol. Fox hunts continued to be pervasive in the United States during the nineteenth century, with hunt clubs forming a social hub in Washington, Baltimore, New York, Brooklyn and many other localities. Hunt clubs continued through the two World Wars, although its popularity in America has waned in the present time.

What is clear about fox hunting is that regardless of when it occurred, the pursuit of the fox has never been connected to sustenance hunting, given that fox are not consumed. Rather, the pastime has been pursued for amusement, for the niceties of its English protocol, and for its social camaraderie.

In nineteenth-century America, people hunted some species nearly to extinction, including mountain lions and bison. The bison, once plentiful in America, exist today only because a few survivors were formed into a breeding herd and carefully preserved. In Europe, the magnificent red deer, brown bear, and roebuck that formerly inhabited the reserved forests of central Europe have been sadly depleted by hunters.

Today, the motivations to hunt are several: for amusement, for mastery of certain skills such as sharp-shooting, for a sense of domination over wild animals, for the satisfaction of showing off "trophies" to friends, and, in the case of consumable animals, to bring home a wild animal for a roast. However, while some species of commonly hunted animals are suitable for eating, such as deer, most others, such as fox, mountain lion, prairie dogs, raccoons, squirrels, bear, and moose, are not. Hunters claim that hunting brings them back to nature. Erich Fromm has said, "In the act of hunting, a man becomes, however, briefly, a part of nature again. He returns to the natural state, becomes one with the animal, and is freed of the existential split: to be part of nature and to transcend it by virtue of his consciousness."[24] Some people associate hunting with the Second Amendment right to bear arms, although many kinds of hunting involve other means of killing, such as bows and arrows. Others claim that men are hunters in their innermost being, that it is an innate feature of human nature to desire to hunt. Others justify hunting on the grounds that hunters harvest excess game animals—those which would die anyway from other causes if not taken in hunting.

■ IV. EVOLVING STANDARDS OF WHAT CONSTITUTES ACCEPTABLE FORMS OF AMUSEMENT, AND THE BASIS OF MORAL CRITICISMS OF HUNTING

What one might regard as a worthy form of amusement in a given time and place in history may be found abhorrent and destructive of public morality in a different time and place. In the history of the world we have witnessed moral growth. While in one period of history slavery had been endorsed by the majority of nations, it became an evil that is now universally condemned. While American Indians were once the object of war and regarded as something less than human, that attitude has long faded into the past.

Moral progress also occurs with respect to the types of activities human beings engage in for amusement. In times past people found it praiseworthy to engage in certain pastimes which, today, we find to be perverse. In ancient Rome and again in eighteenth-century Europe it was considered perfectly moral, under the customs of the time, to provoke and bait animals to fight each other for the amusement of spectators. This was a diversion that was accepted, tolerated, and which attracted great crowds. Today in most cultures, we regard the pitting of animals against one another in fights as a cruel and barbarous practice. Dog fights, cock fights, and other animal fights are outlawed under animal cruelty laws almost universally in the West, and few would disagree that these pastimes are offensive to human sensibilities and demeaning to public morality.

Another form of amusement, once legal, at least in ancient Rome, and now universally condemned, was the activity of famously pitting human beings against each other as gladiators. In addition, the Romans famously forced Christians, prisoners, and foreigners to engage in mortal combat with lions in the Roman Coliseum.

A common mantra among hunters is that the "sport" is not only a permissible pastime under the law, but that it is a morally permissible form of recreation and amusement. However, the criticism of hunting from a moral standpoint appears to have emerged centuries ago in three main strands of argument. The first in time and importance was a humanist opposition, closely related to anti-war sentiments by such figures as Thomas More, Erasmus, and Agrippa. In *Utopia*, the Utopians regard hunting "as a thynge unworthye to be used of free men," relegating the activity to butchers. The so-called pleasure of the hunt, according to Utopians, is no more than a pleasure in killing or mutilation, and it either reveals a cruel disposition or creates one, the hunter losing his humanity "by longe use of so cruell a pleasure."[25] Erasmus takes a similar view in *Praise of Folly*.[26]

Agrippa in *Of the Vanitie and Uncertaintie of Artes and Sciences* (1530) condemned hunting as "detestable" and "cruell Arte," one that leads men to set "all humanitie apart" and "become salvage beastes." Following Augustine, Agrippa located the origin of hunting in the act of Original Sin, which ended forever the peace between men and animals. Agrippa said that when God said to the serpent, " 'I will set hatred betweene thee and the woman, and betweene thy seede and her seede,' of this sentence the battail of huntinge tooke his beginning." Agrippa claimed that throughout history hunting is a "battle" that is a symptom of human depravity, and is linked to "wicked menne and sinners." He made a connection between hunting and tyranny: "Huntinge was the beginninge of Tyrannye, because it findeth no Authoure more meete than him, whiche hathe learned to dispise God, and nature, in the slaughter and boocherie of wilde beastes, and in the spillinge of bloude."[27]

Throughout his plays, Shakespeare draws upon the connection between hunting and human violence. In the midst of Elizabethan England, when the hunt was highly reveered by the aristocracy, Shakespeare, in *Love's Labor's Lost*, expressed the folly of hunting in a scene where the Princess of France, who was waiting, bow in hand, for the hunt to begin, acknowledged the cruelty of her role, that of playing "the murderer" in ambush (4.1.8). She reflected upon the unworthiness of her motives, admitting that she hunts "for praise alone." In lines that resonate throughout the play, she treats the desire for praise in hunting as a symptom of the destructive quest for fame in all human activities:

And out of question so it is sometimes:

> Glory grows guilty of detested crimes,
> When for fame's sake, for praise, an outward part,
> We bend to that the working of the heart;
> As I for praise alone now seek to spill
> The poor deer's blood, that my heart means no ill.

Margaret Cavendish, Duchess of Newcastle, also wrote a powerful antihunting poem, "The Hunting of the Hare" (1653).[28]

The second major strand of moral criticism of hunting was a sentimental type of opposition, led most notably by Montaigne, who issued detailed condemnations of the cruelty of the hunt in the essay "Of Cruelty." Noting that he hates cruelty above all other vices, he admits that he cannot bear even to see "a chickins neck pulld off" or to hear the "groane" of "a seely dew-bedabled hare . . . when she is seized upon by the howndes." Montaigne admitted that there was a certain irresistible excitement of the hunt, but he recoiled at the suffering imposed upon the animal: "As for me, I could never so much as endure, without remorce and griefe, to see a poore, silly, and innocent beast pursued and killed, which is harmeles and voide of defence, and of whom we receive no offence at all."

The third strand was an opposition led by the English Puritans, which developed in the middle and late seventeenth century. John Calvin is quoted as saying that God "will not have us abuse the beasts beyond measure . . . but to nourish them and to have care of them. . . .. If a man spare neither his horse nor his ox nor his ass, therein he betrayeth the wickedness of his nature. And if he say, 'Tush, I care not, for it is but a brute beast,' I answer again, 'Yea, but it is a creature of God.'"[29] This does not appear to condemn hunting itself, but animal cruelty in general. Puritans, however, did protest against hunting not so much because of concern with cruelty to animals but because of the social abuses associated with the hunt—the destruction of property through the wanton pursuit of deer across farmers' fields, the waste of time, and the waste of resources that might have been used to alleviate poverty. Puritan ministers such as Philip Stubbes argued that hunting should be conducted only in necessity, not as a form of recreation:

> If necessitie or want of other meats inforceth us to seek after their [animals'] lives, it is lawfull to use them in the feare of God, with thanks to his name; but for our pastimes and vain pleasures sake, wee are not in any wise to spoyle or hut them. Is he a Christian man or rather a pseudo-christian, that delighteth in blood? . . . Is hee a Christian that buieth up the corne of the poor, turning it into bread (as many doo) to feed dogs for his pleasure? Is hee a Christian that liveth to the hurt of his Neighbour in treading and breaking down his hedges, in casting open his gates in trampling of his corne?[30]

In modern times the idea of autonomy rights for animals was persuasively advanced in 1857, when Henry David Thoreau suggested that nature itself should have legal rights, as do powerless people subject to oppression. He pointed out the inconsistency of the president of an antislavery society wearing a beaverskin coat. For John Muir, not only animals, but plants and even crystals are part of a created community to which human beings, also, belong. He asked rhetorically, "What good are rattlesnakes for?" and answered that they were "good for themselves, and we need not begrudge them their share of life."[31] In 1867, hiking through Florida, he referred to the alligators he encountered as "fellow mortals" filling the "place assigned them by the great Creator of us all" and "beautiful in the eyes of God."[32] The course charted by Thoreau and Muir has been brought into sharper focus in recent years by Tom Regan, Peter Singer, and other able advocates.

Modern anti-cruelty statutes seem to have as their philosophical grounding the idea that cruel treatment of animals is a precursor to the cruel treatment of humans.[33] In other words, it is in the interest of the public welfare to outlaw cruelty to animals because that practice has an antisocial impact on the behavior of human beings. There has been substantial research documenting a correlation between human violence against animals and human violence against humans: "[H]urting animals is one of the earliest reported symptoms of conduct disorder."[34] Twenty-five percent of men incarcerated for violent psychiatric or criminal behavior have a history of engaging in "substantial cruelty" to animals, compared to zero percent of non-incarcerated men.[35] Extensive modern research has revealed that in childhood, serial killers invariably manifest antisocial traits, including acts of cruelty to animals.[36] The child may dream of dominating the family dog, eventually going so far as to kick it. Finding kicking the dog rewarding, the future killer expands his behavior to beating, and eventually killing the dog. The future killer's childhood focus on violence leads to an adulthood oriented around violence.[37]

The conventional wisdom of modern sociology pointing to the link between child animal-abusers and adult sociopathic behavior was intuited long ago by Locke, Kant, and other philosophers. Locke in his *Educational Writings,* said this about animal cruelty:

> One thing I have frequently observed in children, that when they have got possession of any poor creature, they are apt to use it ill; they often torment and treat very roughly young birds, butterflies and such other poor animals which fall into their hands, and that with a seeming kind of pleasure. This, I think, should be watched in them, and if they incline to any such cruelty, they should be taught the contrary usage. For the custom of tormenting and killing of beasts will by degrees harden their minds even towards men; and they who delight in the suffering and destruction of inferior creatures will not be apt to be very compassionate or benign to those of their own kind.[38]

Kant, in his *Duties Towards Animals and Spirits,* said:

> Our duties towards animals are merely indirect duties towards humanity. Animal nature has analogies to human nature, and by doing our duties to animals in respect of manifestations of human nature, we indirectly do our duty towards humanity.[39]

Thomas Aquinas, in his book *Summa Contra Gentiles,* said the following:

> [I]f any passages of Holy Writ seem to forbid us to be cruel to dumb animals, for instance to kill a bird with its young: this is ... to remove man's thoughts from being cruel to other men, and lest through being cruel to animals one become cruel to human beings.[40]

Arthur Schopenhauer said, in a similar vein:

> Boundless compassion for all living beings is the firmest and surest guarantee of pure moral conduct. ... Whoever is inspired with it will assuredly injure no one, will wrong

no one, [and] will encroach on no one's rights. . ... The moral incentive advanced by me as the genuine, is further confirmed by the fact that *the animals* are also taken under its protection.[41]

And in one of many criminal prosecutions for animal cruelty, one judge said: "[H]uman beings should be kind and just to dumb brutes; if for no other reason than to learn how to be kind and just to each other."[42]

Clearly, the purpose of laws that protect against animal cruelty is not only to protect animals, but to preserve public morals. The rationale behind these laws is that there is a relationship between kindness to animals, a decent character, and a decent civilization.

■ V. THE TECHNIQUES COMMONLY EMPLOYED IN HUNTING CONSTITUTE ANIMAL CRUELTY

In this section I will show that the activity of hunting, particularly in light of the techniques commonly employed in hunting, constitute animal cruelty, and are therefore subject to moral criticism because they contribute to the breakdown of human morality. Some of the hunting practices found throughout the world are as follows:

- Aerial hunting, which allows hunters to shoot wolves and other animals from helicopters or planes. This protocol has been approved in Alaska, among other places, ostensibly because predator populations had increased, thus creating a need for aerial hunting.[43]
- "Canned hunts," in which all sorts of animals—from African lions to European boars—are provided as game for fee-paying hunters at private fenced-in shooting preserves. A growing number of people participate in "canned hunting" operations, where they may pursue trophy animals that have no chance in the matter because they are confined in fences.[44] One advertisement reads: "Tired of traveling, spending money and coming home with nothing to show for it? Book your successful trophy hunt today! . . . No license required, no harvest—no charge."[45] Canned hunting is nothing new. In the nineteenth century, there were palatial private railroad cars "fitted up with special reference to shooting expeditions."[46] Railroads built specially constructed hotels for hunters,[47] and produced pamphlets "written as if each railroad had been routed with particular care to pass through famous and well-stocked game haunts."[48]
- "Contest kills," from Pennsylvania's pigeon shoots to Colorado's prairie dog shoots, in which shooters use live animals as targets while competing for money and prizes in front of a cheering crowd.
- "Wing shooting," in which hunters lure gentle mourning doves to sunflower fields and blast the birds of peace into pieces for nothing more than

target practice, leaving more than 20% of the birds they shoot crippled and unretrieved.

- "Baiting," in which trophy hunters litter public lands with piles of rotten food so they can attract unwitting bears or deer and shoot the feeding animals at point-blank range. Some jurisdictions have enacted laws that prohibit or curtail this practice. In November, 1996, voters in Washington State approved an initiative that banned the use of bait to attract black bears, and the use of hounds when hunting black bear, cougar, bobcat, or lynx. Opponents called the initiative "animal rights extremism," and claimed that its proponents were interested in "the total elimination of the use of animals in science; the total dissolution of the use of animals in private and commercial animal agriculture; and the total eradication of all fishing."[49]
- "Hounding," in which hunters unleash packs of radio-collared dogs to chase and tree bears, cougars, racoons, foxes, bobcats, lynx, and other animals in a high-tech search and destroy mission, and then follow the radio signals on a handheld receptor and shoot the trapped animal off the tree branch.
- "Calling," which is commonly practiced in pursuit of deer, consists of waiting in hiding and making noises in imitation of the call of a female during the rutting season, or else of the challenge of a male. In either case a male will answer and will gradually come right up to the "sportsman" believing him to be a possible mate or a probable antagonist. Calling deer is one of the oldest European hunting techniques, dating back long before the introduction of firearms. The technique has also been successfully adopted by moose hunters in North America.
- "Decoys," in which animals are lured by artifacts that look like the targeted animal's own species, while the hunter waits in a concealed and strategic place.[50]
- "Sitting up," which is to wait in hiding over some spot where the animal will probably pass or return, such as a water hole, game trail, crossing point, or a salt lick. It should be noted that sitting up over water or a salt lick is not generally considered a "sportsmanlike" procedure and it is prohibited by law in some localities. In Elizabethan England the most common form of hunting was for deer to be driven before stationary hunters armed with crossbows, who were positioned in ambushes or specially constructed stands. Greyhounds were often used in such hunts, both to chase the deer to the waiting hunters and to run down those that had been wounded. Coursing was a type of hunt that was essentially a spectator "sport," with observers stationed on stands en route or even in rooms with view of the chase, in which game were pursued and attacked by greyhounds.
- Contaminating the burrows of small game, such as rabbits, a day or two before the shoot, with foul-smelling substances such as kerosene and tar,

which the gamekeeper sprinkles into each hole. The rabbits leave their holes at night to feed, but will not return to them, objecting to the smell. On the day of the shoot the rabbits are found laying around undergrowth in the fields, from which they are easily dislodged by beaters with sticks, or by spaniels.

- Pursuit of polar bears with guides in specially designed "tundra buggies."
- At a certain point in the late nineteenth century an archery craze swept the United States.[51] Bow hunters insisted that the bow and arrow was used in hunting not as a superior weapon or equal in destructive power to guns, but "solely for the greater pleasure of its use in pursuit of game."[52]

What is common to each of these practices is that there is a power asymmetry. The hunted animals are lured, tricked, or manipulated in a way that gives them little or no chance of surviving, and then maimed or killed. The methods outlined above also make it the case that the hunter is spared from physical strain, endurance, stamina, fatigue, or other hardship. As discussed in detail below, it is hard to see how these activities qualify as a "sport." In addition, often enough due to inept shooting or inept aiming with a bow and arrow, and coupled with the sheer difficulty of accurately shooting a moving target, animals are maimed rather than killed outright, and then run away, often mortally injured to die a slow agonizing death. This contradicts the "ethic" of a "humane" kill that hunters generally advocate.

■ VI. ASYMMETRIES BETWEEN COMPETITIVE SPORTS AND HUNTING

My principal argument for excluding hunting from the category of sports is that hunting fails to be governed by principles that generally govern sports—that is, agonistic sports. If hunting is a sport, it would have to be a competitive sport, for the activity involves a competitive engagement of some kind, with two or more "players"—the hunter and the hunted subject. There is a particular structure to agonistic sports. Such sports are literally *constituted* by rules that are established by the inventors of the game, and are agreed upon by players who voluntarily play the game (either in teams or in pairs of players). The players compete against each other according to these rules until the winner is declared and the game ends. The players are supposed to be competitively matched so as to allow for a fair game. There are rules against attacking the bodily integrity of other players. There is a certain degree of physical prowess associated with sports. There is frequently an aesthetic component associated with sports. Certain virtues, such as courage, come into focus in sports. Good sportsmanship, which is a term of art, is associated with being a good player in a sport. As I will show, these elements are absent in the activity of hunting. Other authors have offered criteria of their own. The classic, still influential study of agonistic games by Johan Huizinga,

Homo Ludens,[53] describes five elements, some of which I have imported into my criteria.

I should say at the outset of this section that it is not my purpose to articulate criteria that can describe with analytic precision what constitute the asymmetries between sport and hunting. We cannot assume that because some accounts or descriptions of a certain domain are inexact, that inexactness is an impediment to understanding the truth about the subject matter, or that accounts cannot be given that are exacting enough to be action-guiding. Ethics is an inexact discipline. As Aristotle said, in an ethical theory, "it will be satisfactory if we can indicate the truth roughly and in outline."[54] Indeed, inexactness is a phenomenon in all areas outside of natural science. We cannot indicate with precision, for instance, the exact point at which a friendship can be said to start or how many friends one needs in order to have a good life, just as it is not possible to specify the number of people needed to make a city. Not all instances of friendship need exhibit the identical conditions, and so it is a mistake to insist that friendship fit into a neat algorithm and be identical in every instance.

These classifying criteria, although incomplete, have a sufficient degree of precision appropriate to the inquiry. I do not think it is feasible to articulate a single standard that will embrace all relevant factors that everyone can rally around. I have grouped them according to certain features of sport which I consider uncontroversial and salient to this inquiry. While the classifications overlap each other to some extent, they are as distinct as the subject matter admits. This model is useful for the purpose of providing broad criteria that, balanced together, should suffice to determine whether such an activity constitutes a sport. It is a *web,* an intricate network of criteria that are intertwined, so that if seen under a microscope, a complex mesh of unsuspected threads and knots might be seen. As in Mendeleiev's periodic table, each category has its place and there is room set aside to accommodate the unknown in specific positions, which might eventually be filled in. This model anticipates that we might supply the missing details for ourselves, based on our own reflectiveness.

1. Sports are structured around and indeed *constituted* by a set of rules

A key feature of sports is that the activity has its own rules and its own internal systematic relation of these rules that establishes the rights and obligations of the players, the structure of the game, the object of the game, and the method of computing points and penalties so as to ascertain the winner. The rules of a sport literally *constitute* the sport. They are not optional features of the sport. In other words, a sport does not exist without the rules that create the sport, and the sport gets its meaning and value within the parameters of these rules. There is the understanding in sports that each player will obey the rules of the game, or else the integrity of the game is violated. The rules of a sport are universal. That is, the game of baseball has the same rules wherever in the world it is played. The rules of a game are not imposed from outside the game, such as by a governmental authority or by some legislative enactment in the civil law, but are established by the inventor of the game.

Hunting, by contrast, is not constituted by rules. The act of hunting is something that prehistoric mankind undertook as a means of survival, as a means of outwitting wild animals in the wilderness. There were no "rules" that anyone promulgated in order for the activity of hunting to take place. With hunting, there is no "points system" for ascertaining a winner, no "goal" of the game other than to kill the victim, and no system of "rights" and "obligations" of the players. The activity is simply one in which the hunter shoots and kills (or maims) the victim.

A counterargument might be that there are numerous rules that regulate hunting, and that these rules seem to "constitute" hunting, just as any other sport. However, I would argue that these "rules" were enacted to protect hunters, and have no coherence or general design. The history of the hunting regulations shows that they were sponsored by elite hunting clubs, such as the Boone and Crockett Club of New York City, which was devoted to propounding the agenda of hunting. This club created and implemented hunting regulations throughout the country.[55] The hunting magazine *Forest and Stream* announced in 1901 the "basic principle" that "the game of this country belongs to the sportsman. . .. It is his, and he shall have it."[56] According to *Forest and Stream*, "Game laws can benefit the community only as, and in such degree as, they are in the interest of sportsmen."[57] This influential magazine asserted that "[A]ll the best measures for the protection of game . . . must always emanate from those who shoot and fish for their pleasure."[58] Wildlife management laws in fact were socially driven conventions, or indeed,

> were in fact always strategies aimed at regulating people, and oftentimes specific groups of local people who used wildlife in ways that other groups deemed either undemocratic, unsporting or not scientifically grounded. Rural, local, Native, or ethnic Americans usually lost these battles to more politically astute urban elites who had science and/or government on their side.[59]

By contrast, rules that constitute sports originate from the inventor of the sport, not from special interest groups seeking to enact laws through the political process.

When hunting "rules" were enacted, the sporting elite sought to weed out those who hunted for the purpose of marketing their kill: "When sport is enjoyed for its own sake therein is the pleasure, and its tendencies are elevating; but, on the contrary, let profit be connected with our pleasures and how soon they degenerate."[60] Anyone who hunted for a living was a detested rival who was condemned as "persistent, reckless, and morally depraved,"[61] a "despicable wretch who has neither manhood nor money to render him worthy of any consideration";[62] and marketers committed "simply a species of murder."[63] Hunters were concerned that the availability of wild animals would be tarnished by the practices of subsistence hunters, "pot hunters" and others who lived off the wilderness, whom they regarded as living in a savage state, as "vagabonds of the most worthless description . . . a miserable set."[64] In 1894, *Forest and Stream* demanded a total ban on the marketing of hunted animals, so as to exclude its hated rivals from hunting:

> The day of wild game as an economic factor in the food supply of the country has gone by. . . . [W]e can now supply food with the plow and reaper and cattle ranges cheaper than it can be furnished with the rifle and the shotgun. In short, as a civilized people we are no longer in any degree dependent for our sustenance upon the resources and the methods of primitive man.

Why should we not adopt as a plank in the sportsman's platform a declaration to this end—*That the sale of game should be forbidden at all seasons?*[65]

Within six years, anti-marketing hunting "rules" were enacted nationwide.[66] The hypocrisy of the hunting elite is that the push to ban marketing of game was justified on the grounds that no wild species can withstand exploitation for commercial purposes, but in fact "elimination of commercial hunting merely allocated wildlife from one social group to another. Sportsmen simply made their interest and the public interest appear to be the same, and state regulation of wildlife served that part of the public interest represented by upper-class hunters."[67]

Thus, the laws that limited hunting to particular times of the year were motivated not to conserve wildlife, but to end market hunting.[68] Bag limits, which became part of customary hunting regulations, were another way to limit the presence of marketers, although hunters were not generally enthusiastic about such limitations applied to their own endeavors. In 1890 *Forest and Stream* asserted, "[W]e may feel a certain kindly regard for the man who shoots a few birds and then stops for fear of ruining the chances of later arrivals; but we should regard the act rather as a virtue of supererogation than as of ethical obligation."[69]

Today, many jurisdictions have adopted hunting regulations pertaining to the time, manner, and place of hunting, but these are not rules which *constitute* hunting but rather are laws to regulate it, principally for the purpose of minimizing animal cruelty and to protect public safety. Clearly, hunting can exist in the absence of these regulations, while a sport cannot exist in the absence of its rules. And by no means are these regulations "universal," but vary from jurisdiction to jurisdiction.

Other hunting regulations clearly are not rules in the sense that applies to sports in the relevant sense described above. A wide range of hunting regulations are for other purposes, such as to minimize animal cruelty, to provide for the public safety, to curtail certain hunting techniques that are deemed deceitful or unethical, and to protect wild animal populations from being depleted. Hunting regulations invariably require that hunters apply for and obtain a hunting license for the season, and that the hunter be a certain minimum age, usually 16, to qualify for a license. In California, for instance, is it unlawful to take game birds and mammals within 400 yards of any baited area, a practice that many regard as deceitful and unethical.[70] It is prohibited to use electronic or mechanically-operated calling or sound-reproducing devices for luring game birds.[71] Most jurisdictions have a "bag and possession" limit, prescribing the daily bag limit of each kind of game bird and mammal which may be taken. Some jurisdictions prohibit the shooting of birds and mammals while pursuing them from motor-driven air or land vehicles or motorboats.[72] There are prohibitions against night hunting.[73] There are state-imposed restrictions on when and where dogs may be employed for the pursuit and taking of game.[74] Some jurisdictions limit the areas where the use of dogs is permitted for the pursuit and taking of game. There are other regulations on the methods authorized for taking big game,[75] and prescribing the gauge of shotguns and other methods permitted to be used in taking small game, so as to insure that killing happens as humanely as possible.[76]

It was the hunting lobby that was behind levying hunting license fees. The idea was to use the proceeds to hire wardens to enforce other rules such as closed seasons.[77] The hunting lobby eventually succeeded in getting enacted a Federal tax upon arms and ammunition,[78] with the condition that the funds be applied to the states for state wildlife purposes.[79] As a result, hunters scored a coup in their longstanding effort to weed out subsistence hunters and other "vagabonds" who were too poor to pay gun taxes or to even afford guns. Hunters also lobbied for restricting the means of taking game, for specifying the type of firearms to be deployed with specific types of game, and succeeded in banning many practices employed by subsistence hunters, such as laying bird snares—the poor man's method of choice.[80]

Other types of "rules" of hunting are "rules of thumb," or practical safety tips. These clearly are not rules in the sense of constituting sports. Rules of thumb which include, for example, "Make sure your head net doesn't obscure your vision," or "Don't assume you are the only hunter in the area," or "Be certain of a companion's location," or "Know and identify your target and what is beyond," or "Discuss safety techniques with companions," or "One should use a flashlight when walking in the dark," or "Be extremely careful using decoys," "Always keep your gun pointed in a safe direction," "Always keep your finger off the trigger until ready to shoot," "Never use alcohol or drugs before or while hunting," "Respect property rights and secure permission before hunting," or "Whenever you see a rabbit moving through cover, yell out his position to alert other hunters," are not rules that constitute a sport, but are simply practical rules of thumb.[81] Some of these are safety rules to avoid accidents and to avoid shooting other hunters. Other "rules" of hunting pertain to such things as wearing a red hunting coat, or to wear a vest, or a rider's helmet, and other protocol of apparel. Other "rules" might include what the hunting horn musicians are to play, or that you are to never ride too close to the dogs, and the horses should face the dogs, and that there should be provision of water for the dogs to drink and to wet their noses.

Even if we regard these as "rules" of hunting, they are hardly rules in the sense applicable to sports. These "rules" do not *constitute* the hunting in the way that the rules of sports *constitute* the sports to which they pertain. No sport can exist without rules, for it is the rules that literally make up the game, while hunting as an activity can exist without any rules being in place. Hunting has existed for millennia with no rules. Moreover, the "rules" are not internal to hunting but imposed by governmental authorities. The "rules" are not universalizable, but vary from jurisdiction to jurisdiction. Finally, the "rules" are not intended to define what hunting is, but are laws for the public welfare, to minimize animal cruelty, and to aid wildlife management.

2. Sports are competitive games[82] played by human beings against one another, and the players agree to comply with the rules of the game. Also, sports have a certain degree of complexity compared to nonsport activities

Sports are played between individual human beings or between groups of human beings in teams. Animals are sometimes utilized in sports, such as in horse racing, dog racing, Olympic equestrian events such as dressage, and so forth.

Bull-fighting is widely viewed as a "sport," but I would argue that bull-fighting may be equated with the barbaric practices of the Roman Circus. I would reiterate my claim, made in section IV, that evolving standards of what constitute acceptable forms of amusement disqualify bull-fighting as "sport," and that the techniques employed in bull-fighting constitute animal cruelty, along the lines I argued in section V,[83] so that clearly there is a power asymmetry between matador and bull.

The players of a sport agree, expressly or impliedly, to comply with the rules of the game, and it is understood that failure to adhere to the rules will result in penalties or other forfeitures. In order to comprehend the rules of a sport, one must possess rational thinking of a certain degree of development. Children, for instance, might not be able to grasp the rules of, say, football until they reach a certain level of maturity, so that they, therefore, cannot properly engage in that sport. In hunting the opponent is a nonsentient creature, while the hunter is a human being with the power of practical reason. With hunting, the activity pits a human being against a wild animal that is incapable of "consenting" to the "game," rather than a human being against another human being. Even if there were "rules" that constitute hunting, animals do not have the capability of comprehending the rules, and hence they cannot be said to be "participants" in any real sense. The hunted animal does not "understand" or "agree" to any sort of participation in the enterprise, or to make an effort to "win" in the engagement.

Hunted animals do not "choose" to engage in the activity; they are not voluntary participants in the activity, but are lured, baited, and hunted down.

Furthermore, competitive sports have a certain complexity built into their structure, with a structured beginning, middle, and end. The rules of any competitive sport prescribe how to determine which team gets the ball first, how the game starts, what the positioning of the players is, the manner of serving or pitching the ball, what constitutes intermediate achievement of goals or points, and how to determine when the game ends and who is the victor. With hunting, there is little complexity built into the structure of the activity.[84] All there is to the "game" is to aim and shoot, and perhaps to set up beforehand some set of deceptive techniques used to bait or call animals to their death. As underscored below, such practices are antithetical to true sports and to true sportsmanship.

3. Sports have for their end victory in the game

While it is perfectly legitimate to play a sport for its intrinsic worth—for the pleasure and fun that the activity provides as an end in itself—still, in any competitive sport the players have the aim of winning. Players expect each other to pursue their self-interested ends of winning the game. The rules of the game prescribe how to determine who is the winner.

Hunting, by contrast, does not prescribe a system of judging who is the "winner" of the hunt. If a hunter shoots at a deer and misses, and the deer escapes into the woods, are we to say that the "game" has come to an end, and that the deer is the winner of the game? Perhaps, in a sense, if the hunter shoots and misses the target, or maims instead of kills the victim, this can be a deeply humiliating sense of defeat, particularly if one is sensitive about the fact that a maimed animal is likely to suffer an excruciating death rather than be killed cleanly and quickly. But with hunting, there is no such thing as being the "winner" or "loser."

4. The rules of sports prohibit violating the bodily integrity of the players

Directly attacking the bodily integrity of another player is, with few exceptions, strictly prohibited in sports. Even with contact sports such as boxing, where the ultimate objective is to knock out the opponent, there are rules respecting the manner of inflicting blows and prohibitions on attacking an opponent who is down, and it is certainly illegitimate to strike a blow reasonably calculated to kill the opponent. With hunting the reverse is true: Violation of the bodily integrity of the victim indeed is the very goal of the hunter. The hunter's aim is to assault the physical integrity of the "opponent" by killing it.

There are no "rules" to prevent an inept marksman from hunting. Hunting licenses are granted upon paying the applicable fee and qualifying as to age. Due to inept shooting or inept aiming with a bow and arrow, and coupled with the sheer difficulty of accurately shooting a moving target, animals are often maimed rather than killed outright, and then run away, often mortally injured to die a slow agonizing death. When this happens there is no "violation" of any "rules."

5. Physical prowess and skills are associated with sports

Sports involve a variety of physical and mental skills and endurance that the players must develop and work on in order to successfully engage in the sport. In classical Greek athletics, the *agon* or "contest" was very important. There was a sort of heroism of the athletic contest. There was a sense of divine perfection represented in the bodily action of the victor—a strength, nobility, and power from a unique human achievement of prowess and mental acumen.[85]

Each sport has a particular type of athletic accomplishment one must develop. Physical coordination, speed, strength, and endurance are skills invariably needed in competitive sports. In golf, for instance, there is the need to master coordination of the arm and wrist, learning how to hit the ball properly with the proper driving iron and with the right sort of swinging motion, aiming at the goal, maneuvering awkward angles, and many other challenges. In gymnastics there is considerable practice required in developing flexibility of one's entire body, of learning and executing difficult jumps and moves of certain heights, and so on.

With hunting there is often very little by way of physical activity in the first instance, and often the activity has little by way of challenge to the hunter. In the forests during hunting season one sees roads full with RV campers, and in some regions it is permitted to go after animals with aerial shoots or jeeps on roads well kept by park management personnel. While some kinds of hunt entail physical stamina and skill, such as the chase, more commonly the hunt involves lying in wait, which is a nonphysical activity. Theodore Roosevelt referred to the various types of easy hunting as "debased," "contemptible," and "luxurious and effeminate artificiality."[86] Clearly, there is a certain "softness" to contemporary hunting practices and little of discipline or hardship as found in traditional sports. Even in the stark climate of the Arctic, polar bear hunts are conducted, as mentioned above, from the sedentary comfort of "tundra buggies."

There *is* a skill involved in developing the technique of sharpshooting, but how that skill, in and of itself, carried into hunting, would baptize the hunt into becoming a "sport" is far from clear given that the other elements of sports discussed in this paper are lacking.

6. There is an aesthetics component to sports that is absent in hunting

Many if not all sports have an aesthetics component. Spectators may comment on the beauty of a particularly skillful move on the part of a player. In baseball, a batter's swing might be of a certain perfection that spectators will call it "beautiful."

Sometimes the aesthetic component is a principal part of the athlete's objective, such as in gymnastics, ice-skating, diving, and ski-jumping. These sports are keyed to spectators in a unique way, that is, not just the physical skill, but with a regard to the aesthetic appeal of the formal execution of the movement.

With hunting, there is no "aesthetics" component. One might say "that was a beautiful shot," meaning that the hunter made his target, but the use of the word "beautiful" in this context does not carry an aesthetics implication, but instead refers metaphorically to the mechanical precision of the shot. There is nothing beautiful in seeing a pheasant drop down from the sky. Once a wild animal is hit, there is nothing by way of aesthetics, but instead there is a somewhat ugly, brutal, bloody mess to behold.

7. Sports are divided into professional and amateur categories

Most sports have a professional component, where athletes earn a living at the chosen sport, such as in tennis, baseball, hockey, golf, or football. For professional athletes, the activity is instrumental in nature—a means to earning a living, and towards that end the uppermost concern of the player in engaging in the sport is to win.

For nonprofessional or amateur players, one's motivation in the activity is usually the intrinsic value it has; that is, for its direct and immediate end—fun, pleasure, relaxation or delight. There can also be some instrumental value for amateur players, such as to engage in an activity that will benefit one's physical health and stamina, or to gain victories and personal triumph, or as an outlet for one's aggression or competitive nature. An amateur player also has at least in the back of one's mind that the purpose of engaging in the sport is to win. Amateur players often have a kind of compulsion to win even in a friendly game of tennis, and this compulsion is, I think, one of the features that makes for the intrinsic enjoyment of the game.

With hunting, there is no "amateur/professional" divide. There is no such thing as a professional hunter who earns a living competing against other hunters, nor do hunting "teams" exist, except, perhaps for groups licensed by wildlife management to cull excessive herds, but such operations are not regarded by the participants as "sport" or amusement, but as a necessary and regrettable mode of wildlife management. One might refer to the participants in a formal fox hunt as a "team," but in reality they are a social group, and they not competing against another team, but against a fox. Finally, there is no "hunting" event at the Olympics or under the auspices of any other organized commission.

8. In sports players are fairly matched to insure a level playing field

Another element of sports is that the players or teams need to be competitive with one another. That is, they need to be fairly matched as to skill in the particular sport, so that there will be a level playing field. The competing players, if mismatched, will play a noncompetitive game where the outcome can be easily anticipated beforehand. Such a game will not pose much of a challenge to the athletes that outmatch the other side. It will not be much fun for the spectators to see the victors vanquishing the losers with dispatch. The match will be unfair because there will be an asymmetry in the power balance, little of a bona fide engagement, and simply an overwhelming force vanquishing the weak.

With hunting there is no fair matching of the "players." Sports do not condone methods of the play which place the opponent at an unfair advantage, but with hunting the opponent—that is, the animal being hunted—is subjected to techniques that give the hunter a completely asymmetrical power advantage. Some hunting regulations, as mentioned above, attempt to level the playing field, as it were, by prohibiting such practices as lying in wait in baited fields or producing mechanical calls. These are not rules that constitute the "game," but are laws imposed from the outside for the purpose of instilling a modicum of ethics that otherwise would be missing in hunting, and in any event are far from universal in scope. Even with hunting regulations in place there is still a power asymmetry, with hunters lying in wait for an animal which, once in the sites of the hunter's rifle, has little or no chance of "winning." This is exacerbated in the many jurisdictions where decoys or other deceptive modes are employed to lure animals, or by aerial shooting. The victims have no guns with which to shoot back or defend themselves. The hunter is invariably out of range so that the victims cannot even make an effort to fight back.

9. Sports are usually played in clearly demarcated spaces set apart from other activities

There are arenas, stadiums, running tracks, courses, and so on. These spatial arrangements, indeed, are frequently integral to the play, so that particular transgressions, such as a foul ball, pertain to violating the boundaries of the space. By contrast, hunting usually takes place in the wilderness, the forest, the great outdoors, with no particular spatial boundaries other than outposts of parklands circumscribed by roadways.

10. Certain virtues are deployed in playing sports

Certain virtues need to be deployed while participating in competitive sports. Also, participating in sports helps one develop certain moral values, such as respect for others, personal responsibility, fairness, affability, politeness, good humor, self-realization, prudence, friendship, and individuality. Participating in sports fosters a sense of achievement, motivation, and self-esteem,[87] which are valuable goods in other areas of life.

I will concede that participation in both sports and hunting involves the deployment of certain virtues in common. These virtues include patience (being attentive in the face of tedium), prudence, stamina, *sang-froid,* perseverance, self-control, self-reliance, and quickness of mind. Participation in both sports and hunting seems to require one to deal with various emotions and feelings, such as anger, frustration, daring, and hope. Also, sports and hunting involve the struggle to attain a technical achievement that requires some measure of practice, attention to detail, and endurance. In both cases there is some degree of hard work, inevitable misfortune and defeat, and sometimes criticism of one's actions. Common to sports and hunting are other traits, not exactly virtues, but traits that one often needs to deploy in order to succeed at the goal, such as adventuresomeness, the manifestation and control of a predatory temperament, an attitude of ferocity, the ability to inflict "damage" on the opponent, and cunning. Also, both sports and hunting have in common the need to utilize mental capacities such as coordinating strategy with teammates (or fellow hunters), coordinating tactical planning with teammates, anticipating problematic conditions, and exploiting advantageous conditions.

On the other hand, there are certain immoral values associated with hunting, such as power in domination over nonhuman animals, and pleasure in killing. Furthermore, the virtue of courage, usually required in competitive sports, seems to have no place in hunting. With sports, participants usually need to muster courage in facing an adverse team that is apparently better skilled, or in struggling to attain new goals, in learning about strategy, in excelling in whatever skills the game demands, and in facing injuries or facing defeat. Hunters often claim that hunting requires courage because of the fears, dangers and stamina involved. But courage involves risking some harm or danger to oneself. Courage often can require endurance and brute strength as well. Aristotle said that courage involves fear as it is called for by the particular features of the circumstances.[88] Aristotle claimed that courage is always related to fear in that it is invoked in response to fear rationally perceived. If the circumstances are safe enough so that the threat to one's life or safety is minimal, one appropriately feels little or no fear and a robust sense of confidence. If there is absence of fear and a robust sense of confidence, we are not within the sphere of activity pertaining to courage.

Certain wild animals, such as mountain lions, are generally considered to be somewhat cowardly and rarely attack humans. Certainly deer are not menacing creatures, nor are wild duck. Moreover, with such practices as hunting from jeeps, "tundra buggies," and with professional guides or with the aid of dogs, it is not at all obvious how courage enters the picture at all even in the pursuit of "big game." To the contrary, some of the practices of hunting seem to be signs of cowardice, or at least of overweening domination over a weaker protagonist, such as with putting out of "decoys" to attract pheasants, ducks, doves, and other birds, or shooting pheasants with the services of "beaters" employed to put the birds over the guns at a height and pace to test the shooter's skill. Thus, a hunter lying in wait or poised in a jeep or helicopter—cannot be said to be acting out of courage.

Let us suppose for a moment that certain acts of hunting do involve courage. Suppose in circumstances of significant fear and danger, I kill a polar bear. Suppose further that I find it important to bring back a trophy, such as the bear's head and skin, to get acknowledgement, esteem, and praise from friends in response to my courageous act, or to aid in my boasting of prowess and courage. I do this because I want to feel honored when others acknowledge my act. What are we to say about hunters who hunt to gain trophies?

Aristotle claimed that to pursue honor or to seek the esteem of others was, in and of itself, a superficial quest.[89] According to Aristotle, virtues such as courage are acts done for their intrinsic worth, not as a means to some further end. If I am courageous in stalking and killing a polar bear or other big game, but my motive in doing so is to bring back a trophy so as to gain the esteem of my friends, this is seeking out something that depends on the approval of others and implies a lack of self-sufficiency. Thus, if I perform an act of courage *in order to obtain honor rather than the courageous deed being an end in itself,* I am doing it for the wrong reason and intention. I lack the requisite emotional state for my deed to qualify as true courage. It is not an act of true courage because it is motivated by my pursuit of honor rather than for the sake of virtue. The action is superficial, lacking in excellence, and therefore, does not count as truly virtuous.

11. After finishing a game of sports, one can evaluate whether the game was "good" or "bad"

With sports one can always say, after the game is over, "that was [or was not] a good game." To say a game was a good one means that the players were equally matched,[90] that it was competitively challenging, that it was fairly played, and that the winner won through a combination of skill, prowess, endurance, and perhaps a dose of luck. At the end of a hunt, however, none of these criteria comes in for evaluation because none is present.

How is it possible to say that a "game" of hunting was fairly played? The notion of fairness has no place in hunting, where the object of one's hunt is considered "fair game"—that is, available for the taking, with no "rules" of engagement except paying a fee for a hunting license or, perhaps, in some jurisdictions, to use a certain gauge shotgun so as to effect a quick kill. The "players" are not competitively or equally matched. In fact, there is an extreme asymmetry in matching. Wild animals have little or no chance at the end of a sensible shotgun, particularly when there is a group of guns poised, not just one. And there is clearly no "fair chase" when a hunter uses powerful weapons from aerial ambush, or when a fox is being raged at by hounds.

Moreover, as noted above, there are various practices traditionally sanctioned by hunters, outlawed in some jurisdictions, but still permitted in many others, that are not only unethical, but outrightly treacherous. The treacherous means used to lure wild animals, such as decoys, baiting, mating sounds, and so on, pose an extreme disparity in the playing field. And often enough, the hunter will miss the target. Bowhunting yields a rate of about 50% of crippling rather than killing. For every animal killed, one animal is left wounded to suffer—either to bleed to death or to become infested with parasites and diseases.[91]

It is not possible to say that the "best" player won in a hunting "match" because in reality there is only one player, the hunter. The victim is not, by any stretch of the imagination, poised to "compete" in the "sport," and is not even a voluntary "player" in the enterprise.

12. Good sportsmanship is a traditional feature of sports

The notion of good sportsmanship is a product of the fact that sports are *competitive* activities that involve winners and losers who can only be guessed at beforehand, for if the contestants are competitively matched, as they must be in competitive sports, the outcome of a contest may be difficult to predict. With a level playing field the winner is one who won fairly according to the rules in play.

One of the tenets of good sportsmanship is to recognize that although the will to win is important, winning is not all-important. John Rawls said that games are a social union that involves an agreed upon and cooperative "scheme of conduct in which the excellences and enjoyments of each [player] are complementary to the good of all."[92] The idea here is that players need to have a genuine commitment to the values of fellowship and goodwill, which are held more important than winning. Under this notion of good sportsmanship, the fraternal relationships, the mutual affection, camaraderie, and fellowship of engaging in a sport, are sacrosanct, intrinsic to sport itself.

The Sportsmanship Brotherhood, founded in 1926, adopted the slogan, "Not that you won or lost—but that you played the game." This brought home the idea that the *manner* in which a sport is played is no less important than its outcome. Being a good sport means having a concern for a fair and honest competition. Sportsmanship implies not only abiding by the rules of the game, but a kind of spirit in which the players conduct themselves with the best traditions of competitive, but friendly, rivalry, with a regard to keeping intact the social union that empowers the institution of sport itself.

It is hard to see how any of these features of good sportsmanship can possibly fit into the paradigm of hunting. Moreover, it is inconsistent with principles of sportsmanship to inflict suffering and death on one's "opponent," except perhaps *metaphorically* to "kill" and "fight" the other team "to death." It is inconsistent with good sportsmanship to refer to one's opponent as "resources." It is not a practice of sports to be engaged in "culling," "controlling," or "managing" of one's opponent for "maximum sustained yield." That is the province of wildlife management.

■ VII. WILDLIFE MANAGEMENT DISTINGUISHED FROM HUNTING

Wildlife management is a modern practical science devoted to sustaining of forests and their environs with a view towards preserving the ecological balance of species within given regions. Wildlife management, which often involves culling (that is, killing) of wild animals, is not a "sport," but is a practical science. A common problem addressed by wildlife management is how to handle an overabundance of deer, which causes measurable consequences to private and public natural resources, especially in urban and suburban areas. When deer exceed a certain threshold of population, they may interfere with human activities. Deer can easily jump an eight-foot fence and browse in gardens and yards, eat agricultural crops, carry ticks that transmit Lyme disease, and, not infrequently, damage property by doing such things as jumping through plate glass windows. The deer themselves may not be supportable with sufficient food and living space, and may starve or become diseased or be run over by motor vehicles.

Wildlife management will seek to control overpopulation of deer and other animals by trapping them, and then relocating them or euthanizing them. However, the trapping itself is very stressful to the animals and many deer may die during transport or shortly thereafter. To complicate matters, few places are willing to accept relocated deer. And whether the deer are relocated or euthanized, the process is very expensive.

Another herd reduction technique is to hire a team of sharpshooters to kill as many deer as they can as quickly and efficiently as they can. Wildlife management also tries to reduce deer population by advertising an additional hunting season after the regular fall season to further reduce the deer population, or to organize and advertise managed hunts in parks or on large industrial complexes. In a managed hunt, the host invites a limited number of chosen hunters who may be prequalified by experience, formal hunter safety training, or skills testing. The purpose of the hunt is to reduce the deer population in a measured and expedient manner. Those who are hired for the task do not regard it as amusement or sport, but as wildlife management.

I think the humane answer to problems of wildlife management is to develop sound methods of immunocontraception, or birth control, for deer and other species. Immunocontraception involves immunizing deer with a drug that prevents conception. This can be effective in the long run, although it may not solve immediate problems of overpopulation.

■ VIII. CONCLUSION

It should be apparent that the purpose of hunting is to kill animals for pleasure. In what way is watching a fox being mutilated and killed by hounds after a chase a sport? In what way is aerial killing of wolves in Alaska a sport? In what way is it "good sportsmanship" to participate in hunting seasons that often result in the slow death of orphaned offspring of their legally killed lactating mothers? At best, the use of the term "sport" to refer to hunting is a euphemism.

My effort here has been to point out a categorical fallacy—that hunting is not and ought not to be referred to as a "sport," and that those who participate in hunting as "amusement" are subject to moral criticism because of the unethical practices associated with hunting and the inappropriate linkage of killing with amusement. In doing so I hope to accomplish an internal change in the intellectual emphasis and convictions of hunters and non-hunters alike.

The history of moral progress is a history of expanding and shifting perspectives. The beliefs of entire societies can and do change. It was once the case that slavery was an accepted practice in the United States, and little by little a growing sense of discomfort took hold of the population, resulting in a complete reversal of attitude over time. The same can be said of women's rights, which have emerged and continue to capture public awareness.

Incremental change is how the law moves in any area of reform. My purpose here is to take an incremental step to distinguish sports from hunting. Society has come a long way from the time of Descartes, when it was believed that animals could feel no pain and were merely mechanized creatures. Clearly, in the past few decades there has been a shift in societal attitudes to an approach that views animals as worthy of protection against exploitation, and the movement for the ethical treatment of animals appears to be garnering greater momentum. I do not see how it is possible to ban hunting as an activity, but I do think it is important to make a categorical distinction so that hunters will cease referring to their activity with the euphemism, "sport."

Most of us would agree that animals have consciousness, can feel pain, use tools, and can communicate.[93] Clearly, animals, particularly domesticated pets, experience emotions. Clearly, we have feelings and sympathy toward animals that we do not have toward inanimate objects. We may feel badly about a broken antique plate, but not in the same way that we do about the death of a pet, or for that matter, about running over an animal on the road or witnessing an act of animal cruelty.

It is very rarely the case that a hunt will have as its principal aim the gathering of food. Except for remote regions of the world, we do not need to hunt animals for our sustenance because killing is done by the slaughterhouses, and we can go to the market to purchase meat, fish, and poultry. I personally am opposed to hunting in the regions of the world where killing of wild animals is not done for sustenance, but for amusement. I believe that hunting is a form of animal cruelty and, like all animal cruelty, it affects the whole temper of our civilization. It coarsens us, demeans us, makes us less empathetic.

Sports generally prohibit the infliction of serious infringements upon the bodily integrity of the opponent. Moreover, those who partake of a sport are voluntary participants. In contrast, animals who are hunted are not voluntary participants in the "game," but are forced participants, and their bodily integrity is violated—indeed, that is the very purpose and end of the hunter.

I appreciate the words of Albert Schweitzer, who spent much of his life in the wilderness of Africa. Schweitzer made it abundantly clear that his reverence for life did not end with human beings. He commented that "the great fault of all ethics hitherto has been that they believed themselves to have to deal only with the relations of man to man."[94] In 1923 he wrote that the ethical person "shatters no ice crystal that sparkles in the sun, tears no leaf from its trees, breaks off no flower, and is careful not to crush any insect as he walks."[95] For Schweitzer, the privileged status of human beings implied not a right to exploit but a responsibility to protect. Schweitzer said: "Today it is thought an exaggeration to state that a reasonable ethic demands constant consideration for all living things down to the lowliest manifestations of life. The time is coming, however, when people will be amazed that it took so long for mankind to recognize that thoughtless injury to life was incompatible with ethics."[96] Clearly, the idea here is that human beings and the other members of nature are ecological equals, that while human beings have the technological power to affect nature, it is unethical to regard other species of nature as commodities belonging to us.

Today we witness the removal of most peoples' experience with animals from farm animal to pet, the extension of laws to protect endangered species from extinction, the popularity of documentary nature films, the influence of "liberation movements," the pet industry's rise in promoting its own products and awareness, and the rise of anti-cruelty laws all over the world. It is time for hunting to be decommissioned as a "sport."

▦ **NOTES**

1. Quoted in *Peck v. Dunn*, 574 P.2d 367, 369 (Utah, 1978).
2. In my analysis I am referring to competitive, i.e., agonistic, sports (as distinguished from noncompetitive sports), in which players compete against one another in pairs or in teams, towards the goal of winning the game. Noncompetitive sports are usually solitary activities, such as ice skating, surfing, gymnastics, equitation, archery, skiing, yachting, rowing, and do not customarily involve playing against other players with a view towards winning a game. On the other hand, sometimes noncompetitive sports become competitive when played in tournaments, or are official competitive events in the Olympics, where contestants compete against one another and judges tally points to determine the winner, such as with gymnastics or cross-country skiing events.

3. There are complex issues related to the question of autonomy rights of animals, which are well beyond the scope of this essay. For example, once we grant certain liberty and autonomy rights to animals, the question arises whether we should not only outlaw their killing by humans, but whether we should also protect them from being killed by other animals. This becomes a difficult and murky issue when we consider whether a wolf who has stalked and killed a deer has violated that deer's right to life and liberty. In nature when one animal preys upon another, it would be difficult to formulate a coherent argument that a violation of rights has occurred, since events of this kind are a "natural" part of wilderness life. But there is a contrast when the victim is attacked by a human being. The human acts out of rational thinking and practical reason, while the wolf attacks out of instinct. Moreover, the human acts to hunt often enough not for food but for the pleasure of the kill or for its trophy or prestige value.

4. I believe these practices are shifting in response to moral concerns by consumers for more humane treatment of animals raised for slaughter, and as a result we are seeing a trend to enhance the well-being of farm animals through such reforms as "free cage" farming for poultry, transporting animals with greater care, stopping the use of growth hormones and 24-hour lighting to enhance hen-laying, and so on.

5. Some hunting organizations spend a good deal of time, money, and resources in bringing back various animals from the brink of disaster. The Safari Club International, for example, has spend over $10 million on some 600 projects around the world that benefit various animal species and their native stewards. See *Hearing Before the Committee on Resources,* House of Representatives, 105th Cong., 1st Sess., on H.J. Res. 59, Apr. 30, 1997, at 116.

6. Charles Darwin, *The Descent of Man* (London, 1871), at 72, 880.

7. Francis Darwin, ed., *The Life and Letters of Charles Darwin* (New York: Appleton, 1888), at 1:368.

8. See Charles Darwin, *The Descent of Man and Selection in Relation to Sex* (New York: Appleton, 1874), at 140.

9. John Muir, *A Thousand-mile Walk to the Gulf,* ed. William F. Bade (Boston: Houghton Mifflin, 1917), at 356.

10. P. D. Ouspensky, *Tertium Organum: The Third Canon of Thought, a Key to The Enigmas of the World,* trans. E. Kadloubovsky (New York: Knopf, 1981), at 166 (emphasis in original).

11. *The Writings of Henry David Thoreau,* ed. Bradford Torrey (Boston: Houghton Mifflin, 1906), at 9:210.

12. Ibid., at 2:450.

13. See Tom Regan, *The Case for Animal Rights* (1983).

14. For a discussion of how human reason consistently fails to direct sound decision making, see John Alan Cohan, "'I Didn't Know' and 'I Was Only Doing My Job': Has Corporate Governance Careened Out of Control? A Case Study of Enron's Information Myopia," 40 *Journal of Business Ethics* 275 (2002).

15. James M. Jasper and Dorothy Nelkin, *The Animal Rights Crusade* (1992), at 13.

16. For example, peoples who live in the vast archepelago known as the Solomon Islands are almost entirely dependent on hunting and fishing, as well as on horticulture, for their sustenance.

17. Native Americans hunt, but have never regarded themselves as sportsmen. Throughout the nineteenth century, American Indians had treaty guarantees that

insured their hunting rights. "[T]he Indian thinks of wildlife as a utility; the Caucasian regards it primarily as a source of pleasure." Clifford C. Presnall, "Wildlife Conservation as Affected by American Indian and Caucasian Concepts," 24 *J. of Mammology* 458 (1943). The religion of Indians reinforced their inability to kill for pleasure:

> The Indian regards wildlife as necessary to his existence, so much so that he worships it; he propitiates it with prayers before killing it, in order that future success in the hunt may be assured; . . . he objects to killing purely for sport, believing that it will anger the animal deities who will then hinder his business of hunting for food. (462)

18. Sir Thomas Cockaine argued in 1591 as follows in his *A Short Treatise of Hunting* (Oxford: Oxford University Press, 1932):

> And for the first commendation of Hunting, I find (Gentlemen) by my owne experience in Hunting, that Hunters by their continuall travaile, painfull labour, often watching, and enduring of hunger, of heate, and of cold, are much enabled above others to the service of their Prince and Countrey in the warres, having their bodies for the most part by reason of their continuall exercise in much better health, than other men have, and their minds also by this honest recreation the more fit and the better disposed to all other good exercises. (A3–3V)

19. Quoted in Keith Thomas, *Man and the Natural World* (London: Allen Lane, 1983), at 184.

20. See Edward Berry, *Shakespeare and the Hunt* (Cambridge: Cambridge University Press, 2001), at 8–9.

21. Ibid., at 29.

22. William Harrison, *Description of England,* (1577) at 326–329.

23. See Alan Cowell, "Fox Hunting with Dogs: M.P.'s Say No," *N.Y. Times*, July 1, 2003, at A6.

24. Erich Fromm, *The Anatomy of Human Destructiveness* (New York: Holt, Rinehart & Winston, 1973), at 132.

25. Thomas More, *Utopia*, trans. Ralph Robinson (1551; facs. rpt. Amsterdam: Da Capa Press, 1969), at M2–M2V.

26. Desiderius Erasmus, *Chaloner: The Praise of Folie*, ed. Clarence H. Miller, Early English Text Society (London: Oxford University Press, 1965), at 54.

27. Henry Cornelius Agrippa, *Of the Vanitie And Uncertaintie Of Artes And Sciences*, ed. Catherine M. Dunn (Northridge: California State University, 1974), at 260–263.

28. Cavendish's poem is printed in *Kissing the Rod: An Anthology of Seventeenth-Century Women's Verse*, ed. Germaine Greer et al. (London: Virago Press, 1988), at 168–172.

29. Keith Thomas, *Man and the Natural World,* (1983) at 154.

30. Philip Stubbes, *The Anatomie of Abuses* (1583; facs. rpt. Amsterdam: Da Capa Press, 1972), at 5.

31. John Muir, *Our National Parks* (Boston: Houghton Mifflin, 1901), at 57–58.

32. J. Baird Callicott, ed., *Companion to a Sand County Almanac* (Madison: University of Wisconsin Press, 1987), at 67 (quoting from John Muir's 1867 journal).

33. See Gary L. Francione, *Animals, Property and the Law* (1995), at 123.

34. Frank R. Ascione, "Children Who Are Cruel to Animals: A Review of Research and Implications for Developmental Psychopathology," 6 *Anthrozoos* 226, 235 (1993).

35. Ibid., at 231.

36. Albert M. Drukteinis, "Contemporary Psychiatry: Serial Murder—The Heart of Darkness," 22 *Psychiatric Annals*, 532–538, at 532 (1992). In addition to a history of animal cruelty and abuse, children who became serial murderers universally have a history of other antisocial and unusual activities, such as destructive play, cruelty towards other children, a disregard for others, fire setting, theft and property destruction.

37. Ibid.

38. John Locke, *Some Thoughts Concerning Education*, ed. F. W. Garforth (Heinemann Educational Books, 1964[1693]), at 152.

39. Immanuel Kant, "Duties to Animals and Spirits," in *Animal Rights and Human Obligations*, ed. Tom Regan and Paul Singer (1976), at 122.

40. Thomas Aquinas, "Differences between Rational and Other Creatures," in *Animal Rights and Human Obligations,* supra note 39, at 56, 59.

41. Arthur Schopenhauer, "A Critique of Kant," in *Animal Rights and Human Obligations,* supra note 39, at 124, 125–126.

42. *Stephens v. State*, 3 So. 458, 459 (Miss. 1888).

43. See "Alaska: Hunting from Planes is Allowed," *N.Y. Times*, June 19, 2003, at A19.

44. See Wayne Pacelle, "Stacking the Hunt," *N.Y. Times*, Dec. 9, 2003, at A29.

45. Ibid.

46. 13 *Forest and Stream* (1880), at 1030.

47. 17 *Forest and Stream* (1881), at 186.

48. James A. Tober, *Who Owns the Wildlife?* (1981), at 71.

49. Jon M. Akers, "Arguments For and Against Initiative 655," available at http://www.secstate.wa.gov/vote96/measures/i655.htm, cited by Daniel M. Warner, "Environmental Endgame: Destruction for Amusement and a Sustainable Civilization," 9 *S.C. Environ. L. J.*, at 1, 53 (2000).

50. Typical of advice given to hunters on the use of decoys is as follows:

Before you set your decoys out onto a likely field, you should ask yourself, what is your objective? The answer should be, to trick a goose, a pair of geese or a small family of geese to break away from the oncoming flock and get closer to your hiding place and give you an opportunity to shoot your gun. Hunting is about OPPORTUNITIES! By setting out a good spread of decoys in a field that the geese like and by being concealed, you should get 3 to 5 opportunities each morning to harvest Canada geese and 3 to 7 opportunities to get some snow geese. The reason you would get more opportunities to get snow geese is, there are more of them! If your hunting party of 4 gets 3 opportunities to get some Canada's and shoot well, you would end up with 6 to 8 geese each time out. That is a great hunt!

How many decoys do I need? After hunting geese for 35 years, I am convinced that less is better than more. Geese have become very wary and are hard to fool. Canada geese see spreads of 200 in every field while snows see 500 in most fields. Every field looks the same and the geese are not fooled. In recent years, 50 of my most successful goose hunts have been using less than 48 goose decoys. I had some great hunts using 0 decoys because the snow geese knew we were using phony geese to try to kill them. We stayed in the same field with great concealment and "smoked the geese" without using a decoy! (www.eHuntingCentral.com)

51. "The Archery Fever Is Indeed Upon Us," 13 *Forest And Stream* (1879), at 708.

52. "Hunting with the Bow," 13 *Forest And Stream* (1879), at 837.

53. Johan Huizinga, *Homo Ludens: A Study of the Play Element in Culture* (1950). According to Huizinga, first there is the voluntary nature of the activity. Second, play defines its own, specialized domain: "It is rather a stepping out of 'real' life into a temporary sphere with a disposition of its own. . . . It interpolates itself as a temporary activity satisfying in itself and ending there (8–9). Third, play is distinct in location and duration: "It is 'played out' within certain limits of time and place. It contains its own course and meaning" (9). That is, play has an internal structure that is characterized by "repetition and alteration" (9–10). Fourth, there is a special temporary and spatial domain in sport characterized by "an absolute and peculiar order" (10). That is, the game "creates order, *is* order. Into an imperfect world and into the confusion of life it brings a temporary, a limited perfection. The least deviation from it 'spoils the game'" (10, emphasis in original). Fifth, there is an element of tension or doubt:

> Tension means uncertainty, chanciness; a striving to decide the issue and so end it. The player wants something to "go", to "come off"; he wants to "succeed" by his own exertions. . . . It is this element of tension and solution that governs all solitary games of skill and application such as puzzles. . . . Though play as such is outside the range of good and bad, the element of tension imparts to it a certain ethical value in so far as it means a testing of the player's prowess: his courage, tenancity, resources. (10–11)

54. Aristotle, *Nicomachean Ethics,* at 1:1094b.

55. See Thomas Lund, "Nineteenth Century Wildlife Law: A Case Study of Elite Influence," 33 *Arizona State Law Journal* 936, 945 (2001).

56. 57 *Forest and Stream,* Nov. 23, 1901, at 53.

57. 44 *Forest and Stream* (1895), at 121.

58. 3 *Forest and Stream* (1875), at 41.

59. Dan L. Flores and Eric G. Bolen, "Gazing Across the Gulf: Environmental History and American Wildlife Ecology, Special Symposium—Wildlife and American Wildlife History: Insights from the Past," in *Transactions of the Fifty-seventh North American Wildlife and Natural Resources Conference,* at 701, 703–704 (1992).

60. "Sportsman or Pet-Hunter," *The Rod and The Gun,* Nov. 20, 1875, at 114.

61. *American Sportsman,* Feb. 6, 1875, at 299 (letter).

62. "Illegal Transportation of Game," *American Sportsman,* Jan. 10, 1874, at 232.

63. 7 *Forest and Stream* (1876), at 88 (letter).

64. "Protection of Large Game," 18 *Forest and Stream* (1882), at 63.

65. 42 *Forest and Stream* (1894), at 89.

66. See Thomas Lund, supra note 55, at 956.

67. Robert Doherty, *Disputed Waters* (1990), at 49.

68. See Thomas Lund, supra note 55, at 953. Before refrigeration, those who hunted as marketers favored winter taking so that they could easily preserve their stock in trade, and accordingly the hunting lobby pushed for declaring hunting closed in the winter.

69. 35 *Forest and Stream* (1890), at 225.

70. See Title 14 *California Code of Regulations,* §275.5.

71. See, e.g., Title 14 *California Code of Regulations,* §311(h).

72. See, e.g., Title 14 *California Code of Regulations,* §251.

73. See, e.g., Title 14 *California Code of Regulations,* §263.

74. See, e.g., Title 14 *California Code of Regulations,* §265.

75. See, e.g., Title 14 *California Code of Regulations,* §353.

76. See, e.g., Title 14 *California Code of Regulations,* §311.

77. See Thomas Lund, supra note 55, at 980.

78. Federal Air in Wildlife-Restoration (Pittman-Robertson) Act, ch. 899, §§ 1, 3, 50 Stat. 917 (1937).

79. "It was the hunter who applied the political pressure enabling earmarked license funds for the operations of official state resource agencies. The same political force caused the enactment of the Pittman-Robertson and Dingell-Johnson Acts." *Report of the 56th Convention of the Int'l Ass'n of Game, Fish and Conservation Comm'rs* 74 (1966) (Remarks of T. Kimball).

80. See Thomas Lund, supra note 55, at 962.

81. For further practical rules of thumb, See *All Outdoors* ("Dedicated to the enjoyment of Indiana's natural resources"), available at http://bayoubill.com/archives/2003/wildturkeysafety.html

82. My focus in this paper pertains to agonistic sports—that is, competitive sports. I have no objection to noncompetitive sports, such as scuba diving, skiing, rollerblading, being called sports. These noncompetitive sports are often solitary activities and, as such, lack many of the features applicable to agonistic sports.

83. Bullfighters attract the bull with their scarlet capes, and use tiny steel points to which are attached many colored ribbons or papers, which are stuck in the fleshy portion of the bull's neck by the *banderilleros,* who await the bull's coming in the center of the ring, facing him with arms extended. This and other tricks, such as *el salto de la garrocha,* have as their object to weaken the enormous strength of the bull, so as to render possible and less dangerous the work of the *matador.* When the presiding officer gives the signal for the death of the bull, the *matador* draws near the bull with the *muleta* in his left hand and the sword in his right hand; he calls the bull to him, or throws himself upon him, and plunges the sword into the neck of the bull. If he strikes him in the nape of the neck, killing him instantly, it is called *descabellar,* but if the bull is simply wounded the *puntillero* puts an end to his life with a dagger. The music now strikes up, while two little mules, richly caparisoned, drag out the bull and the dead horses. This is repeated again and again, the number of bulls being usually eight for each *corrida.*

The authorities of the Catholic Church have often condemned bull-fighting. St. Pius V (1 November, 1567, Const. "De salute") prohibited this form of amusement everywhere, threatening with many penalties the princes who countenanced it, as well as the performers and spectators, especially clergymen and religious. See *The Catholic Encyclopedia, Volume III* (Robert Appleton, 1908). The following account of bullfighting illustrates the extreme asymmetry of the power between the matador and the bull, and the cruelty of the techniques employed:

The ceremony begins punctually with a parade of participants around the ring. Then the trumpet sounds, the "Gate of Fear" opens, and the leading player—"el toro"—thunders in. An angry half-ton animal is an awesome sight even from the cheap seats.

The fight is divided into three acts. Act I is designed to size up the bull and wear him down. The matador (from the word matar—to kill), with help from his assistants, attracts the bull with the shake of the cape, then directs the bull past his body, as close as his bravery allows. After a few passes, the picadors enter, mounted on horseback, to spear the powerful swollen lump of muscle at the back of the bull's neck. This lowers the bull's head and weakens the thrust of his horns. (In the 19th century horses had no protective pads and were often killed.)

In Act II, the matador's assistants ("banderilleros") continue to enrage and weaken the bull. The unarmed banderillero charges the charging bull, and leaping acrobatically across the bull's path, plunges brightly colored, barbed sticks into the bull's vital neck muscle.

After a short intermission during which the matador may, according to tradition, ask permission to kill the bull and dedicate the kill to someone in the crowd, the final, lethal Act III begins.

The matador tries to dominate and tire the bull with hypnotic capework. A good pass is when the matador stands completely still while the bull charges past. Then the matador thrusts a sword between the animal's shoulder blades for the kill. A quick kill is not always easy, and the matador may have to make several bloody thrusts before the sword stays in.

Throughout the fight, the crowd shows its approval or impatience. Shouts of "Ole!" or "Torero!" mean they like what they see—whistling or rhythmic hand-clapping greets cowardice and incompetence.

You're not likely to see much human blood spilled. In 200 years of bullfighting in Sevilla, only thirty fighters have died (and only one was actually a matador). If a bull does kill a fighter, the next matador comes to kill him. Even the bull's mother is killed since the evil qualities are assumed to come from the mother.

After an exceptional fight, the crowd may wave white handkerchiefs to ask that the matador be awarded the bull's ear or tail. A brave bull, though dead, gets a victory lap from the mule team on his way to the slaughterhouse. Then the trumpet sounds, and a new bull barges in to face a fresh matador. A typical bullfight lasts about three hours and consists of six separate fights—three matadors fighting two bulls each.

For a closer look at bullfighting by an American aficionado, read Ernest Hemingway's classic "Death in the Afternoon." (Rick Steves, *Bullfighting: Culture or Cruelty?*, available at http://www.ricksteves.com/news/archive/0799bullfight.htm)

84. Other activities, such as practicing golf putts, target practice, or practicing pitching a ball, or playing catch—also do not count as "sports" because they are merely exercises or practicing of technique that might go into mastering a sport. Nor do such activities have "rules" or a structured beginning, middle, and end, and there is no winner or loser.

85. Plato said "God alone is worthy of supreme seriousness, but man is God's plaything and that is the best part of him. Therefore every man and woman should live life accordingly, and play the noblest games and be of another mind from what they are at present" (*Laws*, at 803c–d).

86. W. A. Baillie-Grohman and F. Baillie-Grohman, eds., *The Master of Game* (New York: Duffield, 1909), at xxiii.

87. Self-esteem comes into the picture when a youngster of otherwise ordinary and unexciting circumstances can prove himself or herself by excelling in sports. For a brief time, he or she can be an object of admiration and esteem of those who see his prowess.

88. Aristotle said: "The man, then, who faces and who fears the right things and from the right motive, in the right way and at the right time, and who feels confidence under

corresponding conditions, is brave; for the brave man feels and acts according to the merits of the case and in whatever way the rule directs" (*Nicomachean Ethics,* 1115b15).

89. Aristotle observed: "People seem to seek honor in order to convince themselves of their own goodness; at any rate it is by intelligent men, and in a community where they are known, and for their goodness, that they seek to be honored; so evidently in their view goodness is superior to honor" (*Nicomachean Ethics,* 1095b27–30).

90. Arthur Leff also refers to this as a formal quality of sport: "The players in any game are treated for purposes of the game as formally identical. They have each the same access to the field and the mechanisms of play, and the same formal entitlements." Arthur A. Leff, "Law and," 87 *Yale Law Journal* 989, 999–1000 (1978).

91. See Fund for Animals, "Hunting Is Immoral," in *An Overview of Killing for Sport* (1997), available at http://www.fund.org/facts/overview.html.

92. See Peter J. Arnold, "Three Approaches Toward an Understanding of Sportsmanship," 10 *Journal of the Philosophy of Sport* 61–70, 62 (1984).

93. See John Balzar, "Creatures Great and—Equal?," *L.A. Times,* Dec. 25, 1993, at Al.

94. Albert Schweitzer, *Out of My Life and Thought* trans. C. T. Campion, chapter 13, at 188 (London: G. Allen & Unwin, Ltd. 1933).

95. Albert Schweitzer, *Philosophy of Civilization: Civilization and Ethics,* trans. John Naish (London: A. and C. Black, 1923), at 254.

96. Albert Schweitzer, *The Animal World of Albert Schweitzer,* ed. Charles R. Joy (Boston: Beacon, 1950), at 169.

PART VIII

Enhancement and Improvement

As mentioned in part II, competitors are often grouped by characteristics such as age, weight, and gender to promote fairness. These groupings still occasionally result in lopsided outcomes when some participants have far superior combinations of natural ability and training. As long as the rules of preparation and engagement are followed, we cannot claim the winners of a blow-out are cheaters nor can we call the competition unfair—or can we? What happens when one side, which is otherwise evenly matched with another, employs a legal but innovative preparation or uses a piece of equipment that confers a significant advantage? This is where the line between fair improvement and unfair enhancement must be drawn.

The difficulty in drawing this line is demonstrated by two examples from the locker room of the American football team, the New England Patriots. Putting the particular facts of each case aside (partly because they are still disputed), consider the general premises. The first is videotaping an opposing team's coach (2007 "Spygate"). Filming the signals given by an opposing team's coach to predict coming plays is a legal activity with limitations. Those limits include not watching the footage during the game in which it is taped, and not filming an opposing team from the opposing team's own sideline. At some point in the sport's development, rule-makers decided that teams should be allowed to attempt to film the other team's signals and later try to link whatever they caught on tape to the corresponding plays, but that allowing such filming from too short a distance would unreasonably diminish the challenge. Ignoring the limitations by filming from the same sideline violates the fairness contract to which both teams are parties, regardless of whether the filming team intended to cheat or merely to find an edge. In this case, the particulars of how coach-filming fits within the game's constitution were pre-established. Assuming the Patriots did film from the same sideline, according to the rules this was not fair in terms of improvement: it was unfair enhancement.

The second example concerns the inflation level of balls used in games (2015 "Deflategate"). Since 2006, each team on offense uses its own footballs that must be inflated between 12.5 and 13.5 psi. However, the temperature of the environment in which the inflation level is measured was not specified in the rules. Thus, if ball pressure is measured in a hot room before a game, ball pressure will drop on a cold field. Slightly deflated footballs are easier to throw and catch. A team that intentionally measures ball pressure in a hot room so that it might deflate on the field is not necessarily acting outside the explicit rules. Is this an innovation that is consistent with the spirit of the game, or is it a trick that had yet to be tried that now warrants an official rule change? In other words, improvement or unfair enhancement?

To answer questions like this, Thomas Murray, in chapter 23, says we should consider continuity and equal opportunity. Continuity concerns the change's performance consequences. How significant an edge does a slightly deflated football grant? If team A uses it and team B does not, how much do the odds shift in A's favor? If this practice becomes accepted, does it lead to an arms race in which balls are measured in boiler rooms and become floppy bags on the field, thus transforming the entire appearance and strategy of football? The rules of sports should and do evolve to enhance entertainment value and capitalize on innovative strategies, but the consequences of drastic changes are hard to predict. Often, the best adaptations are incremental so they can be redirected or reversed as necessary.

Equal opportunity concerns each team's access to the innovation. Imagine a near future in which gene transfer for pain coping is proved safe and it allows athletes to endure greater physical strain. Soccer players can now sprint at top speed 25 percent longer on average and go whole games without "flopping"—that is, feigning injury to take a break and emphasize an opponent's questionable contact. This might be a tool that would enable a beneficial evolution for the game. However, if the gene-transfer procedure costs an outrageous amount of money, or is only effective in a small subset of the genetic population, then the technology would not be accessible to all players or soccer teams. This would then confer a significant advantage on a few, leading to unfair enhancement.

How are innovations that are only accessible to the rich any less fair than natural conditions that lead to advantages for one athlete or team? For example, teams in higher geographic locations train with thinner air and can achieve greater cardiovascular fitness than their opponents closer to sea level. It would be unreasonable to require all teams to practice within a narrow elevation range. Teams would have to relocate, which would be costly and cause them to lose connection to their home communities. Even if all competitors train equally, some will still have genetically higher peak oxygen uptake (VO2 max) providing greater endurance. It would be unreasonable to disqualify an athlete on the grounds that her VO2 max was abnormally high. The difference between examples like these and limited-access innovations is that natural advantages are often beyond control while tools and techniques are within our control.

Sports participants and spectators expect and appreciate a certain amount of fate. When the lot has been cast and one team's advantage cannot be ascribed to wrongdoing or even just intentional actions, we accept it. These circumstances carry lessons that assist in life: no matter how hard I work, sometimes another will win. I may not always be able to come out on top, but I can learn how to accept my loss and appreciate the intrinsic value of my effort. And occasionally, despite incredible odds, the natural underdog claims victory. This story line undergirds some of our greatest sport memories. Tools and techniques, unlike genetic predisposition and geographic location, can be controlled to promote fairness. Perhaps the best employment of hypoxic environments, as described by Sigmund Loland and Arthur Caplan in chapter 26, is to compensate for natural altitude differences. Allowing only teams that train below a threshold elevation to use hypoxic chambers might be a reasonable rectification of an unfair natural advantage. But this allowance would have to be based on sophisticated research regarding the technology's impact on performance as compared with the impact of altitude on cardiovascular fitness.

Consider each of the techniques and tools described in this chapter—from anabolic steroids, to carbon fiber Cheetah blades, to human growth hormones, to ice vests—in terms of the following questions: Is the innovation safe? How much does the innovation increase the user's ability? Do all participants have access to the innovation? Should the innovation only be available to a specific set of athletes, and if so, why? If the innovation is safe and accessible, does it make the sport more enjoyable for both the fans and the athletes? Faster, stronger, and bigger sports are not necessarily more fun or better sports. If fans cannot relate in any way to the performance of athletes, will they remain fans of sport or become voyeuristic admirers of human engineering? Using these questions to guide the development of safe, fair, and honest sports helps ensure that sports reflect and reinforce the strongest values of the communities in which sports are played. And don't worry, ethical sports can and will continue to set new performance records that give the best reasons to fans to paint their faces, argue on the radio with one another, and bond with their families and coworkers over the teams and players they love and hate.

23 Sports Enhancement

■ THOMAS H. MURRAY

■ FRAMING THE ISSUE

Spring in America brings flowers, sweet warm breezes, and the thwack of a bat striking a baseball. But swings that would once have resulted in a fly ball to the warning track may now, with chemical assistance, deposit the ball in the bleachers. The Mitchell Report, an early Christmas present to baseball fans released in December 2007, confirmed that a number of Major League players have used performance-enhancing drugs.

Athletes using drugs to boost performance is hardly news. Anabolic steroids and stimulants have plagued the Olympics for decades. Professional cycling—including its premier event, the Tour de France—nearly collapsed over reports that drug use was widespread. The 2006 victor, American Floyd Landis, had his title stripped because of evidence that his testosterone levels were abnormally high, an indication that he may have boosted them with injections or patches.

An intriguing split has emerged in the public reaction to baseball's drug problem. For some, there's not much to think about: the rules forbid performance-enhancing drugs; breaking the rules is cheating; cheating is wrong—end of story.

Others are not so sure. They raise a variety of objections. Some claim that athletes are just giving people what they want: fans enjoy home runs, athletes who take drugs such as anabolic steroids hit more home runs, what's all the fuss? Of course the fans in the Roman Coliseum may have loved to see lions tearing the arms off Christians or gladiators hacking each other to death. So "what the fans desire" is not an ethically robust defense.

Others say that athletes should be free to do whatever they want to their own bodies. From this point of view, each athlete is best situated to balance the risks and benefits of using performance-enhancing drugs. The principal flaw in this argument is that it fails to understand that what one athlete chooses to do affects everyone in the competition. The athletes I know all crave a level playing field. If my competition is gaining an edge by using a drug that tilts the field in their favor, then their choice pressures me to do the same. Otherwise I may end up losing to someone who is less talented or less dedicated.

▦ WHY PROHIBIT PERFORMANCE ENHANCERS?

A more subtle and serious question is why we prohibit certain performance aids in the first place. Sure, the rules of sport may ban anabolic steroids or synthetic hormones like human growth hormone (HGH), believed to enhance strength, and erythropoietin (EPO), which stimulates the production of oxygen-carrying cells in the blood and thereby increases endurance (see the following table for a list and history of such substances). But what makes those means for improving performance bad while other things, from better equipment to more sophisticated training methods or nutrition regimens, are perfectly okay? What makes the use of performance-enhancing drugs in sport an ethical problem?

Sport Enhancement: Past, Present, and Future

Product	Purpose
Anabolic steroids	Artificial substances related to male sex hormones that are used to build muscles.
Stimulants	Substances such as amphetamines that act on the brain to increase alertness.
Human growth hormone (HGH)	Believed to enhance strength.
Erythropoietin (EPO)	Believed to increase endurance.
Tetrahydrogestrinone (THG); "the clear"	An anabolic steroid once undetectable by anti-doping labs.
Cheetahs	Carbon fiber blades that replace the amputated lower legs of Oscar Pistorius, a South African sprinter.
Gene therapy	Genetic manipulation may one day improve athletic ability.

One common place to look for a response is the distinction between therapy and enhancement. Therapy is good, enhancement is suspect, right? Unfortunately, it's not so clear or simple. The tools biomedical research creates to treat disease are completely indifferent to the fluid and sometimes disputed boundary between therapy and enhancement. A product like synthetic HGH is in certain cases like insulin for people with diabetes. For children who can't make enough HGH themselves, the synthetic form can help replace what is missing. On the other hand, healthy athletes can use HGH to try to build larger-than-normal muscles. The HGH molecule neither knows nor cares whether it is helping a child inch towards normality or making a hugely muscled athlete even more muscular. Somewhere between the two, we've crossed the border from the friendly, familiar land of therapy to the unmapped, vaguely ominous terrain of enhancement.

Nor is biomedical enhancement obviously bad in all circumstances. Imagine a relatively innocuous drug that steadied a neurosurgeon's hand so that her patients healed more rapidly with fewer complications: the ethics of that sort of performance enhancement would focus on whether neurosurgeons are ethically *required* to use the drug.

So the mere fact that some drugs enhance performance isn't sufficient to decide whether they're good, bad, or otherwise. The context matters. If it's wrong for athletes to use performance-enhancing drugs, there must be something about sport that makes it so. I'll discuss three characteristics of sport that provide the context and plausible justification for banning such drugs:

- The significance of rules in sport
- Natural talents and their perfection
- The prospect of an "arms race" in sport, ending in the triumph of the so-called performance principle.

▪ THE SIGNIFICANCE OF RULES IN SPORT

Every sport has rules (with the possible exception of "Calvinball" from the "Calvin and Hobbes" comic strip, where the only rule is that you can't use the same rule twice). The rules in each sport in effect determine which characteristics among all possible sources of difference influence who wins and who loses. Team A may be wealthier than Team B, but neither is allowed to bribe the umpire—a competition that Team A is likely to win.

Improvements in equipment can transform a sport. When pole-vaulters traded in their wooden poles for fiberglass ones, they were able to leap much higher. Swimmers now have suits available that allow them to slip through the water with a minimum of resistance. Typically, sport deals with innovations in equipment in one of three ways.

Sometimes it embraces the new technology, as track and field did with fiberglass poles. The critical factors here were continuity and equal opportunity. Continuity was assured because the poles still required the same skills from pole-vaulters, such as speed down the runway, strength, and agility. Equal opportunity meant that all athletes had to have access to fiberglass poles. One controversy over the new slippery swimsuits is whether all competitors will be able to use them. Otherwise, an inferior swimmer wearing the suit might beat out the most talented one. Technology would trump ability.

Sometimes a sport accepts technological innovation as a part of the competition. Skiers use special combinations of waxes, bobsled teams compete to come up with the fastest sled. Even then, sports make and enforce rules. Athletes can compete on technology only up to a certain point: no jet engines allowed on bobsleds, for instance.

Many innovations that would surely improve performance are banned outright. An athlete who showed up for the Boston Marathon wearing Rollerblades would be wheeled right off the start line. The marathon is for runners, not skaters. (Of course, one could try to organize a sport where Rollerbladers competed to cover the same course as the Boston Marathon; but that would be a different sport.) The Tour de France insists on a minimum weight for all bikes. As every road cyclist knows, the lighter the bike, the less energy required to climb the mountains that help make the Tour so famous and so difficult. This rule accomplishes two things. It neutralizes one advantage that the wealthiest or best-supported cyclists would gain by using fabulously expensive, custom-made parts of exotic metals or synthetics. It also protects cyclists against the temptation to shave every last gram off of critical components, increasing the risk of catastrophic failures when the bike is screaming down a switchback mountain road at 100 kilometers an hour.

Rules are changed at times to preserve a sport. Basketball banned goaltending—swatting the ball away just as it was about to go into the hoop—when players became so tall and athletic that they could stand by the basket and prevent most shots from having a chance to go in. Later, basketball created the three-second lane to keep offensive players from camping under the basket, and then the three-point line to reward good shooting and force defenders to venture out to the perimeter. These changes opened the game up for rapid cuts, screens, and sharp passes once again.

■ THE POINT OF SPORT: NATURAL TALENTS AND THEIR PERFECTION?

In most sports—including all Olympic events—using performance-enhancing drugs is against the rules. But why? On what grounds does Nordic skiing ban EPO? What gives baseball the right to prohibit anabolic steroids?

If the point of an endurance sport like crosscountry skiing is to see how rapidly you can cover long distances without collapsing, then anything that allows you to go harder and longer would improve your performance, including EPO. Why doesn't Nordic skiing welcome EPO the same way it welcomes synthetic fiber garments and faster skis? To some critics, Nordic skiing is being inconsistent. If the point of the sport is to go faster, then EPO should be treated just like better ski waxes, the critic may argue.

But most aficionados of sport persist in seeing a difference between using drugs to enhance performance and employing other means to the same end. Intensive training, smart tactics, dedication, studying your competitors—all these can improve one's performance and all of them are regarded as admirable ways of perfecting your natural talents.

Those natural talents are, of course, allotted in vastly uneven measure among us all. Some commentators see this as a form of injustice and performance-enhancing drugs as a remedy for nature's cruel inequalities. Why should the race go to the swift? What if I'm a clumsy, slow-footed slogger? Shouldn't I have an equal opportunity to get to the finish line first? If anabolic steroids or stimulants can balance out the uneven shares of talent given by birth, shouldn't I be allowed to use them? Then victory will belong to the one who trains the hardest perhaps, talent be damned—or neutralized, at least.

When performance-enhancing drugs have the power to overcome differences in natural talents and the willingness to sacrifice and persevere in the quest to perfect those talents, we cannot avoid confronting the question: What do we value in sport? Emerging technologies—from hypoxic chambers and carbon fiber prostheses to genetic manipulation—will force us consider what, after all, is the point of sport?

■ SPORT, THE "ARMS RACE," AND THE TRIUMPH OF THE PERFORMANCE PRINCIPLE

When Hastings Center researchers spoke with athletes in the early 1980s about performance-enhancing drugs in sport, they described an intensely competitive world in which tiny differences—fractions of a second in the hundred meter sprint, inches in the discus or shot put—separated the victor from the vanquished. Where a drug could give even a small edge, some athletes would be tempted to use it. And, just as significant, every other athlete in that event would feel enormous pressure to join in. The dynamics of drugs in sport bear more than a superficial resemblance to an arms race: each party drives the other further, lest either be left behind.

Critics of doping control sometimes argue that sport would be better off if athletes were just allowed to take whatever drugs they wanted. Fans would get more dramatic performances. The playing field would be leveled (because every athlete could use the same drugs). We could do away with the cat and mouse game between drug users and testers, saving money and aggravation.

These purported advantages would come at some cost. Sports that revere records and historical comparisons (think of baseball and home runs) would become unmoored by drug-aided athletes obliterating old standards. Athletes, caught in the sport arms race, would be pressed to take more and more drugs, in ever wilder combinations and at increasingly higher doses. While the scientific evidence that the drugs athletes use are harmful is often less conclusive than opponents of drugs in sport portray, that's little reason for comfort.

Athletes often take drugs at multiples of the dosages that have been studied for their benefits and risks, and they take drugs in bizarre combinations. It's unlikely that any research ethics committee would permit a scientifically controlled study that administered such large amounts and odd mixtures of drugs. So, yes, we should be concerned about risks to athletes, and we should perform whatever epidemiological and observational studies are possible under the circumstances. The drug race in sport has the potential to create a slowmotion public health catastrophe. Finally, we may lose whatever is most graceful, beautiful, and admirable about sport, which brings us back to the quintessential American game, baseball.

■ EMERGING CHALLENGES

When I was a kid my father, born in 1917, gave me the baseball glove he'd used as a young man. It was indeed a glove: leather, rather stiff, with short fingers and no webbing. I might has well have worn an oven mitt. Eventually I acquired a fielder's glove more suited for baseball in the 1950s and '60s. The new glove certainly enhanced my performance as an infielder—though not by much, at least not until my late teens when my scrawny body acquired a little muscle and coordination.

Modern baseball gloves—supple, long-fingered, webbed—allow fielders to snatch line drives and scoop up hard grounders with relative ease. They improve performance, no doubt. But infielders still have to get to the ball, catch it, and throw accurately to the base. They need quickness, agility, strength, and extraordinarily swift reaction times, qualities that great infielders have always possessed. This is one technology that has enriched rather than detracted from sport.

Sport as we know it faces emerging challenges on many fronts. To mention just a few:

- Will the underworld of clandestine drug developers, promoters, and enablers overwhelm the drug control apparatus? The synthetic anabolic steroid tetrahydrogestrinone (THG)—now infamous as "the clear" peddled by the Balco lab—was created by an independent chemist. Its selling point was that the processes by which samples were prepared for testing by the anti-doping labs made the drug undetectable. The lab got its hands on a sample of THG, deciphered its chemistry, and adapted their procedures to detect it. Balco was exposed and the chemist went to prison. Is this evidence that doping control can work effectively? Or does it show that ultimately the effort will be futile because other chemists, other labs, and more willing athletes will inevitably pop up?
- Hypoxic chambers permit athletes to mimic what very few would otherwise be able to find: a geography that would enable them to train at low altitude (and therefore train at maximum intensity) but "live" at high altitude, as simulated by the hypoxic chamber (and thereby gain the increased endurance that some athletes develop from spending most of their time in an oxygen-depleted environment). Oscar Pistorius, a South African sprinter, saw both of his lower legs amputated. Yet he can achieve remarkable times in the 400 meters thanks to his talent, his perseverance—and a pair of carbon fiber blades known as Cheetahs. Scientists disagree over whether Cheetahs are more efficient than our flimsy biological equipment. Pistorius wants to run in the Olympics, not the Special Olympics. Technologies like hypoxic chambers and carbon fiber limbs are harbingers of what sport will confront in the future. They will compel us to ask again and again, What is the meaning of this sport? What counts as "fair" competition? What, in

the end, should mark the difference between excellent performance and lesser performances—or something else entirely, like the Rollerblading marathoner?

- A huge volume of hot air is being created around the prospect that athletes will be genetically enhanced. The same techniques being perfected for gene therapy may be used to give athletes a genetically programmed boost. Progress in gene therapy is in a relatively early stage of development, but the doping control agencies have realized that they need to engage the interest and creativity of top scientists, who are now working on a variety of promising strategies to detect gene doping.

▪ CHALLENGES FOR POLICYMAKERS AND JOURNALISTS

For policymakers, two major categories of challenges emerge. The first set of challenges have to do with research. For decades the competition between drug-using athletes and their enablers on the one hand and antidoping workers on the other was uneven. The labs, for example, had to scramble to support their research into new substances and new analytic methods. Dopers could make plenty of money supplying athletes seeking a competitive advantage. Finally, with the advent of new agencies such as the World Anti-Doping Agency (WADA) and the United States Anti-Doping Agency (USADA), a small but reliable stream of funds for research became available. With better funding, much more could be done.

It could be very helpful to learn more about the culture of sports doping—why athletes dope, who influences their decisions, and the like. It would be equally interesting to do research to develop alternative strategies to encourage clean sport and discourage doping. Some promising ideas are being pursued, like the commitment of Team Slipstream (now Team Garmin-Chipotle) and Team High Road (now Team Columbia), professional cycling teams, to test each of their riders regularly. In addition to catching possible drug users, the routine tests establish physiological baselines; sharp departures from them could signal pharmacological tampering and may also prove useful in monitoring the cyclists' health. Other strategies should be encouraged and studied.

I pointed out earlier the difficulty of studying the risks when athletes use drugs in high dosages and novel combinations. We may not be able to construct an ethical clinical trial, but scientists can gather helpful data with other methodologies. Such research should be encouraged and funded.

The second major challenge is nontherapeutic drug use among adolescents. Various reports disagree about the percentages of teens using drugs such as anabolic steroids, but study after study shows alarming high levels of use. The research also reveals that young people may be more eager for the cosmetic effect—looking "buff" on steroids or HGH—than for any impact on performance. How to make such drugs less available and less attractive to adolescents is a significant policy challenge.

Finally, a word of appreciation for journalists, especially sports columnists: My admittedly unscientific impression is that the items in the daily newspaper most likely to be devoted to philosophy are the columns in the sports section. There, grand debates unfold over matters of justice and over the meaning of sport. Should Barry Bonds' home run totals be marked with an asterisk because they may have been drug-assisted? Should he be elected to the Baseball Hall of Fame in Cooperstown? What's fair? What after all is valued most in baseball? What makes it fascinating, regularly frustrating, and occasionally transcendently beautiful? A steady tattoo of monstrous home runs? Or, like the greatest wines, a diverse mix of elements, somehow blending into a harmonious whole?

There are wide and vigorous disagreements on just about every matter I've touched. Let the dialogue flourish, and let the games begin.

◾ RESOURCES

◾ WEB SITES

- www.wada-ama.org—The World Anti-Doping Agency. Includes the complete World Anti-Doping Code, resources, and news.
- www.usantidoping.org—The U.S. Anti-Doping Agency. Includes tools for athletes, resources, and a press kit.

◾ RECENT NEWS

- Joshua Robinson and Alan Schwarz, "Olympic Dream Stays Alive, on Synthetic Legs," *New York Times*, May 17, 2008.
- Duff Wilson and Michael S. Schmidt, "Report Ties Star Players to Baseball's 'Steroids Era,'" *New York Times*, December 14, 2007.
- Michael Hiltzik, "She Did It, But All Will Pay," *Los Angeles Times*, October 6, 2007.
- Randal C. Picker, "Competitive Disadvantage: As Contests Move from Playing Field to Laboratory, Athletes, Sports Would Be Hurt," *Chicago Tribune*, August 22, 2007.
- Joel Garreau, "Is it Time for a Flex Plan?: Techno-Athletes Change the Definition of Natural," *Washington Post*, August 1, 2007.

◾ FURTHER READING

- Thomas H. Murray, "Enhancement," in *The Oxford Handbook of Bioethics*, ed. Bonnie Steinbock (Oxford University Press, 2007).
- Sarah Glazer, *Enhancement* (The Hastings Center, 2006). Primer available at www.the-hastingscenter.org/uploadedFiles/Publications/enh ancement%20primer.pdf.
- Thomas H. Murray, "Gene Doping and Olympic Sport," *Play True*, Spring 2005.

- Don H. Catlin and Thomas H. Murray, "Performance-Enhancing Drugs, Fair Competition, and Olympic Sport." *Journal of the American Medical Association*, July 1996.
- Norman Fost, "Banning Drugs in Sports: A Skeptical View," *Hastings Center Report* July–August 1986.

24 Performance-Enhancing Substances in Sports

A Review of the Literature

■ AMIT MOMAYA, MARC FAWAL, AND REED ESTES

■ 1. INTRODUCTION

Performance-enhancing substances (PESs) have become widespread and a serious issue in sports. Often referred to as "doping," the use of PESs refers to the use or manipulation of substances, synthetic or autologous, with the intention of altering sports performance. Greater media coverage coupled with improved and more frequent testing has brought further attention to the use of PESs by professional athletes over the past few decades. However, athletes at all levels, seeking to attain the highest performance, continue to use PESs despite the potential health risks and penalties [1, 2]. Physicians need to be aware of the prevalence of PESs in sports and their potential deleterious effects. With greater understanding, physicians can better educate athletes on PESs and curb the use of substances that may ultimately harm the athlete.

The concept of PESs has been a part of competitive sport since its inception. Both Greek athletes competing in the ancient Olympics and Roman gladiators used certain wines, herbal teas, and mushrooms to help enhance performance [1, 2]. Since then, PESs have evolved with advances in pharmaceutics. In 1998, a large number of PESs were found during a raid at the Tour de France. This event triggered the creation of the World Anti-Doping Agency (WADA) in 1999 as an independent international agency with the mission to create a doping-free sporting environment. WADA labels a substance as banned in competition if two of the following three criteria are met: (1) enhances sport performance, (2) poses a risk to health, or (3) violates the spirit of the sport [3]. WADA publishes the World Anti-Doping Code, which has been adopted by several sporting organizations across the world, including the International Olympic Committee (IOC). WADA works closely with smaller anti-doping agencies on several fronts, including the implementation of the code and accreditation of testing laboratories. Although WADA may establish guidelines for sanctions, the ultimate decision is left to the specific league in which the athlete participates.

In addition to the Tour de France, recent investigations surrounding Major League Baseball (MLB) have brought greater attention to PESs and drawn attention from the US Congress. The commissioner of the MLB appointed George Mitchell, a former Democratic senator, to investigate the use of PESs in the MLB. After a lengthy investigation, the Mitchell Report was released, which named 89 baseball players alleged to have used PESs [4]. Seeing this issue as a national health policy concern, the US government decided to hold congressional hearings, during which specific high-profile players were interrogated.

The purpose of this article is to summarize the prevalence of PESs among athletes, the physiology and effects of common PESs, and the evolution of drug testing (Table 24.1). Furthermore, we discuss ways to prevent PES use. PubMed searches were performed corresponding to each section in this manuscript with associated keywords such as "anabolic steroids" or "gene doping." An emphasis was placed on highlighting literature published within the last decade to provide readers with current, evidence-based medicine. The authors also cited articles based on the strength of the study design.

▪ 2. EPIDEMIOLOGY

Although numerous studies have attempted to determine the prevalence of PES use, much of the data are limited to self-reported surveys, which are subject to response error. Nonetheless, the overall incidence of PES use among athletes at all levels appears to be high. Current reported rates of PES use among athletes are variable and range from 5 to 31% [5–10].

Dietz et al. [11] conducted an anonymous questionnaire to gauge the rate of use of illicit or banned substances among triathletes in Germany. Among 2,987 respondents, 13.0% reported the use of illicit or banned substances to improve physical performance. Furthermore, the study also reported a 15.1% rate of cognitive doping—that is, the use of substances that enhance focus, learning performance, and memory.

Another study in Germany evaluated the rate of doping and illicit drug use by elite athletes and compared it with outcomes of official doping tests. The athletes were questioned using either an anonymous standardized questionnaire or interviewed using a randomized response technique. The authors reported a 6.8% doping rate, which is in stark contrast to the 0.81% positive test results from official doping tests conducted by the WADA and National Anti-Doping Agency (NADA) [12].

Buckman et al. [10] conducted a study on 234 male student athletes at one university to evaluate the risk profile of those who use PESs. The study based its definition of a PES on a published National Collegiate Athletic Association (NCAA) classification that included both licit and illicit substances. The study reported a 31% usage rate of PES in the year prior to the survey. Among those

TABLE 24.1. *Reference Guide to Performance-Enhancing Substances*

Performance-enhancing substance	Desired effects	Major adverse effects	Minor adverse effects	Status	Route of administration	Testing/detection method	Mechanism of action
Anabolic–androgenic steroids	Increase muscle size, strength, lean body mass; decrease body fat	Testicular atrophy, CV disease, atherosclerosis, myocardial disease, liver dysfunction, cancer	Acne, gynecomastia	Banned by IOC and all major sporting bodies	Oral, topical, injectable	Urine immunoassay, chromatography, mass spectrometry	Upregulation of genes responsible for muscle growth, counteracts catabolic effects of glucocorticoids
Creatine	Increase in strength, power output, sprint performance, total work to fatigue, peak force/power; decrease lactate threshold; increase weight and lean body mass	Heatstroke	Dehydration	Allowed	Oral	N/A	Provides an energy substrate to allow for contraction of skeletal muscle
Human growth hormone	May increase lean body mass and decrease fat mass	Carpal tunnel syndrome, pseudotumor cerebri, CV disease, hyperlipidemia, insulin resistance	Arthralgias	Banned by IOC and International Federations	Injectable	Recombinant hGH: naturally derived hGH ratio	Promotes growth through action of insulin-like growth factor-1, protein anabolism, lipolysis
Amphetamines/stimulants	Increase in alertness and metabolism; may increase strength, muscular power, speed, acceleration, aerobic power, anaerobic capacity, endurance	Arrhythmias, heat exhaustion, seizures, myocardial infarction, sudden death	Agitation, GI upset, nausea, headaches, insomnia, hallucinations	Banned by IOC, NCAA, NFL	Oral, injectable, inhalable	Urine quantitative analysis	Central nervous system stimulant through stimulation of norepinephrine

Substance	Effects	Side effects	Status	Route	Detection	Mechanism
Erythropoietin/ blood doping	Increase in oxygen-carrying capacity, endurance	Hypertension, myocardial infarction, pulmonary embolism, immune reaction	Banned by IOC and all major sporting bodies	Injectable	Athlete biologic passport (hemoglobin mass)	Stimulates increased production of erythrocytes leading to increased hematocrit and higher oxygen-carrying capacity
Beta-hydroxy-beta-methylbutyrate	May increase lean body mass, muscle strength, power; enhance recovery	Unknown	Allowed	Oral	N/A	Upregulation of mTOR/p70S6 K pathway, promoting protein synthesis and muscle hypertrophy, decreased proteolysis, decreased LDH production
Gene doping	Dependent on targeted protein	Immune reaction, cancer, overexpression of gene product, germ line modification	Banned by IOC	Injectable, inhalation	No WADA-approved detection methods exist	Transcription and production of specific targeted protein

using PESs, 31% reported using banned substances. The study concluded that those using PESs were more likely to engage in other substance use behaviors (e.g., binge drinking). The study cited the limited number of subjects as a potential weakness.

PES use has also been examined with respect to sex and sport by a recent NCAA survey study [13]. The percentage of female athletes who reported anabolic steroid use in the previous 12 months was 0.1% during the 2013 year compared with 0.7% of male athletes. Particular substances were found to be associated with certain men's sports: anabolic–androgenic steroids (AAS) with lacrosse (1.7%), American football (0.7%), and baseball (0.7%); human growth hormone (hGH) with baseball (1.3%) and lacrosse (1.1%); and creatine with wrestling (28.5%), baseball (28.1%), and American football (27.5%).

■ 3. SUBSTANCES

Commonly used PESs among athletes include AAS, hGH, creatine, erythropoietin (EPO), blood doping, amphetamines and stimulants, and beta-hydroxy-beta-methylbutyrate (HMB). Gene doping has also received concern recently as technology allows it to become more conceivable.

3.1. Anabolic–Androgenic Steroids

AAS have traditionally received the greatest attention among PESs in sports. Examples of AAS include testosterone, methyltestosterone, and danazol. A recent meta-analysis by Sagoe et al. [14] reported a global lifetime prevalence of the use of AAS of 6.4% for males and 1.6% for females. Moreover, the prevalence of AAS use was highest among recreational and competitive athletes, and the odds of AAS use increased by 91% with participation in at least one sport. The study also found that the prevalence of AAS use was slightly higher in the 2000s than in the 1990s. Even among adolescents, the rate of AAS use is high. In a questionnaire study of high school varsity football players in the USA, 6.3% reported that they were either current or former AAS users, with the average age at first use being 14 years [15].

Designer steroids have also played a greater role in sports medicine over the past two decades [16, 17]. These steroids are chemically modified from known banned anabolic steroids in an attempt to avoid detection. Tetrahy-drogestrinone (THG) has become one of the most popular and widely known designer steroids [14, 15].

Androstenedione, a precursor to testosterone, has also become popular, especially after MLB player Mark McGuire admitted to using it [18]. The mechanism of action is believed to be related to its degradation into testosterone.

3.1.1 Physiology

The human body naturally produces testosterone, an endogenous anabolic steroid responsible for male secondary sexual characteristics and muscle and bone metabolism. AAS are synthetic derivatives of testosterone. AAS bind to an androgen receptor (AR) in the cytoplasm of target tissues, triggering a molecular cascade that results in androgenic and anabolic effects similar to those caused by testosterone. Specifically, the AR is involved in the regulation of transcription of genes responsible for muscle growth. Furthermore, the enzyme 5-alpha-reductase plays a crucial role by converting AAS into dihydrotestosterone, which can also act on the AR. In addition, AAS displace cortisol from its receptors and thus counteract the catabolic effects of glucocorticoids [19].

3.1.2. Performance

Due to the lack of consistency with regard to dosing and methods in previous studies, it is difficult to compare clinical trials studying performance and AAS. Studies have shown that the main benefit of AAS on performance is related to increased muscle size, strength, and lean body mass [20–22].

Bhasin et al. [20] showed that men who took supra-physiologic doses of testosterone, coupled with exercise, increased fat-free mass and muscle size and strength. In another study, Giorgi et al. [22] randomly assigned 21 male weight training subjects to either a testosterone or a placebo group. Over a 12-week period, those in the testosterone group demonstrated significantly greater increases in muscle strength and circumference and decreases in abdominal skinfold measurements than the placebo group. No studies to date have demonstrated beneficial effects of AAS on endurance performance [23].

Specifically, with regard to androstenedione, no studies have demonstrated any significant ergogenic effect. In a double-blind study of 50 men who participated in a 12-week high-intensity resistance program, androstenedione was not shown to enhance adaption to resistance training in terms of body composition or strength [24]. Other studies have reached similar conclusions [25, 26].

3.1.3. Adverse Effects

Common side effects of AAS use include acne, testicular atrophy, gynecomastia, cutaneous striae, and injection site pain. Additionally, life-threatening side effects include cardiovascular disease with impaired diastolic filling, arrhythmias, stroke, blood clots, liver dysfunction, and cancer [27].

The most important cardiovascular changes involve increases in triglyceride levels, increases in concentrations of several clotting factors, and changes in myocardium, including increases in left ventricular mass and dilated cardiomyopathy. These effects vary depending on the type and dose of AAS and may be reversible with cessation of use. Other adverse effects include reductions in endogenous testosterone, gonadotropic hormones, and sex hormone-binding globulin. Reductions in these hormone levels result in decreased testicular size, sperm count, and sperm motility [28]. The physiology of AAS and their downstream effects are shown in Figure 24.1.

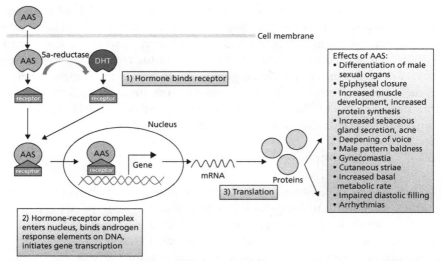

Figure 24.1. The physiology of anabolic–androgenic steroids and their downstream effects. *AAS* anabolic–androgenic steroids, *DHT* dihydrotestosterone, *DNA* deoxyribonucleic acid, *mRNA* messenger ribonucleic acid.

Due to concern for neurotoxic effects from AAS use, a study was conducted to evaluate for cognitive deficits among long-term AAS users when compared with nonusers. A long-term user was defined as an individual who had used AAS for at least 2 years. Long-term users and nonusers did not differ significantly in response speed, sustained attention, and verbal memory. However, visuospatial performance was significantly lower among those who reported long-term use of AAS. Furthermore, within the user group, visuospatial performance negatively correlated with the total lifetime dose of AAS [29].

3.1.4. Testing

Testing for steroids is often performed with a urine immunoassay used to calculate a testosterone: epitestosterone ratio. Epitestosterone is a metabolite that is not affected by exogenous steroids. Increases in this ratio, therefore, help determine AAS use. Ratios are typically less than 2:1; the WADA has set the upper limit at 6:1 [30]. Much of the focus on urinary metabolites has focused on long-term metabolites, which allow for a longer detection window.

Recently, more attention has been directed at chromatographic and mass spectrometric techniques, which can help differentiate natural and synthetic endogenous steroids.

Designer steroids remain difficult to detect. Strategies to combat designer steroid use have focused on two methods. One method centers on a non-targeted approach. The basis for this approach is that designer steroids have common chemical structures to known endogenous steroids. Thus, by searching for these commonalities, one may identify abnormally high levels of certain steroids. Another method involves an indirect approach, examining the effects of exogenous steroids on the profile of endogenous steroids. For example, it is known that the administration of AAS suppresses endogenous steroid concentrations, and such a finding in an athlete may trigger a search for designer steroid use [30].

3.2. Creatine

Creatine is one of the most common sports supplements used today, with sales estimated around $US 400 million annually [31]. Creatine monohydrate is a naturally occurring compound synthesized endogenously and consumed in most diets. It has been studied since the 1920s and gained notoriety by its mainstream use in the 1992 Barcelona Summer Olympics [32].

In a large-scale survey of approximately 21,000 student athletes, the NCAA reported that creatine use in the 12 months prior to the survey was 14.0% among all athletes. Usage rates were highest among wrestlers at 29% [13].

3.2.1. Physiology

Creatine is an amino acid formed from arginine and glycine through a transferase enzyme that produces ornithine and guanidinoacetate. The guanidinoacetate is then methylated by S-adenosyl-L-methionine to form creatine. This process occurs largely in the kidney, except for methylation, which occurs in the liver (Fig. 24.2). A total of 95% of the creatine formed is stored in skeletal muscle, specifically in fast twitch type II fibers [31].

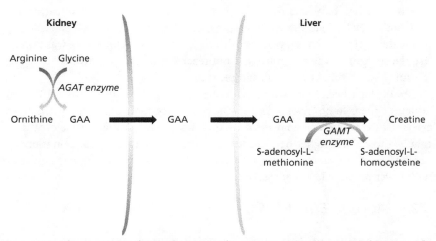

Figure 24.2. The creatine pathway. *GAA* guanidinoacetate, *AGAT* arginine: glycine amidinotransferase, *GAMT* guanidinoacetate methyltransferase.

Creatine serves as an energy substrate for the contraction of skeletal muscle. Those cells with a high energy demand utilize creatine in the form of phosphocreatine, which functions as a donor of phosphate to produce adenosine triphosphate (ATP) from adenosine diphosphate (ADP). Skeletal muscle cells store enough phosphocreatine and ATP for about 10 s of high-intensity action [33].

3.2.2. Performance

Numerous studies have been performed on creatine supplementation and its role in enhancing sports performance. Increases in strength, power output, sprint performance, total work to fatigue, peak force, and peak power performed during multiple sets of maximal-effort contractions have been shown [27].

Specifically, in cyclists, several studies have shown that creatine helps maintain force and power output [34–36]. Oliver et al. [37] examined the effect of creatine on blood lactate levels during cycling. A total of 13 recreationally active men were placed on a 6-day creatine supplementation program and tested before and after with maximal, incremental cycling. Blood tests demonstrated that creatine supplementation decreased lactate levels and tended to raise lactate threshold. The lactate threshold was defined as 4 mmol/L, above which it becomes very difficult to maintain exercise performance.

The beneficial effects of creatine have also been demonstrated in other sports. Weight lifters have reported increased single repetition maximum weight of approximately 20–30% [38, 39]. Track and field athletes have demonstrated a decrease in mean sprint times [40]. However, competitive swimmers did not demonstrate improvements in sprint performance with creatine supplementation [41]. With regard to body composition, weight and lean body mass tend to increase by about 1–2 kg [27, 42, 43].

Most studies have examined short-term (less than 1 week) creatine use. A recent study by Claudino et al. [44] examined chronic (7 weeks) creatine supplementation in elite soccer players. Although jumping performance was lower in the placebo group, the difference did not reach statistical significance. However, the study was limited by a small sample size.

Results have been inconsistent with regard to the effects of creatine [18]. Some athletes appear to be "responders" while others are "nonresponders." These discrepancies can likely be explained by the idea of preloading muscle creatine— that is, those with higher baseline levels of creatine before supplementation will exhibit less of an increase in muscle creatine with supplementation than those with lower baseline levels of creatine [45, 46].

3.2.3. Adverse Effects

Short-term creatine use is regarded as safe and without significant adverse effects [27]. However, the number of long-term studies is limited, and caution should be exercised in the setting of renal and liver disease [27].

There is a theoretical risk of dehydration caused by the use of creatine, as its osmotic effect can lead to water being drawn into muscles. Athletes are encouraged to maintain adequate hydration while using creatine. Bailes et al. [47] postulate that creatine may be linked to subclinical dehydration and heatstroke. Wen et al. [48] report two cases of otherwise healthy athletes sustaining venous thromboembolisms (VTE) and suspect a link to creatine. They report that the dehydration, caused by the creatine, was a precipitating factor for the VTE.

There are also concerns with regard to renal function due to the large creatine load, but one study that monitored creatine supplementation for up to 5 years did not reveal a decrease in glomerular filtration rate [49].

3.2.4. Testing

Creatine is available as an over-the-counter nutritional supplement and is found in various forms. It is not tested for nor banned by any major athletic organization. However, the NCAA does have a policy that none of its member teams will provide creatine to their players [50].

3.3. Human Growth Hormone

The use of hGH as a supplement for performance enhancement has received worldwide attention over the past decade. Athletes from numerous sports have admitted to the use of hGH [13]. Further attention was brought upon hGH after the Mitchell report, which identified numerous MLB players as having used PESs, one of which was hGH [4].

One study published in 1992 surveyed high school students and reported a 5% use of hGH in male students, while 31% of males reported knowing someone who was using hGH. These users also were more likely to abuse anabolic steroids. The average age at first use was between 14 and 15 years [51]. A 2013 NCAA survey study reported that 0.4% of student athletes admitted to using hGH in the previous year [13].

3.3.1. Physiology

hGH is released by the somatotrope cells of the anterior pituitary gland, and it promotes growth through the actions of insulin-like growth factor-1. These hormones cause an increase in lipolysis and protein anabolism, ultimately resulting in a decrease in fat mass and an increase in lean mass [27]. In adolescence, the pulsatile release of hGH is regulated by a number of factors, including growth hormone-releasing hormone, sleep, exercise, L-dopa, and arginine [18].

3.3.2. Performance

Few studies have been conducted regarding performance and hGH use. Postulated benefits include improved athletic performance via increased muscle mass and improved exercise capacity [52]. However, scientific evidence has failed to demonstrate an ergogenic effect with supraphysiologic doses of hGH, although doses studied may be lower than those used by athletes [53].

With regard to body composition, lean body mass increases while fat mass decreases significantly with hGH. However, the overall increase in weight is not significant [52]. One study investigated strength outcomes in 22 healthy men. A double-blind protocol was employed with an hGH group and a placebo group. Urine specimens were tested to ensure no concurrent AAS use. hGH was not shown to increase biceps or quadriceps strength with one repetition maximum strength testing [54]. In another study, changes in muscle circumference between groups treated with hGH versus placebo were not shown to be significant [55]. Furthermore, no benefits in maximal oxygen consumption (VO_{2max}), respiratory exchange ratio, energy expenditure, bicycling speed, or power output have been shown [52]. The major limiting factor in these studies involves the lack of dosing standardization.

Use of hGH appears to continue despite the lack of evidence-based medicine to support its use in athletes. Many of the purported benefits may stem from the theoretical benefits from known physiologic pathways. However, such effects may apply only to those who are growth hormone deficient and not to athletes.

3.3.3. Adverse Effects

Chronic use of hGH can lead to multiple adverse effects. Because hGH activates the renin-angiotensin system, it can cause fluid accumulation, thus leading to arthralgias, carpal tunnel syndrome, and pseudotumor cerebri. Reported effects also include cardiovascular disease, hyperlipidemia, cancer, and insulin resistance [56].

3.3.4. Testing

hGH exhibits a very short half-life in blood and a low concentration in urine, making it difficult to detect. Furthermore, due to the pulsatile nature of hGH secretion, there are wide fluctuations in circulation. hGH is also often affected by sleep, exercise, stress, and nutrition [57].

Nonetheless, the most reliable method that currently exists focuses on the ratio of concentrations of recombinant hGH versus naturally derived isotopes of hGH. Limits are set based upon ratios collected in routine hGH testing of athletes [58].

3.4. Amphetamines and Stimulants

Stimulants have been used in sports to enhance performance throughout history, but in the past decade these drugs have gained attention due to the deaths of two professional athletes who were reportedly using ephedrine [18]. Commonly used stimulants include amphetamines, caffeine, ephedrine, pseudoephedrine, phen-ylephrine, and methamphetamines.

In a recent survey of nearly 21,000 students in grades 8–10 in the USA, an increased use of amphetamines was seen among males who participated in la-crosse (adjusted odds ratio 2.52) and wrestling (adjusted odds ratio 1.74) [59]. In contrast, no association among females and sporting type was found for am-phetamine use. Stimulants have accounted for nearly 10% of adverse analytical findings by the WADA in 2010. Furthermore, they have been the second most common reason for a positive test in recent years [27]. Another study involving drug testing of several high schools in the USA found that 543 (16.6%) of 3,000 samples were positive for drugs of abuse. Most commonly, these positive results were for central nervous system (CNS) stimulants. However, sampling was not limited to athletes [15].

3.4.1. Physiology

Amphetamines are CNS stimulants and chemically related to catecholamines. They exhibit an indirect sympathomimetic action by causing the release of norepinephrine from storage vesicles in the sympathetic nerve endings. Norepinephrine then leads to the classic sympathetic effects, including increased arousal, heart rate, blood pressure, and respiratory rate [27]. Half-lives have been reported in pharmacology studies: 19.4 h for amphetamines [60], 5.7 h for caf-feine [61], 6.1 h for ephedrine [62], and 7 h for pseudoephedrine [63]. The route of administration for these substances is usually oral, but they can also be injected.

3.4.2. Performance

One study that has closely examined amphetamine use and athletic performance is by Chandler and Blair [64]. Six male college students were tested, and am-phetamine use was associated with increased strength, muscular power, speed, acceleration, aerobic power, and anaerobic capacity. There was also an increased time to exhaustion, although no increase in VO_{2max} was seen. In another study, pseudoephedrine was shown to increase maximum torque, peak power, and lung function during a maximal cycle performance [65]. Some studies have demon-strated improved times for medium distance runs with the pre-ingestion of caf-feine and ephedrine [66, 67].

Specifically, caffeine has been widely studied with regard to performance in sports. It has been shown to reduce reaction time and delay fatigue in tae-kwondo [68], improve cycling time trials in triathletes [69], and decrease times in cross country double poling [70]. However, other studies have not shown significant improvement with caffeine. In a study with 11 female athletes per-forming repeated sprint cycling, neither ingestion of caffeine plus placebo nor caffeine plus carbohydrate improved repeated sprint performance with short rest intervals [71]. Many athletes use caffeine to counter sleep deprivation, but a study on semi-professional tennis players showed that caffeine did not make up for lost sleep with regard to serving accuracy [72]. Further studies should be performed to elucidate the prevalence of caffeine use by athletes with respect to insufficient sleep.

Other stimulants such as ephedrine and ephedra alone have shown little efficacy or benefit in athletic performance [73]. Shekelle et al. [74] performed a meta-analysis of 52 controlled trials and 65 case reports regarding ephedrine and ephedra. When examining outcomes as related to athletic performance, there were no significant effects. However, the analysis did find that these drugs promoted a modest short-term weight loss.

3.4.3. Adverse Effects

The side effects of stimulants relate to their effects on increasing CNS stimulation. Common side effects include restlessness, agitation, gastrointestinal upset and nausea, headaches, rebound fatigue; serious adverse effects include heat exhaustion, arrhythmias, seizures, hallucinations, and dependence [27, 75]. From 1994 to 1997, the Food and Drug Administration reviewed over 800 cases of ephedra adverse effects, which included hypertension, myocardial infarction, arrhythmias, anxiety, tremors, stroke, and death [76].

3.4.4. Testing

Several classes of amphetamines are banned by the IOC, and the National Football League (NFL) has banned the use of ephedrine. Testing for amphetamines and stimulants involves quantitative tests to detect their presence in urine. Specifically, the NCAA has limited caffeine levels to 15 μg/ml in urine, which is equivalent to approximately six regular sized cups of coffee [77].

3.5. Erythropoietin and Blood Doping

Athletes, especially endurance athletes, benefit from improved delivery of oxygen to their tissues. Such improved oxygen delivery affords athletes improved aerobic capacity. One method by which athletes attempt this is by living or training at high altitudes, which is often thought of as a natural way to improve oxygen delivery [78]. Another method used involves blood transfusions, most commonly autologous. Such a transfusion would artificially increase hematocrit and thus oxygen-carrying capacity. Another artificial method by which athletes have been known to gain an advantage is through the administration of EPO, which is responsible for erythropoiesis.

The rate of use of EPO or blood doping is difficult to quantify. However, it is estimated that such techniques have been widely used throughout endurance sports [18]. One Spanish doping investigation revealed that several athletes had employed the systematic use of autologous blood transfusions. Officials discovered several frozen blood units in addition to calendars with reinfusion dates [79].

3.5.1. Physiology

EPO is a glycoprotein hormone that plays an important role in the differentiation, survival, and proliferation of erythroid cells. EPO is produced mostly in the kidney. In response to hypoxic stress, the body produces a greater amount of EPO. The EPO then binds to the EPO receptor on the red cell progenitor surface. Such binding stimulates a cascade that leads to the increased production of erythrocytes. Such increases in hematocrit lead to higher oxygen-carrying capacities [80].

3.5.2. Performance

Several studies have documented the performance enhancement benefits of blood doping. In one study, after an autologous transfusion of 750 ml of red blood cells, the VO_{2max} increased by 12.8%, and performance times on a treadmill test to exhaustion improved significantly [81]. Other studies have shown decreased times in cross country skiers [82] and in runners during a 10 km race [83].

A double-blind, placebo-controlled study by Birkeland et al. [84] evaluated cycling performance after administration of recombinant human erythropoietin (rhEPO). Mean VO_{2max} increased by 7% in the EPO group from 63.6 to 68.1 mL kg^{-1} min^{-1}, while mean hematocrit increased from 42.7 to 50.8%. Both of these changes were significant. Another study, by Berglund and Ekblom [85], showed similar results.

3.5.3. Adverse Effects

The side effects of EPO should not be underestimated. These adverse effects include hypertension, headaches, and an increased risk for a thromboembolic event due to the rise in hematocrit and viscosity [77]. Furthermore, with large doses, EPO may cause death [80]. During the first year EPO was released, five Dutch cyclists died of unexplained causes. In a 4-year span, between 1997 and 2000, 18 cyclists died from stroke, myocardial infarction, or pulmonary embolism [18].

With regard to blood transfusions, similar risks may be encountered when elevating hematocrit and thus blood viscosity. When homologous transfusions are employed, there is also the risk for transfer of infection such as hepatitis and HIV and major transfusion reactions from blood type incompatibility [86].

3.5.4. Testing

Testing for autologous blood transfusions remains difficult. No direct detection method has been implemented by the WADA. Sophisticated algorithms help detect possible autologous blood transfusions, and these algorithms are based on the total amount of circulating hemoglobin and the percentage of reticulocytes. Because of lower variability with total hemoglobin mass compared to hemoglobin, it has been proposed as a parameter in the Athlete Biologic Passport (ABP). The ABP entails measuring certain biological parameters over time for an athlete. The assumption is that these variables will remain stable over time. Any changes in the ABP would trigger a suspicion for doping. Thus, instead of solely relying on direct testing for banned substances, organizations can incorporate the ABP to help indirectly identify athletes who may be doping [87].

A number of detection methods for rhEPO exist, but it remains difficult to detect exogenous EPO. Such tests include measurement of hematologic parameters, gene-based detection methods, use of peptide markers, electrophoresis, and isoelectric focusing among numerous other methods [80].

3.6. Beta-Hydroxy-Beta-Methylbutyrate

HMB is a metabolite of the amino acid leucine and is a precursor to cholesterol. It is believed to attenuate protein breakdown after workouts and has recently gained greater attention among athletes [88]. A 2013 NCAA survey study reported a 0.2% rate of use among all student athletes [13]. However, it appears that HMB is increasingly being added to many training regimens [88].

3.6.1. Physiology

There are several proposed mechanisms by which HMB acts. One of the primary mechanisms involves the up-regulation of the mechanistic target of rapamycin/p70S6K signaling pathway, which promotes protein synthesis and muscle hypertrophy [89].

Other studies have focused on the anti-catabolic effects of HMB. Smith et al. [90] demonstrated that HMB preserved lean body mass and decreased proteolysis through the down-regulation of the increased expression of certain components of the ubiquitin–proteasome proteolytic pathway. Some studies have examined HMB and its effect on muscle by measuring markers of muscle breakdown. Wilson et al. [91] demonstrated that when non-resistance-trained males received HMB pre-exercise, the rise of lac-tate dehydrogenase (LDH) levels reduced, and HMB tended to decrease soreness. Knitter et al. [92] showed a decrease in LDH and creatine phosphokinase (CPK), a byproduct of muscle breakdown, by HMB after a prolonged run.

3.6.2. Performance

Several studies have been performed with regard to HMB and performance. However, it is difficult to compare the various studies due to different dosing schedules and amounts of HMB, previous training levels of participants, and different performance outcomes.

Kraemer et al. [93] showed that HMB intake in healthy men who underwent a 12-week course of heavy resistance training increased lean body mass, muscle strength, and power with regard to squatting and bench press when compared with a placebo group. Nissen and Sharp [94] performed a meta-analysis and found that HMB increased strength and lean tissue through resistance training. However, when specifically examining trained subjects, some studies have shown no effect. In one study of American collegiate football players [95], no significant effect of HMB on creatine kinase, power, or muscle soreness was observed. In another study on trained American collegiate football players, no effects were demonstrated by HMB when studying bench press, power cleans, squats, or sprint performance [96].

Despite differences in these studies, it does appear that HMB overall enhances muscular hypertrophy, strength, and power. In fact, the International Society for Sports Nutrition, in a position statement, writes that HMB can be used to enhance recovery by reducing skeletal muscle damage after exercise in athletically trained and untrained people. The utility of HMB does seem to be affected by timing of intake prior to workouts and dosage [97]. Further, chronic consumption of HMB appears safe [97].

3.6.3. Adverse Effects

No serious adverse effects from HMB consumption have been reported. In one study, 37 college males took HMB for an 8-week period during resistance training. No adverse effects were seen with regard to blood glucose, blood urea nitrogen, hemoglobin, hepatic enzymes, lipid profile, leukocytes, urine pH, urine glucose, or urine protein excretion [98]. Similarly, Nissen et al. [99] evaluated nine studies and found that HMB was a safe ergogenic aid. In fact, HMB lowered total cholesterol, low-density lipoprotein cholesterol, and systolic blood pressure, thus demonstrating potential cardioprotective effects.

3.6.4. Testing

Currently, HMB is available as an over-the-counter supplement. The drug is not tested for nor banned by any sporting organization.

3.7. Gene Doping

As the field of genetics continues to advance and techniques to modify human genes become more readily available, gene doping draws closer to reality. Gene doping is defined as the "transfer of nucleic acid sequences or the use of normal or genetically modified cells to enhance sports performance" [100]. To date, there is no evidence that gene doping has been employed for sports enhancement.

3.7.1. Physiology

Numerous proteins have been identified for targets of gene doping based on potential and include EPO, insulin-like growth factor, hGH, myostatin, vascular endothelial growth factor, fibroblast growth factor, endorphin, and encephalin [100].

Methods such as injection or inhalation could be used to deliver genetic material containing specific genes into the athlete's body. Once the genetic material is incorporated into the DNA in the nucleus of the cell, the specific gene sequences would be transcribed, resulting in the increased expression of the specific protein encoded by the delivered gene [101]. Various delivery methods have been proposed and studied for such a process. In general, the athlete's cells are isolated from the body, modified in vitro, and transplanted back into the athlete (direct transplant) [102]. There are two methods to modify the athlete's cells in vitro. One method involves DNA trans-fection, through which non-viral transporters such as liposomes deliver plasmid DNA containing the gene material into the cells. The transfection method would likely have a short duration of action on the order of days to weeks [103]. A second method involves transduction with inactive viral vectors. Such a technique would likely lead to a longer duration of action on the order of months to years (Fig. 24.3) [104].

3.7.2. Adverse Effects

Because gene doping is still in the infancy stage, much of the potential adverse effects are theoretical. Nonetheless, such risks are substantial and may compromise the health of athletes who look to obtain an edge without considering the consequences. One potential adverse effect is an immune reaction. The virus or the protein itself may trigger an immune response, which may even lead to destruction of the endogenous protein. Another problem is that the virus may integrate such that it leads to the increased production of proto-oncogenes, thereby increasing the risk of cancer. Also, gene doping may affect germ cells, and its effects, both intended and unintended, may be passed on to offspring. Finally, the expression of the gene is difficult to control, and overexpression may lead to an overabundance of protein that could reach toxic levels [100].

Direct Transplant

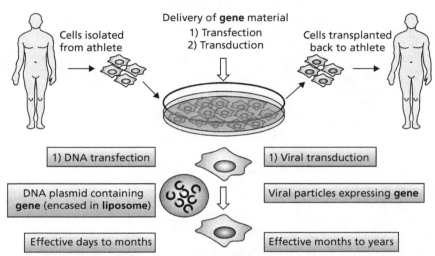

Figure 24.3. Gene doping pathways via transfection or transduction.

3.7.3 Testing

The detection of gene doping will prove to be very difficult. Currently, no WADA-approved detection methods exist for gene doping. The WADA currently prohibits any form of gene or cell doping.

■ 4. THERAPEUTIC USE EXEMPTION

In certain situations, an athlete may require the use of a substance that is banned by WADA for an acute or chronic medical condition. The Therapeutic Use Exemption (TUE) program has been created to allow for athletes to use such substances without facing penalties. In order to meet the requirements for a TUE, four conditions must be met: (1) the banned substance is needed by the athlete for a chronic or acute medical condition and withholding the substance may pose a significant impairment to the health of the athlete, (2) the use of this substance is unlikely to increase athletic performance beyond what is anticipated by the return of the athlete to his or her normal health, (3) no reasonable therapeutic alternative exists, and (4) the need for this banned substance is not the consequence of prior use of a banned substance [105].

In order to obtain a TUE, the athlete and physician must complete appropriate paperwork and submit it to the governing agency. Table 24.2 lists the common substances by class for which athletes sought TUEs in 2013. These data were obtained from the Anti-doping Administration and Management database [106].

TABLE 24.2 *Requests for Therapeutic Use Exemption by Substance Class*

Substance	Percentage
Glucocorticosteroids	36
Stimulants	21
Hormone and metabolic modulators	14
Diuretics and other masking agents	8
Narcotics	6
Beta-2 agonists	5
Peptide hormones, growth factors, and related substances	4
Anabolic agents	3
Chemical and physical manipulation	1
Beta-blockers	1
Cannabinoids	<1
Manipulation of blood and blood components	<1

■ 5. PREVENTION

Despite advances in PES detection, the prevalence of doping persists throughout sports. Some studies have examined preventive techniques, but much work remains in order to protect the health and safety of athletes.

Foremost, education appears to be the keystone to any prevention program. In a 2004 Swedish study, a health promotion program for 16- and 17-year-old adolescents focused on awareness and discussion of attitudes on AAS use over 2 years. The use of AAS tended to decrease after the program [15]. In another study in a low-income community, a short-term nutrition and sport supplement educational program was shown to improve nutrition and sport supplement knowledge [107]. However, these students were not necessarily athletes, and no objective testing data from prior to and after the educational program were available to assess drug use.

Whitaker et al. [108] conducted semi-structured interviews on athletes' perceptions of their role in doping prevention. The study concluded that prevention programs would need to focus on changing the broader group and community norms on doping. Furthermore, anti-doping programs may need to be specialized based on the sport. Harcourt et al. [109] report on a technique by which drug use was reduced in elite Australian football ("Australian Rules"). The authors surmised that player education and a greater number of tests conducted along with a "harm minimization" rather than a "punitive" strategy would lead to a decreased use of prohibited PESs.

Further studies are needed to help formulate an effective program on preventing the use of banned PESs. Such programs will need to start early while the athletes are young and focus on education and awareness. Nevertheless, physicians must be aware of the incidence of PES use despite prevention techniques. When PES use is suspected, the physician must broach the subject with the athlete. Warning signs of PES use may include increased aggressiveness, increased weight, acne, and skin changes from needle marks. Guidelines need to be established to help direct physicians who suspect the use of banned substances by their patients. At this point, testing for banned substances and subsequent reporting should be left to the sport's governing body.

■ 6. CONCLUSION

The current rate of PES use among athletes is disturbing. The majority of studies are limited by response errors, and the true prevalence of PES use may be much higher. Further studies are needed to evaluate the true prevalence of PES use among athletes and differentiate sport-specific rates. Such studies may stem from randomized testing of athletes. Further randomized controlled studies are also needed to resolve conflicting data on specific substances and their effects on sports performance.

As methods of doping continue to advance, the sports medicine physician will need to play an even greater role in protecting athletes from harm. Physicians should be knowledgeable about the types of PESs available and the potential performance benefits and health risks of such substances. Only after the physician gains such knowledge can he or she effectively educate athletes on PESs and effect positive change in the sports community.

■ ACKNOWLEDGMENTS

The authors would like to acknowledge Florence Lee, MD, and Li-yuan Yu-Lee, PhD, for their assistance with the preparation of figures for this manuscript. The authors have no potential conflicts of interest that are directly relevant to the content of this review. No sources of funding were used to assist in the preparation of this review.

■ REFERENCES

1. Botre F, Pavan A. Enhancement drugs and the athlete. Neurol Clin. 2008;26:149–167.
2. De Rose EH. Doping in athletes: an update. Clin Sports Med. 2008;27:107–130.
3. WADA. World anti-doping code (online). 2015. https://wadamain-prod. s3.amazonaws.com/resources/files/wada-2015-world-anti-doping-code.pdf. Accessed 11 Aug 2014.
4. Mitchell G. Report to the Commissioner of Baseball of an independent investigation into the illegal use of steroids and other performance enhancing substances by players in Major League Baseball (online). http://files.mlb.com/mitchrpt.pdf. Accessed 11 August 2014.
5. Nilsson S. Androgenic anabolic steroid use among male adolescents in Falkenberg. Eur J Clin Pharmacol. 1995;48:9–11.
6. Korkia P, Stinson GV. Indication of prevalence, practice and effects of anabolic steroid use in Great Britain. Int J Sports Med. 1997;18:557–562.

7. Simon P, Striegel H, Aust F, et al. Doping in fitness sports: estimated number of unreported cases and individual probability of doping. Addiction. 2006;101:1640–1644.

8. Striegel H, Simon P, Frisch S, et al. Anabolic ergogenic substance users in fitness-sports: a distinct group supported by the health care system. Drug Alcohol Depend. 2006;81:11–19.

9. Kanayama G, Gruber AJ, Pope HG Jr, et al. Over-the-counter drug use in gymnasiums: an unrecognized substance abuse problem? Psychother Psychosom. 2001;70:137–140.

10. Buckman JF, Yusko DA, White HR, et al. Risk profile of male college athletes who use performance-enhancing substances. J Stud Alcohol Drugs. 2009;70:919–923.

11. Dietz P, Ulrich R, Dalaker R, et al. Associations between physical and cognitive doping: a cross-sectional study in 2,997 triathletes. PLoS ONE. 2013;8:e78702.

12. Striegel H, Ulrich R, Simon P. Randomized response estimates for doping and illicit drug use in elite athletes. Drug Alcohol Depend. 2010;106:230–232.

13. Rexroat M. NCAA national study of substance use habits of college student-athletes (online). http://www.ncaa.org/sites/default/files/Substance%20Use%20Final%20Report_FINAL.pdf. Accessed 11 August 2014.

14. Sagoe D, Molde H, Andreassen CS, et al. The global epidemiology of anabolic-androgenic steroid use: a meta analysis and meta-regression analysis. Ann Epidemiol. 2014;24:383–398.

15. Gregory AJ, Fitch RW. Sports medicine: performance-enhancing drugs. Pediatr Clin North Am. 2007;54:797–806.

16. Pereira HM, Padilha MC, Neto FR. Tetrahydrogestrinone analysis and designer steroids revisited. Bioanalysis. 2009;1: 1475–1489.

17. Teale P, Scarth J, Hudson S. Impact of the emergence of designer drugs upon sports doping testing. Bioanalysis. 2012;4:71–88.

18. Tokish JM, Kocher MS, Hawkins RJ. Ergogenic aids: a review of basic science, performance, side effects, and status in sports. Am J Sports Med. 2004;32:1543–1553.

19. Evans N. Current concepts in anabolic-androgenic steroids. Am J Sports Med. 2004;32:534–542.

20. Bhasin S, Storer TW, Berman N, et al. The effects of supra-physiologic doses of testosterone on muscle size and strength in normal men. N Engl J Med. 1996;335:1–7.

21. Forbes GB, Porta CR, Herr BE, et al. Sequence of changes in body composition induced by testosterone and reversal of changes after drug is stopped. JAMA. 1992;267:397–399.

22. Giorgi A, Weatherby RP, Murphy PW. Muscular strength, body composition and health responses to the use of testosterone enanthate: a double blind study. J Sci Med Sport. 1999;2:341–355.

23. Duntas LH, Popovic V. Hormones as doping in sports. Endocrine. 2013;43:303–313.

24. Broeder CE, Quindry J, Brittingham K, et al. The Andro Project: physiological and hormonal influences of androstenedione supplementation in men 35 to 65 years old participating in a high-intensity resistance training program. Arch Intern Med. 2000;160:3093–3104.

25. King DS, Sharp RL, Vukovich MD, et al. Effect of oral androstenedione on serum testosterone and adaptations to resistance training in young men: a randomized controlled trial. JAMA. 1999;281:2020–2028.

26. Wallace MB, Lim J, Cutler A, et al. Effects of dehy-droepiandrosterone vs andro-stenedione supplementation in men. Med Sci Sports Exerc. 1999;31:1788–1792.
27. Liddle DG, Connor DJ. Nutritional supplements and ergogenic AIDS. Prim Care. 2013;40:487–505.
28. Bahrke MS, Yesalis CE. Abuse of anabolic steroids and related substances in sport and exercise. Curr Opin Pharmacol. 2004;4:614–620.
29. Kanayama G, Kean J, Hudson JJ, et al. Cognitive deficits in long-term anabolic-androgenic steroid users. Drug Alcohol Depend. 2013;130:208–214.
30. Geyer H, Schanzer W, Thevis M. Anabolic agents: recent strategies for their detection and protection from inadvertent doping. Br J Sports Med. 2014;48:820–826.
31. Brudnak MA. Creatine: are the benefits worth the risk? Toxicol Lett. 2004;150:123–130.
32. Eichner ER. Ergogenic aids: what athletes are using and why. Phys Sportsmed. 1997;25:70–83.
33. Greydanus DE, Patel DR. Sports doping in the adolescent athlete the hope, hype, and hyperbole. Pediatr Clin North Am. 2002;49:829–855.
34. Balsom PD, Soderlund K, Sjodin B, et al. Skeletal muscle metabolism during short duration high-intensity exercise: influence of creatine supplementation. Acta Physiol Scand. 1995;154:303–310.
35. Birch R, Noble D, Greenhaff PL. The influence of dietary creatine supplementation on performance during repeated bouts of maximal isokinetic cycling in man. Eur J Appl Physiol Occup Physiol. 1994;69:268–276.
36. Dawson B, Cutler M, Moody A, et al. Effects of oral creatine loading on single and repeated maximal short sprints. Aust J Sci Med Sport. 1995;27:56–61.
37. Oliver JM, Joubert DP, Martin SE, et al. Oral creatine supplementation's decrease of blood lactate during exhaustive, incremental cycling. Int J Sport Nutr Exerc Metab. 2013;23:252–258.
38. Earnest CP, Snell PG, Rodriguez R, et al. The effect of creatine monohydrate ingestion on anaerobic power indices, muscular strength and body composition. Acta Physiol Scand. 1995;153:207–209.
39. Stone MH, Sanborn K, Smith LL, et al. Effects of in-season (5 weeks) creatine and pyruvate supplementation on anaerobic performance and body composition in American football players. Int J Sport Nutr. 1999;9:146–165.
40. Aaserud R, Gramvik P, Olsen SR, et al. Creatine supplementation delays onset of fatigue during repeated bouts of sprint running. Scand J Med Sci Sports. 1998;8:247–251.
41. Mujika I, Chatard JC, Lacoste L, et al. Creatine supplementation does not improve sprint performance in competitive swimmers. Med Sci Sports Exerc. 1996;28:1435–1441.
42. Balsom PD, Ekbolm B, Soderlund K, et al. Creatine supplementation and dynamic high-intensity intermittent exercise. Scand J Med Sci Sports. 1993;3:143–149.
43. Balsom PD, Soderlund K, Ekblom B. Creatine in humans with special reference to creatine supplementation. Sports Med. 1994;18:268–280.
44. Claudino JG, Mezencio B, Amaral S, et al. Creatine monohydrate supplementation on lower-limb muscle power in Brazilian elite soccer players. J Int Soc Sports Nutr. 2014;11:e1–e6.
45. Lemon PW. Dietary creatine supplementation and exercise performance: why inconsistent results? Can J Appl Physiol. 2002;27:663–681.

46. Dawson B, Vladich T, Blanksby BA. Effects of 4 weeks of creatine supplementation in junior swimmers on freestyle sprint and swim bench performance. J Strength Cond Res. 2002;16:485–490.
47. Bailes JE, Cantu RC, Day AL. The neurosurgeon in sport: awareness of the risks of heatstroke and dietary supplements. Neurosurgery. 2002;51:283–286.
48. Wen TC, Hae Tha M, Joo Ng H. Creatine supplementation and venous thrombotic events. Am J Med. 2014; 127;e7–e8.
49. Poortmans JR, Francaux M. Long term oral creatine supplementation does not impair renal function in healthy athletes. Med Sci Sports Exerc. 1999;31:1108–1110.
50. NCAA Academic and Membership Affairs Staff. NCAA 2014–2014 division I manual (online). http://www. ncaapublications.com/productdownloads/D114.pdf. Accessed 11 August 2014.
51. Rickert VI, Pawlak-Morello C, Sheppard V, et al. Human growth hormone: a new substance of abuse among adolescents? Clin Pediatr. 1992;31:723–726.
52. Liu H, Bravata DM, Olkin I, et al. Systematic review: the effects of growth hormone on athletic performance. Ann Intern Med. 2008;148:747–758.
53. Baumann GP. Growth hormone doping in sports: a critical review of use and detection strategies. Endocr Rev. 2012;33:155–186.
54. Deyssig R, Frisch H, Blum WF, et al. Effect of growth hormone treatment on hormonal parameters, body composition and strength in athletes. Acta Endocrinol. 1993;128:313–318.
55. Yarasheski KE, Campbell JA, Smith K, et al. Effect of growth hormone and resistance exercise on muscle growth in young men. Am J Physiol. 1992;262:e261–e267.
56. Rennie MJ. Claims for the anabolic effects of growth hormone: a case of the emperor's new clothes? Br J Sports Med. 2003;37:100–105.
57. Saugy M, Robinson N, Saudan C, et al. Human growth hormone doping in sport. Br J Sports Med. 2006;40:135–139.
58. Hanley J, Saarela O, Stephens D, et al. hGH isoform differential immunoassays applied to blood samples from athletes: decision limits for anti-doping testing. Growth Horm IGF Res. 2014;24:205–215.
59. Veliz P, Boyd C, McCabe SE. Adolescent athletic participation and nonmedical Adderall use: an exploratory analysis of a performance-enhancing drug. J Stud Alcohol Drugs. 2013;74:714–719.
60. Ebert MH, Kammen DP, Murphy DL. Plasma levels of amphetamine and behavioral response. In: Gottschalk LA, Merlis S, editors. Pharmacokinetics of psychoactive drugs: blood levels and clinical response. New York: Wiley; 1976: 157–169.
61. Statland BE, Demas TJ. Serum caffeine half-lives: healthy subjects vs. patients having alcohol hepatic disease. Am J Clin Pathol. 1980;73:390–393.
62. Haller CA, Jacob PIII, Benowitz N. Pharmacology of ephedra alkaloids and caffeine after single-dose dietary supplement use. Clin Pharmacol Ther. 2002;71:421–432.
63. Pentel P. Toxicity of over-the-counter stimulants. JAMA. 1984;252:1898–1903.
64. Chandler JV, Blair SN. The effect of amphetamines on selected physiological components related to athletic success. Med Sci Sports Exerc. 1980;12:65–69.
65. Gill ND, Shield A, Blazevich AJ, et al. Muscular and cardiorespiratory effects of pseudoephedrine in human athletes. Br J Clin Pharmacol. 2000;50:205–213.
66. Bell DG, Jacobs I. Combined caffeine and ephedrine ingestion improves run times of Canadian Forces Warrior Test. Aviat Space Environ Med. 1999;70:325–329.

67. Bell DG, McLellan TM, Sabiston CM. Effect of ingesting caffeine and ephedrine on 10-km run performance. Med Sci Sports Exerc. 2002;34:344–349.
68. Santos VG, Santos VR, Felippe LJ, et al. Caffeine reduces reaction time and improves performance in simulated-contest of taekwondo. Nutrients. 2014;6:637–649.
69. Hodgson AB, Randell RK, Jeukendrup AE. The metabolic and performance effects of caffeine compared to coffee during endurance exercise. PLoS One. 2013;8:el–10.
70. Stadheim HK, Kvamme B, Olsen R, et al. Caffeine increases performance in cross-country double-poling time trial exercise. Med Sci Sports Exerc. 2013;45:2175–2183.
71. Lee CL, Cheng CF, Astorino TA, et al. Effects of carbohydrate combined with caffeine on repeated sprint cycling and agility performance in female athletes. J Int Soc Sports Nutr. 2014;11:el–12.
72. Reyner LA, Horne JA. Sleep restriction and serving accuracy in performance tennis players and effects of caffeine. Physiol Behav. 2013;120:93–96.
73. Lattavo A, Kopperud A, Rogers PD. Creatine and other supplements. Pediatr Clin North Am. 2007;54:735–760.
74. Shekelle PG, Hardy ML, Morton SC, et al. Efficacy and safety of ephedra and ephedrine for weight loss and athletic performance: a meta analysis. JAMA. 2003;289:1537–1545.
75. McDuff DR, Baron D. Substance use in athletics: a sports psychiatry perspective. Clin Sports Med. 2005;24:885–897.
76. Greydanus DE, Patel DR. Sports doping in the adolescent: the Faustian conundrum of Hors de Combat. Pediatr Clin North Am. 2010;57:729–750.
77. Spriet LL, Graham TE. Caffeine and exercise performance (online). http://www.acsm.org/docs/current-comments/caffeine andexercise.pdf. Accessed 22 November 2014.
78. McLean BD, Gore CJ, Kemp J. Application of "'live low-train high"' for enhancing normoxic exercise performance in team sport athletes. Sports Med. 2014;44:1275–1287.
79. Morkeberg J. Blood manipulation: current challenges from an anti-doping perspective. Hematol Am Soc Hematol Educ Program. 2013;2013:627–631.
80. Citartan M, Gopinath SC, Chen Y, et al. Monitoring recombinant human erythropoietin abuse among athletes. Biosens Bio-electron. 2014;63:86–98.
81. Robertson RJ, Gilcher R, Metz KF, et al. Effect of induced erythrocythemia on hypoxia tolerance during physical exercise. J Appl Physiol Respir Environ Exerc Physiol. 1982;53:490–495.
82. Berglund B, Hemmingson P. Effect of reinfusion of autologous blood exercise performance in cross-country skiers. Int J Sports Med. 1987;8:231–233.
83. Brien AJ, Simon TL. The effects of red blood cell infusion on 10-km race time. JAMA. 1987;257:2761–2765.
84. Birkeland KI, Stray-Gundersen J, Hemmerbach P, et al. Effect of rhEPO administration on serum levels of s TfR and cycling performance. Med Sci Sports Exerc. 2000;32:1238–1243.
85. Berglund B, Ekblom B. Effect of recombinant human erythropoietin treatment on blood pressure and some haematological parameters in healthy men. J Intern Med. 1991;229:125–130.
86. Leigh-Smith S. Blood boosting. Br J Sports Med. 2004;38:99–101.
87. Morkeberg J. Detection of autologous blood transfusions in athletes: a historical perspective. Transfus Med Rev. 2012;26:199–208.

88. Palisin T, Stacy JJ. Beta-hydroxy-beta-methylbutyrate and its use in athletics. Curr Sports Med Rep. 2005;4:220–223.
89. Pimentel GD, Rosa JC, Lira FS, et al. Beta-hydroxy-beta-methylbutyrate (HMB) supplementation stimulants skeletal muscle hypertrophy in rats via the mTOR pathway. Nutr Metab. 2011;8:e1–e7.
90. Smith HJ, Mukerji P, Tisdale MJ. Attenuation of proteasomeinduced proteolysis in skeletal muscle by beta-hydroxy-beta-methylbutyrate in cancer-induced muscle loss. Cancer Res. 2005;65:277–283.
91. Wilson JM, Kim J, Lee SR, et al. Acute and time effects of beta-hydroxy-beta-methylbutyrate (HMB) on indirect markers of skeletal muscle damage. Nutr Metab. 2009;6:e1–e8.
92. Knitter AE, Panton I, Rathmacher JA, et al. Effects of beta-hydroxy-beta-methylbutyrate on muscle damage after a prolonged run. J Appl Physiol. 2000;89:1340–1344.
93. Kraemer WJ, Hatfield DL, Volek JS, et al. Effects of amino acids supplement on physiological adaptations to resistance training. Med Sci Sports Exerc. 2009;41:1111–1121.
94. Nissen SI, Sharp RL. Effect of dietary supplements on lean mass and strength gains with resistance exercise: a meta-analysis. J Appl Physiol. 2003;94:651–659.
95. Hoffman JR, Copper J, Wendell M, et al. Effects of beta-hydroxy-beta-methylbutyrate on power performance and indices of muscle damage and stress during high-intensity training. J Strength Cond Res. 2004; 18:747–752.
96. Kreider RB, Ferreira M, Greenwood M, et al. Effects of calcium b-HMB supplementation during training on markers of body composition, strength, and spring performance. J Exerc Physiology-online. 2000;3:48–59.
97. Wilson JM, Fitschen PJ, Campbell B, et al. International Society of Sports Nutrition position stand: beta-hydroxy-beta-methylbutyrate (HMB). J Int Soc Sports Nutr. 2013;10:e1–e14.
98. Gallagher PM, Carrithers JA, Godard MP, et al. Beta-hydroxy-beta-methylbutyrate ingestion, part I: effects on strength and fat free mass. Med Sci Sports Exerc. 2000;32:2109–2115.
99. Nissen S, Sharp RL, Panton L, et al. Beta-hydroxy-beta-methylbutyrate (HMB) supplementation in humans is safe and may decrease cardiovascular risk factors. J Nutr. 2000;130:1937–1945.
100. Van der Gronde T, de Hon O, Haisma HJ, et al. Gene doping: an overview and current implications for athletes. Br J Sports Med. 2013;47:670–678.
101. Fischetto G, Bermon S. From gene engineering to gene modulation and manipulation: can we prevent or detect gene doping in sports? Sports Med. 2013;43:965–977.
102. Brill-Almon E, Stern B, Afik D, et al. Ex vivo transduction of human dermal tissue structures for autologous implantation production and delivery of therapeutic proteins. Mol Ther. 2005;12:274–282.
103. Wang W, Li W, Ma N, et al. Non-viral gene delivery methods. Curr Pharm Biotechnol. 2013;14:46–60.
104. Sinn PL, Sauter SL, McCray PBJr. Gene therapy progress and prospects: development of improved lentiviral and retroviral vectors—design, biosafety, and production. Gene Ther. 2005;12:1089–1098.

105. WADA. Therapeutic use exemptions (online). 2015. https://wada-main-prod. s3.amazonaws.com/resources/files/WADA-2015-ISTUE-Final-EN.pdf. Accessed 22 November 2014.
106. Vernec A. Therapeutic use exemptions: principles and practice (online). https://wada-main-prod.s3.amazonaws.com/resources/files/01-_vemec_alan_-_tue_symposium_ paris_vernec_october_23_2014.pdf. Accessed 22 November 2014.
107. Little JC, Perry DR, Volpe SL. Effect of nutrition supplement education on nutrition supplement knowledge among high school students from a low-income community. J Community Health. 2002;27:433–450.
108. Whitaker L, Backhouse SH, Long J. Reporting doping in sport: national level athletes' perceptions of their role in doping prevention. Scan J Med Sci Sports. 2014;24(6):e515–e521.
109. Harcourt PR, Unglik H, Cook JL. Strategy to reduce illicit drug use is effective in elite Australian football. Br J Sports Med0. 2012;46:943–945.

25 Science at the Olympics

Four Selections

Neuroimaging, high-tech materials, new asthma meds, detection-eluding drugs, thermoregulation—will all these make athletes stronger and faster at the 2008 Summer Games in Beijing? *Science* investigates in these four brief articles.*

■ CAN ICE VESTS PROVIDE A COMPETITIVE CHILL?

At the 2004 Athens games, 30 minutes before the women's marathon, Deena Kastor of the United States began her "warm-up." Instead of jogging in the 35°C heat, she donned an ice-filled vest, sat down, and waited for the start of the 42.2-kilometer run. More than 2 hours later, staying cool seemed to pay off. A kilometer from the finish, Kastor pulled into third place to secure a bronze medal. "The vest definitely helps performance because I am delaying the point in the race in which I overheat," says Kastor, who will race in Beijing.

The logic seems unimpeachable. As body temperature climbs to 40°C, strength and endurance evaporate. So cooling off before competition should enable an athlete to push harder and longer. Runners, rowers, cyclists, and others are already using ice vests. But how much does "precooling" help, and for which events? "It definitely lowers body temperature," says Iain Hunter, an exercise scientist at Brigham Young University (BYU) in Provo, Utah. "The question is, does it improve performance? And that's a lot less clear."

Since the 1970s, numerous studies have shown that precooling can dramatically affect some measures of athletic output. A 1995 study of 14 male runners found that if they were first chilled for 30 minutes in a chamber at 5°C, they could run on a treadmill at a certain level of exertion for an average of 26.4 minutes, a whopping 3.8 minutes longer than they averaged otherwise.

Olympic events are typically races over fixed distances, however, and the few studies of race times show much smaller improvements. In 2005, BYU's Hunter and colleagues studied 18 female cross-country runners, who had ingested encapsulated thermometers, as they participated in 4- and 5-kilometer races. Some wore ice vests for an hour before their race, and, on average, their core body temperatures were half a degree lower than those who did not, even at the ends of the

*From *Science Magazine*, 321, no. 5889 (2008). Reprinted with permission from AAAS.

races. But the researchers found only an insignificant difference of a few seconds in the two groups' average times.

Similarly, Kirk Cureton and colleagues at the University of Georgia, Athens, put nine male and eight female runners through simulated 5-kilometer races on treadmills. When the runners wore ice vests during a 38-minute warm-up of jogging and stretching, they finished the time trial 13 seconds faster on average than when they warmed up without them. That was a 57-meter lead over their warmer selves, and "even if it was 10 meters it would be important," Cureton says.

But Cureton and colleagues found that temperature differences vanished by race's end, suggesting that precooling is less valuable for long races like the marathon. It likely helps for races lasting between a minute and an hour, Cureton says. It definitely hurts in sprint events. How it works is a mystery. When the skin is cool, less blood flows to it to carry away heat, leaving more to course through the muscles. Precooling may also change the input from the body's heat sensors to the brain, which regulates pacing, enabling the athlete to push harder, says Rob Duffield, an exercise physiologist at Charles Sturt University in Bathurst, Australia.

This much is certain: Using an ice vest won't make an athlete unbeatable. Paula Radcliffe of the United Kingdom, the world record holder for the women's marathon, wore one before the Athens race. She overheated and dropped out 6 kilometers from the finish.

—Adrian Cho

▪ NAKED TRUTH

- Swimming goggles were first allowed in 1976.
- Some of the first known spiked track shoes were invented by Joseph William Foster in the early 1890s.
- Greek athletes usually competed nude. According to one ancient writer, Pausanias, a competitor deliberately lost his shorts so that he could run more freely during the race in 720 B.C.E., and clothing was then abolished. Other explanations abound.

▪ DO NEW MATERIALS MAKE THE ATHLETE?

In 1960, Ethiopian marathoner Abebe Bikila earned an Olympic gold medal without wearing any shoes. But bare feet on the Olympic track these days are passé, as athletes slip into ever more high-tech gear. Shoes, swimsuits, and clothing are getting lighter and stronger, adhering like glue to athletes' bodies and moving more fluidly through air and water.

In Beijing, U.S. track and field athletes will be wearing Nike shoes and clothing that incorporate threads made of Vectran, a superstrong liquid crystal polymer that withstands high temperatures. The result, according to Nike, is lighter, stiffer shoes to reduce friction and clothes that reduce drag by 7% compared with the Nike outfits worn at the 2004 games in Athens.

Sprinters will also benefit from even tighter compression garments. In theory, these improve performance because of proprioception, that unconscious ability that enables you to pinpoint your nose when your eyes are closed. Physiologist Russ Tucker of the University of Cape Town, South Africa, says that because runners need to contract muscles precisely—at the proper angle, velocity, and time— tight-fitting garments help the brain identify where in space the limb is poised so they know when to activate the muscle.

In the water, the Speedo LZR Racer suit, which debuted in March 2008, is all the buzz. Swimmers donning the suit have broken 46 world records so far. The suit includes polyurethane panels placed strategically around parts of the torso, abdomen, and lower back that experience high amounts of drag in the pool. It also incorporates a corset-like structure that keeps the body in a streamlined position. Raúl Arellano, a biomechanist at the University of Granada, Spain, says the LZR Racer suit could benefit older athletes like 41-year-old Dara Torres of the United States, especially in areas where fat tends to accumulate.

Some of the technologies needed to develop the suit "didn't really exist 10 years ago," says Jason Rance, head of Aqualab in Nottingham, U.K., the division of Speedo that designed the suit. Those include ultrasonic welding that eliminated the need for seams, and technology that allowed parts of the suit to be finely sanded and a water-repellent substance added to prevent water from leaking in.

But the suit has raised eyebrows. "Who's going to win the gold medal, the swimmer or the technician?" asks Huub Toussaint, a biomechanist at the Free University in Amsterdam, who worries that the suit gives swimmers an unfair edge, although the international body governing the sport approved it.

For all the hype surrounding space-age shoes and clothing, there's a flip side: Any boost to performance could just be psychological. South Africa's Tucker, who races for fun, says the compression garments make him feel powerful and secure. Such a superhero aura might give any competitor a mental edge. "It doesn't really matter if the advantages are physically real or not," he says, "as long as the athlete gets some benefit."

—Andrea Lu

■ CAN NEUROSCIENCE PROVIDE A MENTAL EDGE?

For Olympic athletes, physical strength, speed, and stamina are a given. But when elite competitors go head to head, it can be the mind as much as the muscles that determines who wins. A collaboration between sports psychologists and cognitive neuroscientists is trying to figure out what gives successful athletes their mental edge.

One focus is why some athletes rebound better than others after a poor performance. Even at the Olympic level, it's not uncommon for an athlete to blow a race early in a meet and then blow the rest of the meet, says Hap Davis, the team psychologist for the Canadian national swim team. To investigate why—and what might be done about it—Davis teamed up with neuroscientists including Mario Liotti at Simon Fraser University in Burnaby, Canada, and Helen Mayberg at Emory University in Atlanta, Georgia.

The researchers used functional magnetic resonance imaging (fMRI) to monitor brain activity in 11 swimmers who'd failed to make the 2004 Canadian Olympic team and three who made the team but performed poorly. The researchers compared brain activity elicited by two video clips: one of the swimmer's own failed race and a control clip featuring a different swimmer. Watching their own poor performance sparked activity in emotional centers in the brain similar to that seen in some studies of depression, the researchers reported in June in *Brain Imaging and Behavior*. Perhaps more tellingly, the researchers found reduced activity in regions of the cerebral cortex essential for planning movements. Davis speculates that the negative emotions stirred up by reliving the defeat may affect subsequent performances by inhibiting the motor cortex.

Davis and neuroscientist Dae-Shik Kim at Boston University (BU) School of Medicine are now using diffusion tensor imaging to visualize the connections between emotion and motor-planning brain regions. Kim hypothesizes that these connections might differ in athletes who are better able to shake off a bad performance. So far his team has scanned about a dozen BU athletes. Meanwhile, Davis and collaborators have been looking for interventions that would perk up the motor cortex. Additional fMRI studies, as yet unpublished, suggest that positive imagery—imagining swimming a better race, for example—boosts motor cortex activity, even when athletes see a videotaped failure. Jumping exercises have a similar effect, Davis says.

The work has already changed the Canadian team's poolside strategy, he says: "We pickup on [any negativity] right away and intervene." Davis has the swimmers review a video of a bad performance within half an hour and think about how they would fix it. Anecdotally, it seems to be working, he says. "We're seeing more people turn it around."

The fMRI findings suggest that quick, positive intervention helps athletes bounce back, says Leonard Zaichkowsky, a sports psychologist at BU who collaborates with Davis and Kim. But coaches often take a different approach with athletes. "Typically what happens is they've got hard-assed coaches reaming them out for a bad performance," he says. "It's the opposite of what they should be doing."

—Greg Miller

▪ DOES DOPING WORK?

It depends on how much proof you want. By the tough standards of modern medicine, there's little hard evidence for the efficacy of dozens of compounds on the list of the World Anti-Doping Agency (WADA). They are rarely tested in placebo-controlled trials; for most, the evidence is what medical researchers would call "anecdotal."

Many substances on the list are probably useless, most researchers say, if not outright detrimental for athletic prowess. "The science behind it is pretty weak," concedes Swedish oncologist Arne Ljungqvist, a former Olympic high jumper who chairs WADA's Health, Medical & Research Committee.

Not that we don't know anything about what works. Decades ago, double-blind trials for amphetamines and other stimulants showed that they can enhance performance in short, explosive activities, such as sprinting. Anabolic steroids have been proved beyond any doubt to increase muscle mass and enhance performance among male athletes in sports that require strength, such as weight-lifting and shot-putting; in women, they appear to work for endurance sports as well. History provides more circumstantial evidence: In many sports, the amazing rise in performances came to a halt after the crackdown on anabolic steroids began in earnest in the 1980s, and some records have not been broken since then.

But for many other compounds the evidence is thin, says Harm Kuipers, a physician and former speed-skating world champion who studies doping at Maastricht University in the Netherlands. One of the hottest substances of the moment, erythropoietin (EPO), has been tested for performance enhancement in only four double-blind trials, Kuipers says; they showed that it increased maximum oxygen uptake and performance, but apparently for short durations only.

Data are lacking because rigorous trials are expensive, and there's little incentive to fund them. The drugs' target population, top athletes, usually can't be recruited into studies because it might ruin their careers. Also, the list of substances and combinations is endless; cyclists once used a cocktail of strychnine, cognac, and cocaine, for instance. And the risk of side effects can make ethics panels frown.

Still, some say WADA should promote more efficacy studies. The agency is currently spending millions of dollars to improve detection of human growth hormone, a banned substance that appears to be very popular and is very hard to detect. Yet, the "science on efficacy is really soft," says Donald Catlin, who until 2007 led a major antidoping lab at the University of California, Los Angeles. "I'd prefer to have true evidence before we go after it."

If WADA, created in 1999, had a more scientific attitude, it would drop many drugs from the list, which it inherited from the International Olympic Committee, says Kuipers, who sat on the panel for several years. Countless substances—such as beta-agonists, corticosteroids, and narcotics—are listed simply because athletes used them, or were rumored to use them, even though they are widely believed to be useless.

A spot on the list may actually encourage athletes to experiment with a substance, Kuipers says: "The doping list is a shopping list for some." Such experiments can be dangerous. In healthy people, for instance, an overdose of insulin—another listed substance that few believe does athletes any good—can lead to a fatal drop in blood sugar levels.

Ljungqvist takes the opposite view: Removing substances from the list would signal that it's okay to use them, he says. And WADA wants to protect athletes from any drug they don't need, if only to send a message to their young fans. Ljungqvist agrees that this means that practically anything can end up on WADA's list—and that athletes risk ending their careers by taking something that doesn't bring them one bit closer to a gold medal.

—Martin Enserink

26

The Ethics of Technologically Constructed Hypoxic Environments in Sport

■ SIGMUND LOLAND AND ARTHUR CAPLAN

For centuries science, medicine, and technology have provided athletes, both elite and ordinary, with various means to improve their performance. Golf clubs, football helmets, ski waxes, bobsleds, pole vaults, tennis racquets, weight equipment, cricket and baseball bats, archery bows, soccer balls, ice skates, and other equipment have all seen considerable changes in response to scientific knowledge. Training techniques including diet and methods of exercise have rapidly evolved. Nearly all of these changes have contributed to improvements in performance—some of which athletes of earlier eras could not have dreamed of attaining no matter how hard or long they trained.

Now a new generation of technology is upon us. Drugs and pharmaceuticals are available that can improve strength, balance, endurance, and attention. Moreover, technologies that make use of the body's natural adaptive responses to the environment have been developed. For instance, since the early 1990s, athletes have used technologically constructed hypoxic environments (TCHE), such as hypoxic chambers or hypoxic tents, with the intention, at least in part, of increasing red cell mass, maximum oxygen uptake, and thereby endurance and performance.

The use of devices such as TCHE technology has led to debates in the sporting community. Some have focused on biomedical and functional aspects. Is TCHE really performance enhancing? If so, under what conditions, and how can its effects be explained? Are there health risks involved? Other debates raise ethical questions. Is the use of TCHE in line with sporting ideals, or with what the World Anti-Doping Agency (WADA) calls "the spirit of sport," or does it contradict such ideals? (For discussions of the ethics of TCHE-use, see for example 31 *Journal of Medical Ethics* (2005) 112–115, and Loland & Murray, 2007).

How are we to think about these new technologies? What are valuable technologies in sport, what are acceptable technologies, and where ought we to draw the line concerning the unacceptable?

This paper seeks answers to these questions. More specifically, with the use of TCHE as a real case, we develop a framework for thinking about the ethics of performance-enhancing technologies in football and other sports.

▪ A NOTE ON THE NATURE OF ETHICS

It is important to understand that there is no self-evident or obvious answer to the question of whether it is right to use high-altitude simulating tents or any other new technology. The answer to questions concerning the use of technology in sport is not written in some essentialist, platonic form of what sport ought to be, nor is there a "God-given" ethos handed down from on high about what role technology should play. There is no "natural" or "given" answer to be had. Even very dangerous drugs or highly risky training techniques could be permitted if we chose to allow them. The answers to what is allowed, what is permitted, and what is fair in sport are conventional and, as such, must be the subject of critical examination, debate, and rational discourse.

In other words, decisions about technology are in our hands. This is not to say we cannot reach consensus about what to permit and what to exclude. But we need to rely on persuasive arguments about why we compete and what we believe we are trying to accomplish in and with sports.

In order to reach sound conclusions about the limits, if any, to the use of technology in sport, it is necessary to begin with agreement about the facts. Sound normative reasoning relies upon mutual understanding of the facts underlying a particular question (Caplan, 1998). And for any consensus to be effective, it must involve all those with interests in the normative issue—in this case whether TCHE ought to be permitted in football. While some voices merit more respect due to differences in experience or because those who put their bodies on the line in the actual performance of a sport have a greater stake in the answer, seeking consensus requires an effort to solicit a wide variety of opinion. Consensus also requires some effort at consistency with previously established rules and boundaries in that like cases ought to be treated alike if decisions about the use of technologies in sport are to be accepted as fair.

▪ THE SPIRIT OF SPORT

Questions concerning the acceptability of particular performance-enhancing means and methods are related to the discussion of doping due to the consistency required to achieve consensus. Not surprisingly, therefore, the debates on TCHE have attracted the attention of WADA. In 2006, TCHE was reviewed according to existing criteria for substances and the established rationale for being placed on the WADA Prohibited List. These criteria are (1) scientific evidence or experience that demonstrates that the method or substance has the potential to enhance, or enhances, sport performance; (2) medical evidence or experience suggests that the use of the substance or method represents an actual or potential health risk to the athlete; and (3) the use of the substance or the method violates the spirit of sport. (See article 4.3 in the WADA Code, http://www. wada-ama.org/rtecontent/document/code_v3.pdf. Accessed September 30, 2007.)

In terms of criteria (1), WADA's scientific committee stated that TCHE ". . . can significantly enhance performance when properly applied, by increasing the endogenous production of EPO with a subsequent elevation of red blood cell production and a better oxygen transfer to the muscles." When it comes to health issues, the WADA scientific and medical committee concluded that, provided proper medical supervision, moderate altitude simulation, and reliable equipment, ". . . no significant signs of health risks were reported." The key issue then became whether the use of TCHE can be said to be a challenge to what WADA refers to as "the spirit of sport."

In the so-called "fundamental rationale" for the WADA Code, "the spirit of sport" is defined as, ". . . the celebration of the human spirit, body and mind, and is characterized by the following values:

- Ethics, fair play and honesty
- Health
- Excellence in performance
- Character and education
- Fun and joy
- Teamwork
- Dedication and commitment
- Respect for rules and laws
- Respect for self and other participants
- Courage
- Community and solidarity." (http://www.wada-ama. org/rtecontent/document/code_v3.pdf, p. 3. Accessed September 30, 2007.)

These are general references and hard to operationalize when it comes to concrete cases of performance-enhancing technologies. With the strong drive toward maximal performance in elite sport, and with rapid scientific and technological innovation, WADA faces a constant challenge in knowing where to draw the line. In addition to relevant facts about the means under consideration, there is a need for more precise interpretations of the concept of the "spirit of sport." The key issue seems to be what the point is of an athletic performance.

■ ATHLETIC PERFORMANCE

Athletic performances are a complex product of a high number of genetic and extra-genetic factors from the moment of conception to the moment of performance. As with most human phenotypes, the distinction between genetic and environmental influences is hard to uphold. Still, for normative analyses, the distinction may make sense.

Genetic factors can be understood as the predispositions for developing the relevant phenotypes for good athletic performances. A person with predispositions for developing, for instance, unusual speed, endurance, or advanced movement techniques in sports in which these are critical qualities is usually characterized as "talented" at these sports. From the perspective of a population, talent in this sense is distributed in the so-called natural lottery and based on chance.

Athletes develop talent through genes interacting with environment. Environmental influences range from the early nurture and the gradual development of general abilities and skills, to being raised in a particular environment and climate that present particular opportunities to engage in sports, to specific training and the learning of the technical and tactical skills of a particular sport. Environmental influences are based in part on luck; a person with a talent for swimming is born next to a public pool and happens to come under the supervision of a good coach. But, primarily, extraordinary success is based on an athlete's own efforts; the swimmer, runner, or gymnast realizes their talent through hard training over many years.

There are various views on what athletic performances ought to be all about. Below, we discuss a key tension between two sets of interpretations—we will call them "thin" and "thick" interpretations—that seem to be expressions of the basic tension in the normative thinking of competitive sport today.

Thin Interpretations

On what can be labeled the thin interpretation of the point of athletic performance, the definitions of athletic performance as found in the existing competition rules are sufficient. Rules against the use of hands in soccer, or kicking in handball, or pushing other runners in track and field races, are to be kept and honored as they are the constitutive rules that define a framework without which evaluation of performance and the very understanding of the game would not be possible at all. Thin interpretations often include a (Kantian) fairness ethos. Rules are to be kept not only due to the need to define the sport and for valid evaluations of performance and outcome, but out of respect for other competitors as ends in themselves. Outside of competitions, however, thin interpretations reject restrictions on performance-enhancing means and methods other than from what is regulated by general law.

Thin interpretations come in many versions, from what can be labeled harsh realism in which doping is considered a problematic but necessary consequence of the logic of elite sport (Black & Pape, 1997), via versions based on strong antipaternalism that emphasize individual autonomy (Brown, 1990; Tamburrini, 2000), and to so-called neo- or trans-humanistic perspectives that promote radical ideals of human enhancement and performance with the help of modern biotechnology (Fost, 1986; Miah, 2004). From the thin interpretation perspective, appropriate TCHE use is considered a fine-tuning of the human organism and as a reinforcement of the true, transcending spirit of sport.

Counterarguments to thin interpretations are that they are sociologically naïve and contra-productive. Lifting all restrictions on performance-enhancing means and methods may leave athletes in vulnerable positions and reduce their autonomy drastically (Loland, 2001). However, in a situation with fully informed athletes who are capable of free and rational choices, the thin interpretation can be morally defensible. Perhaps visions of elite sport as spheres for human biotechnological self-construction are closer to future realities than many tend to believe? (For discussion of various visions in this respect, see Tamburrini & Tännsjö, 2005.) Still, the thin interpretation of what is permissible in sport is not one that has achieved anything close to consensus in any major sport.

Thick Interpretations

An alternative can be found in thick interpretations in which sport rules are considered to define not just a particular framework for in-competition evaluation of performance but as expressions of ideals with clear and desired implications outside of the competitive setting. Thick interpretations range from the United Kingdom's Ideal's Program, traditional norms of martial arts as exemplified in karate and sumo, Olympic and Paralympic ideology, and WADA's views of "the spirit of sport," to more scholarly treatments of the purpose of sport such as those of Morgan (1994), Loland (2002), and Simon (2004).

The initial core assumptions of the thick interpretation of the spirit of sport are not dissimilar to that of the thin interpretation. Athletes are considered free and responsible moral agents. The consequences drawn, however, are far more extensive.

To realize athlete potential for moral agency, training and competition must cultivate the athlete's responsibility for performance. Performances should be the result of athletic effort. Competitive sport is about individual merit. Only in this way, the thick interpretation argument holds, can sport realize its spirit as a particular sphere for exhibiting human excellence. And, of equal importance, only through rewarding individual effort can sport offer moral lessons to society.

Thick interpretation ideals seem to have a regulative function in the rule systems of most sports. For instance, inequalities that athletes cannot influence with training and for which they cannot be claimed responsible, such as inequalities in sex, age, and body size where these inequalities matter to performance, are eliminated or at least compensated for with the creation of competitive categories.

There is of course much room for improvement here. In some sports, there is a need for more classification; other sports classify too much. For instance, basketball and volleyball, in which body height is crucially important to succeed, there is a rationale for classification according to height. In other sports, such as in rifle shooting or archery, biological sex seems to be irrelevant to performance and sex classification ought to be abandoned. Moreover, the thick interpretation has considerable critical force beyond classification issues. If taken seriously, it would have radical consequences for the regulation of inequalities in financial, scientific, and technological resources behind athletes and teams. But these require more extensive discussion about fairness and justice in sport (see Loland, 2002).

Although significantly challenged by thin interpretations, thick interpretations in one version or the other seem to be generally accepted in the sport community and on the part of the public. The ideal of athletes as moral agents with responsibility for their own performances is widely accepted. If this is so, what are the implications of thick interpretations for performance-enhancing technologies in general and for TCHE use in particular? Four principles can be adduced that seem relevant in answering this question.

I. *The technology must produce verifiable benefit—it must be demonstrably efficacious.* To be utilized and adopted, sport technologies and training techniques must be subject to rigorous scientific analysis. Scientific warrant is the first ethical principle of performance enhancement. No matter how often a technology is used, no matter how many testimonials are given on its behalf, it makes no sense to invest time, money, and sometimes to create inconvenience and risk to pursue ideas that do not work.

Because many more athletes live at low altitudes than very high, the focus on performance impairment tends to be on what happens when competition takes place at an unusually high altitude. As is evident from the papers in this issue, it is clear that altitude inhibits performance. The higher one goes, the more rapidly this is done, the more aerobic capacity is diminished. This has a distinct impact on aerobic sports such as long-distance running and cross-country skiing. It may have a different impact on those who try to play football in that cognition and fine motor-based technique may be impaired, which may limit performance as much as the burden imposed on aerobic performance by a very high altitude. For an individual coming from a low altitude, playing football in locations such as the Bolivian cities of La Paz or Toluca means that the performance is likely to suffer.

One way to compensate for a very high altitude is to use a combination of technology, acclimatization, and training techniques. Interestingly, not every technique used stands up to the test of science. For example, intermittently breathing nitrogen by a mask at sea level does not improve performance. Ultrahigh-altitude training causes harm in some groups susceptible to altitude sickness.

In football, less is known about altitude training and technology than would be ideal. Often limited data are all that are available, derived from small numbers of athletes in a narrow range of sports. The data may not reflect the racial and ethnic diversity present when teams come to play nor do the available data reflect rapidly changing environmental circumstances such as temperature, humidity, shifts in sleep patterns, or diet. This means that caution ought be the order of the day in making recommendations to football players and coaches about the technological benefit to performance they can achieve using TCHE or high-altitude training or both.

II. Safety first

In sport risk is a reality. Many sports are inherently filled with risk and the athletes have the scars, broken bones, and pulled muscles to prove it. And part of the fun of watching sport is to see how athletes face and master risk (or fail to do so).

That said, risk cannot and should not overwhelm the best interests of the athletes who engage in sport. Respect for the health, well-being, and dignity of the athlete must be a paramount consideration in thinking through the ethics of any proposed technological or training innovation. Those performance-enhancing drugs that cause cancer, sterility, or other health problems must be banned because the pressure to use them could lead to situations where the athlete sacrifices his health or a coach or an owner demands such a sacrifice for short-term performance gain. Rules that allow the drama and skill of sport to be in evidence but that also minimize the prospect of serious injury and disability ought to be implemented in every sport be it seatbelts and crash cages in autoracing or keeping athletes adequately hydrated in football and basketball.

Risk can take the form of harms that are emotional, and psychological as well as physical. Having to live in a very confined space for weeks or months to maximize aerobic performance might well violate an athlete's sense of well-being or psychological stability. Asking athletes to wear burdensome equipment at altitude while they engage in football may be both an affront to the elegance and dignity of the athlete as well as a source of very real physical risk in a high-contact sport.

If used properly, TCHE does not seem to imply any direct health risks (Levine, 2006). Still, in thinking about any performance-enhancing technology, all variety of harm must be weighed both short and long term. It is especially important to assess the potential harm done to young athletes and children who often may not have the ability to stand up to parental, peer, or coaching pressures or may simply wish to emulate their heroes despite the fact that they may be more vulnerable to harm.

III. Justice and fairness

Sport competitions ought to be fair and just. Key requirements on fairness concern equality of external conditions, classification of athletes in which inequalities in, for instance, size, age, and sex are eliminated or compensated for, and equal access to technology and training expertise assured. In the context of performance-enhancing technologies, it seems unfair that only some athletes have access to these technologies and not others. The premise, of course, is that the idea in sport is to evaluate an athlete's talent and skills, and not inequalities in their support systems and technologies. Admittedly, this principle is not always honored in the sporting community but deviating too far from it would completely undermine the competitive nature of sport.

The implications of requirements on fairness are obvious. If a performance-enhancing technology is really working and only a few athletes have access, the situation is unfair. In the case of TCHE, it is obvious that if the technology is effective and safe, and if it is considered in line with the spirit of the sport, FIFA has an obligation to provide for equal access both to equipment and to the knowledge about how to use it.

IV. Spirit of sport and rationale for sport

We have proposed two interpretations of the spirit of or the rationale for sport—thin and thick. As a social practice, sport has certain inherent norms and values, developed over decades and even centuries, that indicate its desired significance for individuals and society. In our interpretation, we emphasize the idea of athlete autonomy and responsibility for performance using the thick interpretation of the purpose of sport. What are the implications of this for performance-enhancing technologies in general and for TCHE use in particular?

Many performance-enhancing technologies are of key value and constitutive of sport. Athletes interact in admirable ways with sport equipment such as skis, bikes, skates, and soccer balls. In training and preparation, athletes also interact with a variety of technologies that include weights, training machines, and technological devices that measure air and water resistance as related to movement patterns and body positions, etc. Successful outcomes of these interactions depend on athletic effort and skill. As long as there is equal access among competitors, they are in line with and to a certain extent enforce the spirit of sport.

However, most performance-enhancing technologies, such as the use of most of the substances on WADA's Prohibited List, are considered to provide performance enhancement without athlete effort and skill. Their successful use depends primarily on their correct administration usually guided by external expertise. In addition, most of these means imply significant risks of harm. Upon their use, athletes end up in vulnerable positions in which the nature and consequences of technology use must be carefully overseen by others. Athlete autonomy is threatened. Sport, as a measure of athletic effort and performance, loses its significance. Hence, many argue that potentially harmful expert-administrated performance-enhancing means and methods should be banned. In this interpretation of the spirit of sport, there is strong support for anti-doping.

TCHE is a kind of expert-administered technology. This does not mean that TCHE can be equated with doping. Banned performance-enhancing drugs such as anabolic steroids or EPO meet all three WADA criteria, including the risk of serious harm. TCHE use is reported to create little or no health risk. Some even argue that its performance-enhancing effects are marginal. The physiological adaptive responses to TCHE use is radically different from the workings of doping means such as EPO or blood doping that bypass normal physiological feedback control mechanisms and adaptive responses (Levine, 2006). No athlete or team can perform well without talent and the cultivation of talent through intensive training, but TCHE use can be the significant factor that distinguishes a winner in the end. However, as long as TCHE use does not have strong performance-enhancing effects, the decision of WADA not to ban the technology seems a reasonable one.

However, to protect athlete autonomy and empowerment and encourage athlete responsibility for performance, expert-administered technologies such as TCHE should be continuously and critically discussed and evaluated. The case against a ban at present is not strong. But the case for encouraging, promoting, or demanding the use of TCHE is not strong either.

■ TCHE IN CONTEXTS OTHER THAN PURE PERFORMANCE ENHANCEMENT

Does this mean that there is no place for TCHE in football or other sports? When it comes to football, the consensus statement in this volume is clear: TCHE is not considered to be of any real significance.

If TCHE use exerts only a marginal performance-enhancing effect but is of significance to athlete health and welfare, appropriate use can be within the spirit of sport. If competitions take place in high altitudes, if the use of TCHE is of crucial significance to athlete health and welfare, and if the technology is provided for on an equal access basis, its use should be considered. But again, based on principled concerns about the challenges of performance-enhancing technologies that do not require athlete effort and skill, the thick interpretation of the spirit of sport encourages a restrictive attitude. Indeed, it is problematic whether sport events should take place at altitudes that subtly coerce athletes to use TCHE whether they want to or not.

Should the compensatory use of TCHE be necessary at all in a sport such as football? If there is adherence to the goal that football be played wherever significant human populations dwell, it must be understood that this goal may create the need to use TCHE—a need that could be moderated or eliminated by the thoughtful selection of playing venues. TCHE only activates a (limited) physiological adaptive response and is not recommended as acclimatization for playing football at all.

What can be said of the use of TCHE outside of sports? There is of course nothing wrong with TCHE per se. To the contrary, the technology is crucial in hypoxia research and in providing valuable basic and applied knowledge of the physiology of altitude. Moreover, in a series of applied settings from aviation to physically strenuous work in high altitude as in alpine rescue, the use of TCHE seems both appropriate and important. This underlines a more general ethical point.

To be able to deal in reasonable ways with enhancement technologies in sport and society, it is absolutely necessary to differentiate between the logic and goals of different human practices. The logic of science, aviation, or alpine rescue is primarily an instrumental one. Outcomes in terms of knowledge, or human welfare and human life, justify their existence. The ideal logic (or spirit) of sport is a different one. The rules of sporting games define the removal of the most efficient means to reach a goal in favor of less efficient means (Suits, 1978). Outfield soccer players are not allowed to play the ball with their hands; a handball player cannot kick the ball; a hurdle runner has to run over and not around the hurdles. These obstacles are what make up sporting games and provide them with meaning and value in themselves independent of their outcome, which in this sense is trivial.

■ CONCLUSION

We propose four critical questions as guidelines from which to evaluate new performance-enhancing technologies in sport. These are (I) Is the technology beneficial, (II) Is it safe, (III) Can fairness be assured, and (IV) Is the technology in line with the spirit of or the rationale for sport. The use of TCHE is ambiguous. For the specific case of acclimatization for football in altitude, the consensus statement in this issue does not recommend TCHE use. More generally, in situations in competitions between individuals or teams due to lack of acclimatization, TCHE can be an efficient means to even the playing field and to protect athlete welfare and health. On the other hand, if used as a pure performance-enhancing means to enhance the oxygen carrying capacity of the blood independent of altitude, it belongs to a category of expert-assisted performance enhancement that should be discouraged because it challenges athlete autonomy and responsibility for performance and, thus, the interpretation of the spirit of sport that is currently widely accepted as valid.

Key words: sport, ethics, hypoxic chambers.

Conflict of interest: The authors have declared that they have no conflict of interest.

■ REFERENCES

Black T, Pape A. The ban on drugs in sport: the solution or the problem? J Sport Soc Issues 1997: 21: 83–92.

Brown RM. Practices and prudence. J Philos Sport 1990: XI: 14–22.

Caplan AC. Due consideration. New York: John Wiley & Sons, 1998.

Fost NC. Banning drugs in sport: a skeptical view. Hastings Cent Rep 1986: 16: 5–10.

Levine B. Should "artificial" high altitude environments be considered doping? Scand J Med Sci Sports 2006: 16: 297–301.

Loland S. Technology in sport: three ideal-typical views and their implications. Eur J Sport Sci 2001: 2: 1–10.

Loland S. Fair play in sport. A moral norm system. London: Routledge, 2002.

Loland S, Murray TH. The ethics of the use of technologically constructed high-altitude environments to enhance performances in sport. Scand J Med Sci Sports 2007: 17: 193–197.

Miah A. Genetically modified athletes. Biomedical ethics, gene doping and sport. London: Routledge, 2004.

Morgan WJ. Leftist theories of sport: a critique and reconstruction. Urbana: Illinois University Press, 1994.

Simon RL. Fair play. The ethics of sport, 2nd edn. Boulder: Westview Press, 2004.

Suits B. The Grasshopper. Games, Life and Utopia. Toronto: University of Toronto Press, 1978.

Tamburrini C. 'The hand of god.' Essays in the philosophy of sport. Gothenburg: Acta Universitatis Gothoburgensis, 2000.

Tamburrini C, Tännsjö T, (eds). Genetic technology and sport: ethical questions. London: Routledge, 2005.

27 Gene Transfer for Pain

A Tool to Cope with the Intractable or an Unethical

Endurance-Enhancing Technology?

■ SILVIA CAMPORESI AND
MICHAEL J. MCNAMEE

■ INTRODUCTION

In this paper we consider two plausible scenarios in which an individual is seeking treatment with gene transfer tools to cope better with pain. In the first scenario the individual is a patient, in the second an athlete. The general question explored is whether it is ethically justifiable for the individual to seek an experimental gene transfer treatment in order to raise his/her tolerance to pain. We employ here a comparative strategy to highlight the similarities and dissimilarities between the ethical frameworks used to evaluate the two scenarios, and to reach conclusions regarding the justifiability of the potential practice.

■ GENE TRANSFER FOR PAIN

Untreatable pain represents an enormous problem to society. As estimated by current statistics, approximately 20% of the adult population suffers from chronic pain, and the financial cost to society is estimated at more than €200 billion per annum in Europe, and $150 billion per annum in the USA.[1] Treatment options are limited, with many patients either not responding to them or having incomplete pain reduction.[2]

In the last decade, several translational clinical trials have been carried out that employed gene transfer tools to try to overcome this medical need. Gene transfer trials certainly qualify as translational trials, as they are designed to bring to the bedside the tools developed at the bench of a molecular biology laboratory. We performed a search with keywords 'gene transfer' and 'pain' on the National Health Institutes clinical trials directory, which revealed 20 clinical trials that are either completed or in recruitment.[3] To date nine clinical trials have been completed.[4] Some of these trials are aimed at treating intractable cancer pain, some at treating pain associated with angina pectoris, others at epidermolysis bullosa (a heritable condition where connective tissue disease causes painful blisters in the skin and mucosal membranes), and others to treat the pain associated with peripheral arterial occlusion (a mini-stroke in the leg which causes the necrosis of muscular tissue leading to impaired functionality and chronic pain). This last kind of pain, and the related clinical trial, serves as a case study for our comparative evaluation between a medical context and a sports context, where the former is a traditionally conceived therapeutic intervention, and the latter is one where the intervention rests in the grey zone between therapy and enhancement—or as it has been labelled, therapeutic enhancement.[5] We set out the two scenarios below and evaluate them ethically according to two different frameworks.

Scenario (a): The Medical Context (the Patient)

In scenario (a), in the US TV series *House MD,* the protagonist, Dr Gregory House, has suffered from peripheral ischemia to a leg, which has left him limping and with intractable chronic pain, due to the extensive necrotic muscular tissue in his thigh muscles. He is seeking an alternative solution in a gene transfer clinical trial. Dr House can perhaps be seen as a contemporary instance of the archetypical mythological figure of the 'wounded healer' Chiron, who is able to heal others but unable to heal himself. After having tried many standard and less standard treatments unsuccessfully, our protagonist is now seeking experimental treatments, i.e. treatments that are currently being tested in clinical trials and not yet approved by national regulatory bodies such as the US Food & Drug Administration (FDA) or the European Medicines Agency (EMA), and are unavailable on the market. Among the gene transfer trials currently active or recruiting, one study stands out as the perfect match for a patient like Gregory House.

The trial (Identifier # NCT00304837')[6] is a Phase 1 study that seeks to transfer the DNA codifying for the Vascular Endothelial Growth Factor (VEGF) protein into the legs of patients with peripheral artery disease (PAD). PAD encompasses a range of conditions presenting with blockages in the arteries in the limbs. The nature of the disease is progressive, so that it frequently leads to patients presenting with claudication or critical limb ischemia (CLI).[7] It is this former manifestation of PAD that we are interested to discuss. Most Phase 1 studies are aimed at testing the safety of a new pharmaceutical or treatment in a restricted number of patients, after the treatment has proved efficacious in laboratory testing and animal models, but some—like this one—may also test the efficacy of the agent under study. According to the trial protocol, the DNA codifying for the VEGF protein is injected into the affected legs of the trial subjects on three separate occasions, each two weeks apart. The DNA codifier then directs the cells of the artery wall to increase production of VEGF, which has been shown to cause new blood vessels to grow around the blockages in the leg arteries.[8] It has also been demonstrated that increased VEGF expression through gene transfer techniques improves microcirculation in muscle, and hence increased oxygen and nutrient supply, as well as removal of waste products.[9] Kim et al have observed evidence of growth of new collateral vessels, relief of ischemic pain and ulcer healing in patients with CLI.[10] The trial we are analysing aims not only to test the safety of VEGF-gene transfer, but also to relieve pain and/or heal the ulcers caused by PAD.[11]

Generally speaking, safety concerns about gene transfer are related both to the kind of carrier/vector being used (usually a modified virus) and to the encoded transgene. In our case study, the former are eliminated by injecting the DNA coding for the VEGF protein directly into the patients' leg muscles, without any viral or non-viral carrier, thus eliminating the risks inherent in the vectors and common to many other gene transfer trials. As to the latter risks, it has been shown that overexpression of VEGF causes haemangiomas (benign tumours characterised by an increased number of normal or abnormal vessels filled with blood) in skeletal muscle in mouse animal models.[12] In addition, angiogenesis, can have detrimental consequences in non-target tissues. In particular, the theoretical risk of facilitation of tumour vascularization (and therefore, increased growth) or plaque angiogenesis in non-target tissues must not be ignored.[13] Transient peripheral edema (swelling) due to increased local perfusion is a relatively common and mild side effect.

More serious adverse effects have been rarely observed and are mostly related to the use of viral vectors, therefore are not pertinent to the trial we are discussing which injects DNA in the form of a plasmid (a circular molecule of DNA).[14] A recent study conducted by Muona et al and aimed at assessing the long-term side effects (10+ years) of local VEGF gene transfer to ischemic lower limbs found that adenovirus or plasmid (our case) or liposome mediated intravascular *local* gene transfer does not increase the risk of malignancies, diabetes or any other disease in the long term. The authors also identified as a key element to safe gene transfer the local delivery to the treatment side (as in our case), which reduced the risk of systematic spread of the vector, as well of adverse side-effects to other organs. This suggests that the technique described here could be safely applied both in trial subjects and in healthy individuals (which is pertinent to Scenario (b), below).[15]

As noted by Mughal et al,[16] PAD cannot be attributed to one specific genetic cause, and greater therapeutic efficacy could be obtained by targeted gene transfer using multiple growth factors. Indeed, angiogenic gene transfer strategies such as VEGF-gene transfer are by no means the only ones being explored in the treatment of chronic pain[17] but appear to be among the most advanced at the clinical level, while other strategies are still at the level of animal studies. As a general remark, while we are aware that a certain degree of speculation is necessary when applying our case study to the second scenario (the elite sports context), we think there is sufficient scientific and medical evidence to argue that gene transfer for pain has very plausible applications for enhancing athletic performances.

Scenario (b): The Sports Context (the Elite Athlete)

In scenario (b), the would-be protagonist is an elite athlete competing in an endurance event, such as cross-country skiing, marathon running, tour cycling, triathlon, or an event of similar extended duration, seeking VEGF-gene transfer in order to cope better with the pain inherent in the event as a primary outcome, and as a secondary outcome to perform better as a result. The growth of blood vessels in the limbs, as demonstrated by the clinical trial described above, is likely to aid the athlete in his/her performance by increasing the oxygen-carrying capacity to the limbs (nutrient supply) and the removal of waste products.

It is also obvious that an athlete feeling less pain could perform better, *ceteris paribus,* than other athletes experiencing a greater degree of pain.

■ COMPARING THE SCENARIOS

How are we to understand the similarities and differences these contexts present, and to what extent will the context determine whether it is ethically justifiable for an individual to seek an experimental gene transfer treatment better to cope with pain?

To what extent is the ethical permissibility of the practice dependent upon or independent of the context of gene transfer? We respond to these questions by spelling out two ethical frameworks that might be adopted in order to analyse the two scenarios.

Framework (a): Ethics of Translational Research

With a few relevant exclusions,[18] we do not normally regard pain as an essential or valuable part of our lives. On the contrary, we take measures to diminish or even eliminate pain from our daily lives, and from the lives of those who are dear to us. Even in illnesses where pain is present, we try to eliminate it, although it may not be possible to cure the patient of the underlying cause. Palliative care, which we consider an essential part of treating a sick human being with dignity, is predicated on such an understanding.

The first framework we use to analyse the scenarios is the 'ethics of translational research' approach recently developed by Kimmelman.[19] Kimmelman develops the new concept of 'translational distance', which refers to the space created between cutting-edge biomedical research and clinical applications. It may not be possible in the first in-human studies to apply the concept of 'clinical equipoise', defined by Friedman as "a state of honest, professional disagreement in the community of experts about the preferred treatment".[20] The level of uncertainty is so high in first-in-human research employing gene transfer techniques that robust epistemic thresholds required for clinical equipoise cannot be secured. In its place, the concept of translational distance is a useful and insightful kind of 'epistemic heuristics' to understand the bidirectional flow of knowledge between the bench and the bedside.

While traditionally the value of early clinical trials has been regarded only in terms of their 'progressive value' towards later Phase 2 and Phase 3 studies, such a framework is not applicable when evaluating the social value of first-in-human research as in our case study. In Kimmelman's model, Phase 1 translational studies in between the 'bench and the bedside' are loaded with value if they stimulate preclinical research or if they stimulate further clinical development. In addition, adopting a translational distance model with a non-progressive epistemic value for these trials would help to dispel the 'therapeutic misconception'[21] widespread among (often desperate) first-in clinical trials volunteers. Therapeutic misconception arises where subjects misinterpret the primary purpose of a clinical trial as therapeutic, and conflate the goals of research with the goals of clinical care. As shown in a study of consent documents of gene transfer clinical trials, 20% of consent documents for gene transfer trials fail to explain their purpose as establishing safety and dosage, while only 41% of oncology trials identify palliative care as an alternative to participation. Moreover, the term gene therapy is used with twice the frequency of the term gene transfer.[22]

As defined by Kimmelman, the concept of translational distance "is intended to prompt researchers, review committees, and policy-makers to contemplate the size of the 'inferential gap' separating completed preclinical studies and projected human trial results",[23] and should inform both the design of the studies (that need to incorporate endpoints that make it possible for the knowledge produced to have an impact in terms of further research), and the ethical approval of the trial, that needs to take into account the concept of translational distance rather than that of clinical equipoise. We agree with Kimmelman that the translational research model better captures the reality of how information flows in translational research. As for the individual seeking to be enrolled in such an experimental trial, we recommend that researchers spell out the potential risks and benefits of the experimental procedure to the would-be volunteer; researchers should evaluate the severity of the pre-existing condition in the subject and its refractoriness to other standard treatment; and they should evaluate the subject's decisional autonomy, which will be predicated on reasonable comprehension (and voluntariness) in relation to the foregoing.

Returning to our fictional protagonist, we can see that in this particular case the risks inherent in gene transfer trials due to the viral vectors are eliminated by injecting VEGF directly into the leg muscles of the patients, and therefore the translational distance between the bench and the bedside can also be considered a modest 'inferential gap'. In addition, the pre-existing condition of chronic pain caused by peripheral artery ischemia is severe and refractory to standard treatment. And finally, Dr Gregory House seems to be in a position to make an autonomous decision, one not clouded by therapeutic misconception. As autonomy plays a fundamental role in the ethical framework describing the medical context, there would need to be strong reasons to justify interference with the patient's self-regarding and autonomous choice to participate in the trial, even recognising as we do that the patient may have no available option (apart from palliative care) other than participating in the trial, due to the severity of his condition and the unavailability of therapeutic options. Provided all the above conditions were met, we might reasonably reach the conclusion that his informed consent to participating in the VEGF-clinical trial would be valid.

Framework (b): Ethics of Sports Enhancement

How should we frame the request of an athlete seeking VEGF-gene transfer for the purposes of better coping with pain during a competition? In the first instance, his participation might look like a case of what we could call 'physician-assisted doping'.

The World Anti-Doping Agency (WADA) sets out three criteria used in the decision to call a product or process 'doping'.[24] These pertain to (i) the (potential) performance-enhancing effects; (ii) the potential harm to health; (iii) the violation of the spirit of sport. Only two criteria need apply for a product or process to be prohibited. The Anti-Doping Code recognises the rights of athletes to secure healthcare and that this right supersedes anti-doping regulations. This does not, however, allow the patient-athlete *carte blanche*. Prior to utilising banned products or processes athletes on a registered testing pool (who are on notice that they may be randomly tested) must submit a Therapeutic Use Exemption (TUE) Certificate signed by a relevant medical authority. This certifies that the therapy is necessary for the athlete's condition and that no non-doping alternative is available. Clearly, the process is open to abuse. Moreover, in Paralympic sport, where elite athletes have at least one disabling condition, the problem is even more complex.[25]

Leaving aside for the present the added complexities of unethical behaviour, let us assume that the athlete is asking for a TUE from the relevant authority. In addition to the World Anti-Doping Agency, this might be an International Federation, such as the International Association of Athletics Federations (IAAF), or the Union Cycliste International, or the International Triathlon Union, or an event organiser such as the International Olympic Committee (IOC) or the International Paralympic Committee, who (interestingly) take exclusive charge of in-competition testing during the Olympic and Paralympic Games. There is very little to suggest that a TUE would be achievable in this scenario. Despite TUE precedents for beta-blockers in relation to cardiac patient-athletes in target-accuracy events (such as archery), it is highly unlikely that it would be given for mere pain relief where that pain is simply a marker for injury (and where there may be performance enhancement side effects). The deputy director of the World Anti Doping Laboratory in Cologne, widely recognised as one of the premier testing laboratories, recently remarked upon the practice of using analgesics as analogous to doping:

It is a grey zone. In my opinion pain killers fulfil all requirements of a doping substance because normally pain is a protection mechanism of the body and with pain killers you switch off this protection system.[26]

Given the longstanding routine use and abuse of painkillers in elite sport,[27,28,29] it might be argued that the introduction of VEGF would represent merely an extension of everyday practice. In both the first and also in this second scenario, consideration would have to be given to the autonomy of the decision-making of the individual in arriving at ethically justifiable interventions. In the second scenario this would be thought necessary, while in the first scenario this might be thought both necessary and sufficient, provided that the conditions for a modest translational distance were met, as they are in our case-study. Why then is it insufficient in the context of elite sports? Well, in addition to determining the conditions of consent, additional factors regarding the ethical permissibility of VEGF-gene transfer in an athletic context must be considered.

In contrast to scenario (a), pain can be seen as an essential, integral part of endurance sports. Performing at an elite level in endurance sport and not experiencing pain are mutually exclusive. Indeed, an athlete's ability to tolerate pain is one of the fundamental characteristics that determine athletic performance and provide competitive advantage. Five-times Tour de France winner Lance Armstrong called the event "an exercise in pointless suffering".[30] He and others have talked insightfully about wanting to take opponents (metaphorically) to places that they could not endure. The capacity to endure high levels of pain over significant time (i.e. suffering) is a highly prized trait in multi-day/week Tour event cycling.[31] Indeed one may refer to them as "communities of suffering".[32]

Not only is it the case that we must distinguish the experience of pain from suffering[33] in sports[34] but in addition there are, of course, different kinds of pain an athlete can experience in competition.[35] One is the acute kind that can be defined as an intense and specific pain that occurs suddenly, often a result of injury, often experienced by athletes competing in football or other contact sports. Moreover, one can experience such pain in endurance events too—the cycle crash, the herniated disc in running, and so on. VEGF-gene transfer treatment would be meaningless for this kind of pain so it is irrelevant to this discussion. Rather, we wish to discuss the kind of pain that occurs with endurance exercise. This may include muscle soreness or a burning sensation in the lungs, the feeling that one's heart will explode if the same level of intense effort is maintained much longer, and so forth. The strength of these sensations can range from unpleasant to what is typically thought of as unbearable pain. This second kind of pain is typical of endurance sports such as marathons, triathlon, long distance swimming and cycling, cross-country skiing, and so on. Among athletes, the former kind of pain is often referred to as a 'bad' kind, as it impairs the ability of the athlete to continue playing or competing, while the latter is referred to as a 'good' kind of pain, as it pushes the athlete to compete and perform at a higher level. Indeed, many athletes regard this second or 'good kind' of pain as an achievement and as an essential part of their life and identity as elite athletes.[36]

The level of physical training of an athlete can raise the level of pain that he/she is able to endure, and make a difference in his/her performance. Athletes also report that the level of their 'mental toughness'[37] makes a difference in their ability to cope with pain. Different individuals, though, start from very different baselines in their abilities to endure pain,[38] and this is one of the factors, among many other biological and environmental factors, that affect an athlete's performance. Among these are: their birth place (contrast pre-athletic life at altitude and how this affects phenotypic factors with competitors born at or near sea level); wealth and other non-athletic factors that can enhance the possibilities of success (contrast athletes or teams with and without sports psychological services, or sponsorships that improve equipment access); genetic conditions that may confer an advantage over fellow athletes by increasing the amount of erythrocytes and oxygen supply to muscle cells (consider for example the case of Finnish skier Eero Mäntyranta who won two gold medals in cross-country skiing at the 1964 Winter Olympics. It was later discovered that he had primary familial and congenital polycythemia (PFCP), which causes an increase in red blood cell mass and haemoglobin due to a mutation in the erythropoietin receptor (EPOR) gene).[39]

There is no absolutely agreed upon standard or trigger as to when sports administrators or regulatory bodies like WADA try to even out genetic and biological differences to reach a sufficiently 'level playing field' for all athletes: some inequalities are systematically excluded, while others are ignored.[40] What happens in practice is that we do not usually try to level biological and genetic factors affecting athletic performance, even where we know those factors confer an advantage (as with Mäntyranta), although there is currently a controversy about new IAAF and IOC rules which exclude women athletes with hyperandrogenism from competing in women's events on the basis of a supposed unfair advantage derived from increased levels of testosterone.[41] Typically, philosophers generally agree that the question centres around notions of fairness and equal opportunity, or what Loland calls Fair Opportunity.[42]

Let us think counter-factually here: if we were to try to equalise all the starting conditions (of which tolerance to pain is, again, merely one example) we would move in the direction of having all athletes crossing the finish line at the same point, and then what would be left of the meaning of sport and athletic performance? After all we are precisely interested in distinguishing among excellent performers and performances. Only in certain circumstances, such as horse racing, do sports institutions initiate handicapping systems. And this, it might reasonably be argued, is to keep the competition tight and promote gambling interests. In other scenarios, where a league system—heavily underwritten by commercial media interests—has an incentive to prolong interests and more broadly spread opportunities to win, we find systems like the lower teams gaining access to the best new potential players in a draft system (such as in American Football). But in the main, we would not normally level out the effects of the genetic lottery in sports. If an athlete is 1 metre 40 we steer them away from high jump. If they are 2 metres tall, we do not encourage them to pursue a career as a professional jockey, and so on. Furthermore, a few US companies have started to sell online direct-to-consumer (DTC) genetic tests[43] that aim to exploit the genetic lottery as early as possible, channelling children towards the most 'profitable' athletic future as predicted by the results of the tests.

As mentioned above, different athletes have different baselines and different abilities to cope with pain. While we do try to give people tools better to cope with pain in everyday life, where pain is not—with certain noted exceptions—seen to be an essential or meaningful part of the activity we are performing, in the elite-sports context we do not give people those tools, because pain, as described above, is a fundamental part of practising and competing at an elite level.

Pain can be distinguished from non-relevant inequalities, as for example the kind of shoes or swimsuits or bikes the athletes run, swim, or cycle with, which do not impact upon the mental and physical qualities that are the source of our admiration for athletes and which are instrumental to the securing of victory. For these sorts of products, however, we can and do insist upon degrees of standardisation. Thus, in baseball, cricket, or tennis there are regulations regarding the size and composition of the striking implement and the ball. Curiously, in Formula 1 racing there are prizes for both the best driver *and* the best constructors: the best supporting team of engineers and technologists. But even here there are strict rules about engineering variations. In European football, there are even suggestions that there should be financial fair play, so that team owners cannot 'buy' victory by purchasing sufficiently large numbers of the talent pool.

We cannot, however, 'level-out' the capacity for enduring pain in endurance events without usurping or compromising a key psychological variable inherent within the test. By levelling the ability to endure pain, we would also diminish a substantial part of the meaning of athletic performance, which can be understood as trying to break one's own limits given the starting conditions one has. That is why the toleration of pain qualifies as a relevant inequality that serves *inter alia* to demarcate athletic merit, and we consider that genetically based therapy for pain should not be permitted as it undermines the meaning of sport by interfering significantly with the relationship between natural talents, their virtuous perfection, and athletic success.[44] In other words, our view of the athlete's capacity for pain tolerance could be seen a relevant inequality and essential for the meaning of competition. In the model developed by Loland and Hoppeler that combines a biologically based approach with a Fair Opportunity principle, the use of VEGF transfer could be understood as a way to go beyond human phenotypic plasticity,[45] and thus to go against the Fair Opportunity principle and the idea of the virtuous development of talent.[46]

■ CONCLUSIONS

The differences between the two scenarios we have presented are many and varied. We have focused only on the existence of a fundamental difference between a medical and an elite athletic context of VEGF-gene transfer to tolerate pain. In the latter the choice is fundamentally a self-regarding one, predicated on individual autonomy together with a risk/benefits calculation as the principal factor determining the ethics of that decision. A cautionary note must be struck here. One must be mindful of the areas of uncertainty, the limited evidential base in relation to the experiment[47] and its hoped-for outcomes in scientific and clinical terms. Nevertheless, in elite endurance sports contexts individual autonomy ceases to play the decisive role in the ethical analysis. Sports have traditionally incorporated paternalistic practices regarding the health of competitors but also the fairness of the structuring of competition in order to produce admirable victors. The context of gene-transfer matters for the evaluation of the ethical desirability or permissibility of the experimental practice we are analysing: while in an everyday life scenario, pain does not play a meaningful role (with some noted exceptions), pain does play a meaningful and constitutive role in endurance athletic competition, along with a range of other anatomical, physiological and psychological factors. By increasing the capacity for pain-tolerance, or even subtracting it altogether from the sports picture, we would inevitably subtract also a fundamental part of the meaning of that picture.

We conclude, therefore, that while we would not interfere with the decision of Dr House to be enrolled in a trial for VEGF-gene transfer, we could not justify the request of the athlete seeking VEGF-gene transfer to increase his/her tolerance to pain. As a tool to cope with the intractable pain that visits afflicted patients, VEGF-gene transfer is ethically justifiable and desirable. In endurance sports, the use of VEGF-gene transfer as an endurance enhancement technology is not merely ethically unjustifiable; it compromises an element essential to the activity itself.

What does this comparison tell us about the relationship between the ethics of clinical research (scenario [a]) and the ethics of sports medicine (scenario [b])? We might note that, while the field of clinical research ethics is more established and has a longer history, the field of ethics of sports medicine is a relatively young one, and reflects the underlying tension between the goals of medicine (health) and elite sports (athletic excellence).[48] But the ethics of first-in-human studies, including gene transfer studies, are still largely under-explored. Indeed, Kimmelman's analysis of translational distance is the first and only attempt, to the best of our knowledge, to fill in the void left by the impossibility of applying the concept of clinical equipoise in first-in human gene transfer studies, which are characterised by a level of uncertainty that is simply too high (as we have shown above). Both fields are young and relatively under-explored, and a comparison between the two may highlight insightful similarities, and shed light on problematic aspects of each.[49]

■ ACKNOWLEDGEMENT

McNamee's contribution was supported by the European Commission FP7 Science in Society funded project, *Ethics in Public Policy Making: The Case of Human Enhancement* (EPOCH), grant number SIS-CT-2010-266660 http://epochproject.com.

■ ABOUT THE AUTHORS

Silvia Camporesi is with the Centre for the Humanities and Health, King's College, London, and the Department of Anthropology, History and Social Medicine at the University of California, San Francisco; she can be reached at silvia.camporesi@kcl.ac.uk.

Michael J. McNamee is at the College of Human and Health Sciences, Swansea University; he can be reached at m.j.mcnamee@swansea.ac.uk.

■ NOTES

1. I. Tracey et al. How neuroimaging studies have challenged us to rethink: is chronic pain a disease? *J Pain* 2009;10(11):1113–1120.

2. H. Breivik et al. Survey of chronic pain in Europe: Prevalence, impact on daily life, and treatment, *Eur J Pain* 2006;10(4):287–333.

3. Search on http://Clinicaltrials.gov for "gene transfer AND pain" clinical trials (accessed October 12, 2012). It should be noted that this is accurate at the time of press though the figure appears to be rising sharply month on month.

4. Ibid.

5. T. Tännsjö. Medical enhancement and the ethos of elite sport. In: *Human Enhancement*, ed. J. Savulescu, N. Botrom. Oxford: Oxford University Press; 2010:315–326.

6. Clinicaltrials.gov identifier 'NCT00304837', available at: http://clinicaltrials.gov/ct2/show/NCT00304837?term=pain+gene+therapy&rank=5. Accessed October 12, 2012.

7. N.A. Mughal, D.A. Russell, S. Ponnambalam, et al. Gene therapy in the treatment of peripheral arterial disease. *Br J Surg Soc* 2012;99:6–15.

8. Ibid.

9. M. Giacca, S. Zacchigna. VEGF gene therapy: therapeutic angiogenesis in the clinic and beyond. *Gene Ther* 2012;19(6): 622–629.

10. H.J. Kim et al. Vascular endothelial growth factor-induced angiogenic gene therapy in patients with peripheral artery disease. *Exp Mol Med* 2004;36:336–344.

11. Clinicaltrials.gov, op cit. note 6.

12. M.L. Springer, A.S. Chen, P.E. Kraft, et al. VEGF gene delivery to muscle: potential role for vasculogenesis in adults. *Mol Cell* 1998;2(5):549–558.

13. I. Baumgartner. Therapeutic angiogenesis: theoretic problems using vascular endothelial growth factor. *Curr Cardiol Rep* 2000;2(1):24–28.

14. K. Muona et al. 10-year safety follow-up in patients with local VEGF gene transfer to ischemic lower limb. *Gene Ther* 2012;19:392–395.

15. Ibid.

16. Mughal et al., op.cit note 9.

17. W.F. Goins, J.B. Cohen, J.C. Glorioso. Gene therapy for the treatment of chronic peripheral nervous system pain. *Neurobiol Dis* 2012;48(2):255–270.

18. There are individuals and religions/sects which regard pain as having a high intrinsic value.

19. J. Kimmelman. *Gene Transfer and the Ethics of First-in-Human Research. Lost in Translation.* Cambridge: Cambridge University Press; 2010.

20. B. Fredman. Equipoise and the ethics of clinical research. *New Engl J Med* 1987;317:141–145.

21. G.E. Henderson et al. Therapeutic misconception in early phase gene transfer trials. *Soc Sci Med* 2006;62(1):239–253; S. Horng, C. Grady. Misunderstanding in clinical research: distinguishing therapeutic misconception, therapeutic misestimation, and therapeutic optimism. *IRB* 2003;25(1):11–16.

22. J. Kimmelman, A. Levenstadt. Elements of style: consent form language and the therapeutic misconception in phase 1 gene transfer trials. *Hum Gen Ther* 2005;16(4):502–508.

23. Kimmelman, op. cit. note 21, p. 118.

24. WADA code, 2012, www.wada-ama.org. Accessed October 12, 2012. We note that even though the Code revision process is near completion, each of the three criteria may still apply. It appears that WADA are moving to a position where performance enhancement of a product or process will be a necessary condition for inclusion on their Prohibited list. Nevertheless, and in the face of objections, they have not removed the 'spirit of sport' criterion. See http://www.wadaama.org/Documents/World_Anti-Doping_Program/WADP-The-Code/Code_Review/Code%20Review%202015/Code-Draft-1.0/WADA-Code-2015-Draft-1.0-redlined-to%202009-Code-EN.pdf. Accessed October 13, 2012.

25. P. Van der Vliet. Antidoping in Paralympic sport. *Clin J Sport Med* 2012;22(1):21–25.

26. M. McGrath. Is pain medication in sports a form of legal doping? *BBC News Science and Environment*, June 4, 2012; at http://www.bbc.co.uk/news/science-environment-18282072. Accessed October 12, 2012.

27. R. Huizenga. *You're OK, It's Just a Bruise.* New York. St Martin's Griffin; 1994.

28. H.L. Nixon. A social network analysis of influences on athletes to play with pain and injuries. *J Sport Soc Issues* 1992;13:14–24.

29. H.L. Nixon. Accepting the risks of pain and injury in sports; mediated cultural influences onplaying hurt. *Soc Sport J* 1993;16:127–135.

30. J. Fry. Pain, suffering and paradox in sport and religion. In: *Pain and Injury in Sport: Social and Ethical Analysis,* ed. S. Loland, B. Skirstad, I. Waddington. London: Routledge; 2006:246–259.

31. See most recently the biography of Amstrong's one-time team mate Tyler Hamilton who notes that he was almost singled for a professional contract out by the capacity of

suffer. T. Hamilton, D. Coyle. *The Secret Race*. London: Bantam Press; 2012. Armstrong's own capacity for suffering is the stuff of legend.

32. M.J. McNamee. *Sports, Virtues and Vices*. Abingdon: Routledge; 2008.

33. E. Cassell. *The Nature of Suffering and the Goals of Medicine*. Oxford: Oxford University Press; 2004.

34. Y. Lurie. The ontology of sports injuries. In *Pain and Injury in Sport: Social and Ethical Analysis*, ed. S. Loland, B. Skirstad, I. Waddington. London: Routledge; 2005:200–211; M.J. McNamee. Suffering in and for sport: some philosophical remarks on a painful emotion. In *Pain and Injury in Sport: Social and Ethical Analysis*, ed. S. Loland, B. Skirstad, I. Waddington. London: Routledge; 2005: 229–245.

35. K. Roessler. Sport and the psychology of pain. In *Pain and Injury in Sport: Social and Ethical Analysis*, ed. S. Loland, B. Skirstad, I. Waddington. London: Routledge; 2005:34–48.

36. P.D. Howe. *Sport, Professionalism and Pain*. Abingdon: Routledge; 2003.

37. L. Crust. Mental toughness in sport: a review. *Int J Sport Exer Psych* 2007;5:270–290; D.F. Gucciardi, S. Gordon, J.A. Dimmock. Advancing mental toughness research and theory using personal construct psychology. *Int Rev Sport and Exer Psych* 2009;2:54–72.

38. E. Dolgin. Fluctuating baseline pain implicated in failure of clinical trials. *Nat Med* 2010;16(10):1053.

39. T. Tännsjö. Hypoxic air machines. Commentary. *J Med Ethics* 2004;31(2):113.

40. S. Loland. *Fair Play: A Moral Norm System*. Abingdon: Routledge; 2002.

41. K. Karkazis, R. Jordan-Young, S. Camporesi, et al. Out of bounds? A critique of the new policies on hyperandrogenism in elite female athletes. *Am J Bioethics* 2012;12(7):3–16.

42. S. Loland. Fairness in sport: an ideal and its consequences. In *Performance Enhancing Technologies in Sports*, ed. T.H. Murray, K.J. Maschke, A.A. Wasunna. Baltimore: Johns Hopkins University Press; 2009:175–204. In a notable and carefully articulated review of the essays of the book, Murray argues *inter alia* against the Rawlsian understanding that Loland offers of the Fair Opportunity principle. The precise details are beyond the scope of the present essay. See, however, T.H. Murray. Ethics and endurance-enhancing technologies in sport. In: *Performance Enhancing Technologies in Sports*, ed. T.H Murray, K.J. Maschke, A.A. Wasunna. Baltimore: Johns Hopkins University Press; 2009:141–159.

43. Among these, Atlas Sports Genetics based in Boulder, CO, at http://www.atlasgene.com/ and Sports X Factor at http://www.sportsxfactor.com/. Accessed October 12, 2012.

44. Murray, op cit. note 42, pp. 141–159.

45. Defined as the capacity of a single genotype to exhibit variable phenotypes in different environments, and therefore as the capacity to adapt to different environments.

46. S. Loland, H. Hoppeler, Justifying anti-doping: the fair opportunity principle and the biology of performance enhancement. *Eur J Sports Sci* 2012;12(4):347–353.

47. Kimmelman, op. cit. note 21.

48. M.B. Mathias, The competing demands of sport and health: an essay on the history of ethics in sports medicine. *Clin Sports Med* 2004;23:195–214.

49. See further, S. Camporesi, M.J. McNamee. High risk-acceptance in professional guinea pigs: a comparison between the clinical trial and the doping context. In: *Proceedings of the 40th Annual Conference of the International Association for the Philosophy of Sport*, ed. T. Lacerda, J. Lima, J. Ilundain, S. Soares. Porto: Universidade de Evora Press; 2012:61–62.

◼ PUBLICATION ACKNOWLEDGMENTS

▨ PART I: WHAT IS SPORT?

Chapter 1. Roland Barthes, "What is Sport?" from the book *What is Sport?*. Copyright © 2007, Yale University Press. Reprinted with the permission of Yale University Press.

Barthes, Roland. *What is Sport?*. Yale University Press (2007). ISBN-10: 0300116047 ISBN-13: 978-0300116045.

Chapter 2. "Normative Theories of Sport: A Critical Review," Sigmund Loland, *Journal of the Philosophy of Sport* (2004), Taylor and Francis Ltd. Reprinted with the permission of Taylor and Francis Ltd., http://www.tandfonline.com.

Loland, Sigmund. "Normative Theories of Sport: A Critical Review." *Journal of the Philosophy of Sport* 31, no. 2 (2004): 111–121. DOI: 10.1080/00948705.2004.9714655.

▨ PART II: CATEGORIES AND DISCRIMINATION

A. Professional vs. Amateur

Chapter 3. "Uneven Bars: Age Rules, Antitrust, and Amateurism in Women's Gymnastics," Ryan M. Rodenberg and Andrea N. Eagleman, *University of Baltimore Law Review* (2010). Reprinted with permission from *University of Baltimore Law Review*.

Rodenberg, Ryan M., and Andrea N. Eagleman. "Uneven Bars: Age Rules, Antitrust, and Amateurism in Women's Gymnastics." *University of Baltimore Law Review* 40 (2010): 587–606.

Chapter 4. "Going Pro in Sports: Providing Guidance to Student-Athletes in a Complicated Legal and Regulatory Environment," Glenn M. Wong, Warren Zola, and Chris Deubert, *Cardozo Arts and Entertainment Law Journal* (2010). Reprinted with permission from *Cardozo Arts and Entertainment Law Journal*.

Wong, Glenn M., Warren Zola, and Chris Deubert. "Going Pro in Sports: Providing Guidance to Student-Athletes in a Complicated Legal & Regulatory Environment." *Cardozo Arts and Entertainment Law Journal* 28 (2010): 553–607.

B. Gender

Chapter 5. "Women in Sport: Gender Relations and Future Perspectives," Gertrud Pfister, *Journal of Sport in Society* (2010), Taylor and Francis. Reprinted by permission of Taylor & Francis Ltd, www.tandfonline.com.

Pfister, Gertrud. "Women in Sport: Gender Relations and Future Perspectives 1." *Sport in Society* 13, no. 2 (2010): 234–248.

Chapter 6. Copyright 2012 from "Out of Bounds? A Critique of the New Policies on Hyperandrogenism in Elite Female Athletes," Katrina Karkazis, Rebecca Jordan-Young, Georgiann Davis, and Silvia Camporesi. Reproduced by permission of Taylor and Francis LLC, http://www.tandfonline.com.

Karkazis, Katrina, et al. "Out of Bounds? A Critique of the New Policies on Hyperandrogenism in Elite Female Athletes." *The American Journal of Bioethics* 12, no. 7 (2012): 3–16.

C. Race

Chapter 7. "Race Relations Theories: Implications for Sport Management," Earl Smith and Angela Hattery reprinted, by permission, from *Journal of Sport Management* (2011) 25(2): 107–117. © Human Kinetics, Inc.

Smith, Earl, and Angela Hattery. "Race Relations Theories: Implications for Sport Management." *Journal of Sport Management* 25 (2011): 107–117.

Chapter 8. "'Black Athletes in White Men's Games': Race, Sport, and American National Pastimes," David K. Wiggins, *The International Journal of the History of Sport* (2014), Taylor and Francis. Reprinted by permission of Taylor and Francis Ltd, http://www.tandfonline.com.

Wiggins, David K. "'Black Athletes in White Men's Games': Race, Sport and American National Pastimes." *The International Journal of the History of Sport* 31, nos. 1–2 (2014): 181–202.

D. Disability

Chapter 9. With kind permission from Springer Science+Business Media: *Journal of Science and Engineering Ethics*, "The 'Second Place' Problem: Assistive Technology in Sports and (Re) Constructing Normal," Denise A. Baker (2015) 22(1) : 1–18. Copyright © Springer Science+Business Media Dordrecht 2015.

Baker, Denise A. "The 'Second Place' Problem: Assistive Technology in Sports and (Re) Constructing Normal." *Journal of Science and Engineering Ethics*, 22, no. 1 (2015): 1–18.

Dieffenbach, Kristen D., and Traci A. Statler. "More Similar than Different: The Psychological Environment of Paralympic Sport." *Journal of Sport Psychology in Action* 3, no. 2 (2012): 109–118.

■ **PART III: ATHLETES AS ROLE MODELS**

Lynch, Sandra, Daryl Adair, and Paul Jonson. "Professional Athletes and Their Duty to be Role Models." In *Achieving Ethical Excellence*, edited by Michael Schwartz and Howard Harris, 75–90. Research in Ethical Issues in Organizations, vol. 12. Bingley, UK: Emerald Group Publishing Limited, 2014.

Agyemang, Kwame, and John N. Singer. "An Exploratory Study of Professional Black Male Athletes' Individual Social Responsibility (ISR)." *Spectrum: A Journal on Black Men* 2, no. 1 (2013): 47–71.

■ **PART IV: POWER AND CORRUPTION**

Giroux, Henry A., and Susan Searls Giroux. "Universities Gone Wild: Big Money, Big Sports, and Scandalous Abuse at Penn State." *Cultural Studies ↔ Critical Methodologies*, 12, no. 4 (2012): 267–273.

Jennings, Andrew. "Investigating Corruption in Corporate Sport: The IOC and FIFA." *International Review for the Sociology of Sport*, 46, no. 4 (2011): 387–398.

■ PART V: RISK, CHOICE, AND COERCION

A. Dangerous Sports

Chapter 16. "The Organization and Regulation of Full-Contact Martial Arts: A Case Study of Flanders," Jikkemien Vertonghen, Marc Theeboom, Els Dom, Veerle De Bosscher, and Reinhard Haudenhuyse, *Societies* (2014), an open-access publication of the Multidisciplinary Digital Publishing Institute (MDPI). Reprinted with permission from MDPI.

> Vertonghen, J., et al. "The Organization and Regulation of Full Contact Martial Arts: A Case Study of Flanders." *Societies*, 4, no. 4 (2014): 654–671.

B. Football and Concussions

Chapter 17. "Concussion and Football: Failures to Respond by the NFL and the Medical Profession," David Orentlicher and William S. David, *Florida International University Law Review* (2012). Reprinted with permission from Florida International University Law Review.

> Orentlicher, David, and William S. David. "Concussion and Football: Failures to Respond by the NFL and the Medical Profession." *Florida International University Law Review* 8 (2012): 23–36.

C. Managing Risk

Chapter 18. "Player Safety in Youth Sports: Sportsmanship and Respect as an Injury-Prevention Strategy," Douglas E. Abrams, *Seton Hall Journal of Sports and Entertainment Law* (2012). Reprinted with permission from *Seton Hall Journal of Sports and Entertainment Law*.

> Abrams, Douglas E. "Player Safety in Youth Sports: Sportsmanship and Respect as an Injury-Prevention Strategy." *Seton Hall Journal of Sports and Entertainment Law* 22, no.1 (2012): 1270–1297.

Chapter 19. "Health and Sports Law Collide: Do Professional Athletes Have an Unfettered Choice to Accept Risk of Harm?" Ken Berger, *Medicine and Law* (2011). Reprinted with permission from Medicine and Law.

> Berger, K. J. "Health and Sports Law Collide: Do Professional Athletes Have an Unfettered Choice to Accept Risk of Harm?." *Medicine and Law* 30, no. 1 (2011): 1–22.

■ PART VI: MEDICINE AND SPORTS

Chapter 20. "Ethical Issues in Sports Medicine A Review and Justification for Ethical Decision Making and Reasoning," Bruce Greenfield and Charles Robert

West, *Sports Health: A Multidisciplinary Approach*, 4(6): 475–479. Copyright © 2012 by SAGE Publications. Reprinted by Permission of SAGE Publications.

Greenfield, Bruce H., and Charles Robert West. "Ethical Issues in Sports Medicine A Review and Justification for Ethical Decision Making and Reasoning." *Sports Health: A Multidisciplinary Approach* 4, no. 6 (2012): 475–479.

■ **PART VII: WHAT ABOUT ANIMALS?**

Chapter 21. "Humans, Horses, and Hybrids: On Rights, Welfare, and Masculinity in Equestrian Sports," Kutte Jönsson, *Scandinavian Sports Studies Forum* (2012). Reprinted with permission from *Scandinavian Sports Studies Forum*.

Jönsson, Kutte. "Humans, Horses, and Hybrids: On Rights, Welfare, and Masculinity in Equestrian Sports." *Scandinavian Sport Studies Forum* 3 (2012): 49–69.

Chapter 22. Copyright 2003 from "Is Hunting a "Sport"?" John Alan Cohan. Reproduced by permission of Philosophy Documentation Center, www.pdcnet. org.

Cohan, John Alan. "Is Hunting a "Sport"?." *International Journal of Applied Philosophy* 17, no. 2 (2003): 291–326.

■ **PART VIII: ENHANCEMENT AND IMPROVEMENT**

Chapter 23. "Sports Enhancement," Thomas H. Murray was originally published as a chapter in *From Birth to Death and Bench to Clinic: The Hastings Center Bioethics Briefing Book for Policymakers and Campaigns*, The Hastings Center, Garrison (2008). Reprinted with the permission of the Hastings Center.

Murray, Thomas H. "Sports Enhancement." In *From Birth to Death and Bench to Clinic: The Hastings Center Bioethics Briefing Book for Policymakers and Campaigns*, 153–158. Garrison: The Hastings Center, 2008.

Chapter 24. Springer + Business Media, *Journal of Sports Medicine*, "Performance-Enhancing Substances in Sports: A Review of the Literature," Amit Momaya, Marc Fawal, and Reed Estes (2015) 45(4): 517–531, © Springer International Publishing Switzerland 2015. With permission of Springer Science + Business Media.

Momaya, Amit, Marc Fawal, and Reed Estes. "Performance-Enhancing Substances in Sports: A Review of the Literature." *Sports Medicine* 45, no. 4 (2015): 517–531.

Chapter 25. From *Science* Magazine, "Can Ice Vests Provide a Competitive Chill?," Adrian Cho, *Science* (2008) 321(5889): 625; "Do New Materials Make the Athlete?," Andrea Lu *Science* (2008) 321(5889): 626; "Can Neuroscience Provide a Mental Edge?," Greg Miller, *Science* (2008) 321(5889): 626–627; "Does Doping Work?," Martin Enserink, *Science* (2008) 321(5889): 627. Reprinted with permission from AAAS.

Chapter 26. "Ethics of Technologically Constructed Hypoxic Environments in Sport," Sigmund Loland and Arthur Caplan, *Scandinavian Journal of Medicine & Science in Sports* (2008). Copyright © 2008 The Authors. Journal compilation © 2008 Blackwell Munksgaard. This article is available under a Creative Commons Attribution license, http://onlinelibrary.wiley.com/doi/10.1111/j.1600-0838.2008.00834.x/abstract /.

Loland, Sigmund, and Arthur Caplan. "Ethics of Technologically Constructed Hypoxic Environments in Sport." *Scandinavian Journal of Medicine & Science in Sports* 18, no. s1 (2008): 70–75.

Chapter 27. "Gene Transfer for Pain: A Tool to Cope with the Intractable or an Unethical Endurance Enhancing Technology?" Silvia Camporesi and Michael J. McNamee, *Life Sciences Society and Policy* (2012), a publication of Springer Open Access. This article is reprinted via, and is available under, a Creative Commons license from SpringerOpen. http://lsspjournal.springeropen.com/articles/10.1186/1746-5354-8-1-20.

Camporesi, Silvia, and Michael J. McNamee. "Gene Transfer for Pain: A Tool to Cope with the Intractable or an Unethical Endurance Enhancing Technology?" *Life Sciences Society and Policy* 8, no. 1 (2012): 20–31.

CPSIA information can be obtained
at www.ICGtesting.com
Printed in the USA
BVHW030115201220
595738BV00010B/85